Interpretation of Diagnostic Tests

Interpretation of Diagnostic Tests

A Synopsis of Laboratory Medicine

Fourth Edition

Jacques Wallach, M.D.
Clinical Professor of Pathology,
State University of New York,
Downstate Medical Center;
Attending Pathologist,
Kings County Hospital,
Brooklyn, New York

Little, Brown and Company
Boston/Toronto

INTERPRETATION OF DIAGNOSTIC TESTS: A HANDBOOK SYNOPSIS OF LABORATORY MEDICINE is published in the following translations:

First Edition

INTERPRETACIÓN DE LOS DIAGNÓSTICOS DE LABORATORIO: MANUAL SINÓPTICO DE BIOLOGÍA MÉDICA

Ἑρμηνεία τῶν Διαγνωστικῶν Ἐξετάσεων καὶ Δοκιμασιῶν: Συνοπτικὸν Ἐγχειρίδιον Ἐργαστηριακῆς Ἰατρικῆς

INTERPRETAÇÃO DOS DIAGNÓSTICOS DE LABORATÓRIO

Second Edition

INTERPRETAZIONE DEI TESTS DI LABORATORIO IN MEDICINA

Third Edition

INTERPRETAÇÃO DOS DIAGNÓSTICOS DE LABORATÓRIO, terceira edição

INTERPRETAZIONE DEI TESTS DI LABORATORIO IN MEDICINA

INTERPRETACIÓN DE LOS DIAGNÓSTICOS DE LABORATORIO

MV NY

To Doris
and
To Kim, Lisa, and Tracy

Preface to the Fourth Edition

This new edition was made necessary by the continuing rapid growth of laboratory technologies and further stimulated by the recent emphasis on obtaining the most prompt, expeditious, and cost-effective diagnostic studies while avoiding or curtailing in-hospital studies.

Some significant changes in this edition are

The normal values have been updated and further refined by age and sex.

Important new tests have been included (e.g., assays for therapeutic drug monitoring; serologic tests for HTLV-III, collagen diseases, and hepatitis; steroid receptor assays).

Data on sensitivity, specificity, and predictive value of various tests that allow a comparison of their utility have been added.

Outmoded tests have been deleted (e.g., PBI, colloidal gold, cephalin flocculation, thymol turbidity, BSP).

Many tables and figures have been revised and others have been added.

Recent antibiotic resistance data have been included.

A number of algorithms are presented to illustrate the sequence of tests in some difficult diagnostic areas.

The diagnostic criteria and sequence of laboratory work-up have been changed by the widespread availability of radioimmunoassay methods for hormone assays. Diagnosis of many of these conditions is now within reach of most physicians.

More diagnostic "pearls" are scattered throughout.

Various conditions are included that are newly described or whose importance has been recently realized (e.g., AIDS, chlamydial infections, Legionnaires' disease, campylobacteriosis, toxic shock).

A table of critical values is given.

There is an appendix for the conversion of conventional units to SI units.

While these changes have resulted in a somewhat larger book, I have still maintained the original organization, format, and style of pocket-size portability, ease of use, nominal cost, thoroughness, current information, and other goals of previous editions.

J. W.

Preface to the Previous Editions

Results of laboratory tests may aid in
    Discovering occult disease
    Preventing irreparable damage (e.g., phenylketonuria)
    Early diagnosis after onset of signs or symptoms
    Differential diagnosis of various possible diseases
    Determining the stage of the disease
    Estimating the activity of the disease
    Detecting the recurrence of disease
    Monitoring the effect of therapy
    Genetic counseling in familial conditions
    Medicolegal problems, such as paternity suits

This book is written to help the physician achieve these purposes with the least amount of
    Duplication of tests
    Waste of patient's money
    Overtaxing of laboratory facilities and personnel
    Loss of physician's time
    Confusion caused by the increasing number, variety, and complexity of tests currently available. Some of these tests may be unrequested but performed as part of routine surveys or hospital admission multitest screening.

In order to provide quick reference and maximum availability and usefulness, this handy-sized book features
    Tabular and graphic style of concise presentation
    Emphasis on serial time changes in laboratory findings in various stages of disease
    Omission of rarely performed, irrelevant, esoteric, and outmoded laboratory tests
    Exclusion of discussion of physiologic mechanisms, metabolic pathways, clinical features, and nonlaboratory aspects of disease
    Discussion of only the more important diseases that the physician encounters and should be able to diagnose

This book is not
    An encyclopedic compendium of clinical pathology
    A technical manual
    A substitute for good clinical judgment and basic knowledge of medicine

Deliberately omitted are
    Technical procedures and directions
    Photographs and illustrations of anatomic changes (e.g., blood cells, karyotypes, isotope scans)
    Discussions of quality control
    Selection of a referral laboratory
    Performance of laboratory tests in the clinician's own office
    Bibliographic references, except for the most general reference texts in medicine, hematology, and clinical pathology and for some recent references to specific conditions

The usefulness and need for a book of this style, organization, and content have been increased by such current trends as
    The frequent lack of personal assistance, advice, and consulta-

tion in large commercial laboratories and hospital departments of clinical pathology, which are often specialized and fragmented as well as impersonal

Greater demand for the physician's time

The development of many new tests

The lack of adequate teaching of laboratory medicine in most medical schools. Faculty and administrators still assume that this essential area of medicine can be learned "intuitively" as it was 20 years ago and that it therefore requires little formal training. This attitude ignores changes in the number and variety of tests now available as well as their increased sophistication and basic value in establishing a diagnosis

The contents of this book are organized to answer the questions most often posed by physicians when they require assistance from the pathologist. There is no other single adequate source of information presented in this fashion. It appears from numerous comments I have received that this book has succeeded in meeting the needs not only of practicing physicians and medical students but also of pathologists, technologists, and other medical personnel. It has been adopted by many schools of nursing and of medical technology, physicians assistant training programs, and medical schools. Such widespread acceptance confirms my original premise in writing this book and is most gratifying.

A perusal of the table of contents and index will quickly show the general organization of the material by type of laboratory test or organ system or certain other categories. In order to maintain a concise format, separate chapters have not been organized for such categories as newborn, pediatric, and geriatric periods or for primary psychiatric or dermatologic diseases. A complete index provides maximum access to this information.

Obviously these data are not original but have been adapted from many sources over the years. Only the selection, organization, manner of presentation, and emphasis are original. I have formulated this point of view during 40 years as a clinician and pathologist, viewing with pride the important and growing role of the laboratory but deeply regretting its inadequate utilization.

This book was written to improve laboratory utilization by making it simpler for the physician to select and interpret the most useful laboratory tests for his clinical problems.

J. W.

Acknowledgments

I thank my colleagues in various parts of the world who have shared their clinical and laboratory problems with me. The universal need to convert an ever-expanding mass of raw laboratory data into accessible, clinically usable information has become a matter of increasing significance throughout the medical community and a chief concern of mine in producing this book and in other teaching and research efforts. This need for expeditious, unencumbered information has been repeatedly confirmed during teaching of medical students and house officers, the daily practice of clinical pathology, by discussions with physicians in many countries that I have visited or in which I have taught, and by the translation of these volumes into various languages. I am rewarded by numerous instances of friendship, criticism, kindness, and help and by learning far more than I could include in this small volume. I have been gratified and stimulated beyond any expectation.

My thanks to the staff of Little, Brown and Company, especially to Katherine Arnoldi and her assistant, Jonathan Sarner. Debra Corman and Sandra McLean performed meticulous, difficult work. Betty Herr Hallinger again prepared an outstanding index that greatly facilitates the use of this book. George McKinnon provided special help with the rough manuscript.

The love, generosity, patience, and friendship of my wife Doris can never be sufficiently acknowledged.

Contents

III. Diseases of Organ Systems

IV. Effects of Drugs on Laboratory Test Values

Tables

Normal Values

Notice

The indications and dosages of all drugs in this book have been recommended in the medical literature and conform to the practices of the general medical community. The medications described do not necessarily have specific approval by the Food and Drug Administration for use in the diseases and dosages for which they are recommended. The package insert for each drug should be consulted for use and dosage as approved by the FDA. Because standards for usage change, it is advisable to keep abreast of revised recommendations, particularly those concerning new drugs.

Blood

INTRODUCTION TO NORMAL VALUES

In the majority of laboratory measurements, the combination of short-term physiologic variation and analytic error is sufficient to render the interpretation of single determinations difficult when the concentrations are in the marginal range.

The reader must always keep in mind that all values given in this book are to be used as general guidelines rather than rigid separations of normal from abnormal or diseased from healthy. Considerable variation in test results is due not only to instrumentation, methodology, and other laboratory techniques but also to more subtle preanalytic factors such as position or condition of patient (e.g., supine or upright, fasting or postprandial), time of day, age, sex, climate, effect of diet or drug, characteristics of test population. It is therefore essential that the clinician use the normal values from the laboratory that is performing those particular tests and which it has determined for its own procedures, patient population, etc. Too many misunderstandings result from attempts to apply normal ranges of one laboratory to test results from another laboratory. Misinterpretation of laboratory data due to this error, as well as from overemphasizing the significance of borderline values, has caused immeasurable emotional pain and economic waste for innumerable patients. The clinician is referred elsewhere for a more detailed discussion of this topic.

Special notation should be made when it is particularly germane to that test, e.g., time when blood is drawn is important when the tested component is subject to marked diurnal variation (cortisol, iron), relation to meals (glucose) or IV infusions (electrolytes), source of specimen (arterial or capillary rather than venous blood). Many tests can be properly interpreted only when such information is known.

Some tests are performed too infrequently to be included in this list; other tests have such wide reference ranges that interlaboratory utility is limited.

A review of the texts, reference books, and current literature in clinical pathology often reveals surprising and considerable discrepancy between well-known sources. The following pages of normal laboratory values were summarized from what seemed to be the best and most current sources of data available.

I have used my own experience and clinical judgment in selecting the most useful data to be included.

Table 1-1. Normal Leukocyte Differential Count in Peripheral Blood

Age	Segmented Neutrophils		Band* Neutrophils		Eosinophils		Basophils		Lymphocytes		Monocytes	
	%	No./cu mm	%	No./cu mm	%	No./cu mm	%	No./cu mm	%	No./cu mm	%	No./cu mm
At birth	47 ± 15	8400	14.1 ± 4	2540	2.2	400	0.6	100	31 ± 5	5500	5.8	1050
12 hr	53	12,100	15.2	3460	2.0	450	0.4	100	24	5500	5.3	1200
24 hr	47	8870	14.2	2680	2.4	450	0.5	100	31	5800	5.8	1100
1 wk	34	4100	11.8	1420	4.1	500	0.4	50	41	5000	9.1	1100
2 wk	29	3320	10.5	1200	3.1	350	0.4	50	48	5500	8.8	1000
4 wk	25 ± 10	2750	9.5 ± 3	1150	2.8	300	0.5	50	56 ± 15	6000	6.5	700
2 mo	25	2750	8.4	1100	2.7	300	0.5	50	57	6300	5.9	650
4 mo	24	2730	8.9	1000	2.6	300	0.4	50	59	6800	5.2	600
6 mo	23	2710	8.8	1000	2.5	300	0.4	50	61	7300	4.8	580
8 mo	22	2680	8.3	1000	2.5	300	0.4	50	62	7600	4.7	580

10 mo	22	2600	8.3	1000	2.5	300	0.4	50	63	7500	4.6	550
12 mo	23	2680	8.1	990	2.6	300	0.4	50	61	7000	4.8	550
2 yr	25	2660	8.0	850	2.6	280	0.5	50	59	6300	5.0	530
4 yr	34 ± 11	3040	8.0 ± 3	710	2.8	250	0.6	50	50 ± 15	4500	5.0	450
6 hr	43	3600	8.0	670	2.7	230	0.6	50	42	3500	4.7	400
8 yr	45	3700	8.0	660	2.4	200	0.6	50	39	3300	4.2	350
10 yr	46 ± 15	3700	8.0 ± 3	645	2.4	200	0.5	40	38 ± 10	3100	4.3	350
12 yr	47	3700	8.0	640	2.5	200	0.5	40	38	3000	4.4	350
14 yr	48	3700	8.0	640	2.5	200	0.5	40	37	2900	4.7	380
16 yr	49 ± 15	3800	8.0 ± 3	620	2.6	200	0.5	40	35 ± 10	2800	5.1	400
18 yr	49	3800	8.0	620	2.6	200	0.5	40	35	2700	5.2	400
20 yr	51	3800	8.0	620	2.7	200	0.5	40	33	2500	5.0	380
21 yr	51 ± 15	3800	8.0 ± 3	620	2.7	200	0.5	40	34 ± 10	2500	4.0	300

*Note that these values are higher than those found in other references. They have been obtained by using strict criteria in differentiating segmented from band forms. I do not classify a neutrophil as a segmented form unless a typical threadlike filament is visible.

Source: Data from J. B. Miale, *Laboratory Medicine—Hematology* (6th ed.). St. Louis: Mosby, 1982; average values based on the average leukocyte counts taken from E. C. Albritton, *Standard Values in Blood*. Philadelphia: Saunders, 1952.

Table 1-2. Normal Values for Red Corpuscles at Various Ages

Age	Red Cell Count (millions/cu mm)	Hemoglobin (gm/dl)	Vol. Packed RBC (ml/dl)	Corpuscular Values			
				MCV (cu μ)	MCH (γγ)	MCHC (%)	MCD (μ)
First day	5.1 ± 1.0	19.5 ± 5.0	54.0 ± 10.0	106	38	36	8.6
2–3 days	5.1	19.0	53.5	105	37	35	
4–8 days	5.1	18.3 ± 4.0	52.5	103	36	35	
9–13 days	5.0	16.5	49.0	98	33	34	8.1
14–60 days	4.7 ± 0.9	14.0 ± 3.3	42.0 ± 7.0	90	30	33	7.7
3–5 mo	4.5 ± 0.7	12.2 ± 2.3	36.0	80	27	34	7.4
6–11 mo	4.6	11.8	35.5 ± 5.0	77	26	33	7.3
1 yr	4.5	11.2	35.0	78	25	32	
2 yr	4.6	11.5	35.5	77	25	32	
3 yr	4.5	12.5	36.0	80	27	35	7.4
4 yr	4.6 ± 0.6	12.6	37.0	80	27	34	
5 yr	4.6	12.6	37.0	80	27	34	
6–10 yr	4.7	12.9	37.5	80	27	34	7.4
11–15 yr	4.8	13.4	39.0	82	28	34	
Adults							
Females	4.8 ± 0.6	14.0 ± 2.0	42.0 ± 5.0	87 ± 5	29 ± 2	34 ± 2	7.5 ± 0.3
Males	5.4 ± 0.8	16.0 ± 2.0	47.0 ± 5.0	87 ± 5	29 ± 2	34 ± 2	7.5 ± 0.3

MCV = mean corpuscular volume; MCH = mean corpuscular hemoglobin; MCHC = mean corpuscular hemoglobin concentration; MCD = mean corpuscular diameter.

Source: Data from M. M. Wintrobe et al., *Clinical Hematology* (8th ed.). Philadelphia: Lea and Febiger, 1981. P. 1891.

NORMAL HEMATOLOGIC VALUES

Methemoglobin	<3% of total
Carboxyhemoglobin	<5% of total
Haptoglobins	Genetic absence in 1% of population
Newborns	Absent in 90%; 10 mg/dl in 10%
Age 1–6 months	Gradual increase to 30 mg/dl
Adults	60–270 mg/dl
Osmotic fragility of RBC	Begins in 0.45–0.39% NaCl
	Complete in 0.33–0.30% NaCl
Erythrocyte sedimentation rate	
Wintrobe	
Males	0–10 mm in 1 hour
Females	0–15 mm in 1 hour
Westergren	
Males	0–13 mm in 1 hour
Females	0–20 mm in 1 hour
Blood volume	
Males	75 ml/kg body weight
Females	67 ml/kg body weight (8.5–9.5% body weight in kg)
Plasma volume	
Males	44 ml/kg body weight
Females	43 ml/kg body weight
RBC volume	
Males	30 ml/kg body weight
Females	24 ml/kg body weight
RBC survival time (^{51}Cr)	Half-life: 25–35 days
Reticulocyte count	0.5–1.5% of erythrocytes
Plasma iron turnover rate	38 mg/24 hours (0.47 mg/kg)
Delta-aminolevulinic acid	1.5–7.5 mg/24-hour urine
Ferritin	
Newborns	25–200 ng/ml
1 month	200–600 ng/ml
2–5 months	50–200 ng/ml
6 months–15 years	7–142 ng/ml
Adult males	20–300 ng/ml
Adult females	20–120 ng/ml
Borderline (males or females)	10–20 ng/ml
Hemoglobin electrophoresis	Hgb A = >95%
	Hgb A_2 = 2.5–4.0%
	Hgb F = <2%
	No abnormal variants
Hemoglobin F, RBC	Hemoglobin F remaining in <1% of RBC
Hemoglobin, plasma	<15 mg/dl
Hemosiderin, urine	Negative
Iron, liver tissue	530–900 µg/gm dry weight
Iron, urine	<200 ng/24 hours
Iron, serum	
Children	50–150 µg/dl
Adults	40–175 µg/dl
Iron-binding capacity	250–410 µg/dl
% saturation	20–55%

Transferrin	205–374 mg/dl
Ceruloplasmin	27–37 mg/dl
Copper	70–150 µg/dl
Leukocyte alkaline phosphatase (LAP) score	Score of 40–100
Lysozyme (muramidase), plasma	0.2–15.8 µg/ml
Lysozyme (muramidase), urine	<3 mg/24 hours
Myoglobin, serum	30–90 ng/ml
Myoglobin, urine	0–2 Mb/ml
Pyruvate kinase, erythrocyte	2.0–8.8 units/gm hemoglobin
Folate	Low: <2.0 ng/ml
	Normal: 2.0–20.0 ng/ml
	Elevated: >20.0 ng/ml
Vitamin B_{12} assay (cyanocobalamin)	Low: >100 pg/ml
	Indeterminate: 100–200 pg/ml
	Normal: 200–1100 pg/ml
	Elevated: >1100 pg/ml
Unsaturated vitamin B_{12}–binding capacity	870–1800 pg/ml
Urobilinogen, urine	<4 mg/24 hours
Urobilinogen, stool	50–300 mg/24 hours

BLOOD COAGULATION TESTS

Platelet count	140,000–340,000/cu mm (Rees-Ecker)
	200,000–350,000/cu mm (Coulter counter)
Bleeding time (Simplate)	3–8 minutes
Clot retraction, qualitative	Begins in 30–60 minutes; complete within 24 hours, usually within 6 hours
Coagulation time (Lee-White)	6–17 minutes (glass tubes)
	19–60 minutes (siliconized tubes)
Fibrinogen split products	Positive at >1:8 dilution
Fibrinolysins	No clot lysis in 24 hours
Partial thromboplastin time (activated) (aPTT)	25–37 seconds
Prothrombin time (PT) (one stage)	± 2 seconds of control (control should be 11–16 seconds)
Thrombin time (TT)	± 5 seconds of control
Fibrinogen	150–400 mg/dl
Coagulation factor assay	
II	100 ± 40%
V	100 ± 50%
VII	100 ± 35%
VIII	100 ± 35%
IX	100 ± 40%
X	100 ± 55%
XI	100 ± 35%
XII	100 ± 50%
XIII	100 ± 50%
Factor VIII related antigen	45–185%
Coagulator factor VIII inhibitor	Negative
Platelet antibody	Negative

Ristocetin-Willebrand factor	45–140%
Antithrombin III, plasma	
Immunologic	17–30 mg/dl
Functional	80–120%

BLOOD CHEMISTRIES

The lists of normal blood chemistries are arranged both alphabetically and by type of chemical component (e.g., enzymes, electrolytes, blood gases, pH) for greatest convenience.

The normal values will vary, depending on the individual laboratory as well as the methods used.

Acetone	0.3–2.0 mg/dl
Aldolase	
Newborns	<32 units/L
Children	<16 units/L
Adults	<8 units/L
Ammonia	80–110 µg/dl
Amylase	600–1600 units/L
Base, total	145–160 mEq/L
Base, excess	
Newborns	− 10 to − 2 mmol/L
2 months–2 years	− 6.6 to 0.2 mmol/L
2 years to adult	− 2.3 to 2.3 mmol/L
Bicarbonate, standard	
Premature	18–26 mmol/L
Full term to 2 years	20–26 mmol/L
2 years to adult	22–26 mmol/L
Bicarbonate, actual (calculated from pH and PCO_2)	
Newborns	17–24 mmol/L
Infants	19–24 mmol/L
2 months–2 years	16–24 mmol/L
Children	21–27 mmol/L
Adult males	20–29 mmol/L
Adult females	18–29 mmol/L

Bilirubin (mg/dl)	**Premature**	**Full-term**
Total		
Cord	<2.8	<2.8
24 hours	1–6	2–6
48 hours	6–8	6–7
3–5 days	10–12	4–6
1 month to adult	<1.5	<1.5
Direct		
1 month to adult	<0.5	<0.5

Calcium	8.5–10.5 mg/dl (higher in children)
Carbon dioxide	
Content	24–30 mEq/L Infants: 20–26 mEq/L
Tension	
PCO_2 arterial	35–45 mmHg Newborns: 26–40 mmHg

	PCO$_2$ venous	40–50 mm Hg
Ceruloplasmin		20–40 mg/dl
Chloride		100–106 mEq/L
Cholesterol, total		

	Males (mg/dl)	Females (mg/dl)
Cord	45–98	45–98
3 days–1 year	65–175	65–175
1–19 years	120–200	120–217
20–29 years	120–240	120–218
30–39 years	140–270	140–240
40–49 years	150–280	150–265
50–59 years	160–290	160–290
≥60 years	160–300	160–320

Cholesterol esters	60–75% of total
Cholinesterase	
Plasma	7–19 units
RBC	0.65–1.3 pH units
Copper	70–150 μg/dl
Creatine kinase (CK)	Varies with method
Creatinine	
1 year	≦0.6 mg/dl
2–3 years	≦0.7 mg/dl
4–7 years	≦0.8 mg/dl
8–10 years	≦0.9 mg/dl
11–12 years	≦1.0 mg/dl
13–17 years	≦1.2 mg/dl
18–20 years	≦1.3 mg/dl
Values for females are 0.1 mg/dl lower	
Cryoglobulins	0
Fibrinogen	150–400 mg/dl
Gamma-glutamyl transpeptidase (GGTP)	
Cord	19–270 units/L at 37°C
1–3 days	56–233 units/L at 37°C
4–21 days	0–130 units/L at 37°C
3–12 weeks	4–120 units/L at 37°C
3–12 months, males	5–65 units/L at 37°C
3–12 months, females	5–35 units/L at 37°C
1–15 years	0–23 units/L at 37°C
Adult males	9–69 units/L at 37°C
Adult females	3–33 units/L at 37°C
Glucose (fasting)	60–100 mg/dl (depends on method)
Iron	
Children	50–150 μg/dl
Adults	40–175 μg/dl
Iron-binding capacity	250–410 μg/dl
% saturation	20–55%
Isocitric dehydrogenase (ICD)	50–180 Sigma units/ml
Lactic acid	
Venous	5–20 mg/dl
Arterial	3–7 mg/dl

Lactic dehydrogenase
  (LDH)
  Adults   100–190 units/L at 37°C
  At birth   Up to 3–9 times adult level
  1 day–1 month   Up to 2–5 times adult level
  1 month–2 years   Up to 2–3 times adult level
  3–17 years   1–2 times adult level
Lead   0–40 µg/dl
Leucine aminopeptidase
  (LAP)
  Males   80–200 (Goldbarg-Rutenburg) units/ml
  Females   75–185 units/ml
Lipase   <1.5 units/ml
Lipids, total   450–1000 mg/dl
Lipid fractionation

	Cholesterol (mg/dl)		Triglycerides (mg/dl)	
	Males	**Females**	**Males**	**Females**
Cord	45–98	45–98		
3 days–1 year	65–175	65–175		
1–19 years	120–200	120–217	10–103	10–121
20–29 years	120–240	120–218	10–157	10–100
30–39 years	140–270	140–240	10–182	10–110
40–49 years	150–280	150–265	10–193	10–122
50–59 years	160–290	160–290	10–197	10–134
≥60 years	160–300	160–320	10–199	10–147

  Cholesterol esters   60–75% of total
  Phospholipids   60–350 mg/dl
Magnesium   1.3–2.1 mEq/L
Osmolality   280–295 mOsm/L
Oxygen content, arterial   15–23 vol%
  Saturation, arterial   96–100% of capacity
  Tension, PO_2 arterial
    (while breathing
    room air)
    Newborns   60–75 mmHg
    <60 years   >85 mmHg
    60 years   >80 mmHg
    70 years   >70 mmHg
    80 years   >60 mmHg
    90 years   >50 mmHg
pH, arterial   7.35–7.45
Phenylalanine   0–2 mg/dl (<1 month old)
Phosphatase, acid
  Newborns   7.4–19.4 units/L
  2–23 years   6.4–15.2 units/L
  Adult males   0.5–11.0 units/L
  Adult females   0.2–9.5 units/L
Phosphatase, alkaline
  2–10 years   100–350 units/L
  10–13 years, females*   110–400 units/L
  13–15 years, males*   125–500 units/L

*Periods of accelerated bone growth.

20–60 years	25–100 units/L
Newborns	1–4 times adult values
Children	1–3 times adult values
	Transient 5–7 times adult values

Phosphorus
  Children   4.0–7.0 mg/dl
  Adults   2.3–4.7 mg/dl
Potassium   3.5–5.0 mEq/L
Proteins, serum
  Total   6.0–8.0 gm/dl
    Albumin   3.5–5.5 gm/dl
    Globulin   2.3–3.5 gm/dl
  Electrophoresis
    Albumin   52–65% of total
    Globulin
      Alpha$_1$ 2.5–5.0% of total
      Alpha$_2$ 7–13% of total
      Beta   8–14% of total
      Gamma   12–22% of total
      Alpha$_1$ antitrypsin   >180 mg/dl
                             Z heterozygotes:
                                79–171 mg/dl
                             Z homozygotes:
                                19–31 mg/dl
    Haptoglobin   60–270 mg/dl
    Transferrin   205–374 mg/dl
    C3   100–200 mg/dl
  Immunoglobulins

	IgG (mg/dl)	IgA (mg/dl)	IgM (mg/dl)
Newborns	900–1500	0–5	5–20
1–3 months	250–550	5–50	20–40
4–6 months	300–600	10–55	30–60
7–12 months	400–900	20–60	35–75
2 years	550–1000	35–75	40–80
3 years	550–1100	50–110	40–85
4–5 years	550–1100	60–150	40–95
6–8 years	550–1200	60–170	40–95
12 years	550–1400	60–200	40–110
Adults	550–1900	60–330	45–145

	IgE (mean units/ml)	IgE (range units/ml)
Cord serum	1.6	0.7–3.4
6 weeks–3 months	4.4	1.1–17
3–9 months	16.0	4.2–60
9 months–2 years	18.0	6.4–53
2–5 years	65.0	21–198
5–10 years	89.0	18–451
10–20 years	86.0	12–618
20–70 years	71.0	10–506

The level of IgE in normal sera is extremely low. For the Phadebas IgE test, the normal values shown above have been recorded.

Sodium	136–145 mEq/L
Transaminase	
SGOT (AST)	
<2 years	20–55 units/L
2–5 years	20–50 units/L
5–8 years	20–45 units/L
8–12 years	15–40 units/L
12–14 years	15–35 units/L
14–16 years	15–30 units/L
Adult males	8–46 units/L
Adult females	7–34 units/L
SGPT (ALT)	
Infants	0–54 units/L
<2 years	3–37 units/L
2–8 years	3–30 units/L
8–16 years	3–28 units/L
Adult males	7–46 units/L
Adult females	4–35 units/L
Urea nitrogen (BUN)	5–25 mg/dl
Uric acid	
Males	4.0–8.5 mg/dl
Females	3.0–7.5 mg/dl

BLOOD CHEMISTRIES BY TYPE OF COMPONENT

The normal values will vary, depending on the individual laboratory as well as on the method used.

General

Glucose (fasting)	60–100 mg/dl (depends on method)
Uric acid	
Males	4.0–8.5 mg/dl
Females	3.0–7.5 mg/dl
Urea nitrogen (BUN)	5–25 mg/dl

Bilirubin (mg/dl)

	Premature	**Full-term**
Total		
Cord	<2.8	<2.8
24 hours	1–6	2–6
48 hours	6–8	6–7
3–5 days	10–12	4–6
1 month to adult	<1.5	<1.5
Direct		
1 month to adult	<0.5	<0.5

Creatinine

1 year	$\leq$0.6 mg/dl
2–3 years	$\leq$0.7 mg/dl
4–7 years	$\leq$0.8 mg/dl
8–10 years	$\leq$0.9 mg/dl
11–12 years	$\leq$1.0 mg/dl
13–17 years	$\leq$1.2 mg/dl
18–20 years	$\leq$1.3 mg/dl

Values for females are 0.1 mg/dl lower

Ammonia	80–110 µg/dl
Lipids, total	450–1000 mg/dl

Lipid fractionation

	Cholesterol (mg/dl)		Triglycerides (mg/dl)	
	Males	**Females**	**Males**	**Females**
Cord	45–98	45–98		
3 days–1 year	65–175	65–175		
1–19 years	120–200	120–217	10–103	10–121
20–29 years	120–240	120–218	10–157	10–100
30–39 years	140–270	140–240	10–182	10–110
40–49 years	150–280	150–265	10–193	10–122
50–59 years	160–290	160–290	10–197	10–134
≥60 years	160–300	160–320	10–199	10–147

Cholesterol esters	60–75% of total
Phospholipids	60–350 mg/dl

Enzymes

Amylase	600–1600 units/L
Lipase	<1.5 units/ml
Transaminase	
SGOT (AST)	
<2 years	20–55 units/L
2–5 years	20–50 units/L
5–8 years	20–45 units/L
8–12 years	15–40 units/L
12–14 years	15–35 units/L
14–16 years	15–30 units/L
Adult males	8–46 units/L
Adult females	7–34 units/L
SGPT (ALT)	
Infants	0–54 units/L
<2 years	3–37 units/L
2–8 years	3–30 units/L
8–16 years	3–28 units/L
Adult males	7–46 units/L
Adult females	4–35 units/L
Phosphatase, acid	
Newborns	7.4–19.4 units/L
2–13 years	6.4–15.2 units/L
Adult males	0.5–11.0 units/L
Adult females	0.2–9.5 units/L
Phosphatase, alkaline	
2–10 years	100–350 units/L
10–13 years, females*	110–400 units/L
13–15 years, males*	125–500 units/L
20–60 years	25–100 units/L
Newborns	1–4 times adult values
Children	1–3 times adult values
	Transient 5–7 times adult values

*Periods of accelerated bone growth.

Gamma-glutamyl trans-
  peptidase (GGTP)

Cord	19–270 units/L at 37°C
1–3 days	56–233 units/L at 37°C
4–21 days	0–130 units/L at 37°C
3–12 weeks	4–120 units/L at 37°C
3–12 months, males	5–65 units/L at 37°C
3–12 months, females	5–35 units/L at 37°C
1–15 years	0–23 units/L at 37°C
Adult males	9–69 units/L at 37°C
Adult females	3–33 units/L at 37°C

Leucine aminopeptidase (LAP)

Males	80–200 (Goldbarg-Rutenburg) units/ml
Females	75–185 units/ml

Lactic dehydrogenase (LDH)

Adults	100–190 units/L at 37°C
At birth	Up to 3–9 times adult level
1 day–1 month	Up to 2–5 times adult level
1 month–2 years	Up to 2–3 times adult level
3–17 years	1–2 times adult level

Hydroxybutyric dehydrogenase (α-HBD)	120–260 Rosalki units/ml
Isocitric dehydrogenase (ICD)	50–180 Sigma units/ml
Creatine kinase (CK)	Varies with method

Cholinesterase

Plasma	7–19 units
RBC	0.65–1.3 pH units

Aldolase (ALD)

Newborns	<32 units/ml
Children	<16 units/ml
Adults	<8 units/ml

Malic dehydrogenase (MDH)	25–100 units/ml
Ornithine carbamyl transferase (OCT)	0–500 Sigma units/ml
5′-Nucleotidase	0.3–3.2 Bodansky units

Electrolytes

Sodium	136–145 mEq/L
Potassium	3.5–5.0 mEq/L
Chloride	100–106 mEq/L
Calcium	8.5–10.5 mg/dl (higher in children)

Phosphorus

Children	4.0–7.0 mg/dl
Adults	2.3–4.7 mg/dl
Magnesium	1.3–2.1 mEq/L

Blood Gases and pH

Base, total	145–160 mEq/L

Carbon dioxide

Content	24–30 mEq/L
	Infants: 20–26 mEq/L

Tension
  PCO₂ arterial — PCO_2 arterial   35–45 mmHg
                                                  Newborns: 26–40 mmHg
  PCO_2 venous   40–50 mmHg
Base, excess
  Newborns   −10 to −2 mmol/L
  2 months–2 years   −6.6 to 0.2 mmol/L
  Children to adults   −2.3 to 2.3 mmol/L
Bicarbonate, standard
  Premature   18–26 mmol/L
  Full term to 2 years   20–26 mmol/L
  2 years to adult   22–26 mmol/L
Bicarbonate, actual
  (calculated from
  pH and PCO_2)
  Newborns   17–24 mmol/L
  Infants   19–24 mmol/L
  2 months–2 years   16–24 mmol/L
  Children   21–27 mmol/L
  Adult males   20–29 mmol/L
  Adult females   18–29 mmol/L
Oxygen
  Content, arterial   15–23 vol%
  Saturation, arterial   96–100% of capacity
  Tension, PO_2 arterial (while
    breathing room air)
    Newborns   60–75 mmHg
    <60 years   >85 mmHg
    60 years   >80 mmHg
    70 years   >70 mmHg
    80 years   >60 mmHg
    90 years   >50 mmHg
Osmolality   280–295 mOsm/L
Arterial pH   7.35–7.45
Lactic acid
  Venous   5–20 mg/dl
  Arterial   3–7 mg/dl

Blood Proteins
Proteins, serum
  Total   6.0–8.0 gm/dl
    Albumin   3.5–5.5 gm/dl
    Globulin   2.3–3.5 gm/dl
    Electrophoresis
    Albumin   52–65% of total
    Globulin
      Alpha₁ — $Alpha_1$ 2.5–5.0% of total
      $Alpha_2$ 7–13% of total
      Beta   8–14% of total
      Gamma   12–22% of total
Fibrinogen   150–400 mg/dl
Cryoglobulins   0
$Alpha_1$ antitrypsin   >180 mg/dl
                                                  Z heterozygotes: 79–171 mg/dl
                                                  Z homozygotes: 19–31 mg/dl
Haptoglobin   60–270 mg/dl

| | Transferrin | 205–374 mg/dl |
| | C3 | 100–200 mg/dl |

Immunoglobulins*

	IgG (mg/dl)	IgA (mg/dl)	IgM (mg/dl)
Newborns	900–1500	0–5	5–20
1–3 months	250–550	5–50	20–40
4–6 months	300–600	10–55	30–60
7–12 months	400–900	20–60	35–75
2 years	550–1000	35–75	40–80
3 years	550–1100	50–110	40–85
4–5 years	550–1100	60–150	40–95
6–8 years	550–1200	60–170	40–95
12 years	550–1400	60–200	40–110
Adults	550–1900	60–330	45–145

	IgE (mean units/ml)	IgE (range units/ml)
Cord serum	1.6	0.7–3.4
6 weeks–3 months	4.4	1.1–17
3–9 months	16.0	4.2–60
9 months–2 years	18.0	6.4–53
2–5 years	65.0	21–198
5–10 years	89.0	18–451
10–20 years	86.0	12–618
20–70 years	71.0	10–506

The level of IgE in normal sera is extremely low. For the Phadebas IgE test, the normal values shown above have been recorded.

NORMAL BLOOD LEVELS FOR SEROLOGY TESTS

Amebiasis antibody	<1:64
Aspergillosis antibody	Negative
Blastomycosis antibody	Negative; test is positive in <50% of proven cases
Brucellosis antibody	<1:80
Candidosis antibody	Test positive in 25% of normal population
Chlamydia serology (lymphogranuloma venereum, psittacosis)	Not generally useful for diagnosis of ocular or genital infection in adults
	High levels (1:256) in lymphogranuloma venereum
	Highest levels (1:256–1:8192) in infant pneumonitis
	Low titers may be found in psittacosis. A fourfold increase in titer indicates recent infection with psittacosis.
Cold agglutinin titer	<1:16
Cryptococcosis antigen, serum or CSF	Negative

*Age-related normal values should be established by each laboratory that measures immunoglobulins.

Cytomegalovirus antibody	*
Echinococcosis antibody	Negative

Epstein-Barr virus antibody
  (VCA = viral capsid antigens;
  NA = nuclear antigen)
	Positive VCA/IgG titers indicate infection some time in the past. VCA/IgM antibodies indicate recent primary infection with EBV.
	Antibodies to EBNA develop 6–8 weeks after primary infection and remain positive for life.
	Normal values:
	  <1:10 anti-VCA/IgG
	  <1:5 anti-EBNA
	  <1:10 anti-VCA/IgM
	Recommended only if negative heterophil but infectious mononucleosis still suspect

Hepatitis	See p. 148.
Herpes zoster antibodies	*
Heterophil antibody	Titer 1:56 or absorption pattern showing no twofold titer reduction (see p. 137)
Histoplasmosis antibody, serum, or CSF	Negative
Influenza A or B antibodies	*
Monospot screen	Negative
Mumps antibodies	*
Q fever antibodies	*
Rickettsial antibody (Proteus OX-19, OX-K, OX-2)	<1:40
Rubella	≦1:8 indicates little or no immunity.
Rubeola antibodies	*
St. Louis encephalitis antibodies	*
Sporotrichosis antibody	<1:80

Streptococcal antibodies

	ASO	Anti- DNase-B
Preschool	<85 units	<60 units
School age	<17 units	<17 units
Adults	<85 units	<85 units

Syphilis serology	See p. 138.
Toxoplasmosis antibodies	Titer <1:4 no previous infection. Titer 1:4–1:256 prevalent in general population. Titer >1:256 suggests recent infection. Rising titer is of greatest significance.

*Difference ≧ fourfold using CF or HAI methods between acute and convalescent phase sera drawn within 30 days of each other is indicative of infection with that virus. Congenital infections require serial sera from both mother and infant. Passively acquired antibodies in infant will decay in 2–3 months. Antibody levels that are unchanged or increased in 2–3 months indicate active infection. Absence of antibody in mother rules out congenital infection in infant.

Trichinosis antibody	Negative
Tularemia antibody	<1:40

NORMAL BLOOD ANTIBODY LEVELS

Anti-DNA antibodies	<0.9 μg of native DNA/ml plasma
Antiextractable nuclear antigens*	Negative
Antiglomerular basement membrane antibody	Negative
Antimitochondrial antibodies	Negative at 1:5 dilution
Antinuclear antibodies (ANA)	Negative at 1:32 dilution
Anti—smooth muscle antibody	>1:20
C1 esterase inhibitor	16–33 mg/dl
C3 complement component (beta$_{1c}$-globulin)	
Males	88–252 mg/dl
Females	88–206 mg/dl
C4 complement component	
Males	12–72 mg/dl
Females	13–75 mg/dl
Complement, total serum	41–90 hemolytic units
HLA-B27	Present in: Whites: 6–8% Blacks: 3–4% Orientals: 1%
Intrinsic factor blocking antibody	Negative
Rheumatoid factor	Negative

NORMAL LEVELS FOR METABOLIC DISEASES
(blood, urine, RBC, skin)

Acid mucopolysaccharides	Age dependent
Alpha$_1$ antitrypsin	>180 mg/dl Z heterozygotes: 79–171 mg/dl Z homozygotes: 19–31 mg/dl
Alpha-galactosidase, plasma (Fabry's disease)	0.029–0.88 units/L
Alpha-L-iduronidase (Hurler's syndrome)	3.0–27.4 units/gm skin biopsy
Alpha-mannosidase	0.76–5.92 units/gm skin biopsy
Alpha-N-acetylglucosaminidase (Sanfilippo Type B)	0.092–0.575 units/L (serum)
Arylsulfatase A, serum (mucolipidosis, Type II and III)	0.619–1.99 units/L
Arylsulfatase A, urine	>1.0 units/L
Beta-glucosidase (Gaucher's disease)	0.28–4.71 units/gm skin biopsy
Carbohydrate, urine	Negative
Cystine	
Children <8 years	2–13 mg/24 hours
Children >8 years and adults	7–28 mg/24 hours
Fatty acid profile of serum lipids	Linoleate ≥ 10% of fatty acids in serum lipids

*Includes anti-RNP, anti-Sm, anti-SSB.

	Arachidonate $\geq 6\%$ of fatty acids in serum lipids
	Phytanate $< 0.3\%$ of fatty acids in serum lipids
Free fatty acids	239–843 μEq/L
Galactose, urine	Not detectable
Galactose 1-phosphate (galactosemia)	18.5–28.5 units/gm hemoglobin
Galactosylceramide–beta-galactosidase	0.77–6.92 units/gm skin biopsy
Glucose 6-phosphate dehydrogenase (G-6-PD), RBC	8.6–18.6 units/gm hemoglobin
Glucose phosphate isomerase	14.7–42.2 units/gm hemoglobin
Hexosaminidase A and B, serum	Total: 10.4–23.8 units/L
Hexosaminidase A	Normal: 56–80% of total
	Indeterminate (repeat): 50–55%
	Abnormal: $< 50\%$
Homogentisic acid, urine	Negative
Hydroxyproline, total	
Children	No normals
Adults	15–45 mg/24 hours
Hydroxyproline, urine, 2-hour	
Males	0.4–5.0 mg/2-hour specimen
Females	0.4–2.9 mg/2-hour specimen
25-Hydroxyvitamin D, plasma	15–45 ng/ml
	Values obtained during summer may be higher than during winter. Values < 15 ng/ml may be due to vitamin D deficiency.
^{35}S Mucopolysaccharide turnover	Normal or abnormal turnover
Phenylalanine	
< 1 month of age	0.9–2.0 mg/dl
> 1 month of age	0.9–3.4 mg/dl
Porphyrins, erythrocyte	
total	≤ 30 μg/dl cells
	Borderline: 30–50 μg/dl cells
Porphyrins, stool, 24-hour	
Coproporphyrin	< 200 μg/24 hours
Protoporphyrin	< 1500 μg/24 hours
Uroporphyrin	< 1000 μg/24 hours
Porphyrins, urine, quantitative	
Uro (octacarboxylic)	
Males	0–42 μg/24 hours
Females	1–22 μg/24 hours
Hepatocarboxylic	
Males	1–13 μg/24 hours
Females	1–9 μg/24 hours
Hexacarboxylic	
Males	1–5 μg/24 hours
Females	0–4 μg/24 hours
Pentacarboxylic	
Males	0–4 μg/24 hours
Females	0–3 μg/24 hours
Copro (tetracarboxylic)	
Males	0–96 μg/24 hours
Females	1–57 μg/24 hours

Porphobilinogen

Normal: <1.5 mg/24 hours
Marginal: 1.5–2.0 mg/24 hours
Excess: >2.0 mg/24 hours

Sphingomyelinase
  (Niemann-Pick disease)

1.53–7.18 units/gm skin biopsy

Tyrosine
  Infants (≦ 6 weeks)
  Adults

0.6–2.2 mg/dl
0.6–1.6 mg/dl

Uroporphyrinogen-I-synthase
  Males
  Females

7.9–14.7 nM/L/sec
8.0–16.8 nM/L/sec
Marginal values 6.0–8.0 nM/L/sec
  are suggestive but indeterminate. Values <6.0 nM/L/sec
  are definite for acute, intermittent porphyria.

2

Urine

Specific gravity	1.003–1.030
pH	4.6–8.0 (average = 6.0), depending on diet
Total solids	30–70 gm/L (average = 50). To estimate, multiply last two figures of specific gravity by 2.66 (Long's coefficient).
Osmolality	500–1200 mOsm/L
Volume	600–2500 ml/24 hours (average = 1200)
	Night volume usually < 700 ml with specific gravity > 1.018 or osmolality > 825 mOsm/kg of body weight in children
	Ratio of night to day volume 1:2–1:4
Protein	Qualitative = 0
	0–0.1 gm/24 hours
Glucose	Qualitative = 0
	≦0.3 gm/24 hours
Ketones	Qualitative = 0
Chloride	140–250 mEq/L
Calcium	<150 mg/24 hours on low-calcium (Bauer-Aub) diet
Phosphorus	1 gm/24 hours (average), depending on diet
Urobilinogen	0–4 mg/24 hours
Porphobilinogen	0–2 mg/24 hours
Uroporphyrin	0
Coproporphyrin	50–300 μg/24 hours; 0–75 μg/24 hours in children weighing <80 pounds
Amylase	260–950 Somogyi units/24 hours
Lead	<0.08 μg/ml or 120 μg/24 hours
Delta-aminolevulinic acid	1.5–7.5 mg/24 hours
Homogentisic acid	0
Hemoglobin and myoglobin	0
Creatinine	1.0–1.6 gm/24 hours (15–25 mg/kg of body weight/24 hours)
Creatine	<100 mg/24 hours (<6% of creatinine); higher in children (<1 year: may = creatinine; older children: ≦30% of creatine) and during pregnancy (≦12% of creatinine)
Cystine or cysteine	0
Phenylpyruvic acid	0

Microscopic examination	$\leq$ 1–2 RBC, WBC, epithelial cells/hpf; occasional hyaline cast/lpf
Addis count	
RBC	$\leq$ 1,000,000/24 hours
Casts	$\leq$ 100,000/24 hours
WBC + epithelial cells	$\leq$ 2,000,000/24 hours

3

Stool

Bulk	100–200 gm
Water	Up to 75%
Total osmolality	200–250 mOsm/L
Color	Normally brown
	Clay color (gray-white) in biliary obstruction
	Tarry if >100 ml of blood in upper GI tract
	Red: blood in large intestine or undigested beets or tomatoes
	Black: blood or iron or bismuth medication
	Various colors, depending on diet
pH	7.0–7.5 (may be acid with high lactose intake)
Microscopic examination	RBCs absent
	Epithelial cells present (increased with GI tract irritation); absence of epithelial cells in meconium of newborn may aid in diagnosis of intestinal obstruction in the newborn
	Few WBCs present (increased with GI tract inflammation)
	Crystals of calcium oxalate, fatty acid, and triple phosphate commonly present
	Hematoidin crystals sometimes found after GI tract hemorrhage
	Charcot-Leyden crystals sometimes found in parasitic infestation (especially amebiasis)
	Some undigested vegetable fibers and muscle fibers sometimes found normally
	Neutral fat globules (stained with Sudan), normal 0–2+
Nitrogen	<2.5 gm/day
Urobilinogen	50–300 mg/24 hours (100–400 Ehrlich units/100 gm)
Coproporphyrin	400–1000 mg/24 hours
Fat	<5 gm/24 hours (<4% of measured fat intake) during 3-day period
	<30% of dry weight (on diet of >50 gm of fat/day)
Calcium	≅0.6 gm/24 hours
Sodium and chloride	Variable but considerably lower than simultaneous concentrations in serum
Trypsin	20–950 units/gm

Cerebrospinal Fluid

Simultaneous measurement of blood level should always be performed.

Appearance	Clear, colorless: no clot
Total cell count	0–5/cu mm (all mononuclear cells)
Glucose	45–80 mg/dl (20 mg/dl less than blood level)
	Ventricular fluid 5–10 mg/dl higher than lumbar
Total protein	Lumbar: 15–45 mg/dl
	Cisternal: 15–25 mg/dl
	Ventricular: 5–15 mg/dl
Albumin	10–30 mg/dl
Protein electrophoresis	
Prealbumin	2–7%
Albumin	56–76%
Alpha$_1$ globulin	2–7%
Alpha$_2$ globulin	4–12%
Beta globulin	8–18%
Gamma globulin	3–12%
IgG	<10% of total CSF protein
Chloride	120–130 mEq/L (20 mEq/L higher than serum)
Sodium	142–150 mEq/L
Potassium	2.2–3.3 mEq/L
Carbon dioxide	25 mEq/L
pH	7.35–7.40
Transaminase (GOT)	7–49 units
Lactic dehydrogenase (LDH)	Approximately 10% of serum level
Creatine kinase (CK)	0–3 IU
Bilirubin	0
Urea nitrogen	5–25 mg/dl
Amino acids	30% of blood level
Xanthochromia	0

Serous Fluids (Pleural, Pericardial, and Ascitic)

Specific gravity	1.010–1.026
Total protein	0.3–4.1 gm/dl
Albumin	50–70%
Globulin	30–45%
Fibrinogen	0.3–4.5%
pH	6.8–7.6

See also Table 17-2, pp. 182–185.

Synovial Fluid

Volume	1.0–3.5 ml
pH	Parallels serum
Appearance	Clear, pale yellow, or straw-colored
	Viscous, does not clot
Fibrin clot	0
Mucin clot	Good
WBC (per cu mm)	<200 (even in presence of leukocytosis in blood)
Neutrophils	<25%
Crystals	
Free	0
Intracellular	0
Fasting uric acid, bilirubin	Approximately the same as serum
Total protein	≅25–30% of serum protein
	Mean = 1.8 gm/dl
	Abnormal if >2.5 gm/dl; inflammation is moderately severe if >4.5 gm/dl
Culture	0
Glucose	<10 mg/dl lower than simultaneously drawn serum level

Semen

Volume	1.5–5.0 ml
Liquefaction	Complete in 15–30 minutes
pH	7.2–8.0 (average = 7.8)
Sperm count	60–150 million/ml; 250 million/ejaculation
Motility	≧70% 1 hour after ejaculation
	≧60% 3 hours after ejaculation
Morphology	≧70% of normal morphology
Smear	Usually no RBCs or WBCs present

Liver Function Tests

Cholinesterase (pseudocholines-
    terase)

$\geqq 0.5$ pH units/hour

Galactose tolerance test (GTT)

Excretion of $\leqq 3$ gm galactose in urine 5 hours after ingestion of 40 gm galactose

Prothrombin time

Same as control; if increased, IV administration of synthetic vitamin K returns prothrombin time to normal in obstructive liver disease (or other causes of malabsorption of vitamin K) but not in parenchymal liver disease

Serum bilirubin, serum enzymes (e.g., SGOT, SGPT, LDH, alkaline phosphatase), urine bile, and urobilinogen (see data on differential diagnosis of liver disease, Chap. 24)

Serum proteins, protein electrophoresis, lipoprotein electrophoresis, fractionation of lipids, etc. (see Chap. 24)

Renal Function Tests

Concentration, dilution — Specific gravity > 1.025, specific gravity < 1.003

Phenolsulfonphthalein (PSP) excretion — > 25% in urine in 15 minutes; 55–75% in 2 hours

Clearances (corrected to 1.73 sq m body surface area)

To measure glomerular filtration rate (GFR)

Endogenous creatinine*

Age (years)	Mean Creatinine Clearance (ml/min/1.73 sq m body surface area)
0–1	72
1	45
2	55
3	60
4	71
5	73
6	64
7	67
8	72
9	83
10	89
11	92
12	109
13–14	86
Adults	90–130

Inulin†
Males — 110–150 ml/minute
Females — 105–132 ml/minute
Urea‡
Maximum — 60–100 ml/minute
Standard — 40–65 ml/minute

* *Creatinine clearance* is independent of rate of urine flow. Low concentration of creatinine in serum of infants and young children makes laboratory test difficult and inaccurate. Is excreted by tubules as well as filtered by glomeruli and therefore may overestimate GFR; but is widely used and best measurement of GFR in most clinical instances.
† Normal *inulin clearance* = 25–30 ml/minute during first few days of life; about 50 ml/minute by end of first month. Considerable individual variation makes interpretation difficult unless clearly abnormal. Is best determinant of GFR but requires continuous infusion to maintain adequate blood concentration during test.
‡ *Urea clearance:* marked variability in contributing factors (e.g., BUN, diet, urine flow) makes interpretation difficult and not useful in most clinical situations.

Usually there is good correlation between urine concentrating function and GFR. A normal GFR in association with impaired concentrating ability may be found in sickle cell anemia, diabetes insipidus, nephronophthisis, and various acquired disorders (e.g., pyelonephritis, potassium deficiency, hypercalciuria).

To measure effective plasma flow (RPF) and tubular function

Para-aminohippurate
  (PAH)
    Males   560–800 ml/minute
    Females   500–700 ml/minute
Diodrast   600–800 ml/minute
Filtration fraction (FF) =
  GFR/RPF
    Males   17–21%
    Females   17–23%
Maximal Diodrast excretory
  capacity, Tm_D
    Males   43–59 mg/minute
    Females   33–51 mg/minute
BUN, creatinine (see pp. 42–43)

See also pp. 102–109

Blood and Urine Hormone Levels

Triiodothyronine (T-3), total, serum	90–230 ng/dl
Thyroxine (T-4), total, serum	5.0–13.5 μg/dl
T-4, free, serum	0.8–2.5 ng/dl
	Patients on Synthroid: up to 3.1 ng/dl
Thyroid antiglobulin and microsomal antibodies, serum	Titer < 1:100 for both
Thyroid-stimulating hormone (TSH), serum	0–7 μU/ml Borderline: 7–10 μU/ml
Thyroxine-binding globulin (TBG), serum	16–24 μg/dl (binding capacity for T-4)
Long-acting thyroid-stimulating hormone (LATS), serum	0
Radioactive iodine uptake (RAIU)	9–19% in 1 hour 7–25% in 6 hours
Radioactive iodine excretion, urine	40–70% of administered dose in 24 hours
Calcitonin, plasma	
Basal	
Males	≦ 0.155 ng/ml
Females	≦ 0.105 ng/ml
4-hour calcium infusion of 15 mg calcium/kg	
Males	≦ 0.265 ng/ml
Females	≦ 0.120 ng/ml
Pentagastrin injection of 5 μg/kg	
Males	≦ 0.210 ng/ml
Females	≦ 0.105 ng/ml
Estradiol, serum	
Children	< 1 ng/dl
Adult males	1–5 ng/dl
Premenopausal adult females	3–40 ng/dl
Postmenopausal females	< 3 ng/dl
Estrogens, total (nonpregnant), urine	
Children	< 10 μg/24 hours
Adult males	15–40 μg/24 hours

Data from L. T. Wegener, *Mayo Medical Laboratories Handbook*. Rochester, MN: Mayo Medical Laboratories, 1984; and J. B. Henry (Ed.), *Todd-Sanford-Davidson Clinical Diagnosis by Laboratory Methods* (17th ed.). Philadelphia: Saunders, 1984.

Premenopausal adult females	15–80 µg/24 hours	
Postmenopausal females	<20 µg/24 hours	
Testosterone, serum	**Total**	**Free**
Males	300–1200 ng/dl	9–30 ng/dl
Females	20–80 ng/dl	0.3–1.9 ng/dl

Follicle-stimulating hormone (FSH), serum

Children	<10 IU/L
Adult males	<22 IU/L
Adult females, non-midcycle	<20 IU/L
Adult females, midcycle	<40 IU/L
Postmenopausal females	40–160 IU/L

Luteinizing hormone (LH), serum

Children	<15 IU/L
Adult males	4–24 IU/L
Adult females, non-midcycle	<30 IU/L
Adult females, midcycle	30–150 IU/L
Postmenopausal females	30–120 IU/L

Progesterone, serum

Males	<100 ng/dl
Premenopausal females	
Follicular phase	<70 ng/dl
Luteal phase	200–2000 ng/dl

Chorionic gonadotropins, beta-subunit, serum   <5 IU/L

Chorionic gonadotropins, beta-subunit, serum   <9 IU/L postmenopausal

Males	Undetectable
Pregnancy	
1st trimester	<500,000 IU/24 hours
2nd trimester	10,000–25,000 IU/24 hours
3rd trimester	5,000–15,000 IU/24 hours
Postpartum	Negative within 2 weeks

Prolactin, serum

Males	0–20 ng/ml
Females	0–23 ng/ml

Aldosterone, serum   1–21 ng/dl (A.M.)

Aldosterone, urine   2–16 µg/24 hours

Catecholamine fractionation (free), plasma

Norepinephrine	Supine: 70–750 pg/ml
	Standing: 200–1700 pg/ml
Epinephrine	Supine: <110 pg/ml
	Standing: <140 pg/ml
Dopamine	<30 pg/ml (any posture)

Catecholamine fractionation, urine

Epinephrine	
<1 year	<2.5 µg/24 hours
1–2 years	<3.5 µg/24 hours
2–4 years	<6.0 µg/24 hours

Table10-1. 17-Ketosteroids (Fractionation), Urine (mg/24 hours)

	Adult Females	Adult Males	Males 10–15 yr	Females 10–15 yr	6–9 yr	3–5 yr	1–2 yr	0–1 yr
Pregnanediol	0–4.5	0–1.9	0.1–1.2	0.1–0.7	<0.5	<0.3	<0.1	<0.1
Androsterone	0–3.1	0.9–6.1	0.2–2.0	0.5–2.5	0.1–1.0	<0.3	<0.3	<0.1
Etiocholanolone	0.1–3.5	0.9–5.2	0.1–1.6	0.7–3.1	0.3–1.0	<0.7	<0.4	<0.1
Dehydroepiandrosterone	0–1.5	0–3.1	<0.4	<0.4	<0.2	<0.1	<0.1	<0.1
Pregnanetriol	0–1.4	0.2–2.0	0.2–0.6	0.1–0.6	<0.3	<0.1	<0.1	<0.1
Δ5-Pregnanetriol	0–0.4	0–0.4	<0.3	<0.3	<0.2	<0.2	<0.1	<0.1
11-Ketoandrosterone	0–0.3	0–0.5	<0.1	<0.1	<0.1	<0.1	<0.1	<0.1
11-Ketoetiocholanolone	0–1.0	0–1.6	<0.3	0.1–0.5	0.1–0.5	<0.4	<0.1	<0.1
11-Hydroxyandrosterone	0–1.1	0.2–1.6	0.1–1.1	0.2–1.0	0.4–1.0	<0.4	<0.3	<0.3
11-Hydroxyetiocholanolone	0.1–0.8	0.1–0.9	<0.3	0.1–0.5	0.1–0.5	<0.4	<0.1	<0.1
11-Ketopregnanetriol	0–0.5	0–0.5	<0.3	<0.2	<0.2	<0.2	<0.2	<0.2

Source: L. T. Wegener, *Mayo Medical Laboratories Handbook*. Rochester, MN: Mayo Medical Laboratories, 1984.

4–10 years	0.2–10 µg/24 hours
10–15 years	0.5–20 µg/24 hours
Adults	0–20 µg/24 hours
Norepinephrine	
<1 year	<10 µg/24 hours
1–2 years	1–17 µg/24 hours
2–4 years	4–29 µg/24 hours
4–7 years	8–45 µg/24 hours
7–10 years	13–65 µg/24 hours
10–15 years	15–80 µg/24 hours
Adults	15–80 µg/24 hours
Dopamine	
<1 year	<85 µg/24 hours
1–2 years	10–140 µg/24 hours
2–4 years	40–260 µg/24 hours
4–15 years	65–400 µg/24 hours
Adults	65–400 µg/24 hours
Metanephrines, urine	<1.3 mg/24 hours
Growth hormone (hGH), serum	
Male	0–5 ng/ml
Females	0–10 ng/ml
Vanillylmandelic acid (VMA), urine	
<1 year	<27 µg/mg creatinine
1 year	<18 µg/mg creatinine
2–4 years	<13 µg/mg creatinine
5–9 years	<8.5 µg/mg creatinine
10–14 years	<7 µg/mg creatinine
15–18 years	<5 µg/mg creatinine
Adults	<9 mg/24 hours
Homovanillic acid (HVA), urine	
<1 year	<35 µg/mg creatinine
1 year	<23 µg/mg creatinine
2–4 years	<13.5 µg/mg creatinine
5–9 years	<9 µg/mg creatinine
10–14 years	<12 µg/mg creatinine
15–18 years	<2 µg/mg creatinine
Adults	<8 mg/24 hours
5-Hydroxyindoleacetic acid (5-HIAA) (serotonin), urine	<6 mg/24 hours
Pregnanetriol, pregnanediol, urine	See Table 10-1.
17-Ketogenic steroids, urine	
0–10 years	0.1–4.0 mg/24 hours
11–14 years	2–9 mg/24 hours
Adult males	4–14 mg/24 hours
Adult females	2–12 mg/24 hours
17-Ketosteroids, urine	
0–10 years	0.1–3.0 mg/24 hours
11–14 years	2–7 mg/24 hours
Adult males	6–21 mg/24 hours
Adult females	4–17 mg/24 hours
17-Ketosteroids (fractionation), urine	See Table 10-1.
Adrenocorticotropic hormone (ACTH), plasma	≤120 pg/ml at 9 A.M.
	0–35 pg/ml at midnight

Corticoids (includes cortisol, corticosterone, 11-deoxycortisol) (for general screening), plasma	A.M.: 7–28 µg/dl P.M.: 2–18 µg/dl
Cortisol, free, urine	24–108 µg/24 hours
Cortisol (not for general screening), plasma	A.M.: 7–25 µg/dl P.M.: 2–14 µg/dl
Deoxycorticosteroids (for metyrapone test), plasma	A.M.: 0–5 µg/dl P.M.: 0–3 µg/dl
Renin activity (peripheral vein specimen), plasma	
Na-depleted, upright	
20–39 years	2.9–24.0 ng/ml/hour
≧40 years	2.9–10.8 ng/ml/hour
Na-replete, upright	
20–39 years	≦0.6–4.3 ng/ml/hour
≧40 years	≦0.6–3.0 ng/ml/hour
Insulin, serum	0–25 µU/ml
Gastrin, serum	<300 pg/ml
Angiotensin converting enzyme, serum (not done if < 20 years old)	18–67 units/ml

Blood Vitamin Levels

Vitamin A	20–100 µg/dl
Carotene	
0–6 months	0–40 mg/dl
6 months to adult	40–180 mg/dl
Vitamin C (ascorbic acid)	0.2–2.0 mg/dl
Vitamin D	16–120 ng/ml (procedure not generally available)
	Indirect estimate by measuring serum alkaline phosphatase, calcium, and phosphorus
Vitamin E (alpha-tocopherol)	
Children	3.0–15.0 µg/ml
Adults	5.0–20.0 µg/ml
Vitamin B_1 (thiamine)	5.3–7.9 µg/dl
Vitamin B_2 (riboflavin)	3.7–13.7 µg/dl
Vitamin B_{12} (cobalamin)	
Low	<100 pg/ml
Indeterminate	100–200 pg/ml
Normal	200–1100 pg/ml
Elevated	>1100 pg/ml
Unsaturated vitamin B_{12}-binding capacity	870–1800 pg/ml
Folate (serum)	>2.0 ng/ml
Folate (RBC)	>140 ng/ml

Critical Values

These levels may indicate the need for prompt clinical intervention.

	Low	**High**
Packed cell volume (hematocrit)	<15 vol%	>55 vol%
Hemoglobin	<5 gm/dl	>18 gm/dl
Platelet count	<30,000/cu mm	>1,000,000/cu mm
Platelet count (pediatric)	<20,000/cu mm	>1,000,000/cu mm
Prothrombin time	None	>40 seconds
Total serum bilirubin (newborns)	None	>18 mg/dl (see p. 63)
Serum calcium	<6 mg/dl	>14 mg/dl
Serum glucose	<40 mg/dl	>700 mg/dl
Serum glucose (newborns)	<30 mg/dl	>300 mg/dl
Serum phosphorus	<1 mg/dl	None
Serum potassium	<2.5 mEq/L	>6.5 mEq/L
Serum potassium (newborns)	<2.5 mEq/L	>8.0 mEq/L
Serum sodium	<120 mEq/L	>160 mEq/L
Serum bicarbonate	<10 mEq/L	>40 mEq/L
Blood PCO_2	<20 mmHg	>70 mmHg
Blood pH	<7.2 units	>7.6 units
Blood PO_2	<40 mmHg	None
Positive blood culture		
Positive CSF Gram stain		
Positive CSF culture		

CRITICAL VALUES FOR THERAPEUTIC DRUGS

These levels may indicate the need for prompt clinical intervention.

	Blood Levels
Tobramycin	>12 μg/ml (peak)
Carbamazepine	>20 μg/ml
Ethosuximide	>200 μg/ml
Phenobarbital	>60 μg/ml
Phenytoin	>40 μg/ml
Primidone	>24 μg/ml
Lithium	>2 mEq/L
Lidocaine	>9 μg/ml
Quinidine	>10 μg/ml
Theophylline	>25 μg/ml
Digoxin	>2.5 ng/ml
Digitoxin	>35 ng/ml

Specific Laboratory Examinations

13

Blood

Chemistries

SERUM GLUCOSE

May Be Increased In

Diabetes mellitus, including
    Hemochromatosis
    Cushing's syndrome (with insulin-resistant diabetes)
    Acromegaly and gigantism (with insulin-resistant diabetes in early stages; hypopituitarism later)

Increased circulating epinephrine
    Adrenalin injection
    Pheochromocytoma
    Stress (e.g., emotion, burns, shock, anesthesia)

Acute pancreatitis

Chronic pancreatitis (some patients)

Wernicke's encephalopathy (vitamin B_1 deficiency)

Some CNS lesions (subarachnoid hemorrhage, convulsive states)

Effect of drugs (e.g., corticosteroids, estrogens, alcohol, phenytoin, thiazides, propranolol, chronic hypervitaminosis A)

Fasting hyperglycemia is defined as serum (or plasma) glucose $\geqq$ 140 mg/dl on more than one occasion.

May Be Decreased In

Pancreatic disorders
    Islet cell tumor, hyperplasia
    Pancreatitis
    Glucagon deficiency

Extrapancreatic tumors
    Carcinoma of adrenal gland
    Carcinoma of stomach
    Fibrosarcoma
    Other

Hepatic disease
    Diffuse severe disease (e.g., poisoning, hepatitis, cirrhosis, primary or metastatic tumor)

Endocrine disorders
    Hypopituitarism and Addison's disease
    Hypothyroidism
    Adrenal medulla unresponsiveness
    Early diabetes mellitus

Functional disturbances
    Postgastrectomy
    Gastroenterostomy
    Autonomic nervous system disorders

Pediatric anomalies
    Prematurity

Infant of diabetic mother
Ketotic hypoglycemia
Zetterstrom's syndrome
Idiopathic leucine sensitivity
Spontaneous hypoglycemia in infants
Enzyme diseases
von Gierke's disease
Galactosemia
Maple syrup urine disease
Fructose intolerance
Other
Exogenous insulin (factitious)
Oral hypoglycemic medications (factitious)
Leucine sensitivity
Malnutrition
Hypothalamic lesions
Alcoholism

Blood samples in which serum is not separated from blood cells will show glucose values decreasing at rate of 7 mg/dl/hour at room temperature.

SERUM UREA NITROGEN (BUN)

Increased In

Impaired kidney function (see Serum Creatinine, p. 43)
Prerenal azotemia—any cause of reduced renal blood flow
Congestive heart failure
Salt and water depletion (vomiting, diarrhea, diuresis, sweating)
Shock
Postrenal azotemia—any obstruction of urinary tract (ratio of BUN-creatinine increases above normal of 10:1)
Increased protein catabolism (serum creatinine remains normal)
Hemorrhage into gastrointestinal tract
Acute myocardial infarction
Stress

Decreased In

Severe liver damage (liver failure)
Drugs
Poisoning
Hepatitis
Other
Increased utilization of protein for synthesis
Late pregnancy
Infancy
Acromegaly
Diet
Low-protein and high-carbohydrate
IV feedings only
Impaired absorption (celiac disease)
Nephrotic syndrome (some patients)

A low BUN of 6–8 mg/dl is frequently associated with states of overhydration.
A BUN of 10–20 mg/dl almost always indicates normal glomerular function.

A BUN of 50–150 mg/dl implies serious impairment of renal function.

Markedly increased BUN (150–250 mg/dl) is virtually conclusive evidence of severely impaired glomerular function.

In chronic renal disease, BUN correlates better with symptoms of uremia than does the serum creatinine.

SERUM NONPROTEIN NITROGEN (NPN)

NPN is not as useful as BUN as an index of renal function because it represents a heterogeneous group of substances not all of which are excreted by the kidney. The increase parallels that of BUN.

SERUM CREATININE

Increased In
Diet
   Ingestion of creatinine (roast meat)
Muscle disease
   Gigantism
   Acromegaly
Prerenal azotemia (see Serum Urea Nitrogen [BUN], p. 42)
Postrenal azotemia (see Serum Urea Nitrogen [BUN], p. 42)
Impaired kidney function

Serum creatinine is a more specific and sensitive indicator of renal disease than BUN. Use of simultaneous BUN and creatinine determinations provides more information.

Decreased In
Not clinically significant
Artifactual (e.g., marked increase of serum bilirubin)

BUN-CREATININE RATIO
(see also Table 30-3, pp. 526–527)
Generally supports clinical impressions, but the effect of many factors decreases diagnostic value, especially in acute renal failure.
Normal = 10:1; in acute and chronic renal failure ≅ 10:1

Increased In
Prerenal azotemia (typically ≥ 15:1) (e.g., heart failure, salt depletion, dehydration, blood loss)
Postrenal azotemia (typically ≥ 15:1) (e.g., obstructive uropathy)
Impaired renal function plus
   Excess protein intake or production or tissue breakdown (e.g., GI bleeding, thyrotoxicosis, infection, Cushing's syndrome, high-protein diet, surgery, burns, cachexia, high fever)
   Urine reabsorption (e.g., ureterocolostomy)
Patients with reduced muscle mass (subnormal creatinine production)
Certain drugs (e.g., tetracycline, glucocorticoids)

Decreased In
Renal dialysis
Muscular patients who develop renal failure

Other causes of decreased urea production (e.g., hepatic insufficiency, low protein intake, severe diarrhea or vomiting)

Increased Ratio
Inadequate renal blood flow (e.g., prerenal congestive heart failure, dehydration, shock, glomerular disease)

Decreased Ratio
Low protein intake (e.g., starvation, renal failure)
Chronic renal failure
Repeated dialysis (urea rather than creatinine diffuses out of extracellular fluid)
Severe hepatic insufficiency
Inherited hyperammonemias (urea is virtually absent in blood)
Syndrome of inappropriate secretion of antidiuretic hormone (due to tubular secretion of urea)
Phenacemide therapy (accelerates conversion of creatine to creatinine)
Rhabdomyolysis (releases muscle creatinine)

Inappropriate Ratio
Diabetic ketoacidosis (acetoacetate causes false increase in creatinine with certain methodologies resulting in normal ratio when dehydration should produce an increased BUN-creatinine ratio)
Cephalosporin therapy (interferes with creatinine measurement)

SERUM CREATINE

Increased In
High dietary intake (meat)
Destruction of muscle
Hyperthyroidism (this diagnosis almost excluded by normal serum creatine)
Active rheumatoid arthritis
Testosterone therapy

Decreased In
Not clinically significant
Drugs (e.g., TMP/SMX, cimetidine, cefoxitin)
Artifactual (e.g., diabetic ketoacidosis)

SERUM URIC ACID

Levels are very labile and show day-to-day and seasonal variation in same person; also increased by emotional stress, total fasting.

Increased In
Gout
25% of relatives of patients with gout
Renal failure (does not correlate with severity of kidney damage; urea and creatinine should be used)
Increased destruction of nucleoproteins
    Leukemia, multiple myeloma
    Polycythemia
    Lymphoma, especially postirradiation
    Other disseminated neoplasms

Cancer chemotherapy (e.g., nitrogen mustards, vincristine, mercaptopurine)

Hemolytic anemia

Sickle cell anemia

Resolving pneumonia

Toxemia of pregnancy (serial determinations to follow therapeutic response and estimate prognosis)

Psoriasis (one-third of patients)

Diet

High-protein weight reduction diet

Excess nucleoprotein (e.g., sweetbreads, liver)

Asymptomatic hyperuricemia (e.g., incidental finding with no evidence of gout; clinical significance not known but people so afflicted should be rechecked periodically for gout). The higher the level of serum uric acid, the greater the likelihood of an attack of acute gouty arthritis.

Miscellaneous

von Gierke's disease

Lead poisoning

Lesch-Nyhan syndrome

Maple syrup urine disease

Down's syndrome

Polycystic kidneys

Calcinosis universalis and circumscripta

Some drugs (e.g., thiazides, furosemide, ethacrynic acid, and all diuretics except spironolactone, mercurials, and ticrynafen; small doses of salicylates [< 4 gm/day])

Hypoparathyroidism

Primary hyperparathyroidism

Hypothyroidism

Sarcoidosis

Chronic berylliosis

Some patients with alcoholism

Patients with arteriosclerosis and hypertension. (*Serum uric acid is increased in 80% of patients with elevated serum triglycerides.*)

Certain population groups (e.g., Blackfoot and Pima Indians, Filipinos, New Zealand Maoris)

Decreased In

Administration of ACTH

Administration of uricosuric drugs (e.g., high doses of salicylates, probenecid, cortisone, allopurinol, coumarins)

Wilson's disease

Fanconi's syndrome

Acromegaly (some patients)

Celiac disease (slightly)

Pernicious anemia in relapse (some patients)

Xanthinuria

Administration of various other drugs (x-ray contrast agents, glyceryl guaiacolate)

Neoplasms (occasional cases) (e.g., carcinomas, Hodgkin's disease)

Healthy adults with isolated defect in tubular transport of uric acid (Dalmatian dog mutation)

Unchanged In
Colchicine administration

SERUM CHOLESTEROL
(see also Serum Lipoproteins, p. 77)

Increased In
Idiopathic hypercholesterolemia
Hyperlipoproteinemias
Biliary obstruction
 Stone, carcinoma, etc., of duct
 Cholangiolitic cirrhosis
 Biliary cirrhosis
 Cholestasis
von Gierke's disease
Hypothyroidism
Nephrosis (due to chronic nephritis, renal vein thrombosis, amyloidosis, systemic lupus erythematosus, periarteritis, diabetic glomerulosclerosis)
Pancreatic disease
 Diabetes mellitus
 Total pancreatectomy
 Chronic pancreatitis (some patients)
Pregnancy

Decreased In
Severe liver cell damage (due to chemicals, drugs, hepatitis)
Hyperthyroidism
Malnutrition (e.g., starvation, terminal neoplasm, uremia, malabsorption in steatorrhea)
Chronic anemia
 Pernicious anemia in relapse
 Hemolytic anemias
 Marked hypochromic anemia
Cortisone and ACTH therapy
Hypobeta- and abetalipoproteinemia
Tangier disease

SERUM HDL CHOLESTEROL

Increased In
Vigorous exercise
Increased clearance of triglyceride (VLDL)
Moderate consumption of alcohol
Insulin treatment
Estrogen

Decreased In
Starvation
Obesity
Cigarette smoking
Diabetes mellitus
Hypothyroidism
Liver disease
Nephrosis
Uremia

Progesterone
Elevated serum triglyceride

SERUM SODIUM
(see also Table 13-2; pp. 54–55)

Increased In
(virtually always means lack of water)

Excess loss of water
    Conditions that cause loss via gastrointestinal tract (e.g., in vomiting), lung (hyperpnea), or skin (e.g., in excessive sweating)
    Conditions that cause diuresis
        Diabetes insipidus
        Nephrogenic diabetes insipidus
        Diabetes mellitus
        Diuretic drugs
        Diuretic phase of acute tubular necrosis
        Diuresis following relief of urinary tract obstruction
        Hypercalcemic nephropathy
        Hypokalemic nephropathy
Excess administration of sodium (iatrogenic), e.g., incorrect replacement following fluid loss
"Essential" hypernatremia due to hypothalamic lesions (see p. 508)

Decreased In
(serum osmolality is decreased) (see below)

Dilutional (e.g., congestive heart failure, nephrosis, cirrhosis with ascites)
Sodium depletion
    Loss of body fluids (e.g., vomiting, diarrhea, excessive sweating) with incorrect or no therapeutic replacement, diuretic drugs (e.g., thiazides)
    Adrenocortical insufficiency
    Salt-losing nephropathy
    Inappropriate secretion of antidiuretic hormone
Spurious (serum osmolality is normal or increased)
    Hyperlipidemia (also causes spurious hyperchloremia)
    Hyperglycemia (serum sodium decreases 3 mEq/L for every increase of serum glucose of 100 mg/dl)
    Administration of mannitol
    Hyperproteinemia (e.g., multiple myeloma)

SERUM OSMOLALITY
(freezing point determination)

Hyperosmolality
Due To
Hyperglycemia
    Diabetic ketoacidosis
    Nonketotic hyperglycemic coma
        Clinical picture: A middle-aged or older person with diabetes of recent onset or unrecognized diabetes, who shows neurologic symptoms (e.g., convulsions or hemiplegia) and then becomes stuporous or comatose.
        Serum glucose is very high but, contrary to expectation in

diabetic coma, ketosis is minimal and plasma acetone is not found.

Increased serum osmolality (normal = 280–300 mOsm/L). In mildly drowsy patients, mean is 320 mOsm/L. At level of 350 mOsm/L, there will be some confusion or some stupor. At 400 mOsm/L, most patients are obtunded. State of consciousness does not correlate with height of acidemia.

Osmolality should be determined routinely in grossly unbalanced diabetic patients.

Determinations of blood sodium and potassium levels are not useful in diagnosis or in estimating net ion losses but are performed to monitor changes in sodium and potassium during therapy.

Laboratory findings are those due to complications or precipitating factors (e.g., pneumonia, pancreatitis, stroke).

Some precipitating factors

Drugs (e.g., thiazides, steroids, phenytoin, propranolol)

Glucose overloading (e.g., hyperalimentation, dialysis, IV infusions in treatment of burns)

Dehydration

Pancreatitis with major shift of fluids

Cerebral or cardiovascular accident

Hypernatremia with dehydration

Diarrhea, vomiting, fever, hyperventilation, inadequate water intake

Diabetes insipidus—central

Nephrogenic diabetes insipidus—congenital or acquired (e.g., hypercalcemia, hypokalemia, chronic renal disease, sickle cell disease, effect of some drugs)

Osmotic diuresis—hyperglycemia, administration of urea or mannitol

Hypernatremia with normal hydration—due to hypothalamic disorders

Insensitivity of osmoreceptors (essential hypernatremia)—water loading does not return serum osmolality to normal; chlorpropamide may lower serum sodium toward normal

Defect in thirst (hypodipsia)—forced water intake returns serum osmolality to normal

Hypernatremia with overhydration—iatrogenic or accidental (e.g., infants given feedings with high sodium concentrations or given $NaHCO_3$ for respiratory distress or cardiopulmonary arrest)

Alcohol ingestion is the commonest cause of hyperosmolar state and of coexisting coma and hyperosmolar state.

Hyposmolality

Due To

Hyponatremia with hypovolemia

Adrenal insufficiency (e.g., salt-losing form of congenital adrenal hyperplasia, congenital adrenal hypoplasia, hemorrhage into adrenals, inadequate replacement of corticosteroids, inappropriate tapering of steroids)

Renal losses
GI tract loss (e.g., vomiting, diarrhea)
Other losses (e.g., burns, peritonitis, pancreatitis)
Hyponatremia with normal volume or hypervolemia (dilutional syndromes)
Congestive heart failure, cirrhosis, nephrotic syndrome
Syndrome of inappropriate secretion of antidiuretic hormone (SIADH)

Urine and plasma osmolality are more useful to diagnose state of hydration than changes in hematocrit, serum proteins, and BUN, which are more dependent on other factors than hydration.

Changes in serum sodium most often reflect changes in water balance rather than sodium balance. If patient has not received large load of sodium, hypernatremia suggests need for water and values < 130 mEq/L suggest overhydration.

Formula for *calculation* or *prediction* of serum osmolality:

$$\text{mOsm/L} = (2 \times \text{serum Na}) + \frac{\text{serum glucose}}{18} + \frac{\text{BUN}}{2.8}$$

Difference between measured and calculated values is < 10 in healthy persons.
If measured − calculated osmolality > 10 (osmotic gap), one of the following is present:
Laboratory analytic error
Decreased serum water content
Hyperlipidemia (serum will appear lipemic)
Hyperproteinemia (total protein > 10 gm/dl)
Additional low-molecular weight substances are in serum (measured osmolality will be > 300 mOsm/kg water):
Ethanol
Methanol
Isopropyl alcohol
Ethylene glycol (when large amounts are ingested)
Acetone
Ethyl ether
Paraldehyde
Mannitol

Difference between measured and calculated values can be used to estimate the blood alcohol. Since serum osmolality increases 22 mOsm/kg for every 100 mg/dl of ethanol

Estimated blood alcohol (mg/dl) = osmotic gap $\times \dfrac{100}{22}$

Osmotic gap can also be used to detect accumulation of infused mannitol in serum.

Serum osmolality is also used to determine serum water deviation from normal for evaluation of hyponatremia (see Hyponatremia, pp. 507, 509).

SERUM POTASSIUM
(see also Table 13-2, pp. 54–55)

Increased In
Renal failure
    Acute with oliguria or anuria
    Chronic end-stage with oliguria (glomerular filtration rate
        <3–5 ml/minute)
    Chronic nonoliguric associated with dehydration, obstruction,
        trauma, or excess potassium
Decreased mineralocorticoid activity
    Addison's disease
    Hypofunction of renin-angiotensin-aldosterone system (see p.
        491)
    Pseudohypoaldosteronism
    Aldosterone antagonist (e.g., spironolactone)
Increased supply of potassium
    Red blood cell hemolysis (transfusion reaction, hemolytic
        anemia)
    Excess dietary intake or rapid potassium infusion
    Striated muscle (status epilepticus, periodic paralysis)
    Potassium-retaining drugs (e.g., triamterene)
    Fluid-electrolyte imbalance (e.g., dehydration, acidosis)
    Sudden cell breakdown (e.g., crush injury, major surgery, burns)
    Adynamia episodica hereditaria (transient during attack)
    Laboratory artifacts (e.g., hemolysis during venipuncture, con-
        ditions associated with thrombocytosis, incomplete separa-
        tion of serum and clot)

Decreased In
(see Table 28-2, p. 410)
Renal and adrenal conditions with metabolic alkalosis
    Administration of diuretics
    Primary aldosteronism
    Pseudoaldosteronism
    Salt-losing nephropathy
    Cushing's syndrome
Renal conditions associated with metabolic acidosis
    Renal tubular acidosis
    Diuretic phase of acute tubular necrosis
    Chronic pyelonephritis
    Diuresis following relief of urinary tract obstruction
Gastrointestinal conditions
    Vomiting, gastric suctioning
    Villous adenoma
    Cancer of colon
    Chronic laxative abuse
    Zollinger-Ellison syndrome
    Chronic diarrhea
    Ureterosigmoidostomy
Familial periodic paralysis (during attack)

SERUM CHLORIDE

Increased In
Metabolic acidosis associated with prolonged diarrhea with loss of
    $NaHCO_3$

Renal tubular diseases with decreased excretion of H^+ and decreased reabsorption of HCO_3^- ("hyperchloremic acidosis")
Respiratory alkalosis (e.g., hyperventilation, severe CNS damage)
Excessive administration of certain drugs (e.g., NH_4Cl, IV saline, steroids, salicylate intoxication; acetazolamide therapy)
Some cases of hyperparathyroidism
Diabetes insipidus, dehydration
Sodium loss > chloride loss (e.g., diarrhea, intestinal fistulas)
Bromism
Ureterosigmoidostomy

Decreased In

Prolonged vomiting or suction (loss of HCl)
Metabolic acidoses with accumulation of organic anions (see Anion Gap, pp. 409–412)
Salt-losing renal diseases
Adrenocortical insufficiency
Primary aldosteronism
Expansion of extracellular fluid (e.g., syndrome of inappropriate secretion of antidiuretic hormone, hyponatremia, water intoxication)

HYPOXEMIA

(arterial blood PO_2 75–100 mmHg at rest at sea level while breathing room air; decreases with age and higher altitude)

Due To

Generalized alveolar hypoventilation
    Skeletal abnormalities (e.g., kyphoscoliosis, flail chest due to trauma)
    Neuromuscular conditions affecting respiration (e.g., phrenic nerve paralysis, tetanus, acute poliomyelitis, status epilepticus; depression of respiratory centers of brain by drugs, head injury, cerebrovascular accident)
    Pickwickian syndrome of massive obesity
    Restricted diaphragmatic breathing (e.g., abdominal distention or pain)
    Environmental (e.g., carbon monoxide exposure, smoke inhalation, anesthesia, near drowning)
Decreased pulmonary diffusing capacity
    Alveolar block syndrome (e.g., lymphangitic carcinomatosis, pulmonary adenomatosis, sarcoidosis, berylliosis, Hamman-Rich syndrome, pulmonary hemosiderosis secondary to mitral stenosis)
    Decreased alveolocapillary membrane surface area by restricted expansion or destruction or loss of lung tissue (e.g., resection), compression of lung (e.g., pneumothorax)
Right-to-left cardiac shunt (e.g., congenital heart disease) or increased venous admixture (e.g., pulmonary hemangioma)

Very often, more than one of these mechanisms is operative simultaneously.

Ventilation-perfusion abnormality or mismatched distribution of inspired air with pulmonary blood flow causing regional hypoventilation

Diffuse bronchopulmonary disease (chronic and acute) (e.g., bronchitis, asthma, emphysema, bronchiectasis, atelectasis, pneumoconiosis, granulomata, neoplasm, infarction, pneumonia, mucoviscidosis)

Airway obstruction (e.g., foreign body, croup, neoplasm, retained secretions)

HYPOCAPNIA
(see Tables 13-1 and 13-2, pp. 53, 54–55)

Due To Any Mechanism of Hyperventilation
Physiologic (e.g., pregnancy, high altitude)
Psychogenic
Mechanically controlled
Compensatory secondary to metabolic acidosis
Compensatory secondary to anoxemia (e.g., severe anemia, pneumonia, asthma) (see Hypoxemia, p. 51)
Drugs (e.g., salicylate poisoning)
Central nervous system lesion
Liver failure
Gram-negative sepsis

Arterial PCO_2 promptly reflects changes in depth and rate of ventilation.

HYPERCAPNIA

Due To
Severe electrolyte disturbances
Acute intermittent porphyria
Severe hypothyroidism

See also causes of hypoxemia, p. 51.

BLOOD pH
(normal arterial pH at sea level is 7.40 ± 0.05) (see Table 13-1, p. 53)

Decreased In
Metabolic acidosis (see p. 411)
Respiratory acidosis (see p. 414 and Table 13-1, p. 53)

Increased In
Metabolic alkalosis (see p. 413)
Respiratory alkalosis (see p. 415 and Table 13-1, p. 53)

SERUM MAGNESIUM

Increased In
Renal failure
Diabetic coma before treatment
Hypothyroidism
Addison's disease and after adrenalectomy
Controlled diabetes mellitus in older patients
Administration of antacids containing magnesium

Decreased In
GI disease showing malabsorption and abnormal loss of GI fluids (e.g., nontropical sprue, small bowel resection, biliary and intes-

Table 13-1. Summary of Pure and Mixed Acid-Base Disorders

	Decreased pH	Normal pH	Increased pH
Increased PCO_2	Respiratory acidosis with or without incompletely compensated metabolic alkalosis or coexisting metabolic acidosis	Respiratory acidosis and compensated metabolic alkalosis	Metabolic alkalosis with incompletely compensated respiratory acidosis or coexisting respiratory acidosis
Normal PCO_2	Metabolic acidosis	Normal	Metabolic alkalosis
Decreased PCO_2	Metabolic acidosis with incompletely compensated respiratory alkalosis or coexisting respiratory alkalosis	Respiratory alkalosis and compensated metabolic acidosis	Respiratory alkalosis with or without incompletely compensated metabolic acidosis or coexisting metabolic alkalosis

Source: Adapted from H. H. Friedman, *Problem-Oriented Medical Diagnosis* (3rd ed.). Boston: Little, Brown, 1983.

tinal fistulas, abdominal irradiation, prolonged aspiration of intestinal contents, celiac disease and other causes of steatorrhea)

Prolonged parenteral fluid administration without magnesium (usually > 3 weeks)

Acute alcoholism and alcoholic cirrhosis

Insulin treatment of diabetic coma

Hyperthyroidism

Aldosteronism

Hyperparathyroidism

Hypoparathyroidism

Lytic tumors of bone

Diuretic drug therapy (e.g., ethacrynic acid, furosemide)

Some cases of renal disease (e.g., glomerulonephritis, pyelonephritis, renal tubular acidosis, gentamicin-induced injury)

Acute pancreatitis

Excessive lactation

Idiopathic disorders

Magnesium deficiency may cause apparently unexplained hypocalcemia and hypokalemia; the patients may have neurologic and GI symptoms.

Table 13-2. Urine and Blood Changes in Electrolytes, pH, and Volume in Various Conditions

Measurement	Pulmonary Emphysema	Congestive Heart Failure	Excessive Sweating	Diarrhea	Pyloric Obstruction	Dehydration	Starvation	Malabsorption	Salicylate Intoxication	Primary Aldosteronism
Blood										
Sodium	N	N or D	D	D	D	I	N	D	N	I
Potassium	N	N	N	D	D	N	D	D	N or D	D
Bicarbonate	I	N	N	D	I	N or D	D	N or D	D	I
Chloride	D	D	D	D	D	I	N	N	I	D
Volume	N or I	I	N	D	D	D	N or D	D	N	N
Urine										
Sodium	D	D	D	D	D	I	N or I	D	I	D
Potassium	N	N	N	N or D	N	I	I or N	D	N or I	I
pH	D	N	N	D	I	D	D	N or D	I	N or D
Volume	N	D	N	D	D	D	I	N	N	I

N = normal; D = decreased; I = increased; V = variable.

Table 13-2 (continued)

Measurement	Adrenal Cortical Insufficiency	Diabetes Insipidus	Diabetic Acidosis	Mercurial Diuretic Administration	Thiazide Diuretic Administration	Ammonium Chloride Administration	Diamox Administration	Renal Tubular Acidosis	Chronic Renal Failure	Acute Renal Failure
Blood										
Sodium	D	N or I	D	D	D	D	D	D	D	D
Potassium	I	N	N or I	D	D	D	D	D	N or D	I
Bicarbonate	N or D	N	D	I	D	D	D	D	D	D
Chloride	D	I	D	D	D	I	I	I	D or N	I
Volume	D	D	D	D	D	D	D	D	V	I
Urine										
Sodium	I	N	I	I	I	I	I	I	I	D
Potassium	N or D	N	I	I	I	I	I	I	I	D
pH	N or I	N	D	D	N or I	I	I	I	I	N or I
Volume	N or D	I	I	I	I	I	I	I	V*	D

*Usually increased.

SERUM CALCIUM
(see also p. 90; Table 29-4, pp. 462–463; Fig. 29-1, p. 466; and Table 29-5, pp. 466–467)

Increased In
Hyperparathyroidism, primary or secondary

Malignant tumors (especially breast, lung, kidney)

    Due to ectopic secretion of parathormone-like substance (>60% of these cases are due to squamous cell cancer of lung or renal cancer)

    Due to bone metastases

    Hematologic malignancies (e.g., myeloma, lymphoma, leukemia)

Vitamin D intoxication

Milk-alkali (Burnett's) syndrome

Acute osteoporosis (e.g., immobilization of young patients or in Paget's disease)

Hyperproteinemia (e.g., one-third of patients with sarcoidosis)

Drugs

    Diuretics thiazide and chlorthalidone (rarely increase serum calcium > 1.0 mg/dl)

    Others (e.g., vitamin A, lithium, estrogen, thyroid hormone)

Some endocrine conditions

    Hyperthyroidism (in 20–40% of patients; usually < 14 mg/dl)

    Some patients with myxedema, Cushing's syndrome, Addison's disease, acromegaly)

    (see also Multiple Endocrine Neoplasia [MEN], pp. 513–514)

Granulomatous disease (e.g., tuberculosis, mycoses, berylliosis)

Artifactual (e.g., venous stasis during blood collection by prolonged application of tourniquet, use of cork-stoppered test tubes)

Renal transplantation

Recovery phase of acute renal failure

Miscellaneous

    Familial hypocalciuric hypercalcemia

    Rhabdomyolysis

    Porphyria

Hypercalcemia of sarcoidosis, adrenal insufficiency, and hyperthyroidism tends to be found in clinically evident disease.

Decreased In
Hypoparathyroidism

    Surgical

    Idiopathic

    Pseudohypoparathyroidism

Chronic therapeutic use of anticonvulsant drugs (e.g., phenobarbital, phenytoin)

Total serum protein and albumin should always be measured simultaneously for proper interpretation since 0.8 mg of calcium is bound to 1.0 gm of albumin in serum.

Malabsorption of calcium and vitamin D

    Obstructive jaundice

Hypoalbuminemia

    Cachexia

Nephrotic syndrome
Sprue
Celiac disease
Cystic fibrosis of pancreas
Chronic renal disease with uremia and phosphate retention
Acute pancreatitis with extensive fat necrosis
Insufficient calcium, phosphorus, and vitamin D ingestion
Bone disease (osteomalacia, rickets)
Starvation
Late pregnancy

SERUM PHOSPHORUS

(see also Table 29-4, pp. 462–463)

Increased In
Hypoparathyroidism
Idiopathic
Surgical
Pseudohypoparathyroidism
Excess vitamin D intake
Secondary hyperparathyroidism (renal rickets)
Bone disease
Healing fractures
Multiple myeloma (some patients)
Paget's disease (some patients)
Osteolytic metastatic tumor in bone (some patients)
Addison's disease
Acromegaly
Childhood
Myelogenous leukemia
Acute yellow atrophy
High intestinal obstruction
Sarcoidosis (some patients)
Milk-alkali (Burnett's) syndrome (some patients)
Neoplasms
Excessive breakdown of tissue
Phosphate enemas or infusions
Massive blood transfusions
Magnesium deficiency

Serum magnesium should always be measured in any patient with hypocalcemia.

Artifactual increase by hemolysis of blood.

Decreased In
Alcoholism*
Diabetes mellitus*
Hyperalimentation*

*Indicates conditions associated with severe hypophosphatemia.

Nutritional recovery syndrome* (rapid refeeding after prolonged starvation)

Alkalosis, respiratory (e.g., gram-negative bacteremia) or metabolic

Acute gout

Salicylate poisoning

Administration of glucose intravenously (e.g., recovery after severe burns, hyperalimentation)

Administration of anabolic steroids, androgens, epinephrine, glucagon, insulin

Cushing's syndrome (some patients)

Acidosis (especially ketoacidosis)

Primary hyperparathyroidism

Renal tubular defects (e.g., Fanconi's syndrome)

Hypokalemia

Hypomagnesemia

Administration of diuretics

Prolonged hypothermia (e.g., open heart surgery)

Malabsorption

Vitamin D deficiency and/or resistance, osteomalacia

Malnutrition, vomiting, diarrhea

Administration of phosphate-binding antacids*

Primary hypophosphatemia

Mechanisms of hypophosphatemia are intracellular shift of phosphate, increased loss (via kidney or intestine), or decreased intestinal absorption, usually associated with prior phosphorus depletion. Often, more than one mechanism is operative.

SERUM ALKALINE PHOSPHATASE
(see also Table 29-4, pp. 462–463)

Increased In
Increased deposition of calcium in bone
    Osteitis fibrosa cystica (hyperparathyroidism)
    Paget's disease (osteitis deformans)
    Healing fractures (slightly)
    Osteoblastic bone tumors (osteogenic sarcoma, metastatic carcinoma)
    Osteogenesis imperfecta
    Familial osteoectasia
    Osteomalacia
    Rickets
    Polyostotic fibrous dysplasia
    Late pregnancy; reverts to normal level by 20th day postpartum
    Children
    Administration of ergosterol
Liver disease—any obstruction of biliary system (see pp. 253–255)
    Nodules in liver (metastatic tumor, abscess, cyst, parasite, amyloid, tuberculosis, sarcoid, or leukemia)
    Biliary duct obstruction (e.g., stone, carcinoma)
    Cholangiolar obstruction in hepatitis

*Indicates conditions associated with severe hypophosphatemia.

Adverse reaction to therapeutic drug (e.g., chlorpropamide) (progressive elevation of serum alkaline phosphatase may be first indication that drug therapy should be halted)

Chronic therapeutic use of anticonvulsant drugs (e.g., phenobarbital, phenytoin)

Placental origin—appears 16–20th week of normal pregnancy, increases progressively up to onset of labor, disappears 3–6 days after delivery of placenta. May be increased during complications of pregnancy (e.g., hypertension, preeclampsia, eclampsia, threatened abortion) but difficult to interpret without serial determinations.

Intestinal origin—is a component in ≅25% of normal sera; increases after eating in these persons. Has been reported to be increased in cirrhosis, various diseases of GI tract, chronic hemodialysis.

Ectopic production by neoplasm without involvement of liver or bone (e.g., Hodgkin's disease, cancer of lung or pancreas)

Marked hyperthyroidism in some patients (bone origin)

Some patients with myocardial, pulmonary, renal (one-third of cases), or splenic infarction, usually during phase of organization

Intravenous injection of albumin; sometimes marked increase (e.g., 10 times normal level) lasting for several days (placental origin)

Hyperphosphatasia (liver and bone isoenzymes)

Primary hypophosphatemia (often increased)

Alkaline phosphatase isoenzyme determinations are not clinically useful; heat inactivation may be more useful to distinguish bone from liver source of increased alkaline phosphatase.

Increase in cases of metastases to bone is marked only in prostate carcinoma. Increase > 2 times upper limit of normal in patients with primary breast or lung tumor with osteolytic metastases is more likely due to liver than bone metastases.

Marked elevation in absence of liver disease is most suggestive of Paget's disease of bone or metastatic carcinoma from prostate.

Normal In

Inherited metabolic diseases (Dubin-Johnson, Rotor's, Gilbert's, Crigler-Najjar syndromes; types I–V glycogenoses, mucopolysaccharidoses; increase in Wilson's disease and hemochromatosis related to hepatic fibrosis)

Consumption of alcohol by healthy persons (in contrast to gamma-glutamyl transpeptidase); may be normal even in alcoholic hepatitis.

In acute icteric viral hepatitis, increase is < 2 times normal in 90% of cases, but when alkaline phosphatase is high and serum bilirubin is normal, should rule out infectious mononucleosis as cause of hepatitis.

Decreased In

Excess vitamin D ingestion

Milk-alkali (Burnett's) syndrome

Scurvy

Hypophosphatasia

Hypothyroidism

Pernicious anemia in one-third of patients
Celiac disease
Malnutrition
Collection of blood in EDTA, fluoride, or oxalate anticoagulant

SERUM LEUCINE AMINOPEPTIDASE (LAP)

Parallels serum alkaline phosphatase except that

> LAP is usually normal in the presence of bone disease or malabsorption syndrome.
> LAP is a more sensitive indicator of choledocholithiasis and of liver metastases in anicteric patients.

When serum LAP is increased, urine LAP is almost always increased; but when urine LAP is increased, serum LAP may have already returned to normal.

5'-NUCLEOTIDASE (5'-N)

Increased Only In

Obstructive type of hepatobiliary disease

May be an early indication of liver metastases in the cancer patient, especially if jaundice is absent.

Normal In

Pregnancy and postpartum period (in contrast to serum LAP and alkaline phosphatase); therefore may aid in differential diagnosis of hepatobiliary disease occurring during pregnancy.

Whenever the alkaline phosphatase is elevated, a simultaneous elevation of 5'-N establishes biliary disease as the cause of the elevated alkaline phosphatase. If the 5'-N is not increased, the cause of the elevated alkaline phosphatase must be found elsewhere, e.g., bone disease.

SERUM GAMMA-GLUTAMYL TRANSPEPTIDASE (GGTP)

Increased In

Liver disease. Generally parallels changes in serum alkaline phosphatase, LAP, and 5'-nucleotidase but is more sensitive.

> Acute hepatitis. Elevation is less marked than that of other liver enzymes, but it is the last to return to normal and therefore is useful to indicate recovery.
> Chronic hepatitis. Increased more than in acute hepatitis. More elevated than SGOT and SGPT. In dormant stage, may be the only enzyme elevated.
> Cirrhosis. In inactive cases, average values are lower than in chronic hepatitis. Increases greater than 10–20 times in cirrhotic patients suggest superimposed primary carcinoma of the liver.
> Primary biliary cirrhosis. Elevation is marked.
> Fatty liver. Elevation parallels that of SGOT and SGPT but is greater.
> Obstructive jaundice. Increase is faster and greater than that of serum alkaline phosphatase and LAP.
> Liver metastases. Parallels alkaline phosphatase; elevation precedes positive liver scans.

Cholestasis. In mechanical and viral cholestasis, GGTP and LAP are about equally increased, but in drug-induced cholestasis, GGTP is much more increased than LAP.

Children. Much more increased in biliary atresia than in neonatal hepatitis (300 units/L is useful differentiating level). Children with alpha$_1$ antitrypsin deficiency have higher levels than other patients with biliary atresia.

Pancreatitis. Always elevated in acute pancreatitis. In chronic pancreatitis is increased when there is involvement of the biliary tract or active inflammation.

Renal disease. Increased in lipoid nephrosis and some cases of renal carcinoma.

Acute myocardial infarction. Increased in 50% of the patients. Elevation begins on fourth to fifth day, reaches maximum at 8–12 days. With shock or acute right heart failure, may have early peak within 48 hours, with rapid decline followed by later rise.

Heavy use of alcohol, barbiturates, or phenytoin (Dilantin). Is the most sensitive indicator of alcoholism, since elevation exceeds that of other commonly assayed liver enzymes.

Gross obesity (slight increase)

Normal In

Women during pregnancy (in contrast to serum alkaline phosphatase and LAP) and children over 3 months of age; therefore may aid in differential diagnosis of hepatobiliary disease occurring during pregnancy and childhood.

Bone disease or patients with increased bone growth (children and adolescents); therefore useful in distinguishing bone disease from liver disease as a cause of increased serum alkaline phosphatase.

Renal failure

Strenuous exercise

SERUM ACID PHOSPHATASE

Increased In

Carcinoma of the prostate (see p. 557)

Infarction of the prostate (sometimes to high levels)

Operative trauma or instrumentation of the prostate (may cause transient increase)

Gaucher's disease (only when certain substrates are used in the laboratory determination)

Excessive destruction of platelets, as in idiopathic thrombocytopenic purpura *with* megakaryocytes in bone marrow

Thromboembolism, hemolytic crises (e.g., sickle cell disease) due to hemolysis (only when certain substrates are used in the laboratory determination)

Leukemic reticuloendotheliosis ("hairy") cells using a specific assay

In the absence of prostatic disease, increased acid phosphatase is seen occasionally in

    Partial translocation trisomy 21

    Diseases of bone

        Advanced Paget's disease

        Metastatic carcinoma of bone

        Multiple myeloma (some patients)

        Hyperparathyroidism

        Other

Various liver diseases ($\leqq 9$ King-Armstrong units)
    Hepatitis
    Obstructive jaundice
    Laennec's cirrhosis
    Other
Acute renal impairment (not related to degree of azotemia)
Other diseases of the reticuloendothelial system with liver or
    bone involvement (e.g., Niemann-Pick disease)

Decreased In
Not clinically significant

SERUM AMYLASE

Increased In*
Acute pancreatitis. Increase begins in 3–6 hours; reaches max-
    imum in 20–30 hours; may persist for 48–72 hours. May increase
    up to 40 times normal. Level should be at least 500 Somogyi
    units/dl to be significant evidence of acute pancreatitis. Urine
    levels reflect serum changes by a time lag of 6–10 hours.
Acute exacerbation of chronic pancreatitis
Perforated or penetrating peptic ulcer, especially with involvement
    of pancreas
Postoperative upper abdominal surgery, especially partial gastrec-
    tomy (up to 2 times normal in one-third of patients)
Obstruction of pancreatic duct by
    Stone or carcinoma
    Drug-induced spasm of sphincter (e.g., opiates, codeine, methyl
      choline, chlorothiazide) to levels 2–15 times normal
    Partial obstruction + drug stimulation (see Pancreozymin-
      Secretin Test, p. 175)
Acute alcohol ingestion or poisoning
Salivary gland disease (mumps, suppurative inflammation, duct ob-
    struction due to calculus)
Advanced renal insufficiency. Often increased even without
    pancreatitis
Macroamylasemia

*Increased serum amylase with low urine amylase may be seen in
renal insufficiency and macroamylasemia.*

May also be increased in acute cholecystitis, intestinal obstruction
with strangulation, mesenteric thrombosis, ruptured aortic aneurysm, ruptured tubal pregnancy, viral hepatitis, carcinoma of
lung

Decreased In
Extensive marked destruction of pancreas (e.g., acute fulminant
pancreatitis, advanced chronic pancreatitis, advanced cystic
fibrosis)

---

*It has been suggested that a level of > 1000 Somogyi units is usually due to
surgically correctable lesions (most frequently stones in biliary tree), the pancreas
either being negative or showing only edema; but 200–500 units is usually associated with pancreatic lesions that are not surgically correctable (e.g., hemorrhagic
pancreatitis, necrosis of pancreas).

Severe liver damage (e.g., hepatitis, poisoning, toxemia of pregnancy, severe thyrotoxicosis, severe burns)

Decreased levels are clinically significant only in occasional cases of fulminant pancreatitis.

Amylase-creatinine clearance ratio

$$= \frac{\text{urine amylase concentration}}{\text{serum amylase concentration}} \times \frac{\text{serum creatinine concentration}}{\text{urine creatinine concentration}} \times 100$$

Normal: 1–5%
Macroamylasemia: <1%
Acute pancreatitis: >5%

False Positives

Burns, chronic renal failure, pregnancy, diabetic ketoacidosis, duodenal perforation, recent thoracic surgery, myoglobinuria, or presence of myeloma proteins

SERUM LIPASE

Increased In

Acute pancreatitis. May remain elevated for as long as 14 days after amylase returns to normal

Perforated or penetrating peptic ulcer, especially with involvement of pancreas

Obstruction of pancreatic duct by
    Stone
    Drug-induced spasm of sphincter (e.g., by opiates, codeine, methyl choline) to levels 2–15 times normal
    Partial obstruction + drug stimulation

Usually Normal In

Mumps

SERUM BILIRUBIN

Increased In

(see also Chap. 24, Hepatobiliary Disease and Disorders of the Pancreas)

Hepatic cellular damage
Biliary duct obstructions
Hemolytic diseases
Prolonged fasting
Direct (conjugated) bilirubin
    <20% of total: due to hemolysis or constitutional hyperbilirubinemia (e.g., Gilbert's disease, Crigler-Najjar syndrome)
    20–40% of total: more suggestive of hepatic than posthepatic jaundice
    40–60% of total: occurs in either hepatic or posthepatic jaundice
    >50% of total: more suggestive of posthepatic than hepatic jaundice

Increased conjugated bilirubin may be associated with normal total bilirubin in up to one-third of patients with liver diseases.

Total serum bilirubin > 40 mg/dl indicates hepatocellular rather than extrahepatic obstruction.

A 48-hour fast produces a mean increase of 240% in normal patients and 194% in those with hepatic dysfunction.

SERUM TRANSAMINASE (SGOT)

Increased In
Acute myocardial infarction
Liver diseases, with active necrosis of parenchymal cells
Musculoskeletal diseases, including trauma and intramuscular injections
Acute pancreatitis
Other
> Myoglobinuria
> Intestinal injury (e.g., surgery, infarction)
> Local irradiation injury
> Pulmonary infarction (relatively slight increase)
> Cerebral infarction (increased in following week in 50% of patients)
> Cerebral neoplasms (occasionally)
> Renal infarction (occasionally)

"Pseudomyocardial infarction" pattern. Administration of opiates to patients with diseased biliary tract or previous cholecystectomy causes increase in LDH and especially SGOT. SGOT increases by 2–4 hours, peaks in 5–8 hours; increase may persist for 24 hours; elevation may be 2½–65 times normal.

Falsely Increased In
(because enzymes are activated during test)
Therapy with Prostaphlin, Polycillin, opiates, erythromycin
Calcium dust in air (e.g., due to construction in laboratory)

Falsely Decreased In
(because of increased serum lactate–consuming enzyme during test)
Diabetic ketoacidosis
Beriberi
Severe liver disease
Chronic hemodialysis (reason unknown)
Uremia—proportional to BUN level (reason unknown)

Normal In
Angina pectoris
Coronary insufficiency
Pericarditis
Congestive heart failure without liver damage

Varies < 10 units/day in the same person

SGPT generally parallels SGOT, but the increase is less marked in myocardial necrosis, chronic hepatitis, cirrhosis, hepatic metastases, and congestive changes in liver and is more marked in liver necrosis and acute hepatitis.

SERUM LACTIC DEHYDROGENASE (LDH)

Increased In

Acute myocardial infarction. Serum LDH is almost always increased, beginning in 10–12 hours and reaching a peak (of about 3 times normal) in 48–72 hours. The prolonged elevation of 10–14 days is particularly useful for late diagnosis when the patient is first seen after sufficient time has elapsed for CK and SGOT to become normal. Levels > 2000 units suggest a poorer prognosis. Because many other diseases may increase the LDH, isoenzyme studies should be performed. Increased serum LDH, with a ratio of $LDH_1/LDH_2 > 1$ ("flipped" LDH), occurs in acute renal infarction, pernicious anemia, and hemolysis associated with hemolytic anemia or prosthetic heart valves as well as in acute myocardial infarction. In acute myocardial infarction, flipped LDH usually appears between 12 and 24 hours and is present within 48 hours in 80% of patients; after 1 week it is still present in < 50% of patients, even though total serum LDH may still be elevated; flipped LDH never appears before CK MB isoenzyme. LDH_1 may remain elevated after total LDH has returned to normal; with small infarcts, LDH_1 may be increased when total LDH remains normal. (See Serum Creatine Phosphokinase [CK] Isoenzymes, pp. 68–69.)

Acute myocardial infarction with congestive heart failure. May show increase of LDH_1 and LDH_5.

Congestive heart failure alone. LDH isoenzymes are normal.

Insertion of intracardiac prosthetic valves consistently causes chronic hemolysis with increase of total LDH and of LDH_1 and LDH_2. This is also often present before surgery in patients with severe hemodynamic abnormalities of cardiac valves.

Cardiovascular surgery. LDH is increased up to 2 times normal without cardiopulmonary bypass and returns to normal in 3–4 days; with extracorporeal circulation, it may increase up to 4–6 times normal; increase is more marked when transfused blood is older.

Hepatitis. Most marked increase is of LDH_5, which occurs during prodromal stage and is greatest at time of onset of jaundice; total LDH is also increased in 50% of the cases. LDH_5 is also increased with other causes of liver damage (e.g., chlorpromazine hepatitis, carbon tetrachloride poisoning, exacerbation of cirrhosis, biliary obstruction) even when total LDH is normal. Liver disease, per se, does not produce marked increase of total LDH or LDH_5. If liver disease is suspect but total LDH is very high and isoenzyme pattern is nonspecific, rule out cancer.

Untreated pernicious anemia. Total LDH (chiefly LDH_1) is markedly increased, especially with hemoglobin < 8 gm/dl. Hemolytic anemia can probably be ruled out if LDH_1 and LDH_2 are not increased in an anemic patient. Normal in iron deficiency anemia, even when very severe.

Malignant tumors. Increased in $\cong 50\%$ of patients with carcinoma, especially in advanced stages. In patients with cancer, a higher LDH level generally indicates a poorer prognosis. Whenever the total LDH is increased and the isoenzyme pattern is nonspecific or cannot be explained by obvious clinical findings (e.g., myocardial infarction, hemolytic anemia), cancer should always be ruled out.

Increased in $\cong 60\%$ of patients with lymphomas and lymphocytic leukemias. Increased in $\cong 90\%$ of patients with acute leukemia; degree of increase is not correlated with level of WBC; relatively low levels in lymphatic type of leukemia. Increased in 95% of patients with myelogenous leukemia. (See also Chap. 27, Hematologic Diseases.)

Disease of muscle (see pp. 303–305, 307). Marked increase of LDH_5 is likely due to anoxic injury of striated muscle.

Electrical and thermal burns and trauma. Marked increase of total LDH (about the same as in myocardial infarction) and LDH_5

Pulmonary embolus and infarction (see Serum Lactic Dehydrogenase [LDH] Isoenzymes, below)

Renal diseases. LDH_4 and LDH_5 may be increased in nephrotic syndrome. LDH_1 and LDH_2 may be increased in nephritis. In renal cortical infarction, total LDH may be increased with $LDH_1 > LDH_2$. Rule out renal infarction if LDH_1 is increased in the absence of myocardial infarction or anemia. Generally not clinically useful but may mimic pattern of acute myocardial infarction.

Other causes of hemolysis

Artifactual (e.g., poor venipuncture, failure to separate clot from serum, heating of blood)

Various hemolytic conditions in vivo (e.g., hemolytic anemias)

Decreased In

X-ray irradiation

SERUM LACTIC DEHYDROGENASE (LDH) ISOENZYMES

Interpretation of this test must be correlated with clinical status of the patient. Do serial determinations to obtain maximum information.

Condition	LDH Isoenzyme Increased
Acute myocardial infarction	I and II (see pp. 65–66)
Acute renal cortical infarction	I and II
Pernicious anemia	I
Sickle cell crisis	I and II
Electrical and thermal burn, trauma	V
Mother carrying erythroblastotic child	IV and V
Acute myocardial infarction with acute congestion of liver	I and V
Early hepatitis	V (may become normal even when SGPT is still rising)
Malignant lymphoma	III and IV (may even increase II) (reflects effect of chemotherapy)
Disseminated lupus erythematosus	III and IV
Dermatomyositis	V
Carcinoma of prostate	V
Pulmonary embolus and infarction	II and III
Pulmonary embolus with acute cor pulmonale causing acute congestion of liver	III and V

Increased total LDH with normal distribution of isoenzymes may be seen in myocardial infarction, arteriosclerotic heart disease with chronic heart failure, various combinations of acute and chronic diseases (this may represent a general stress reaction).

About 50% of patients with carcinoma have altered LDH patterns. This change often is nonspecific and of no diagnostic value.

In pernicious anemia, hemolysis, and renal cortical infarction, the isoenzyme pattern may mimic myocardial infarction but the time to peak value and the increase help to differentiate.

SERUM ALPHA-HYDROXYBUTYRIC DEHYDROGENASE (α-HBD)

Increased In

Acute myocardial infarction. Is more specific than SGOT and LDH but less specific than CK and LDH isoenzymes.

Other conditions that cause elevation of fast-moving LDH in serum (e.g., muscular dystrophy, megaloblastic anemia)

Increase is always accompanied by increased LDH activity.

May Be Slightly Increased In
Heart failure
Nephrosis

Normal In
Angina pectoris

SERUM CREATINE KINASE (CK)

Increased In

Necrosis or acute atrophy of striated muscle
    Acute myocardial infarction
    Severe myocarditis
    Progressive muscular dystrophy
    Amyotrophic lateral sclerosis ($>40\%$ of cases)
    Polymyositis
    Myoglobinuria
    Thermal and electrical burns (values usually higher than in acute myocardial infarction)
    Traumatic injury of muscle. Increase may last for 2 weeks, especially if associated with arterial obstruction.
    Severe or prolonged exercise (transient increase, some patients)
    Status epilepticus
    Postoperative state. Increase may last up to 5 days. Greater increase with use of electrocautery in surgery
Half of patients with extensive brain infarction. Maximum levels in 3 days; increase may not appear before 2 days; levels usually less than in acute myocardial infarction and remain increased for longer time; return to normal within 14 days; high mortality associated with levels > 300 IU. Elevated serum CK in brain infarction may obscure diagnosis of concomitant acute myocardial infarction.
Parturition and frequently the last few weeks of pregnancy
Malignant hyperthermia

Hypothyroidism—becomes normal within 6 weeks of replacement therapy

Slight Increase Occasionally In

Intramuscular injections. Variable increase after intramuscular injection to 2–6 times normal level. Returns to normal 48 hours after cessation of injections.

Muscle spasms or convulsions in children

Electrical cardiac defibrillation or countershock in 50% of patients; returns to normal in 48–72 hours.

Normal In

Angina pectoris

Pericarditis

Pulmonary infarction

Renal infarction

Liver disease

Biliary obstruction

Neurogenic muscle atrophy

Pernicious anemia

Malignancies

Following cardiac catheterization and coronary arteriography unless myocardium has been injured by catheter

SERUM CREATINE KINASE (CK) ISOENZYMES

MB Isoenzyme Increased In

Acute myocardial infarction. MB isoenzyme is evident at 4–8 hours, peaks at 24 hours, is present in 100% of patients within the first 48 hours; by 72 hours, two-thirds of patients still show some elevation. CK isoenzyme studies provide the best laboratory discrimination between the presence or absence of myocardial necrosis. Increase of CK-MB and $LDH_1 > LDH_2$ has sensitivity of 90% and specificity of 95% for acute myocardial necrosis.

Cardiac trauma

Myocarditis (some cases)

Congestive heart failure (moderate)

Coronary angiography (transient)

Cardiac surgery (transient) and heart valve replacement

Muscular dystrophy, polymyositis, collagen vascular diseases (especially systemic lupus erythematosus), massive myoglobinuria or rhabdomyolysis

Electrical and thermal burns and trauma ($\cong$ 50% of patients; but not supported by $LDH_1 > LDH_2$)

Rocky Mountain spotted fever

Reye's syndrome

Hyperthermia, hypothermia

Hypothyroidism (some cases)

MB Isoenzyme Not Increased In

Angina

Cardiac arrest or cardioversion not due to myocardial infarction

Cardiac hypertrophy or cardiomyopathy unless there is myocarditis or heart failure

Cardiac pacemaker or catheterization (including Swan-Ganz)

Cardiopulmonary bypass
IM injections (total CK may be increased)
Seizures (total CK may be markedly increased)
Brain infarction or injury (total CK may be increased)
Pulmonary embolism

BB Isoenzyme May Be Increased In

Malignant hyperthermia, uremia, brain infarction (see Serum Creatine Kinase, p. 67) or anoxia, necrosis of intestine, various neoplasms, biliary atresia. It is rarely encountered clinically.

SERUM ISOCITRATE DEHYDROGENASE (ICD)

Increased In
Liver disease
    Early viral hepatitis, hepatitis of infectious mononucleosis and of liver poisons—ICD > 25 IU, becomes normal in 2–3 weeks
    Metastatic carcinoma—ICD < 20 IU
    Cirrhosis—normal or slightly increased
    Extrahepatic biliary obstruction—normal
    Neonatal biliary atresia—may be increased
    With protein malnutrition—may be increased
Active placental degeneration
    Placental infarction
    Preeclampsia

Normal In
Acute myocardial infarction
Pregnancy

SERUM ALDOLASE (ALD)

Increased In
Cell destruction
    Acute myocardial infarction
    Burns
    Acute hepatitis
    Muscular dystrophies (especially Duchenne type), myopathies, polymyositis
    Carcinoma of prostate
    20% of cancer patients—more frequent with liver involvement

Normal In
Neurogenic muscle atrophy
Cirrhosis (or may be slightly increased)
Obstructive jaundice (or may be slightly increased)

SERUM ORNITHINE CARBAMYL TRANSFERASE (OCT)

Increased In
Liver cell damage (e.g., hepatitis, metastatic carcinoma, cirrhosis, acute cholecystitis)
Alcohol consumption
Prolonged exercise (some patients)

Table 13-3. Serum Protein Electrophoretic Patterns in Various Diseases*

Condition	Total Protein	Albumin	Alpha$_1$ Globulin	Alpha$_2$ Globulin	Beta Globulin	Gamma Globulin	Comment
Multiple myeloma	I	D	Dyscrasia of beta$_{2A}$ or gamma$_2$ Ig				Total globulin, marked I Variable location of M globulin
Macroglobulinemia	I	D	Dyscrasia of beta$_{2M}$			Marked I	Electrophoresis same as multiple myeloma
Hodgkin's disease	D	D	I	I		V	
Lymphatic leukemia and lymphoma	D	D			D	D	
Myelogenous and monocytic leukemia	D	D			D	I	Gamma globulin to differentiate types of acute leukemias
Hypogammaglobulinemia	D	N	N	N	N	D	
Analbuminemia	Marked D	Marked D	N	I	I	I	
Gastrointestinal diseases Peptic ulcer	D	D	May be I	May be I			

Condition							
Ulcerative colitis	D	D	May be I	May be I	I	D	
Protein-losing enteropathy	Marked D	D	I	I	N	D	
Acute cholecystitis	D	D				N	
Nephrosis	D	D	N	I	N	D	Typical pattern.
Chronic glomerulonephritis	D	D	N	N	N	N	
Laennec's cirrhosis	D	D	N	N	N	I	Characteristic pattern of beta-gamma "bridging"
Acute viral hepatitis	D	D (means acute hepatocellular damage)	N	N	N	V	
Stress	D	D	I	I	I	I	"Three-fingered" pattern
Hypersensitivity						I	
Sarcoidosis	I	D	Stepwise increase of α_2, beta, and gamma				"Sarcoid steps" help differentiate from other lung disease

I = increased or elevated; D = decreased or diminished; V = variable; N = normal; blank = no significant change.

*Nonspecific changes of decreased albumin and increased globulin occur in many conditions (e.g., infections, neoplasms, metabolic diseases).

Table 13-3 (continued)

Condition	Total Protein	Albumin	Alpha$_1$ Globulin	Alpha$_2$ Globulin	Beta Globulin	Gamma Globulin	Comment
Collagen disease Lupus erythematosus (SLE)		D		I		I	Gamma globulin levels of prognostic value
Polyarteritis nodosa		D		I		N	
Rheumatoid arthritis		D		I	I	I	
Scleroderma						V	No significant changes
Acute rheumatic fever		D		I	No significant changes		Albumin D due to hemodilution
Essential hypertension Congestive heart failure	D	D	No significant changes				(Hemodilution, diminished hepatic synthesis, and possible excessive enteric loss)

Metastatic carcinomatosis	D	I	I	D	Nonspecific pattern
Certain infections (meningitis, pneumonia, osteomyelitis)	D	I	I		
Myxedema					Changes due to hemodilution
Hyperthyroidism	D	N	N	N	
Diabetes mellitus	D	I	I	N	

I = increased or elevated; D = decreased or diminished; V = variable; N = normal; blank = no significant change.
*Nonspecific changes of decreased albumin and increased globulin occur in many conditions (e.g., infections, neoplasms, metabolic diseases).
Source: Adapted from F. W. Sunderman, Jr., Recent Advances in Clinical Interpretation of Electrophoretic Fractionations of the Serum Proteins. In F. W. Sunderman and J. C. Sunderman (Eds.), *Serum Proteins and the Dysproteinemias*. Philadelphia: Lippincott, 1964.

SERUM CHOLINESTERASE

Decreased In

Poisoning with organic phosphate insecticides

Liver diseases

> Especially hepatitis. Lowest level corresponds to peak of disease and becomes normal with recovery.

> Cirrhosis with ascites or jaundice. Persistent decrease may indicate a poor prognosis.

> Some patients with metastatic carcinoma, obstructive jaundice, congestive heart failure

Congenital decrease. Such patients are particularly sensitive to administration of succinylcholine during anesthesia.

Some conditions that may have decreased serum albumin (e.g., malnutrition, anemias, infections, dermatomyositis, acute myocardial infarction, liver diseases—see above)

SERUM FRUCTOSE 1-PHOSPHATE ALDOLASE

Decreased In

Heterozygous carrier state for Tay-Sachs disease

SERUM ALBUMIN

Increased In

Dehydration (relative increase)

Decreased In

Inadequate intake (e.g., malnutrition)

Decreased absorption (e.g., malabsorption syndromes)

Increased need (e.g., hyperthyroidism, pregnancy)

Impaired synthesis (e.g., liver diseases, chronic infection, congenital analbuminemia)

Increased breakdown (e.g., neoplasms, infection, trauma)

Increased loss (e.g., edema, ascites, burns, hemorrhage, nephrotic syndrome, protein-losing enteropathy)

SERUM PROTEIN GAMMOPATHIES
(localized or general increase in immunoglobulins demonstrated by serum immunoelectrophoresis)

Monoclonal
(hyperproteinemia very frequent)

IgG gammopathy with or without Bence Jones protein (60% of patients

IgA gammopathy (16% of patients)

IgM gammopathy (15% of patients)

Bence Jones gammopathy (light-chain disease) (9% of patients)

IgE gammopathy (heavy-chain disease), very rare

IgD gammopathy, very rare

Only two-thirds of patients with monoclonal gammopathy are symptomatic (IgG, IgA, IgD, and Bence Jones gammopathies are associated with classic picture of multiple myeloma—see pp. 370–374; IgM gammopathy is associated with classic picture of macroglobulinemia—see pp. 374–375).

Classic (associated with increased serum M protein > 3 gm/dl and increased number of plasma cells in marrow > 25%)
  Multiple myeloma
  Waldenström's macroglobulinemia
  Certain malignant lymphomas
Idiopathic (not associated with diseases in classic group) (serum M protein usually < 2 gm/dl; plasma marrow cells usually 5–25% of total marrow white cells)
  In apparently healthy persons
  Associated with various diseases (e.g., diabetes mellitus, cirrhosis, abnormalities of lipid metabolism, chronic infections, collagen diseases, myeloproliferative diseases, and neoplasms not of lymphocyte or plasma cell origin)

Either type may be familial.

Polyclonal Gammopathy with Hyperproteinemia
Collagen diseases (e.g., systemic lupus erythematosus, rheumatoid arthritis, scleroderma)
Liver disease (e.g., chronic hepatitis, cirrhosis)
Chronic infection (e.g., chronic bronchitis and bronchiectasis, lung abscess, tuberculosis, osteomyelitis, subacute bacterial endocarditis, infectious mononucleosis, malaria)
Miscellaneous (e.g., sarcoidosis, malignant lymphoma, acute myeloid and monocytic leukemia, diabetes mellitus)
Idiopathic (family of patients with lupus erythematosus)

SERUM BETA$_{2M}$ GLOBULIN
(gamma$_{1M}$ globulin; 19S gamma globulin; gamma$_1$ globulin; beta$_2$ macroglobulin)

Increased In
Waldenström's macroglobulinemia (marked increase)
Symptomatic macroglobulinemia
  Cirrhosis
  Nephrosis
  Rheumatoid arthritis
  Eosinophilic granulomatosis
  Hyperglobulinemic purpura
  Other

SERUM BETA$_{2A}$ GLOBULIN
(gamma$_{1A}$ globulin)

Increased In
Multiple myeloma (occasionally)

Decreased In
Multiple myeloma
Lipoid nephrosis
Macroglobulinemia

SERUM ALPHA$_1$ ANTITRYPSIN
Decreased In
Alpha$_1$ antitrypsin deficiency (see p. 379 and Table 13-5, p. 79)

Increased In
Infections
Neoplasia
Pregnancy and use of birth control pills

IMMUNODIFFUSION OF SERUM PROTEIN

Diagnosis of Specific Diseases
Multiple myeloma
Waldenström's macroglobulinemia
Hypogammaglobulinemia
    Agammaglobulinemia
    Agamma-A-globulinemia
Analbuminemia
Bisalbuminemia
Afibrinogenemia
Atransferrinemia
Wilson's disease

Other Changes
Nonspecific changes in serum proteins
Protein pattern changes in urine, cerebrospinal fluid, peritoneal
    fluid, etc.

IMMUNOGLOBULIN A (IgA)

Increased In
(in relation to other immunoglobulins)
γA myeloma (M component)
Cirrhosis of liver
Chronic infections
Rheumatoid arthritis with high titers of rheumatoid factor
Systemic lupus erythematosus (some patients)
Sarcoidosis (some patients)
Wiskott-Aldrich syndrome
Other

Decreased In
(alone)
Normal persons (1:700)
Hereditary telangiectasia (80% of patients)
Type III dysgammaglobulinemia
Malabsorption (some patients)
Systemic lupus erythematosus (occasionally)
Cirrhosis of liver (occasionally)
Still's disease (occasionally)
Recurrent otitis media (occasionally)

Decreased In
(combined with other immunoglobulin decreases)
Agammaglobulinemia
    Acquired
        Primary
        Secondary (e.g., multiple myeloma, leukemia, nephrotic
          syndrome, protein-losing enteropathy)
    Congenital
Hereditary thymic aplasia

Type I dysgammaglobulinemia (decreased IgG and IgA and increased IgM)

Type II dysgammaglobulinemia (absent IgA and IgM and normal levels of IgG)

IMMUNOGLOBULIN E (IgE)

Increased In
Atopic diseases
   Exogenous asthma in ≅60% of patients
   Hay fever in ≅30% of patients
   Atopic eczema

Influenced by type of allergen, duration of stimulation, presence of symptoms, hyposensitization treatment

Parasitic diseases (e.g., ascariasis, visceral larva migrans, hookworm disease, schistosomiasis, *Echinococcus* infestation)
E-myeloma

Normal or Low
Asthma

A normal serum IgE level excludes the diagnosis of bronchopulmonary aspergillosis.

IMMUNOGLOBULIN D (IgD)

Increased In
Chronic infection (moderately)
IgD myelomas (greatly)

IMMUNOGLOBULIN M (IgM)

Increased In
Liver disease
Chronic infections
Waldenström's macroglobulinemia

SERUM LIPOPROTEINS

Decreased In
Abetalipoproteinemia (Bassen-Kornzweig syndrome): Chylomicrons, low-density lipoproteins (LDL), and very-low-density lipoproteins (VLDL) are absent; high-density lipoproteins (HDL) are normal. Marked decrease in plasma triglycerides (<30 mg/dl) and cholesterol (<100 mg/dl). Patients also have acanthotic RBCs and low serum carotene levels (see p. 295). (The condition is an autosomal recessive trait.)

Tangier disease: There is a marked decrease (heterozygous) or absence (homozygous) of HDL. Pre-beta lipoprotein is absent. Serum cholesterol (<100 mg/dl) and phospholipid are decreased; triglycerides are normal or increased (100–250 mg/dl).

Hypobetalipoproteinemia: Low-density lipoproteins are 10–20% of normal. Plasma triglycerides are normal; cholesterol is decreased (≅50–60 mg/dl). May be caused by malabsorption of fats, infection, anemia, hepatic necrosis, hyperthyroidism, acute myocar-

Table 13-4. Serum Immunoglobulin Changes in Various Diseases

Disease	IgG	IgA	IgM
Immunoglobulin disorders			
(see Table 27-15, pp. 382–383)			
Lymphoid aplasia	D	D	D
Agammaglobulinemia	D	D	D
Type I dysgammaglobulinemia	D	D	N or I
(selective IgG and IgA deficiency)			
Type II dysgammaglobulinemia	N	D	D
(absent IgA and IgM)			
IgA globulinemia	N	D	N
Ataxia-telangiectasia	N	D	N
Multiple myeloma, macroglobulinemia,			
lymphomas (see pp. 370–375)			
Heavy-chain disease	D	D	D
IgG myeloma	I	D	D
IgA myeloma	D	I	D
Macroglobulinemia	D	D	I
Acute lymphocytic leukemia	N	D	N
Chronic lymphocytic leukemia	D	D	D
Acute myelogenous leukemia	N	N	N
Chronic myelogenous leukemia	N	D	N
Hodgkin's disease	N	N	N
Liver diseases			
Hepatitis	I	I	I
Laennec's cirrhosis	I	I	N
Biliary cirrhosis	N	N	I
Hepatoma	N	N	D
Miscellaneous			
Rheumatoid arthritis	I	I	I
Systemic lupus erythematosus	I	I	I
Nephrotic syndrome	D	D	N
Trypanosomiasis	N	N	I
Pulmonary tuberculosis	I	N	N

N = normal; I = increased; D = decreased.

dial infarction, acute trauma; or may be familial, i.e., absence of causative disease and presence of a similar pattern in first-degree relatives. (It is an autosomal dominant trait.)

Increased In

Hyperbetalipoproteinemia: See Table 28-5, pp. 424–427.

Hyperalphalipoproteinemia: This disorder may be caused by alcoholism, extensive exposure to chlorinated hydrocarbon pesticides, exogenous estrogen supplementation; or it may be familial (it is an autosomal dominant trait). High-density lipoproteins (alphalipoproteins) are increased (> 70 mg/dl). Total serum cholesterol is somewhat increased; triglycerides are normal (see Table 28-5, pp. 424–427.)

Table 13-5. Changes in Serum Immunoproteins in Various Conditions

Condition	Albumin	Alpha$_1$ Antitrypsin	Haptoglobin	Transferrin	C3
Acute inflammation	D	I	I	D	Slight I
Chronic inflammation	D	V–I	V–I	D	Slight I
Chronic liver disease	D	V–I	V	D	V–D
Obstructive jaundice	N	N	V–I	N	I
Hemolytic anemia	N	N	D	N	N
Iron deficiency	N	N	N	I	N
Acute glomerulonephritis	N	N	N	N	D
Systemic lupus erythematosus	D	I	D[a]	D	V–D[b]
Alpha$_1$ antitrypsin deficiency	N	D	N	N	N
Analbuminemia	D	N	N	N	N
Agammaglobulinemia	N	N	N	N	N
IgG myeloma	D	N	N	N	N
IgA myeloma	D	N	N	N	N
Waldenström's macroglobulinemia	D	N	N	N	N

N = normal; D = decreased; I = increased; V = variable.
[a] D with associated hemolytic anemia.
[b] N if immunosuppressive treatment is effective.

TRIGLYCERIDES
(see Serum Lipoproteins, preceding section)

Increased In
(see section on lipoprotein electrophoresis in Table 28-5, pp. 424–427)
Familial hyperlipidemia
Liver diseases
Nephrotic syndrome
Hypothyroidism
Diabetes mellitus (higher values correlate with hyperglycemia and poorer control of diabetes; reduced by insulin therapy)
Alcoholism
Gout
Pancreatitis
von Gierke's disease
Acute myocardial infarction (rise to peak in 3 weeks; increase may persist for 1 year)

Decreased In
Congenital abetalipoproteinemia
Malnutrition

SERUM TRIIODOTHYRONINE (T-3) UPTAKE
(see Table 29-2, pp. 455–457)

This test should be used only with a simultaneous measurement of serum T-4 to exclude the possibility that an increased T-4 is due to an increase in T-4–binding globulin. Measurement of serum T-3 concentration should be done by radioimmunoassay for diagnosis of hyperthyroidism (see p. 450).

Increased In
See causes of *decreased* serum thyroxine-binding globulin, p. 82.

Decreased In
See causes of *increased* serum thyroxine-binding globulin, p. 82.

Normal In
Pregnancy with hyperthyroidism
Nontoxic goiter
Carcinoma of thyroid
Diabetes mellitus
Addison's disease
Anxiety
Certain drugs (mercurials, iodine)

Variable In
Liver disease

SERUM TOTAL THYROXINE ASSAY (T-4)
(see Table 29-2, pp. 455–457)

Increased In
Hyperthyroidism
Pregnancy
Certain drugs (estrogens, birth control pills, *d*-thyroxine, thyroid extract, TSH, heroin, methadone)

Table 13-6. Free Thyroxine Index in Various Conditions

Condition	T-3	T-4	Free Thyroxine Factor (T-7) (T-3 Uptake × T-4)
Normal			
Range	24–36	4–11	96–396
Mean	31	7	217
Hypothyroid	22	3	66
Hyperthyroid	38	12	456
Pregnancy, estrogens (especially birth control pills)	20	12	240*

*Normal even though T-3 and T-4 alone are abnormal.

"Euthyroid sick" syndrome
Increase in thyroxine-binding globulin (see p. 82)

Decreased In
Hypothyroidism
Hypoproteinemia (e.g., nephrosis, cirrhosis)
Certain drugs (phenytoin [Dilantin], triiodothyronine, testosterone, ACTH, corticosteroids)
"Euthyroid sick" syndrome
Decrease in thyroxine-binding globulin (see p. 82)

Not Affected By
Radiopaque substances for x-ray studies
Mercurial diuretics
Nonthyroidal iodine

FREE THYROXINE INDEX (T-7)
This is the product of T-3 uptake and T-4 (or T-3 uptake and protein-bound iodine).
It permits correction of misleading results of T-3 and T-4 determinations caused by pregnancy, estrogens (especially birth control pills), and other conditions that alter the thyroxine-binding protein concentration.

FREE THYROXINE ASSAY (NORMALIZED THYROXINE)
(see Table 29-2, pp. 455–457)
This determination gives corrected values in patients in whom the total thyroxine (T-4) is altered on account of changes in serum proteins or in binding sites.
    Pregnancy
    Drugs (e.g., androgens, estrogens, birth control pills, phenytoin [Dilantin])
    Altered levels of serum proteins (e.g., nephrosis)

Increased In
Hyperthyroidism
Hypothyroidism treated with thyroxine
"Euthyroid sick" syndrome

Decreased In
Hypothyroidism
Hypothyroidism treated with triiodothyronine
"Euthyroid sick" syndrome

SERUM THYROXINE-BINDING GLOBULIN (TBG)
(see Table 29-2, pp. 455–457)

Increased In
Pregnancy
Excess TBG, genetic or idiopathic
Hypothyroidism (some patients)
Certain drugs (estrogens, birth control pills, perphenazine [Trilafon])
Acute intermittent porphyria
Acute hepatitis

Decreased In
Nephrosis and other causes of marked hypoproteinemia such as liver disease, severe illness, stress (thyroxine-binding-prealbumin [TBPA] also decreased)
Deficiency of TBG, genetic or idiopathic
Hyperthyroidism
Acromegaly (TBPA also decreased)
Certain drugs
    Androgens, anabolic steroids
    Glucocorticoids (TBPA is increased)

Decreased Binding of T-3 and T-4 Due to Drugs
Salicylates
Phenytoin
Orinase, Diabinase
Penicillin, heparin, barbital

An increased TBG is associated with increased serum T-4 and decreased T-3 resin uptake; a converse association exists for decreased TBG.

SERUM TSH (THYROID-STIMULATING HORMONE; THYROTROPIN)
(hormone secreted by anterior pituitary)
Primary usefulness is in diagnosis of hypothyroidism and in differentiation of primary and secondary hypothyroidism.

Increased In
Primary untreated hypothyroidism. Increase is proportionate to the degree of hypofunction, varying from 3 times normal in mild cases to 100 times normal in severe myxedema. A single determination is usually sufficient to establish the diagnosis. Especially useful

in early or subclinical hypothyroidism before the patient develops clinical findings, goiter, or abnormalities of routine laboratory thyroid tests. In very early cases with only marginal elevation, the thyroid-releasing hormone stimulation test offers a more refined diagnostic procedure. Serum TSH suppressed to normal level is the best monitor of dosage of thyroid hormone for treatment of hypothyroidism, but it does not indicate overtreatment.

Hashimoto's thyroiditis, including those with clinical hypothyroidism and about one-third of those patients who are clinically euthyroid

Other conditions (test is not clinically useful)
  Iodide deficiency goiter
  Iodide-induced goiter or lithium treatment
  External neck irradiation
  Post-subtotal thyroidectomy
  Neonatal period

Decreased In

Secondary (pituitary) hypothyroidism

Hypothalamic hypothyroidism

Hyperthyroidism. Some patients have normal levels, and it may not be possible to differentiate low range of normal from an abnormally decreased value. A TRH stimulation test may be required to establish the diagnosis (see following section).

Normal In

Cushing's syndrome

Acromegaly

Pregnancy at term

TRH (THYROID-RELEASING HORMONE) STIMULATION TEST (TRF [THYROTROPIN-RELEASING FACTOR])
(see Fig. 13-1)

Serum TSH is measured before and after the intravenous administration of TRH (usually 500 or 200 μg).

The TSH response to TRH is modified by thyroxine, antithyroid drugs, corticosteroids, estrogens, and levodopa. Response is increased during pregnancy.

Normal response—a significant rise from a basal level of about 1 μU/ml by 8 μU/ml at 20 minutes and return to normal by 120 minutes. Response is usually greater in women than in men.

Blunted TSH response may also occur in uremia, Cushing's syndrome, acromegaly, administration of certain drugs (corticosteroids, levodopa, large amounts of salicylates).

Hyperthyroidism—shows no rise in the depressed TSH level. A normal rise virtually excludes hyperthyroidism. This test may be particularly useful in T-3 toxicosis in which the other tests are normal or in patients clinically suspicious for hyperthyroidism with borderline serum T-3 levels. When serum TSH measurements are available, the TRH stimulation test is superior to the T-3 suppression test of RAIU (see p. 86).

Primary hypothyroidism—an exaggerated rise of an already increased TSH level.

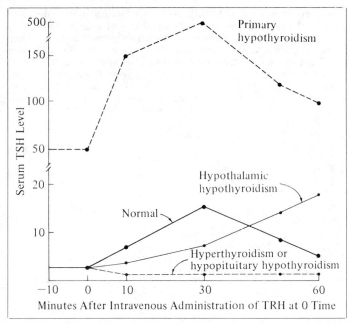

Fig. 13-1. Sample curves of serum TSH response to administration of TRH in various conditions.

Secondary (pituitary) hypothyroidism—no rise in the decreased TSH level.

Hypothalamic hypothyroidism—low serum T-3 and T-4 and TSH levels, with a TRH response that may be exaggerated or normal or (most characteristically) with a peak delay 45–60 minutes. Diagnosis must be based on clinical studies that exclude the pituitary gland as the site of the disease.

TSH response to TRH may also be suppressed in nonthyroidal conditions (e.g., starvation, renal failure, elevated levels of glucocorticoids, and depression).

Has largely replaced the T-3 suppression test, as TRH test is simpler, more convenient, less expensive.

	Baseline TSH (μU/ml)	Change in TSH 30 Minutes After TRH Administration (μU/ml)
Euthyroidism	< 10	> 2 (95% of cases)
Hyperthyroidism	< 10	< 2
Primary hypothyroidism	> 10	> 2 (exaggerated)
Secondary hypothyroidism	< 10	< 2
Tertiary hypothyroidism	< 10	> 2 (delayed or exaggerated or N)

TRH test may remain abnormal even after successful therapy of Graves' disease.

Abnormal TSH response to TRH administration does not definitely establish the diagnosis of hyperthyroidism (because autonomous production of normal or slightly increased amounts of thyroid hormones causes pituitary suppression).

THYROID AUTOANTIBODY TESTS

Antithyroglobulin Antibodies

Precipitin test

Frequently negative in juvenile form and in the oxyphil variant

Positive in 96% of fibrous variant (which is more common in middle-aged and elderly patients)

Newer tests are more sensitive (see below).

Immunofluorescence test is used as research and specialty tool.

Indirect hemagglutination (using tanned RBCs) is most widely used.

Positive (1:10–1:640) in 4% of normal population; gradually increases in frequency with age in females

Positive in 70% of fibrous and oxyphil variant of Hashimoto's disease

Frequently absent or present only in low titers in juvenile form

Occasionally positive in carcinoma of thyroid, subacute thyroiditis, and Graves' disease

Absence does not exclude Hashimoto's thyroiditis.

>1:1000 occurs virtually only in Graves' disease or Hashimoto's thyroiditis.

Thyroid Microsome Antibodies

Largely supplanted by indirect hemagglutination

Positive (1:100–1:1600) in 7% of normal population, reaching peak of 15% in females in sixth decade

Positive in 60–70% of patients with Hashimoto's thyroiditis

Second Colloid Antigen (CA-A)

Immunofluorescence test against colloid protein

Available only in specialty laboratories

Present in 50% of patients with subacute thyroiditis

Present in some cases of Hashimoto's thyroiditis without other antibodies

Thyroid Membrane Receptors
(a group of serum IgG that stimulate thyroid gland)

Includes long-acting thyroid stimulator (LATS), long-acting thyroid stimulator protector (LATS-P), thyroid-stimulating immunoglobulin (TSI), thyroid-stimulating antibody (TSAb), thyrotropin-binding inhibition activity (TBIA).

LATS-P assay is positive in > 75% of patients with Graves' disease and 50% of patients with euthyroid Graves' ophthalmoplegia.

High titer in last trimester of pregnancy predicts neonatal thyrotoxicosis even if mother is euthyroid.

High titer of TSI in presence of HLA-DR3 strongly predicts poor response to antithyroid medication, and therefore some authorities recommend RAIU treatment for adults with these findings.

Useful to distinguish subacute thyroiditis and Hashimoto's thyroiditis, as antibodies are more common in the latter.

Hashimoto's thyroiditis is very unlikely cause of hypothyroidism in the absence of thyroglobulin and microsome antibodies.

Significant titer of thyroglobulin and microsome antibodies in euthyroid patient with unilateral exophthalmos suggests the diagnosis of euthyroid Graves' disease.

Graves' disease with elevated titers of antimicrosome antibodies should direct surgeon to perform a more limited thyroidectomy to avoid late postthyroidectomy hypothyroidism.

THYROID UPTAKE OF RADIOACTIVE IODINE (RAIU)

A tracer dose of radioactive iodine (^{131}I or ^{123}I) is administered orally, and the radioactivity over the thyroid is measured at specific time intervals (e.g., 2–6 hours and again at 24 hours). The percent of administered iodine in the thyroid is an index of thyroid trapping and organification of iodide.

Because of widespread dietary use of iodine in the United States, RAIU should not be used to evaluate euthyroid state.

Indications for test:

Detection of hyperthyroidism associated with low RAIU, e.g., factitious hyperthyroidism, subacute thyroiditis, struma ovarii.

Evaluate use of radioiodine therapy.

Determine presence of an organification defect in thyroid hormone production.

Contraindicated in pregnancy, lactation, childhood. It is invalidated for 2–4 weeks after administration of antithyroid drugs, thyroid, or iodides; the effect of organic iodine (e.g., x-ray contrast media) may persist for a much longer time.

T-3 suppression test. Administration of triiodothyronine causes less suppression in the hyperthyroid patient than in the normal person; has been replaced by the TRH stimulation test (see pp. 83–85).

Increased In

Hyperthyroidism (Graves' disease, toxic nodule)

Thyroiditis (early Hashimoto's; recovery stage of subacute thyroiditis)

TSH excess (TSH administration, TSH production by neoplasm, defective thyroid hormone synthesis)

Withdrawal rebound (thyroid hormones, propylthiouracil)

Increased iodine excretion (e.g., diuretics, nephrotic syndrome, chronic diarrhea)

Decreased iodine intake (salt restriction, iodine deficiency)

Decreased In

Hypothyroidism (tertiary, secondary, late primary)

Thyroiditis (late Hashimoto's; active stage of subacute hyroiditis*)

Thyroid hormone administration (T-3 or T-4) (therapeutic, factitious†)

Antithyroid medication

---

*RAIU does not usually respond to TSH administration in subacute thyroiditis.
†RAIU is augmented after TSH administration in factitious thyrotoxicosis.

Increased iodine intake (e.g., x-ray contrast media, iodine-containing drugs, iodized salt)

BLOOD AMMONIA

Increased In
Liver failure (e.g., acute hepatic necrosis, terminal cirrhosis, hepatectomy)

In cirrhosis, blood ammonia may be increased after portacaval anastomosis.
Not all cases of hepatic coma show increased blood ammonia.

Some aminoacidurias (see Table 28-6, pp. 428–430)

BLOOD LACTIC ACID
(see Lactic Acidosis, pp. 412–413)

SERUM CAROTENOIDS

Increased In
Excessive intake (especially carrots)
Postprandial hyperlipemia
Hyperlipemia (e.g., essential hyperlipemia)
Diabetes mellitus
Hypothyroidism

Decreased In
Carotenoid-poor diet—blood level falls within 1 week (*vitamin A level unaffected by dietary change for 6 months because of much larger body stores*)
Malabsorption syndromes (*a very useful screening test for malabsorption*)
Liver disease
High fever

PLASMA RENIN ACTIVITY (PRA)

Blood should be drawn in an ice-cold tube and the plasma immediately separated in a refrigerated centrifuge. Renin level should be indexed against 24-hour level of sodium in urine.

PRA is particularly useful to diagnose curable hypertension (e.g., unilateral renal artery stenosis, primary aldosteronism).

Increased In
15% of patients with essential hypertension
Renal hypertension (see below)
Renin-producing tumors of the kidney (see p. 554)
Reduced plasma volume due to low-sodium diet, diuretics, hemorrhage, Addison's disease
Secondary aldosteronism (usually very high levels) (see p. 489)
10% of patients with chronic renal failure
Normal pregnancy
Pheochromocytoma
Last half of menstrual cycle (twofold increase)

Erect posture for 4 hours (twofold increase)
Ambulatory patients compared to bed patients
Bartter's syndrome
Various drugs (guanethidine, minoxidil, hydralazine, diazoxide, thiazides, furosemide, spironolactone, nitroprusside, saralasin, estrogens). *Antihypertensive drugs should be discontinued for at least 2 weeks before measurement of PRA; spironolactone may cause an increase for up to 6 weeks; estrogens may cause an increase for up to 6 months (see p. 680).*

In diagnosis of renal hypertension, renin is assayed in blood from each renal vein, inferior vena cava, and aorta. The test is considered diagnostic when the level from the ischemic kidney is at least 1½ times greater than the level from the normal kidney (which is equal to or less than the level in the aorta that serves as the standard). This is due to high PRA in the peripheral blood, increase in PRA in the renal vein compared to the renal artery of the affected kidney, and suppression of PRA in other kidney. Maximum renin stimulation accentuates the difference between the two kidneys and should *always* be obtained by pretest conditions (avoid antihypertensive, diuretic, and oral contraceptive drugs for at least 1 month if possible; low-salt diet for 7 days; administer thiazide diuretic for 1–3 days; upright posture for at least 2 hours). This is the most useful diagnostic test in renovascular hypertension as judged by surgical results but is not a sufficiently reliable guide to nephrectomy in patients with hypertension due to parenchymal renal disease. *In renovascular hypertension, if renal plasma flow is impaired in the "normal" kidney, surgery often fails to cure the hypertension.*

Decreased In

Increased plasma volume due to high-sodium diet, administration of salt-retaining steroids
20% of patients diagnosed at the present time as having "essential hypertension"
Advancing age in both normal and hypertensive patients (decrease of 35% from the third to the eighth decade)
Primary aldosteronism. Usually absent or low and can be increased less or not at all by sodium depletion and ambulation in contrast to secondary aldosteronism. *PRA may not always be suppressed in primary aldosteronism; repeated testing may be necessary to establish the diagnosis.*
Adrenocortical hypertension
Various drugs (propranolol, clonidine, reserpine; slightly with methyldopa) (see p. 680)

PLASMA INSULIN

Not clinically useful for diagnosis of diabetes mellitus because of the very wide range in both normal and diabetic patients and because results may be influenced by many other factors.

Increased In

Insulinoma. Fasting blood insulin level over 50 μU/ml in presence of low or normal blood glucose level. Intravenous tolbutamide or administration of leucine causes rapid rise of blood insulin to very high levels within a few minutes with rapid return to normal.

Untreated obese diabetics (mild cases). The fasting level is often increased.

Acromegaly (especially with active disease) after ingestion of glucose

Reactive hypoglycemia after glucose ingestion, particularly when diabetic type of glucose tolerance curve is present

Absent In
Severe diabetes mellitus with ketosis and weight loss. In less severe cases, insulin is frequently present but only at lower glucose concentrations.

Normal In
Hypoglycemia associated with nonpancreatic tumors

Idiopathic hypoglycemia of childhood, except after administration of leucine

SERUM C-PEPTIDE
C-peptide is formed during conversion of proinsulin to insulin; C-peptide serum levels correlate with insulin levels in blood, except in islet cell tumors and possibly in obese patients. Therefore test is useful for estimating insulin levels in the presence of circulating insulin antibodies that interfere with insulin assay. Also useful in factitious hypoglycemia due to surreptitious administration of insulin in which high serum insulin levels will occur with low C-peptide levels.

PLASMA CATECHOLAMINES (NOREPINEPHRINE, EPINEPHRINE)

Increased In
Pheochromocytoma

Neural crest tumors (neuroblastoma, ganglioneuroma, ganglioblastoma)

Diabetic ketoacidosis (markedly elevated)

Acute myocardial infarction (markedly elevated)

Heavy exercise

After surgery

Hypothyroidism

Thyrotoxicosis

Volume depletion (induced by diuretics)

Renal disease

Heavy alcohol intake

Hypoglycemia

Various drugs (see p. 665)

PLASMA TESTOSTERONE
Male hypogonadism—levels lower than in normal male

Klinefelter's syndrome—levels lower than in normal male but higher than in normal female and orchiectomized male

Stein-Leventhal syndrome—variable; increased when virilization is present

Adrenogenital syndrome—with virilization (due to tumor or hyperplasia), level is much higher than in normal female; decreases following adrenal suppression

Idiopathic hirsutism—inconclusive
Ovarian stromal hyperthecosis

PLASMA ACTH

Decreased In
Cushing's syndrome due to adrenal tumor
Secondary hypoadrenalism

Increased In
Pituitary Cushing's syndrome
Primary adrenal insufficiency
Ectopic ACTH syndrome (e.g., carcinoma of lung)—levels very
  high, with no diurnal variation

SERUM PARATHYROID HORMONE
(see Fig. 29-1, p. 466)

	Parathyroid Hormone Elevated	Parathyroid Hormone Not Increased
Serum calcium low	Secondary hyperparathyroidism (chronic renal disease Pseudohypoparathyroidism (or normal hormone level	Hypoparathyroidism (surgical or idiopathic)
Serum calcium high	Primary hyperparathyroidism Familial hypocalciuric hypercalcemia Lithium-induced hypercalcemia Some neoplasms with ectopic production of parathyroid hormone (e.g. hypernephroma)	Hypercalcemia not due to hyperparathyroidism (e.g., various malignancies, milk-alkali syndrome, thiazide diuretics, vitamin D intoxication, sarcoidosis, hyperthyroidism, immobilization)
Serum calcium normal	Pregnancy Nephrolithiasis Secondary hyperparathyroidism (chronic renal disease)	Normal

There is considerable overlap of serum parathyroid hormone levels
  in normal patients and those with proven hyperparathyroidism.
  "Normal" level depends on the serum calcium level, which should
  always be determined simultaneously. Selective catheterization
  of veins draining the thyroid-parathyroid region for determination
  of parathyroid hormone levels may confirm the diagnosis of

hyperparathyroidism by showing a significant elevation at one site compared to at least one other site.

SERUM PROLACTIN

Increased In

Hypothalamic lesions (e.g., sarcoidosis, eosinophilic granuloma, histiocytosis X, tuberculosis, glioma, craniopharyngioma)

Pituitary lesions (e.g., prolactinoma, section of pituitary stalk, empty-sella syndrome, 20–40% of patients with acromegaly, up to 80% of patients with chromophobe adenomas)

Other endocrine diseases (e.g., hypothyroidism, Addison's disease, polycystic ovaries)

Ectopic production of prolactin (e.g., bronchogenic carcinoma, renal cell carcinoma)

Neurogenic causes (e.g., nursing and breast stimulation, spinal cord lesions, chest wall lesions such as herpes zoster)

Stress (e.g., surgery, hypoglycemia, vigorous exercise)

Pregnancy (rise to 10–20 times level before pregnancy); decreases during postpartum unless nursing occurs

Chronic renal failure (becomes normal after successful renal transplant but not hemodialysis)

Galactorrhea and/or amenorrhea (see pp. 501–502)

Idiopathic causes (some probably represent early cases of microadenoma too small to be detected by radiology

Drugs

Neuroleptics (e.g., phenothiazines, thioxanthenes, butyrophenones)

Opiates (morphine, methadone)

Reserpine

Alpha-methyldopa

Estrogens

Thyrotropin-releasing hormone

Amphetamines

Isoniazid

Decreased In

Drugs

Dopamine agonists

Ergot derivatives (bromocriptine mesylate, gergotrile mesylate, lisuride hydrogen maleate)

Levodopa, apomorphine, clonidine

SERUM ALPHA-FETOPROTEIN (AFP)

Normal ($<$ 40 ng/ml)

Absent after first weeks of life

Increased In

Primary cancer of liver (hepatoma) in 50% of whites and 75–90% of nonwhites; levels may be markedly elevated ($>$ 1000 ng/ml). Elevated in almost 100% of cases in children and young adults.

Some patients with liver metastases from carcinoma of stomach or pancreas

Embryonal carcinoma (in 27% of cases) or malignant teratoma (in 60% of cases) of ovary and testis

Neonatal hepatitis. Most patients with this disorder have levels > 40 ng/ml, but in neonatal biliary atresia most patients have levels < 40 ng/ml.

Pregnancy; increased above normal level in fetal open spina bifida or anencephaly. *(Increased blood levels of AFP in pregnancy is a valuable screening test, but diagnosis should be confirmed by finding of increased levels in amniotic fluid; serum should be drawn after the 15th week of gestation.)*

Ataxia-telangiectasia

Absent In

Various types of cirrhosis and hepatitis in adults

Seminoma of testis

Choriocarcinoma, adenocarcinoma, and dermoid cyst of ovary

SERUM CARCINOEMBRYONIC ANTIGEN (CEA)

There is a wide overlap in values between benign and malignant disease.

The following limitations must be remembered:

CEA test is not a screen for the detection of early cancer.

CEA titers < 2.5 ng/ml do not rule out malignant disease (primary, metastatic, or recurrent).

CEA is not an absolute test for malignant disease or for a specific type of malignancy.

CEA level should never be used as the sole criterion for diagnosis.

Summary of current data:

97% of healthy nonsmokers have plasma CEA levels < 2.5 ng/ml.

19% of heavy smokers and 7% of former smokers have CEA levels > 2.5 ng/ml.

75% of patients with carcinoma of entodermal origin (colon, stomach, pancreas, lung) have CEA titers > 2.5 ng/ml, and two-thirds of these titers are > 5 ng/ml.

Titers > 20 ng/ml are usually associated with metastatic disease or with a few types of cancer (e.g., cancer of the colon or pancreas); however, metastases may occur with levels < 20 ng/ml.

50% of patients with carcinoma of nonentodermal origin (especially cancer of the breast, head, and neck) have CEA titers > 2.5 ng/ml, and 50% of the titers are > 5 ng/ml.

40% of patients with noncarcinomatous malignant disease have increased CEA levels, usually 2.5–5.0 ng/ml.

Active cases of nonmalignant inflammatory diseases (especially of the digestive tract, e.g., ulcerative colitis, regional enteritis, diverticulitis, cirrhosis) frequently have elevated levels that decline when the disease is in remission.

In patients with carcinoma of entodermal origin, a CEA level > 5 ng/ml before therapy suggests localized disease and a favorable prognosis, but a level > 10 ng/ml suggests extensive disease and a poor prognosis. A fall of CEA to < 2.5 ng/ml after the therapy suggests adequate treatment, but persistent elevation may indicate residual tumor. A rising CEA level may indicate recurrent carcinoma of entodermal origin, even if the pretreatment level was normal. However, for an individual patient, it is difficult to predict the outcome on the basis of these data. The carcinoma may precede clinical evidence of recurrence.

With values > 20 ng/ml, plasma CEA correlates with tumor volume in breast and colon cancer; is useful for monitoring tumor response or progression; 20% change in plasma level is concordant with change in the tumor.

Change in CEA level precedes clinical changes by 2–6 months in advanced breast and colon cancer.

In ≅ 50% of patients with advanced breast or colon cancer, there may be a latent phase of 4–6 weeks from onset of therapy to change in CEA level.

Do not test heparinized patients or collect plasma in heparinized tubes, since this may interfere with accuracy of CEA assay.

SERUM GASTRIN

Normal levels: from absent to ≦ 200 pg gastrin/ml serum
Elevated levels: > 500 pg/ml

Condition	Serum Gastrin	Serum Gastrin After Intragastric Administration of 0.1N HCl
Peptic ulcer without Zollinger-Ellison syndrome	Normal range	—
Zollinger-Ellison syndrome	Very high	No change
Pernicious anemia	High level may approach that in Zollinger-Ellison syndrome	Marked decrease

Calcium infusion (IV calcium gluconate, 5 mg/kg body weight/hour for 3 hours) with preinfusion blood specimen compared to specimens every 30 minutes for up to 4 hours. Normal patients show minimal serum gastrin response to calcium. Patients with Zollinger-Ellison syndrome show excessive increase in serum gastrin.

Secretin infusion (IV of 9 units/kg body weight for 1 hour) with blood specimens drawn before and at 15-minute intervals. Normal patients and patients with duodenal ulcer show no increase in serum gastrin. Patients with Zollinger-Ellison syndrome show increased serum gastrin that usually peaks in 45–60 minutes.

Indications for measurement of serum gastrin and gastric analysis include:

Atypical peptic ulcer of stomach, duodenum, or proximal jejunum, especially if multiple, unusual location, poorly responsive to therapy, or multiple, rapid, or severe recurrence after adequate therapy

Unexplained chronic diarrhea with or without peptic ulcer

Marked gastric acid hypersecretion (e.g., > 100 ml/hour or > 10 mM/hour)

Peptic ulcer disease with associated endocrine conditions (see MEN, pp. 513–514).

Measurement for screening of all peptic ulcer patients would not be practical or cost-effective.

Increased Serum Gastrin Without Gastric Acid Hypersecretion

Atrophic gastritis, especially when associated with circulating parietal cell antibodies

Pernicious anemia in $\cong$ 75% of patients

Some patients have carcinoma of body of stomach, a reflection of the atrophic gastritis that is present.

Chronic renal failure with serum creatinine > 3 mg/dl; occurs in 50% of patients

Increased Serum Gastrin with Gastric Acid Hypersecretion

Zollinger-Ellison syndrome (gastrinoma) (see pp. 475–476)

Hyperplasia of antral gastrin cells

Isolated retained antrum—a condition of gastric acid hypersecretion and recurrent ulceration following antrectomy and gastrojejunostomy that occurs when the duodenal stump contains antral mucosa

Pyloric obstruction with gastric distention

Short-bowel syndrome due to massive resection or extensive regional enteritis

SERUM CALCITONIN

Basal fasting level may be increased in patients with medullary carcinoma of the thyroid even when there is no palpable mass in the thyroid.

Calcium infusion and/or pentagastrin injection are used as provocative tests in patients with normal basal levels who have a family history of thyroid carcinoma, a calcified thyroid mass, pheochromocytoma, hyperparathyroidism, hypercalcemia, amyloid-containing metastatic carcinoma of unknown origin, or facial characteristics of the mucosal neuroma syndrome.

Serum calcitonin levels are also useful to detect recurrence of medullary carcinoma or metastases after the primary tumor has been removed or to confirm complete removal of the tumor.

Increased levels have also been reported in some patients with

Carcinoma of lung, breast, islet cell, or ovary and carcinoid due to ectopic production

Hypercalcemia of any etiology stimulating calcitonin production

Zollinger-Ellison syndrome (hypergastrinemia)

Pernicious anemia

Acute or chronic thyroiditis

Chronic renal failure

Basal calcitonin levels

> 2000 pg/ml are almost always associated with medullary carcinoma of thyroid with rare cases due to obvious renal failure or ectopic production of calcitonin.

500–2000 pg/ml generally indicate medullary carcinoma, renal failure, or ectopic production of calcitonin.

100–500 pg/ml should be interpreted cautiously with repeat assays and provocative tests; if these and repeat tests in 1–2 months are still abnormal, some authors recommend total thyroidectomy.

SERUM THYROGLOBULIN
(normal < 60 ng/ml)

Increased in most patients with differentiated thyroid carcinoma but not with undifferentiated or medullary thyroid carcinomas.

May be useful to assess the presence and possibly the extent of residual or recurrent or metastatic carcinoma.

In differentiated thyroid carcinoma treated with total thyroidectomy or radioiodine and taking thyroid hormone therapy, plasma thyroglobulin levels are undetectable if functional metastases are absent but elevated if functional metastases are present. (See also p. 460.)

Is not useful for screening high-risk groups (e.g., neck radiation in childhood) because

   May not be increased in patients with small occult thyroid carcinomas

   Increased levels may also be found in patients with nontoxic nodular goiter

   Presence of autoantibodies interferes with the test procedure for which the patients' serum must first be screened.

In differential diagnosis of hyperthyroidism, level is very low or not detectable in factitious hyperthyroidism and high in all other types of hyperthyroidism (e.g., thyroiditis).

GLYCOHEMOGLOBIN
(may be reported as Hb A_{1c} hemoglobin or as A_{1b}, A_{1a}, A_{1c}) (values may not be comparable with different methodologies and even different laboratories using same methodology)

Glucose combines with hemoglobin continuously and nearly irreversibly during life span of RBC; thus glycosylated hemoglobin will be proportional to mean plasma glucose level during previous 1–3 months. Therefore, is better monitor of patient compliance and long-term blood glucose level control in diabetes mellitus. Does not require dietary preparation or fasting. Has low sensitivity but high specificity compared to oral GTT, which has high sensitivity but low specificity in diagnosis of diabetes mellitus. Increased level almost certainly means diabetes mellitus if other factors (see list below) are absent, but a normal level does not rule out impaired glucose tolerance.

Normal (A_{1a}, A_{1b}, A_{1c}) = 4–8%

In known diabetics

   7% indicates good diabetic control

   10% indicates fair diabetic control

   13–20% indicates poor diabetic control

For level of 4–20%, this formula may estimate daily average plasma glucose:

Mean daily plasma glucose (mg/dl)
= 10 × (glycohemoglobin level + 4)

Increased In
HbF > normal or 0.5% (e.g., fetomaternal transfusion during pregnancy)
Chronic renal failure with or without hemodialysis
Iron deficiency anemia
Splenectomy
Increased serum triglycerides
Alcohol
Lead toxicity

Decreased In
Hemolytic anemias
Presence of Hb S, Hb C, Hb D
Congenital spherocytosis
Acute or chronic blood loss
Pregnancy

Functional Tests

ORAL GLUCOSE TOLERANCE TEST (OGTT)*
Prior diet of > 250 gm of carbohydrate daily and no alcohol for 3
    days before test. Fasting for 10–16 hours before test. No medica-
    tion, smoking, or exercise during test. Not to be done during re-
    covery from acute illness, emotional stress, surgery, pregnancy.
    Certain drugs should be stopped several weeks before the test
    (e.g., oral diuretics, oral contraceptives, phenytoin).
Loading dose of glucose for adults is 75 gm, 100 gm during preg-
    nancy, 1.75 gm/kg for children (flavored solution). Draw blood at
    fasting, 30, 60, 90, 120 minutes; in pregnancy extend test to 3
    hours; 30-minute sample offers little additional information but
    can confirm adequate gastric absorption when patient is nau-
    seous.
For diagnosis of diabetes mellitus, at least two values should be
    increased.
OGTT should be reserved principally for patients with "borderline"
    fasting plasma glucose levels.
OGTT is not indicated in
        Persistent fasting hyperglycemia
        Persistent fasting normoglycemia
        Suspected gestational diabetes
        Secondary diabetes (e.g., genetic hyperglycemic syndromes, fol-
            lowing administration of certain hormones)
        Patients with typical clinical findings of diabetes mellitus and
            random plasma glucose > 200 mg/dl
Test is of limited value for diagnosis of diabetes mellitus in children
    and is rarely indicated for that purpose.

Decreased Tolerance In
Excessive peak
        Increased absorption (normal IV GTT curve) with normal re-
            turn to fasting level

*Data from National Diabetes Group, 1978.

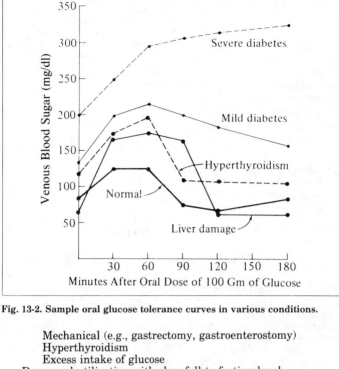

Fig. 13-2. Sample oral glucose tolerance curves in various conditions.

    Mechanical (e.g., gastrectomy, gastroenterostomy)
    Hyperthyroidism
    Excess intake of glucose
Decreased utilization with slow fall to fasting level
    Diabetes mellitus
    Hyperlipidemia, types III, IV, V
    Hemochromatosis
    Steroid effect (Cushing's disease, administration of ACTH
       or steroids)
    CNS lesions
Decreased formation of glycogen with low fasting levels and
    subsequent hypoglycemia
    von Gierke's disease
    Severe liver damage
    Hyperthyroidism (normal return to fasting level)
    Increased epinephrine (stress, pheochromocytoma) (normal
       return to fasting level)
    Pregnancy (normal return to fasting level)

Increased Tolerance In
Flat peak
    Pancreatic islet cell hyperplasia or tumor
    Poor absorption from GI tract (normal IV GTT curve)
       Intestinal diseases (e.g., steatorrhea, sprue, celiac disease,
         Whipple's disease)
       Hypothyroidism
       Addison's disease
       Hypoparathyroidism

Table 13-7. Criteria for Diagnosis of Glucose Intolerance

	Plasma Glucose (mg/dl)			
Condition	Fasting	1 Hour	2 Hours	3 Hours
Normal	<115	<200	<140	
Impaired glucose tolerance	115–140	>200	140–200	
Diabetes mellitus	>140	>200	>200	
Gestational diabetes mellitus	>105	>190	>165	>145

Late hypoglycemia
    Pancreatic islet cell hyperplasia or tumor
    Hypopituitarism
    Liver disease

See Serum Glucose, p. 41, and Table 34-1, pp. 672–677, for effect of drugs.

Difficulty in interpretation has caused abandonment of other GTTs, such as IV GTT, cortisone GTT.

TOLBUTAMIDE TOLERANCE TEST

Administer 1 gm sodium tolbutamide intravenously within 2 minutes. *Always keep IV glucose available to prevent severe reaction.*

Adrenal insufficiency—normal or low curve

Severe liver disease—low curve

Test is most useful for diagnosis of secreting islet cell tumor and to rule out functional hyperinsulinism.

In normal persons, glucose is a more potent stimulus for insulin release than tolbutamide, but the opposite is true in insulinoma, which shows an exaggerated early insulin peak (3–5 minutes after injection) with a sustained elevation of insulin and depression of glucose at 150 minutes.

In islet cell tumor, the fall in blood sugar is usually more marked than in functional hypoglycemia; more important, the blood sugar fails to recover even after 2–3 hours.

In functional hypoglycemia, return of blood sugar to normal is usually complete by 90 minutes.

It has been suggested that

serum glucose (mg/dl) minus ½ serum insulin (μU/ml)

< 43 indicates insulinoma but ≧43 excludes diagnosis of insulinoma.

INSULIN TOLERANCE TEST

Administer 0.1 unit insulin/kg body weight intravenously. *Use smaller dose if hypopituitarism is suspected. Always keep IV glucose available to prevent severe reaction.*

Normal

Blood glucose falls to 50% of fasting level within 20–30 minutes; returns to fasting level within 90–120 minutes.

Table 13-8. Serum Glucose Change Induced by Tolbutamide in Various Conditions

	% of Fasting Serum Glucose At	
Disease	20 Minutes	30 Minutes
Islet cell tumor	17–50	40–60
Normal functional hyperinsulinism	50–80	60–76
Borderline diabetes	80–84	77–81
Probable diabetes	85–89	82–86
Diabetes	$\geqq 90$	$\geqq 87$

Increased Tolerance
Blood glucose falls < 25% and returns rapidly to fasting level.
Hypothyroidism
Acromegaly
Cushing's syndrome
Diabetes mellitus (some patients; especially older, obese ones)

Decreased Tolerance
Increased sensitivity to insulin (excessive fall of blood glucose)
Hypoglycemic irresponsiveness (lack of response by glycogenolysis)
        Pancreatic islet cell tumor
        Adrenocortical insufficiency
        Adrenocortical insufficiency secondary to hypopituitarism
        Hypothyroidism
        von Gierke's disease (some patients)
        Starvation (depletion of liver glycogen)

INSULIN GLUCOSE TOLERANCE TEST
Administer simultaneously 0.1 unit insulin/kg body weight intravenously and 0.8 gm glucose/kg body weight orally.
Insulin-sensitive diabetics show little change in blood sugar.
Insulin-resistant diabetics show a diabetic glucose tolerance curve.
Other changes parallel those in the insulin tolerance test.

ORAL DISACCHARIDE TOLERANCE TEST
Administer 1 gm/kg body weight of the test carbohydrate (disaccharide). Determine blood glucose at fasting, ½-, 1-, 2-, and 3-hour intervals.
Normal: Blood glucose increases > 24 mg/dl above fasting level.
Abnormal in disaccharide malabsorption: Blood glucose increases 0–21 mg/dl above fasting level. False abnormal test may be due to delayed gastric emptying or delayed blood collection.
Confirm disaccharide malabsorption by
        Repeating tolerance test using constituent monosaccharides
        Testing stool for
                pH: $\leqq 5$ is abnormal
                Sugar: >0.5% is abnormal; 0.25–0.5% is suspicious; 0.25% is normal.

Taking intestinal biopsy for histologic study and disaccharidase activity assay

D-XYLOSE TOLERANCE TEST

Give 25 gm D-xylose in water orally. Collect a total 5-hour urine specimen (normal is >5 gm in 5 hours). Blood may also be taken at fasting, ½-, 1-, and 2-hour intervals (normal is > 25 mg/dl). The test reflects intestinal malabsorption.

Chief value is in distinguishing small intestinal malabsorption, which has decreased values, from pancreatic steatorrhea, which has normal values (see p. 237).

Decreased In

Malabsorption in jejunum (e.g., celiac disease, sprue, some patients with *Giardia lamblia* infestation, small-intestine bacterial overgrowth, viral gastroenteritis)—<4 gm in 5-hour urine

Elderly persons

Normal absorption but decreased urinary excretion (e.g., renal insufficiency, myxedema, vomiting, dehydration)

Patients with ascites (urine values are low)

Normal In

Steatorrhea due to pancreatic disease

Cirrhosis of liver

Postgastrectomy state

Malnutrition

TRIOLEIN ^{131}I ABSORPTION TEST

The patient fasts overnight after taking 30 drops of Lugol's iodine solution on the previous day.

Administer 15–20 μc of triolein [131]I. Collect blood every 1–2 hours for the next 6–8 hours.

Collect stools for 48–72 hours until radioactivity disappears.

Normal: ≥10% of administered radioactivity appears in the blood within 6 hours; <5% appears in the feces.

The test is useful for screening patients with steatorrhea. Normal values indicate that digestion of fat in the small bowel and absorption of fat in the small bowel are normal.

If results are abnormal, do an oleic acid ^{131}I absorption test.

OLEIC ACID ^{131}I ABSORPTION TEST

Methodology and normal values are the same as for the triolein absorption test.

An abnormal result indicates a defect in small bowel mucosal absorption function (e.g., sprue, Whipple's disease, regional enteritis, tuberculous enteritis, collagen diseases involving the small bowel, extensive resection). Abnormal pancreatic function does not affect the test.

POLYVINYLPYRROLIDONE (PVP-^{131}I)

Give 15–25 μc of PVP-^{131}I intravenously, and collect all stools for 4–5 days.

Normal: <2% is excreted in feces when the mucosa of the GI tract is intact.

In protein-losing enteropathy, >2% of administered radioactivity appears in the stool.

^{51}Cr TEST FOR GASTROINTESTINAL BLEEDING

Tag 10 ml of the patient's blood with 200 μc of ^{51}Cr, and administer it intravenously. Collect daily stools for radioactivity measurement and also measure simultaneous blood samples.

Radioactivity in the stool establishes GI blood loss. Comparison with radioactivity measurements of 1 ml of blood indicates the amount of blood loss.

The test is useful in ulcerative diseases (e.g., ulcerative colitis, regional enteritis, peptic ulcer).

GALACTOSE TOLERANCE TEST

Use an oral dose of 35 gm of galactose/sq m body area.

Normal: Serum galactose increases to 30–50 mg/dl; returns to normal within 3 hours.

Galactosemia: Serum increase is greater, and return to baseline level is delayed.

Heterozygous carrier: Response is intermediate.

The test is not specific or sensitive enough for genetic studies.

Beware of hypoglycemia in von Gierke's disease.

CAROTENE TOLERANCE TEST

Low values for serum carotene levels are usually associated with steatorrhea.

Measure serum carotene following daily oral loading of carotene for 3–7 days.

Normal

Increase of serum carotene by > 35 μg/dl indicates previously low dietary intake of carotene and/or fat.

Decreased In

Steatorrhea. Serum carotene increases > 30 μg/dl. Patients with sprue in remission with normal fecal fat excretion may still show low carotene absorption.

Mineral oil interferes with carotene absorption. On a fat-free diet only 10% is absorbed.

IODINE TOLERANCE TEST

A fasting patient who has received no iodine for 1 week is given 0.3–0.5 ml of strong iodine solution in milk. Blood iodine determinations are made every half hour for 2½ hours.

Normal: Blood iodine increases from 10 to ≦ 160 or 170 μg/dl in half an hour; by 2½ hours it decreases to only 150 μg.

Hyperthyroidism: Blood iodine increases from 15 μg to only 40 μg after 1 hour.

CREATINE TOLERANCE TEST
(ingestion of 1–3 gm creatine)

Normal: Creatine is not increased in blood or urine.

Decreased muscle mass: Blood and urine creatine increases in

  Neurogenic atrophy
  Polymyositis
  Addison's disease

Hyperthyroidism
Male eunuchoidism
Other

TRYPTOPHAN TOLERANCE TEST
The test demonstrates pyridoxine deficiency. It may be positive in pyridoxine-responsive anemia, or it may be normal.
A positive test produces abnormally large urinary excretion of xanthurenic acid.

ELLSWORTH-HOWARD TEST
Determine urinary phosphorus before and after injection of *potent* parathyroid extract.
Hypoparathyroidism: Urinary phosphorus is increased > 10 times.
Pseudohypoparathyroidism: Urinary phosphorus is increased < 2 times (i.e., poor or no response to parathormone injection).
Pseudopseudohypoparathyroidism: Response to parathormone injection is normal. Urinary phosphorus is increased 5–6 times.
Basal cell nevus syndrome: Decreased response to parathormone injection is often shown.

RESPONSE OF ELEVATED SERUM CALCIUM TO CORTICOIDS
Corticoids do not suppress elevated serum calcium in hyperparathyroidism.
Corticoid administration does suppress the elevated serum calcium level in
Sarcoidosis
Metastatic neoplasm
Vitamin D excess
Multiple myeloma
Hyperthyroidism

CALCIUM TOLERANCE
Constant diet: Measure phosphorus in three 24-hour urines. On second day, administer calcium intravenously (15 mg/kg body weight).
Normal: Calcium infusion causes marked decrease in urine phosphorus on second day, followed by rebound increase on third day.
Hyperparathyroidism: Only slight changes appear in urine phosphorus.

PHOSPHATE DEPRIVATION
After a diet of 800 mg phosphate/day, determine serum phosphorus and BUN and 12-hour urine phosphorus.
Normal: 6–17 ml/minute
Hyperparathyroidism: higher (even with renal dysfunction)
Hypoparathyroidism: lower (e.g., < 6 ml/minute), even when hypocalcemia has been corrected

TUBULAR REABSORPTION OF PHOSPHATE (TRP)
After a constant dietary intake of moderate calcium and phosphorus for 3 days, phosphorus and creatinine are determined in fasting blood and 4-hour urine specimens to calculate TRP.

$$TRP = 100 \left(1 - \frac{\text{urine phosphorus} \times \text{serum creatinine}}{\text{urine creatinine} \times \text{serum phosphorus}} \right)$$

Normal: TRP is >78% on normal diet; higher on low-phosphate diet (430 mg/day).

Hyperparathyroidism: TRP is <74% on normal diet; <85% on low-phosphate diet.

False-positive result may occur in uremia, renal tubular disease (some patients), osteomalacia, sarcoidosis.

URINE CONCENTRATION TEST

Restrict water intake for 14–16 hours; then collect three urines at 1-, 2-, and 4-hour intervals, and measure specific gravity.

Normal: Urine specific gravity is ≧1.025.

With decreased renal function, specific gravity is <1.020. As renal impairment is more severe, specific gravity approaches 1.010.

The test is sensitive for early loss of renal function, but a normal finding does not necessarily rule out active kidney disease.

The test is unreliable in the presence of any severe water and electrolyte imbalance (e.g., adrenal cortical insufficiency, edema formation), low-protein or low-salt diet, chronic liver disease, pregnancy, lack of patient cooperation.

Fluid deprivation may be contraindicated in heart disease or early renal failure.

VASOPRESSIN (PITRESSIN) CONCENTRATION TEST

The bladder is emptied, and urine is collected 1 and 2 hours after subcutaneous injection of 10 units of vasopressin. Water intake is not restricted, but no diuretics should be administered.

Normal: The specific gravity should reach ≧1.020.

Interpretation is the same as in the urine concentration test.

In diabetes insipidus, urine specific gravity becomes normal after vasopressin administration but not after fluid restriction.

The test may be used in the presence of edema or ascites. It is contraindicated in coronary artery disease and pregnancy.

See Diabetes Insipidus, pp. 508, 510.

URINE OSMOLALITY

Measurement of urine osmolality during water restriction is an accurate, sensitive test of decreased renal function.

The patient is on a high-protein diet for 3 days; has a dry supper and no fluids on the evening before the test; empties the bladder at 6 A.M., discards urine, and returns to bed. Test urine specimen is collected at 8 A.M.

Normal: concentration of >800 mOsm/kg

Minimal impairment of renal concentrating ability: 600–800 mOsm/kg

Moderate impairment: 400–600 mOsm/kg

Severe impairment: <400 mOsm/kg

Urine osmolality may be impaired when other tests are normal (Fishberg concentration test, BUN, PSP excretion, creatinine clearance, IV pyelogram); may be especially useful in diabetes mellitus, essential hypertension, silent pyelonephritis.

It may be well also to measure serum osmolality and calculate urine-serum ratio (normal = >3).

See Diabetes Insipidus, pp. 508, 510.

URINE DILUTION TEST

No breakfast is allowed; 1500 ml of water is taken within 30–45 minutes, and urine is collected every hour for 4 hours.

Normal: Urine volume is >80% of ingested amount (1200 ml). Specific gravity is 1.003 in at least one specimen.

With decreased renal function there is a smaller volume of urine. Specific gravity may not fall below 1.010.

Loss of dilution ability occurs later than loss of concentrating ability.

Water loading may be contraindicated in kidney and heart disease.

PHENOLSULFONPHTHALEIN (PSP) EXCRETION TEST

Administer an IV injection of 1 mg/kg body weight or usually 6 mg in 1-ml volume. Collect urine and (sometimes) blood samples at 15-, 30-, and 60-minute intervals.

The test is useful to detect slight to moderate decrease in renal function. It is not useful in chronic azotemia with fixed specific gravity (serum creatinine and creatinine clearance are more useful then).

It is hazardous in severe renal insufficiency or heart failure because adequate prior hydration is required to obtain sufficient urine volume. Using small urine volumes magnifies errors.

The test is distorted by residual bladder urine, abnormal drainage sites (e.g., fistulas), and interfering substances (e.g., hematuria).

Hepatic disease may give falsely elevated values (because 20% of the dye is normally removed by the liver). False results may also occur in multiple myeloma (because of excessive protein binding) and in hypoalbuminemia. Certain drugs may interfere with PSP excretion (e.g., salicylates, penicillin, some diuretic and uricosuric drugs, and some x-ray contrast media).

The 15-minute PSP excretion correlates with the glomerular filtration rate (GFR); a normal 15-minute value indicates normal GFR. Progressive decrease of 15-minute value is proportional to decreased GFR (e.g., 15% PSP excretion in 15 minutes approximates a 45% GFR). If the GFR is normal, the PSP test indicates renal blood flow or tubular function; there are better tests available for measuring these two functions, and the PSP test is now rarely used.

Increased dye excretion in later time periods compared to the initial 15-minute period suggests increased residual urine due to obstructive uropathy or incomplete bladder emptying; the latter can be ruled out by indwelling catheterization during the test.

PSP that is normal with increased BUN and serum creatinine and decreased GFR suggests acute glomerulonephritis. PSP parallels these parameters in most chronic renal diseases.

GLOMERULAR FILTRATION RATE (GFR)

Serum creatinine increase occurs in 10–20% of patients taking aminoglycosides and up to 20% of patients taking penicillins (especially methicillin). Elderly patients with a normal serum creatinine and diminished muscle mass may have a 30% decrease in GFR.

To estimate GFR from serum creatinine, this equation may be used:

$$\text{GFR} = \frac{(140 - \text{age in years})\ (\text{weight in kg})}{72 \times \text{serum creatinine}}$$

Glomerular filtration rate (GFR) is measured with urea clearance, creatinine clearance, or inulin clearance.

OTHER RENAL FUNCTION TESTS*

Renal plasma flow (RPF) is measured with para-aminohippurate (PAH) clearance or Diodrast clearance.

$$\text{Filtration fraction (FF)} = \frac{\text{GFR}}{\text{RPF}} \qquad (\text{normal} = 0.2)$$

Urea clearance is normal until >50% of renal parenchyma is inactivated. With renal insufficiency, the clearance test parallels the parenchymal destruction.

Urinary acidification is impaired in chronic renal disease with azotemia. It is decreased without parallel impairment of GFR in renal tubular acidosis, some cases of Fanconi's syndrome, and some cases of acquired nephrocalcinosis.

Proximal tubular malfunction is indicated by urinary excretion of substances normally reabsorbed by tubules: in renal glycosuria (blood glucose < 180 mg/dl as in Fanconi's syndrome, heavy-metal poisoning), aminoaciduria, phosphaturia.

See also Serum Urea Nitrogen (BUN) (p. 42), Serum Creatinine (p. 43), Phenolsulfonphthalein (PSP) Excretion Test (p. 104), Urine Concentration Test (p. 103), and Urine Dilution Test (p. 104).

Serum creatinine and BUN are not useful in discovering early renal insufficiency because they do not become abnormal until 50% of renal function has been lost. The creatinine clearance test, particularly serial measurements, is the most reliable test of renal function. After baseline measurements have been obtained, serum creatinine levels can be evaluated.

If there is a discrepancy between these two tests, additional studies may be performed (e.g., concentration and dilution tests, urinalyses, biochemical studies of serum and urine, urine cultures, renalgrams and scans, biopsy).

Impairment may be more severe than indicated by laboratory studies if signs and symptoms are more disabling.

Estimate of creatinine clearance from single serum creatinine clearance may be required for prompt therapy of nephrotoxic drug reaction or because of difficulty of accurate 24-hour urine collection. This estimate may be obtained by the following formulas or by the nomogram (Fig. 13-3).

---

*See standard laboratory texts for information on the technical performance of clearance tests.

Table 13-9. Laboratory Guide to Evaluation of Renal Impairment

Condition	Renal Clearance of Endogenous Creatinine[a] (glomerular filtration rate)	Urinary Excretion of IV PSP[b] in 15 Minutes (renal tubular transport mechanisms)
Normal	Men: 130–200 L/24 hours (90–139 ml/min) Women: 115–180 L/24 hours (80–125 ml/min)	≧ 25%
Slight impairment	75–90 L/24 hours (52.0–62.5 ml/min)	15–25%
Mild impairment	60–75 L/24 hours (42–52 ml/min)	10–15%
Moderate impairment	40–60 L/24 hours (28–42 ml/min)	5–10%
Marked impairment	<40 L/24 hours (<28 ml/min)	<5%

[a] Creatinine clearance is normally less in women than men, and it usually decreases with age, starting at age 20.
[b] Phenolsulfonphthalein.

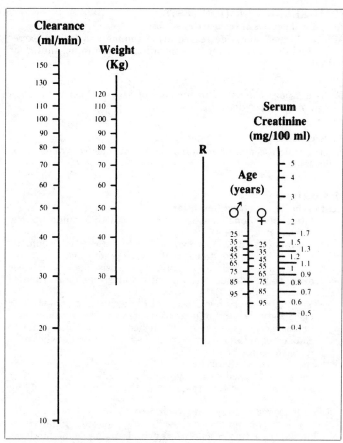

Fig. 13-3. Nomogram for rapid estimation of endogenous creatinine clearance. With a straightedge, join weight to age. Keep straightedge at crossing point of line marked "R." Then move the right-hand side of the straightedge to the appropriate serum creatinine value and read the patient's clearance from the left side of the nomogram. (From G. B. Appel and H. C. Neu, Antimicrobial agents in patients with renal disease. *Medical Times* 105(9):116, Sept. 1977.)

Creatinine clearance (ml/min/1.73 sq m)

$$= \frac{(98 - 0.8) \times (\text{age} - 20)}{\text{serum creatinine}}$$ Values for women are 90% of predicted

or

$$= \frac{(140 - \text{age}) \times \text{body weight (kg)}}{72 \times \text{serum creatinine}}$$ Values for women are 85% of predicted

SPLIT RENAL FUNCTION TESTS
(for aid in diagnosis of renal artery stenosis)
Affected kidney shows decreased urine volume and sodium excretion and decreased urine concentration of creatinine, inulin, or
  PAH.

*These tests are not useful in presence of urinary tract obstruction
  (e.g., in men over age 50).*

RENAL BIOPSY
Electron microscopy and immunofluorescent microscopy should be
  available.

May Be Indicated In
Acute renal failure to differentiate
> Acute glomerulonephritis—to be treated with immunosuppres-
>   sive agents and dialysis
> Drug-induced (e.g., methicillin) acute interstitial nephritis
>   with eosinophilia—to be treated with prednisone
> Interstitial nephritis and papillary necrosis due to analgesic
>   drug abuse—to be treated with dialysis and cessation of
>   analgesics (see p. 648)
> Systemic lupus erythematosus (SLE), necrotizing angiitis, and
>   Goodpasture's syndrome (to be treated with prednisone or hy-
>   drocortisone) are to be distinguished from ischemic or neph-
>   rotoxic renal failure (to be treated with dialysis; does not need
>   drug therapy).

Lipoid nephrosis to differentiate
> SLE—to be treated with prednisone
> Amyloid nephropathy—to be treated by therapy of underlying
>   infection
> Occult bacterial endocarditis—to be treated with antibiotics
> Renal vein thrombosis—to be treated with anticoagulants
> Characteristic lipoid nephrosis of children and young adults is
>   prednisone-responsive.
> Diffuse generalized membranous glomerulonephritis is steroid-
>   resistant.
> Proliferative glomerulonephritis (e.g., poststreptococcal, ana-
>   phylactoid purpura) is to be treated with immunosuppressive
>   agents.

Fixed and persistent proteinuria that does not respond to trial of
  prednisone therapy; routine biopsy not indicated in children or
  adolescents
In adults, corticosteroid treatment should not be instituted until a
  responsive disease has been diagnosed by biopsy.
Diagnosis of unsuspected disease (e.g., nephrocalcinosis of hyper-
  parathyroidism)
Diagnosis of renal disease of unknown etiology
Evaluation of therapeutic effect (e.g., SLE, polyarteritis nodosa)
Complete diagnosis prior to renal transplantation or chronic dialy-
  sis
Culture of organism in some cases of pyelonephritis
Other

Contraindicated In
Patient with bleeding tendencies
Patient with unilateral kidney
Uncooperative patient

CYTOLOGIC EXAMINATION OF VAGINAL SMEAR (PAPANICOLAOU SMEAR) FOR EVALUATION OF OVARIAN FUNCTION

Maturation index (MI) is the proportion of parabasal, intermediate, and superficial cells in each 100 cells counted.

Lack of estrogen effect shows predominance of parabasal cells (e.g., MI = 100/0/0).

Low estrogen effect shows predominance of intermediate cells (e.g., MI = 10/90/0).

Increased estrogen effect shows predominance of superficial cells (e.g., MI = 0/0/100), as in hormone-producing tumors of ovary, persistent follicular cysts.

Some Patterns of Maturation Index in Different Conditions

	Index
Childhood	
Normal	80/20/0
Cortisone therapy	0/98/2
Childbearing years	
Preovulatory (late follicular) phase	0/40/60
Premenstrual (late luteal) phase	0/70/30
Pregnancy (second month)	0/90/10
Cortisone therapy	0/85/15
Amenorrhea after ovarian irradiation	0/30/70
Surgical oophorectomy	0/80/20–0/90/10
Bilateral oophorectomy and adrenalectomy	0/98/2
Postmenopausal years, early (age 60)	65/30/5
Postmenopausal years, late (age 75)	
Untreated	100/0/0
Moderate estrogen treatment	0/50/50
High-dose estrogen treatment	0/0/100
Years after bilateral oophorectomy	100/0/0
Postadrenalectomy, bilateral	6/94/0

Karyopyknotic index (KI) is the percent of cells with pyknotic nuclei.

Increased estrogen effect (e.g., KI = >85%) is seen, as in cystic glandular hyperplasia of the endometrium.

Eosinophilic index is the percent of cells showing eosinophilic cytoplasm; it may also be used as a measure of estrogen effect.

Combined progesterone-estrogen effect: No quantitative cytologic criteria are available. Endometrial biopsy should be used for this purpose.

The pattern may be obscured by cytolysis (e.g., infections, excess bacilli), increased red or white blood cells, excessively thin or thick smears, or drying of smears before fixation (artificial eosinophilic staining).

Hematology

CAUSES OF LEUKOPENIA
Infections, especially
    Bacterial (e.g., overwhelming bacterial infection, septicemia, miliary tuberculosis, typhoid, paratyphoid, brucellosis, tularemia)
    Viral (e.g., infectious mononucleosis, hepatitis, influenza, measles, rubella, psittacosis)
    Rickettsial (e.g., scrub typhus, sandfly fever)
    Other (e.g., malaria, kala-azar)
Drugs and chemicals, especially
    Sulfonamides
    Antibiotics
    Analgesics
    Marrow depressants
    Arsenicals
    Antithyroid drugs
    Many others
Ionizing radiation
Hematopoietic diseases
    Pernicious anemia
    Aleukemic leukemia
    Aplastic anemia and related conditions
    Hypersplenism
    Gaucher's disease
    Felty's syndrome
Anaphylactic shock
Cachexia
Miscellaneous
    Disseminated lupus erythematosus
    Severe renal injury
    Various neutropenias
Artifactual associated with automated WBC counters (artifact is corrected when manual WBC counts are performed)
    Leukocyte fragility due to immunosuppressive and antineoplastic drugs
    Lymphocyte fragility in lymphocytic leukemia
    Excessive clumping of leukocytes in monoclonal gammopathies (e.g., multiple myeloma), cryofibrinogenemia (e.g., SLE), in presence of cold agglutinins

CAUSES OF LEUKOCYTOSIS
Acute infections
    Localized (e.g., pneumonia, meningitis, tonsillitis, abscess)
    Generalized (e.g., acute rheumatic fever, septicemia, cholera)
Intoxications
    Metabolic (uremia, acidosis, eclampsia, acute gout)
    Poisoning by chemicals, drugs, venoms, etc. (e.g., mercury, epinephrine, black widow spider)
    Parenteral (foreign protein and vaccines)
Acute hemorrhage
Acute hemolysis of red blood cells

Myeloproliferative diseases
Tissue necrosis
    Acute myocardial infarction
    Necrosis of tumors
    Burns
    Gangrene
    Bacterial necrosis, etc.
Physiologic conditions (e.g., exercise, emotional stress, menstruation, obstetrical labor)
Steroid administration (e.g., prednisone 40 mg orally or hydrocortisone 100–200 mg IV) causes increased polymorphonuclear neutrophil leukocytes of 1700–7500 (peak in 4–6 hours and return to normal in 24 hours); no definite shift to left. Lymphocytes decrease 70% and monocytes decrease 90%.

CAUSES OF LYMPHOCYTOSIS
Infections
    Pertussis
    Infectious lymphocytosis
    Infectious mononucleosis
    Infectious hepatitis
    Mumps
    German measles
    Chronic tuberculosis
    Undulant fever
    Convalescence from acute infection
    Thyrotoxicosis (relative)
    Neutropenia with relative lymphocytosis
    Lymphatic leukemia

CAUSES OF ATYPICAL LYMPHOCYTES
Lymphatic leukemia
Viral infections
    Infectious lymphocytosis
    Infectious mononucleosis
    Infectious hepatitis
    Viral pneumonia and other exanthems of childhood
    Mumps
    Chickenpox
    German measles
Pertussis
Brucellosis
Syphilis (in some phases)
Toxoplasmosis
Drug reactions and serum sickness
Normal persons may show up to 12% atypical lymphocytes.

CLUES TO DIAGNOSIS OF ATYPICAL OR LEUKOPENIC LEUKEMIA
Peripheral monocytosis
Peripheral cytopenia with normoblasts
Hypercellular marrow with hyperplasia of myeloid and/or erythroid elements
Acquired Pelger-Huët anomaly (see p. 366)

Table 13-10. Some Common Causes of Leukemoid Reaction

Cause	Myelocytic	Lymphocytic	Monocytic
Infections	Endocarditis Pneumonia Septicemia Leptospirosis Other	Infections mono- nucleosis Infectious lym- phocytosis Pertussis Chickenpox Tuberculosis	Tuberculosis
Toxic conditions	Burns Eclampsia Poisoning (e.g., mercury)		
Neoplasms	Carcinoma of colon Embryonal car- cinoma of kid- ney	Carcinoma of stomach Carcinoma of breast	
Miscellaneous	Treatment of megaloblastic anemia (of pregnancy, pernicious anemia) Acute hemor- rhage Acute hemolysis Recovery from agranulocy- tosis	Dermatitis her- petiformis	
Myeloprolifer- ative dis- eases			

BASOPHILIC LEUKOCYTES

Increased In
Chronic myelogenous leukemia
Polycythemia
Myeloid metaplasia
Hodgkin's disease
Postsplenectomy
Chronic hemolytic anemia (some patients)
Chronic sinusitis
Chickenpox
Smallpox
Myxedema
Nephrosis (some patients)
Foreign protein injection

Decreased In

Hyperthyroidism

Pregnancy

Period following irradiation, chemotherapy, and glucocorticoids

Acute phase of infection

CAUSES OF MONOCYTOSIS

(> 10% of differential count; absolute count > 500/cu mm)

Monocytic leukemia, other leukemias

Myeloproliferative disorders (myeloid metaplasia, polycythemia vera)

Hodgkin's disease and other malignant lymphomas

Lipid storage diseases (e.g., Gaucher's disease)

Tetrachlorethane poisoning

Recovery from agranulocytosis and subsidence of acute infection

Many protozoan infections (e.g., malaria, kala-azar, trypanosomiasis)

Some rickettsial infections (e.g., Rocky Mountain spotted fever, typhus)

Certain bacterial infections (e.g., subacute bacterial endocarditis, tuberculosis, brucellosis)

Chronic ulcerative colitis and regional enteritis

Sarcoidosis

Collagen diseases (e.g., rheumatoid arthritis, SLE)

PLASMA CELLS

Increased In

Plasma cell leukemia

Multiple myeloma

Hodgkin's disease

Chronic lymphocytic leukemia

Other neoplasias (cancer of liver, kidney, breast, prostate)

Cirrhosis

Rheumatoid arthritis

SLE

Serum reaction

Bacterial infections (e.g., syphilis, tuberculosis)

Parasitic infections (e.g., malaria, trichinosis)

Viral infections (e.g., infectious mononucleosis, rubella, measles, chickenpox, benign lymphocytic meningitis)

Decreased In

Not clinically significant

CAUSES OF EOSINOPHILIA

Allergic diseases (e.g., bronchial asthma, hay fever, urticaria, drug therapy)

Parasitic infestation, especially with tissue invasion (e.g., trichinosis, echinococcus disease) (see Pulmonary Infiltrations Associated with Eosinophilia, p. 222)

Some infectious diseases (e.g., scarlet fever, erythema multiforme)

Some skin diseases (e.g., pemphigus, dermatitis herpetiformis)

Some hematopoietic diseases (e.g., pernicious anemia, chronic myelogenous leukemia, polycythemia, Hodgkin's disease); postsplenectomy

Some gastrointestinal diseases (e.g., eosinophilic gastroenteritis, ulcerative colitis, regional enteritis)
Postirradiation
Miscellaneous conditions
    Polyarteritis nodosa
    Certain tumors (ovary, involvement of bone or serosal surfaces)
    Sarcoidosis
    Löffler's parietal fibroplastic endocarditis (see p. 214)
    Familial condition
    Poisoning (e.g., phosphorus, black widow spider bite)

LEUKOCYTE ALKALINE PHOSPHATASE STAINING REACTION
(in untreated diseases)

Usually Increased In
Leukemoid reaction
Polycythemia vera
Lymphoma (including Hodgkin's, reticulum cell sarcoma)
Acute and chronic lymphatic leukemia
Multiple myeloma
Myelosclerosis
Aplastic anemia
Agranulocytosis
Bacterial infections
Cirrhosis
Obstructive jaundice
Pregnancy and immediate postpartum period
Administration of Enovid
Mongolism (trisomy 21)
Klinefelter's syndrome (XXY)

Usually Decreased In
Chronic myelogenous leukemia
Paroxysmal nocturnal hemoglobinuria
Hereditary hypophosphatasia
Nephrotic syndrome
Progressive muscular dystrophy
Refractory anemia (siderotic)
Sickle cell anemia

Usually Normal In
Secondary polycythemia
Hemolytic anemia
Infectious mononucleosis
Viral hepatitis
Lymphosarcoma

Usually Variable In
Pernicious anemia
Idiopathic thrombocytopenic purpura
Iron deficiency anemia
Acute myelogenous leukemia
Acute undifferentiated leukemia

This test is clinically most useful in differentiating chronic myelogenous leukemia from leukemoid reaction.

NITROBLUE TETRAZOLIUM (NBT) REDUCTION IN NEUTROPHILS

Increased In
Bacterial infections, including miliary tuberculosis and tuberculous meningitis
Nocardia and other systemic fungal infections
Various parasitic infections
Malaria
Chédiak-Higashi syndrome
Idiopathic myelofibrosis
Normal infants up to age 2 months
Pregnancy
Patients taking birth control pills
Some patients with lymphoma suppressed by chemotherapy

Decreased or Normal
(in absence of bacterial infection)
Normal persons
Postpartum state
Postoperative state (after 7–10 days)
Cancer
Tissue transplantation
Other conditions with fever or leukocytosis not due to bacterial infection (e.g., rheumatoid arthritis)

Decreased or Normal
(in presence of bacterial infection)
Antibiotic therapy—effectiveness of treatment indicated by reduction of previous elevation, sometimes in < 6 hours
Localized infection
Administration of corticosteroids and immunosuppressive drugs (contrary findings with corticosteroids have also been reported)
Miscellaneous conditions, probably involving metabolic defects of neutrophil function
  Chronic granulomatous disease
  Neutrophilic deficiency of glucose 6-phosphate dehydrogenase or myeloperoxidase
  SLE
  Sickle cell disease
  Chronic myelogenous leukemia
  Lipochrome histiocytosis
  Congenital and acquired agammaglobulinemia
  Other

Increased
(from previously determined normal level)
May be used before other clinical parameters to monitor development of infection in chronically ill patients
  Development of wound sepsis in burn patients

Development of infection in uremic patients on chronic hemodialysis

Other

Usual normal values reported are < 10%, but there is considerable variation (≦ 14%), and each laboratory should establish its own normal range.

NBT test has been used principally in differentiating untreated bacterial infection from other conditions that may simulate it and for the diagnosis of poor neutrophilic function, particularly in chronic granulomatous disease. In many studies, few patients are included, considerable variation in technical performance occurs, or inadequate data are presented for comparison. Further evaluation of the clinical usefulness of the test in many of the conditions in which contradictory findings have been reported must await more definitive studies.

PLATELET COUNT

May Be Increased In
(>500,000/cu mm)

Malignancy, especially disseminated, advanced, or inoperable

Myeloproliferative disease (e.g., polycythemia vera, chronic myelogenous leukemia)

Patients recently having surgery, especially splenectomy

Collagen disorders, usually rheumatoid arthritis

Iron deficiency anemia

Pseudothrombocytosis

    Cryoglobulinemia

    Malaria parasites

    Fragments of RBCs or WBCs

    Microspherocytes

    Howell-Jolly bodies, nucleated RBCs, Heinz bodies, clumped Pappenheimer bodies

Miscellaneous disease states (e.g., acute infection, cardiac disease, cirrhosis of the liver, chronic pancreatitis)

Approximately 50% of patients with "unexpected" increase of platelet count are found to have a malignancy.

Decreased In

Thrombocytopenia (see p. 385)

Pseudothrombocytopenia (laboratory artifact; diagnosis by examination of stained peripheral blood smear)

    Platelet clumping induced by EDTA blood collection tubes is the most common cause.

    Platelet satellitosis

    Platelet cold agglutinins

    Giant platelets

    RBC count > 6,500,000/cu mm

MEAN PLATELET VOLUME
(measured by certain automated hematology instruments)

Increased In

Immune thrombocytopenic purpura

Thrombocytopenia due to sepsis (recovery phase)

Myeloproliferative disorders
Massive hemorrhage
Prosthetic heart valve
Splenectomy
Vasculitis

Decreased In
Reactive thrombocytosis
Megaloblastic anemia
Acute leukemia
Antileukemic chemotherapy
Aplastic anemia
Hypersplenism
Thrombocytopenia due to sepsis

ERYTHROCYTE SEDIMENTATION RATE (ESR)
(see Table 13-11)
ESR is useful to
>   Detect occult disease (e.g., screening program)
>   Follow course of a certain disease (e.g., tuberculosis, rheumatic fever, myocardial infarction)
>   Confirm a diagnosis or a differential diagnosis (e.g., acute myocardial infarction as opposed to angina pectoris; early acute appendicitis versus ruptured ectopic pregnancy or acute pelvic inflammatory disease; rheumatoid arthritis as opposed to osteoarthritis; acute versus quiescent gout)

May Be "Falsely" Low In
Polycythemia vera
Secondary polycythemia
Sickle cell anemia
Hereditary spherocytosis
Disseminated intravascular coagulopathy
Cachexia
Massive hepatic necrosis

Formula for normal range Westergren ESR:

Men: $\text{ESR} = \dfrac{\text{age (years)}}{2}$

Women: $\text{ESR} = \dfrac{\text{age (years)} + 10}{2}$

Hyperviscosity syndrome should be suspected in patients with hyperproteinemia (e.g., multiple myeloma, Waldenström's macroglobulinemia) with rouleaux formation but no increase of ESR.

SERUM C-REACTIVE PROTEIN (CRP)

Increased In
Any acute inflammatory change or necrosis: CRP precedes the rise in ESR; with recovery, disappearance of CRP precedes the return to normal of ESR. CRP disappears when inflammatory process is suppressed by steroids or salicylates.
Acute myocardial infarction: CRP appears within 24–48 hours, be-

Table 13-11. Changes in Erythrocyte Sedimentation Rate*

Disease	Increased In	Not Increased In
Infectious	Tuberculosis (especially) Acute hepatitis Many bacterial infections	Typhoid fever Undulant fever Malarial paroxysm Infectious mononucleosis Uncomplicated viral diseases
Cardiac	Acute myocardial infarction Active rheumatic fever After open-heart surgery	Angina pectoris Active renal failure with heart failure
Abdominal	Acute pelvic inflammatory disease Ruptured ectopic pregnancy Pregnancy—third month to about 3 weeks postpartum Menstruation	Acute appendicitis (first 24 hours) Unruptured ectopic pregnancy Early pregnancy
Joint	Rheumatoid arthritis Pyogenic arthritis	Degenerative arthritis
Miscellaneous	Significant tissue necrosis especially neoplasms (most frequently malignant lymphoma, cancer of colon and breast) Increased serum globulins (e.g., myeloma, cryoglobulinemia, macroglobulinuria) Decreased serum albumin Hypothyroidism Hyperthyroidism Acute hemorrhage Nephrosis, renal disease with azotemia Arsenic and lead intoxication Dextran and polyvinyl compounds in blood	Peptic ulcer Acute allergy

*Extreme elevation of ESR is found particularly in association with malignancy (most frequently malignant lymphoma, carcinomas of colon and breast), hematologic diseases (most frequently myeloma), collagen diseases (e.g., rheumatoid arthritis, SLE), renal diseases (especially with azotemia), infections, drug fever, and other conditions (e.g., cirrhosis). Westergren method is more accurate; Wintrobe method is more convenient.

gins to fall by third day, and becomes negative after 1–2 weeks; correlates with peak CK-MB levels, but CRP peak occurs 1–3 days later. Failure of CRP to return to normal indicates tissue damage in heart or elsewhere.

Following surgery: CRP increases within 4–6 hours to peak at 48–72 hours (usually at 25–35 mg/dl). Begins to decrease after third postoperative day. Said to be more sensitive to monitor complications (e.g., infection, pulmonary infarction) than WBC, ESR, temperature, pulse rate.

May be useful to monitor disease activity in bacterial and viral infections, rheumatic diseases, myocardial infarction, burns.

May be useful in differential diagnosis (e.g., acute myocardial infarction versus angina).

Useful for diagnosis of intercurrent infection

> Active severe SLE: Produces almost no increase of CRP but CRP increases with infection.
>
> Leukemia: Fever, blast crisis, or cytotoxic drugs cause only modest elevation of CRP, but intercurrent infection stimulates significantly higher CRP levels and is particularly useful to monitor response to antibiotic therapy.

CRP is significantly higher in Crohn's disease than in ulcerative colitis and corresponds to relapse, remission, and response to therapy in Crohn's disease.

Erythrocyte Indices
(see pp. 329–330)

MEAN CORPUSCULAR VOLUME (MCV)
(hematocrit divided by RBC count)

Decreased In
Microcytic anemias, especially iron deficiency, anemia of chronic disease, and certain hemoglobinopathies
Marked leukocytosis (> 50,000/cu mm)*
In vitro hemolysis or fragmentation of RBCs*
Warm autoantibodies*

Increased In
Macrocytic anemias
Chronic alcoholism (may be a useful screening test for this)
Infants and newborns
Methanol poisoning*
Marked hyperglycemia (> 600 mg/dl)*
Marked reticulocytosis (> 50%) due to any cause*
Marked leukocytosis (> 50,000/cu mm)*

MEAN CORPUSCULAR HEMOGLOBIN (MCH)
(hemoglobin divided by RBC count)

Decreased In
Microcytic and normocytic anemias

*Due to methodologic interference

Increased In
Macrocytic anemias
Infants and newborns
Conditions with cold agglutinins*
In vivo hemolysis*
Monoclonal proteins in blood*
High heparin concentration*

MEAN CORPUSCULAR HEMOGLOBIN CONCENTRATION (MCHC)
(hemoglobin divided by hematocrit)

Decreased In
(< 30.1 gm/dl)
Microcytic anemias. *Normal value does not rule out any of these anemias. Low MCHC may not occur in iron deficiency anemia when performed with automated instruments.*
Marked leukocytosis (> 50,000/cu mm)*

Increased In
Hereditary spherocytosis should be considered whenever MCHC > 36 gm/dl.
Infants and newborns
In vivo hemolysis*
Conditions with cold agglutinins or severe lipemia of serum*
High heparin concentration*

PERIPHERAL BLOOD SMEAR IN DIFFERENTIAL DIAGNOSIS OF ANEMIAS
The smear may also indicate leukemia, other conditions. Confirm the RBC indices.
Basophilic or polychromatophilic macrocytes—shows increased erythropoiesis in hemorrhage or hemolysis
Oval macrocytes with increased number of lobules of polynuclear leukocytes—in megaloblastic anemia
Target cells—in hemoglobinopathies (especially Hb C); also thalassemia, iron deficiency anemia, liver disease
Abnormally shaped RBCs—ovalocytes, sickle cells, spherocytes, poikilocytes, schistocytes
Microcytes with stippling—in thalassemia, lead poisoning

CONDITIONS ASSOCIATED WITH RBC INCLUSIONS

Reticulocytes†	Any condition with increased reticulocyte count
Basophilic stippling (multiple dark dots)	Lead poisoning, heavy metal poisoning, and severe anemia
Cabot's rings	Occasionally seen in severe hemolytic anemias and pernicious anemia
Howell-Jolly bodies (dark purple spherical bodies)	Occasionally seen in severe hemolytic anemias and pernicious anemia
	Occasionally seen in leukemia, thalassemia, postsplenectomy

*Due to methodologic interference
†Not seen with Wright's stain; requires supravital cresyl violet stain.

Pappenheimer bodies (siderotic granules) (purple coccoid granules at periphery)	Anemias with defect of incorporating iron into hemoglobin; show hypochromic microcytic anemia with increased serum iron and total iron-binding capacity (e.g., thalassemia, lead poisoning, di Guglielmo's disease, pyridoxine-responsive anemia, pyridoxine-unresponsive anemia)
Heinz-Ehrlich bodies*	Congenital glucose-6-PD deficiencies; other drug-induced hemolytic anemias
Plasmodium trophozoites	Malaria

RETICULOCYTES

Increased In
After blood loss or increased RBC destruction: normal response is three- to sixfold increase
After iron therapy for iron deficiency anemia
After specific therapy for megaloblastic anemias

Increase indicates effective RBC production mechanisms. It is a useful index of therapeutic response in these diseases.

Possibly other hematologic conditions (e.g., polycythemia, metastatic carcinoma in bone marrow, di Guglielmo's disease)

Increased reticulocyte count can elevate MCV in hemolytic disorders, hemorrhage, treatment of vitamin B_{12} deficiency.

Decreased In
Ineffective erythropoiesis or decreased RBC formation
    Severe autoimmune type of hemolytic disease
    Aregenerative crises
    Megaloblastic disorders
Alcoholism
Myxedema

SICKLING OF RBCs

Occurs In
Sickle cell disease
Sickle cell trait

False Positive In
First 4 months after transfusion with RBCs having sickle cell trait
Mixture on slide with fibrinogen, thrombin, gelatin (glue)
Excessive concentration of sodium metabisulfite (e.g., $\geq 4\%$ instead of 2%)
Drying of wet coverslip preparation
Poikilocytosis

*Not seen with Wright's stain; requires supravital cresyl violet stain.

False Negative In

First 4 months after transfusion with normal RBCs

Heating, bacterial contamination, or prolonged washing with saline of RBCs

Newborn

Sickling should be confirmed with hemoglobin electrophoresis and genetic studies.

SOME CAUSES OF POIKILOCYTOSIS

Round

Spherocytes	Congenital spherocytosis
	Warm autoimmune hemolytic anemia
	Cold autoimmune hemolytic anemia
Stomatocytes	Acute alcoholism (transient)
	Certain drugs (e.g., phenothiazines)
	Neoplastic, cardiovascular, hepatobiliary diseases
	Hereditary stomatocytosis (see p. 353)
	Artifactual
Target cells	Hemoglobin C disease or trait
	Thalassemia minor
	Iron deficiency anemia
	Liver disease
	Postsplenectomy state
	Artifactual

Elongated

Ovalocytes, elliptocytes	Hereditary (>25% in smear) (see p. 352)
	Microcytic anemia (<25% in smear) (see Table 27-5, p. 338)
	Megaloblastic anemias
Teardrop	Spent polycythemia vera
	Myelofibrosis
	Thalassemia (especially homozygous beta)
Sickle cell	Sickle cell anemia
	Sickle cell–beta thalassemia
Hemoglobin C crystalloids	Hemoglobin C trait or disease
	Sickle cell–hemoglobin C disease

Spiculated

Acanthocytes	Abetalipoproteinemia (many present) (see p. 77)
	Postsplenectomy state (few present)
	Fulminating liver disease (variable number present)
Helmet, triangle	DIC
	Severe valvular heart disease or prosthetic heart valves
	Microangiopathic hemolytic anemia
	Snakebite (see p. 655)

"Bite" cells   Hemolysis due to certain drugs with or
                                without glucose-6-PD deficiency

OSMOTIC FRAGILITY

Increased In

Hereditary spherocytic anemia (*can be ruled out if there is a normal fragility after 24-hour sterile incubation*)
Hereditary nonspherocytic hemolytic anemia
Acquired hemolytic anemia (*usually normal in paroxysmal nocturnal hemoglobinuria*)
Hemolytic disease of newborn due to ABO incompatibility
Some cases of secondary hemolytic anemia (usually normal)
After thermal injury
Symptomatic hemolytic anemia in some cases of
> Malignant lymphoma
> Leukemia
> Carcinoma
> Pregnancy
> Cirrhosis
> Infection (e.g., tuberculosis, malaria, syphilis)

Decreased In

Early infancy
Iron deficiency anemia
Thalassemia
Sickle cell anemia
Homozygous hemoglobin C disease
Nutritional megaloblastic anemia
Postsplenectomy
Liver disease
Jaundice

SERUM IRON

Increased In

Idiopathic hemochromatosis
Hemosiderosis of excessive iron intake (e.g., repeated blood transfusions, iron therapy)
Decreased formation of RBCs (e.g., thalassemia, pyridoxine-deficiency anemia, pernicious anemia in relapse)
Increased destruction of RBCs (e.g., hemolytic anemias)
Acute liver damage (degree of increase parallels the amount of hepatic necrosis); some cases of chronic liver disease
Progesteronal birth control pills
Falsely increased by hemolysis

Decreased In

Iron deficiency anemia
Normochromic (normocytic or microcytic) anemias of infection and chronic diseases (e.g., neoplasms, active collagen diseases)
Nephrosis (due to loss of iron-binding protein in urine)
Pernicious anemia at onset of remission
Falsely decreased in lipemic specimens

Diurnal variation with 6–7 A.M. specimen up to 50 µg/dl > 6–8 P.M. specimen

SERUM TOTAL IRON-BINDING CAPACITY (TIBC)

Increased In
Iron deficiency anemia
Acute and chronic blood loss
Acute liver damage
Late pregnancy

Decreased In
Hemochromatosis
Cirrhosis of the liver
Thalassemia
Anemias of infection and chronic diseases (e.g., uremia, rheumatoid
   arthritis, some neoplasms)
Nephrosis

SERUM TRANSFERRIN

Increased In
Iron deficiency anemia
Pregnancy, estrogen therapy, hyperestrogenism

Decreased In
Hypochromic microcytic anemia of chronic disease
Acute inflammation
Thermal burns
Chronic infections
Chronic diseases (e.g., various liver and kidney diseases,
   neoplasms)
Nephrosis
Malnutrition
Genetic deficiency

SERUM TRANSFERRIN SATURATION

Increased In
Hemochromatosis
Hemosiderosis
Thalassemia

Decreased In
Iron deficiency anemia
Anemias of infection and chronic diseases (e.g., uremia, rheumatoid
   arthritis, some neoplasms)

SERUM FERRITIN
Chief iron-storage protein in the body
Reflects reticuloendothelial storage of iron
Correlates with total body iron stores

Decreased In
Iron deficiency anemia. *May be decreased before anemia and other
   changes occur. No other condition causes a low level. Is more sensitive test than percent iron saturation (iron × 100 divided by TIBC)
   and/or RBC zinc protoporphyrin. Returns to normal range within
   few days after onset of oral iron therapy; failure to produce serum*

ferritin level > 50 μg/L suggests noncompliance or continued iron loss.

Increased In

Anemias other than iron deficiency (e.g., megaloblastic, hemolytic, sideroblastic, thalassemia major and minor)

Many patients with various acute and chronic liver diseases, malignancies (e.g., leukemia, Hodgkin's disease), chronic inflammation (e.g., arthritis), hyperthyroidism. *Serum ferritin may not be decreased when these conditions coexist with iron deficiency, and bone marrow stain for iron may be the only way to detect the iron deficiency.*

Iron overload (e.g., hemosiderosis, idiopathic hemochromatosis) (can be used to monitor therapeutic removal of excess storage iron). Percent saturation is more sensitive to detect early iron overload in hemochromatosis.

Indications for Serum Ferritin Measurements

Detect iron deficiency

Determine response to iron therapy

Differentiate iron deficiency from chronic disease as cause of anemia

Monitor iron status in patients with chronic renal disease with or without dialysis

Detect iron overload states and monitor rate of iron accumulation and response to therapy

Population studies of iron levels and response to iron supplement

STAINABLE IRON (HEMOSIDERIN) IN BONE MARROW

Increased In

Hemolytic anemias (decrease or absence may signify acute hemolytic crisis)

Megaloblastic anemias in relapse

Hemochromatosis and hemosiderosis

Uremia (some patients)

Chronic infection (some patients)

Chronic pancreatic insufficiency

Decreased In

Iron deficiency anemia (e.g., inadequate dietary intake, chronic bleeding, malignancy, acute blood loss)

Polycythemia vera (usually absent in polycythemia vera but usually normal or increased in secondary polycythemia)

Pernicious anemia in early phase of therapy

Collagen diseases (especially rheumatoid arthritis, systemic lupus erythematosus)

Infiltration of marrow (e.g., malignant lymphomas, metastatic carcinoma, myelofibrosis, miliary granulomas)

Uremia

Chronic infection (e.g., pulmonary tuberculosis, bronchiectasis, chronic pyelonephritis)

Miscellaneous conditions (e.g., old age, diabetes mellitus)

The absence of iron in marrow is the most reliable index of iron deficiency; its presence almost invariably rules out iron deficiency

anemia. Only individuals with decreased marrow iron are likely to benefit from iron therapy.

Marrow iron disappears before the peripheral blood changes. It rapidly disappears after hemorrhage.

One may have a normal serum iron and TIBC in iron deficiency anemia, especially if Hb is < 9 gm/dl.

EXCESSIVE IRON DEPOSITION IN DISEASES ASSOCIATED WITH IRON OVERLOAD
Idiopathic hemochromatosis
Hemochromatosis secondary to
    Increased intake (e.g., Bantu siderosis, excessive medicine ingestion)
    Anemias with increased erythropoiesis (especially thalassemia major; also thalassemia minor, some other hemoglobinopathies, paroxysmal nocturnal hemoglobinuria, "sideroachrestic" anemias, refractory anemias with hypercellular bone marrow, etc.)
    Liver injury (e.g., following portal shunt surgery)
    Atransferrinemia

SERUM CERULOPLASMIN

Decreased In
Wilson's disease (deficient or absent in early stages) (*may be normal in 2–5% of patients*)
Moderate transient deficiencies in some patients with
    Nephrosis
    Sprue
    Kwashiorkor
Normal infants

Increased In
Pregnancy
Patients taking estrogen or birth control pills
Rheumatoid arthritis (may cause green color of plasma)
Thyrotoxicosis
Cancer
Cirrhosis
Infection

Measure ceruloplasmin in any patient under age 30 with hepatitis, hemolysis, or neurologic symptoms to allow early diagnosis and treatment of Wilson's disease.

SERUM COPPER

Increased In
Anemias
    Pernicious anemia
    Megaloblastic anemia of pregnancy
    Iron deficiency anemia
    Aplastic anemia
Leukemia, acute and chronic
Infection, acute and chronic

Malignant lymphoma
Biliary cirrhosis
Hemochromatosis
Collagen diseases (including SLE, rheumatoid arthritis, acute rheumatic fever, glomerulonephritis)
Hypothyroidism
Hyperthyroidism
Frequently associated with increased C-reactive protein
Ingestion of oral contraceptives and estrogens

Decreased In

Nephrosis (ceruloplasmin lost in urine)
Wilson's disease
Acute leukemia in remission
Some iron deficiency anemias of childhood (that require copper as well as iron therapy)
Kwashiorkor

SERUM VITAMIN B$_{12}$

Increased In

Leukemia—acute and chronic myelogenous; about one-third of the cases of chronic lymphatic; some cases of monocytic. Normal in stem cell leukemia, multiple myeloma, Hodgkin's disease.
Leukocytosis
Polycythemia vera
Some cases of carcinoma (especially with liver metastases)
Liver disease (acute hepatitis, chronic hepatitis, cirrhosis, hepatic coma)

Decreased In

Inadequate absorption
    Lack of intrinsic factor
        Pernicious anemia (usually <100 ng/L; 100–150 ng/L usually signifies early vitamin B$_{12}$ deficiency even without neuropathy or macrocytosis)
        Loss of gastric mucosa (e.g., gastrectomy, cancer of stomach)
        Primary hypothyroidism. (Almost 50% of patients have serum achlorhydria with intrinsic factor failure and low vitamin B$_{12}$; rarely megaloblastic anemia develops.)
    Malabsorption (e.g., sprue, celiac disease, idiopathic steatorrhea, regional ileitis, fistulas, resection of bowel)
    Loss of ingested vitamin B$_{12}$; fish tapeworm (*Diphyllobothrium latum*) infestation
    Inadequate intake due to severe dietary restrictions
Pregnancy—progressive decrease during pregnancy (*normal serum B$_{12}$ level in megaloblastic anemia of pregnancy*)
Some drugs (e.g., anticonvulsants, oral contraceptives)
Dietary folic acid deficiency
One-third of patients with multiple myeloma

SCHILLING TEST

Differentiates pernicious anemia from other causes of vitamin B$_{12}$ deficiency (*commonplace injection of vitamin B$_{12}$ by physicians may make serum level temporarily normal for many weeks*) and can establish the functional absence of intrinsic factor before serum B_{12} deficiency or anemia is present or after patient has received vitamin B_{12} treatment.

Fasting patient is given oral ^{58}Co B_{12} and ^{57}Co B_{12} bound to intrinsic factor. In 1–2 hours, a flushing dose of 1 mg of nonradioactive B_{12} is injected IM or subcutaneously, and a 24-hour urine specimen is collected.

In pernicious anemia, the ^{58}Co in the urine is low (usually <5% of the administered dose), but the ^{57}Co B_{12} bound to intrinsic factor is normally absorbed and excreted (>10% of the administered dose).

In intestinal malabsorption, ^{57}Co and ^{58}Co in the urine are equally low (<5%). Both become normal if underlying cause is treated (e.g., administer exogenous pancreatic enzyme in patients with pancreatic insufficiency, antibiotic treatment in patients with bacterial overgrowth).

SERUM FOLIC ACID

Decreased In

Inadequate intake (e.g., megaloblastic anemia of pregnancy, megaloblastic anemia of infancy, nutritional megaloblastic anemia, some cases of liver disease)

Malabsorption (e.g., sprue, celiac disease, idiopathic steatorrhea)

Folic acid antagonist drugs (e.g., Aminopterin for treatment of leukemia, anticonvulsant drugs)

Excessive utilization due to marked cellular proliferation (e.g., hemolytic anemias, myeloproliferative diseases, carcinomas)

Serum folic acid activity <3 ng/ml is associated with a positive formiminoglutamic acid (FIGLU) test and positive hematologic findings.

Serum folic acid activity 3–6 ng/ml is associated with a variable FIGLU test and variable hematologic findings.

Serum folic acid activity >6 ng/ml is associated with a normal FIGLU test and normal hematologic findings.

Decreased serum folate (<3 ng/ml) occurs after 3 weeks of a low-folate diet (<5 μg folate/day; daily requirement is 100–200 μg/day) before other evidence of deficiency. Is not evidence of tissue deficiency. May also be decreased with phenytoin (Dilantin) therapy, high serum alcohol levels, 10% of patients with vitamin B_{12} deficiency.

3–6 months of low folate diet

Hypersegmentation of PMNs (>1% with 6 lobes); persists for 2 weeks after folate therapy. May also occur on chemotherapy and as a congenital anomaly.

Macroovalocytosis; MCV may be normal in presence of concomitant disease (e.g., iron deficiency, thalassemia minor, anemia of chronic disease). Round macrocytosis without hypersegmentation of PMNs is usually not due to folate deficiency; is common in liver disease, marked reticulocytosis, hypothyroidism, malignancy, use of antimetabolites, well-nourished alcoholics.

Megaloblastic marrow. May also occur in refractory macrocytic anemias, preleukemias, acute myelocytic leukemia, erythroleukemia but without hypersegmented PMNs and giant band cells and metamyelocytes.

Low RBC folate. Is low in 60% of patients with vitamin B_{12} deficiency so cannot be interpreted without a vitamin B_{12} level. Is increased in iron deficiency; hence, may not be reduced in combined folate and iron deficiency.
Anemia

Increased In
Period following folic acid administration
Vegetarians
Some cases of blind loop syndrome (due to folate synthesis by bacteria in intestine)
A few patients with pure vitamin B_{12} deficiency anemia

FETAL HEMOGLOBIN
(alkali denaturation method; confirmed by examination of hemoglobin bands on electrophoresis)

Normal
<2% over age 2
>50% at birth; gradual decrease to $\cong 5\%$ by age 5 months

Increased In
Various hemoglobinopathies (see Table 27-9, pp. 348–349). $\cong 50\%$ of patients with thalassemia minor have high levels of Hb F; even higher levels are found in virtually all patients with thalassemia major. In sickle cell disease, Hb F >30% protects the cell from sickling; therefore, even infants with homozygous S have few problems before age 3 months.
Hereditary persistence of fetal hemoglobin
Nonhereditary refractory normoblastic anemia (one-third of patients)
Pernicious anemia (50% of untreated patients); increases after treatment and then gradually decreases during next 6 months; some patients still have slight elevation thereafter. Minimal elevation occurs in $\cong 15\%$ of patients with other types of megaloblastic anemia.
Some patients with leukemia, especially juvenile myeloid leukemia with Hb F of 30–60%, absence of Philadelphia chromosome, rapid fatal course, more pronounced thrombocytopenia, and lower total WBC count
Multiple myeloma
Molar pregnancy
Patients with an extra D chromosome (trisomy 13–15, D_1 trisomy) or an extra G chromosome (trisomy 21, Down's syndrome, mongolism)
Acquired aplastic anemia (due to drugs, toxic chemicals, or infections, or idiopathic); returns to normal only after complete remission and therefore is reliable indicator of complete recovery. Better prognosis in patients with higher initial level.

Decreased In
A rare case of multiple chromosome abnormalities (probably C/D translocation)

SERUM HEMOGLOBIN

Slight Increase In
Sickle cell thalassemia
Hemoglobin C disease

Moderate Increase In
Sickle cell–hemoglobin C disease
Sickle cell anemia
Thalassemia major
Acquired (autoimmune) hemolytic anemia

Marked Increase In
Any rapid intravascular hemolysis

SERUM HAPTOGLOBINS

Increased In
One-third of patients with obstructive biliary disease
Conditions associated with increased ESR and alpha$_2$ globulin
  (infection; inflammation; trauma; necrosis of tissue; collagen
  diseases such as rheumatic fever, rheumatoid arthritis, and
  dermatomyositis, scurvy, amyloidosis; nephrotic syndrome; dis-
  seminated neoplasms such as Hodgkin's disease, lymphosarcoma)
Therapy with steroids or androgens
Aplastic anemia (normal to very high)
Diabetes mellitus

Decreased In
Parenchymatous liver disease (especially cirrhosis)
Hemoglobinemia (related to the duration and severity of hemolysis)
Due To
    Intravascular hemolysis (e.g., hereditary spherocytosis with
      marked hemolysis, pyruvate kinase deficiency, autoimmune
      hemolytic anemia, some transfusion reactions)
    Extravascular hemolysis (e.g., large retroperitoneal hemor-
      rhage)
    Intramedullary hemolysis (e.g., thalassemia, megaloblastic
      anemias, sideroblastic anemias)
Genetically absent in 1% of general population
Infancy

Haptoglobin determinations are useful
    When splenectomy is being considered. Patients with chronic
      hemolysis (e.g., hereditary spherocytosis, pyruvate kinase
      deficiency) should not have splenectomy when serum hapto-
      globin is >40 mg/dl if infection and inflammation have been
      ruled out. Increased haptoglobin level following splenectomy
      for these conditions indicates success of surgery; haptoglobin
      reappears at 24 hours and becomes normal in 4–6 days in
      hereditary spherocytosis treated with splenectomy.
    In diagnosis of transfusion reaction by comparison of pretrans-
      fusion and posttransfusion levels. Posttransfusion reaction

serum haptoglobin level decreases in 6–8 hours; at 24 hours it is <40 mg/dl or <40% of pretransfusion level.
In paternity studies. May aid by determination of haptoglobin phenotypes.

BONE MARROW ASPIRATION

May Be Useful In
Nonhematologic diseases
- Metastatic tumor
- Parasitic infestations (e.g., malaria, kala-azar, histoplasmosis)
- Infections (e.g., tuberculosis, brucellosis)
- Granulomas (e.g., sarcoidosis, Hodgkin's disease)
- Histiocytoses (Gaucher's disease, Niemann-Pick disease)

Hemosiderin staining of bone marrow
Hematologic diseases
- With normal myeloid-erythyroid ratio (in normal adult it is 3:1–4:1)
    - Aplastic anemia
    - Myelosclerosis
    - Multiple myeloma
    - Diseases of megakaryocytes
- With increased myeloid-erythyroid ratio
    - Most infections
    - Leukemoid reaction
    - Myeloid leukemias
    - Decreased number of nucleated red cells
- With decreased myeloid-erythyroid ratio
    - Decreased number of myeloid cells (agranulocytosis)
    - Hyperplasia of erythyroid cells
        - Megaloblastic anemias (see, e.g., pernicious anemia, sprue, steatorrhea)
        - Normoblastic anemias (see, e.g., iron deficiency anemia, hemorrhage, hemolysis, thalassemia)
        - Normoblastic hyperplasia (e.g., polycythemia vera)

NEEDLE ASPIRATION OF SPLEEN

May Be Useful In
Differential diagnosis of
- Lymphocytic leukemia (>90% lymphocytes, many of which are abnormal and have increased number of mitoses)
- Myelocytic leukemia (20–60% of cells are myelocytes)
- Myeloid metaplasia of spleen with myelofibrosis (50–60% of cells are lymphocytes that still persist)
- Chronic inflammatory splenomegaly (myelocytes are < 5% of cells)
- Leukemoid reaction and leukemia

Parasitic infestations (e.g., malaria, leishmaniasis)
Infections (e.g., tuberculosis, brucellosis)
Histiocytoses
Hodgkin's disease

See Some Causes of Splenomegaly, p. 368.

Coagulation

BLEEDING TIME
(Mielke modification of Ivy method)
Should use a standardized technique: blood pressure cuff on upper
   arm inflated to 40 mmHg; two small skin incisions are made on
   volar surface of forearm using a specially calibrated template.
Normal = 4–7 minutes.

Usually Prolonged In
Symptomatic patients with von Willebrand's disease (see p. 394),
   especially 2 hours after ingestion of 300 mg of aspirin
Thrombocytopenia
Myeloproliferative diseases
Uremia
Recent ingestion of certain anti-inflammatory drugs (e.g., aspirin,
   indomethacin, phenylbutazone)
Various thrombocytopathies and congenital platelet defects

Usually Normal In
Hemophilia
Severe hereditary hypoprothrombinemia
Severe hereditary hypofibrinogenemia
Scurvy
Other

**COAGULATION (CLOTTING) TIME (CT) ("LEE-WHITE
CLOTTING TIME")**

Prolonged In
Severe deficiency of any known plasma clotting factors except Fac-
   tors XIII (fibrin-stabilizing factor) and VII
Afibrinogenemia
Marked hyperheparinemia

Normal In
Thrombocytopenia
Deficiency of Factor VII
von Willebrand's disease
Mild coagulation defects due to any cause

This is the routine method for control of heparin therapy. It is not a
   reliable screening test for bleeding conditions because it is not
   sensitive enough to detect mild conditions but will only detect
   severe ones. Normal CT does not rule out a coagulation defect.
   There are many variables in the technique of performing the test.

TOURNIQUET TEST

Positive In
Thrombocytopenic purpuras
Nonthrombocytopenic purpuras
Thrombocytopathies
Scurvy

PROTHROMBIN TIME (PT)

Prolonged By Defect In
Factor I (fibrinogen)
Factor II (prothrombin)
Factor V (labile factor)
Factor VII (stable factor)
Factor X (Stuart-Prower factor)

Prolonged In
Inadequate vitamin K in diet
> Premature infants
> Newborn infants of vitamin K–deficient mothers (hemorrhagic disease of the newborn)

Poor fat absorption (e.g., obstructive jaundice, fistulas, sprue, steatorrhea, celiac disease, colitis, chronic diarrhea)
Severe liver damage (e.g., poisoning, hepatitis, cirrhosis)
Drugs (e.g., coumarin-type drugs for anticoagulant therapy, salicylates)
Idiopathic familial hypoprothrombinemia
Circulating anticoagulants
Hypofibrinogenemia (acquired or inherited)

The test is very useful for control of long-term oral anticoagulant therapy with coumarins.

PARTIAL THROMBOPLASTIN TIME (PTT)

Prolonged By Defect In
Factor I (fibrinogen)
Factor II (prothrombin)
Factor V (labile factor)
Factor VIII
Factor IX
Factor X (Stuart-Prower factor)
Factor XI
Factor XII (Hageman factor)

Normal In
Thrombocytopenia
Platelet dysfunction
von Willebrand's disease (may be prolonged in some patients)
Isolated defects of Factor VII

PTT is the best *single screening* test for disorders of coagulation; it is abnormal in 90% of patients with coagulation disorders when properly performed.
The test may not detect mild clotting defects (25–40% of normal levels), which seldom cause significant bleeding.

PROTHROMBIN CONSUMPTION

Impaired by any defect in phase I or phase II of blood coagulation
> Thrombocytopathies
> Thrombocytopenia
> Hypoprothrombinemia
> Hemophilias
> Circulating anticoagulants
> Other

Table 13-12. Thromboplastin Generation Test

Components	Mixtures
BaSO$_4$-adsorbed plasma (Factors V, VIII present; VII, IX, X absent) from	P P N N
Serum (VII, IX, X present; V, VII absent) from	P N P N
Washed platelets from	N N N P
Abnormality	
Normal	+ + + +
Thrombocytopenia, thrombasthenia	+ + + 0
von Willebrand's disease	0 0 + +
Factor V deficiency (severe)	0 0 + +
Factor VII deficiency	+ + + +
Factor VIII deficiency (hemophilia)	0 0 + +
Factor IX deficiency (Christmas disease)	0 + 0 +
Factor X deficiency	0 + 0 +
Factor XI (PTA) deficiency	0 + + +
Factor XII deficiency	0 + + +
Circulating anticoagulant	0 0 0 +

P = patient; N = normal control; + = thromboplastin is generated (i.e., fibrin clot forms); 0 = thromboplastin is not generated (i.e., fibrin clot does not form).

THROMBOPLASTIN GENERATION TEST (TGT)
(Table 13-12)

This test uses three components (BaSO$_4$-adsorbed plasma, serum, washed platelets) that are individually substituted in turn to mixtures of patient's blood to localize the defect in thromboplastin generation. It can be used to localize coagulation defects due to

    Factor VIII
    Factor IX (may not detect mild deficiencies)
    Factor X
    Factor V
    Factor VII
    Thrombasthenia
    Circulating anticoagulant

It may not detect disease after recent blood or plasma transfusion.

POOR CLOT RETRACTION
Various thrombocytopenias
Thrombasthenia

COAGULATION TESTS
See Table 27-18, pp. 388–390, for specific diseases and altered test results.

BLOOD VOLUME
Blood volume determination is usually done using albumin tagged with ^{125}I or ^{131}I; red cell mass may be measured by labeling RBCs with ^{51}Cr.

May Be Useful To

Determine the most appropriate blood component (whole blood, plasma, or packed cells) for replacement therapy. For example, normal total blood volume and decreased red cell mass indicate the need for packed red cell transfusion.

Evaluate the clinical course. For example, immediately after acute severe hemorrhage, the hemoglobin concentration, hematocrit value, and RBC may be normal and not indicate the severity of blood loss, whereas appropriate measurements will show decreased blood volume, plasma volume, and red cell mass. After hemorrhage, the subsequent fluid shift from extravascular to intravascular space may produce a "falling" value for hemoglobin concentration, hematocrit, and RBC and falsely suggest continuing hemorrhage.

Assess the real degree of anemia in chronic conditions in which other mechanisms may disguise or accentuate the extent of RBC deficiency. For example, anemia and hemoconcentration together may produce an apparently normal hemoglobin concentration, hematocrit reading, and RBC. Hemodilution in uremia may make the anemia more marked and apparently more severe.

Alert the surgeon who compares the preoperative and postoperative values in surgical patients to
    Unexpected blood loss
    Need for replacement of the appropriate blood component, which may vary with the surgical procedure (e.g., in thoracoplasty the blood loss may be 900 ml, representing approximately equal red cell and plasma losses; in gastrectomy the blood loss may be 1800 ml, representing an RBC loss of 400 ml and a plasma loss of 1400 ml)

Differentiate polycythemia vera (increased total blood volume, plasma volume, red cell mass) and secondary polycythemia (normal or decreased total blood volume and plasma volume) in most cases

Radioisotopes should not be administered to children or pregnant women. In the presence of active hemorrhage, the isotope is lost via the bleeding site, and a false value will be produced.

RBC UPTAKE OF RADIOACTIVE IRON (^{59}Fe)

^{59}Fe is injected intravenously, and blood samples are drawn in 3, 7, and 14 days for measurement of radioactivity.

In pure red cell anemia, the rate of uptake of ^{59}Fe is markedly decreased.

PLASMA IRON ^{59}Fe CLEARANCE

^{59}Fe is injected intravenously, and blood samples are drawn in 5, 15, 30, 60, and 120 minutes for measurement of radioactivity.

ERYTHROCYTE SURVIVAL IN HEMOLYTIC DISEASES (^{51}Cr)

Increased In

Thalassemia minor

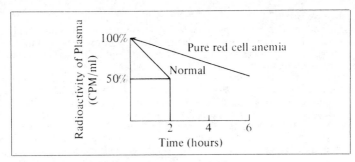

Fig. 13-4. RBC uptake of radioactive iron (^{59}Fe).

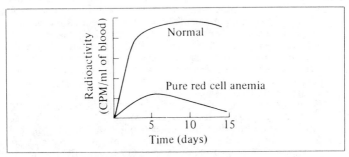

Fig. 13-5. Plasma iron (^{59}Fe) clearance.

Decreased In
Idiopathic acquired hemolytic anemia
Paroxysmal nocturnal hemoglobinuria
Association with chronic lymphatic leukemia
Association with uremia
Congenital nonspherocytic hemolytic anemia
Hereditary spherocytosis
Elliptocytosis with hemolysis
Hemoglobin C disease
Sickle cell–hemoglobin C disease
Sickle cell anemia
Pernicious anemia
Megaloblastic anemia of pregnancy
In the normal person, half of the radioactivity of plasma disappears in 1–2 hours.
In pure red cell anemia, half of the plasma radioactivity may not disappear for 7–8 hours.

Normal In
Sickle cell trait
Hemoglobin C trait
Elliptocytosis without hemolysis or anemia

Serology

"PREGNANCY" TEST
(immunoassay detection of human chorionic gonadotropin [HCG] in urine, serum, plasma)

Positive In
Pregnancy. Test becomes positive as early as 4 days after expected date of menstruation; it is > 95% reliable by 10th–14th day. HCG increases to peak at 60th–70th day, then drops progressively.

Hydatidiform mole, choriocarcinoma. Test negative 1 or more times in > 60% and negative at all times in > 20% of these patients, for whom more sensitive methods (e.g., radioimmunoassay) should be used. Quantitative titers should be performed for diagnosis and for following the clinical course of patients with these conditions.

False negative results may occur with dilute urine or in cases of missed abortion, dead fetus syndrome, ectopic pregnancy. False positive results may occur with bacterial contamination or protein or blood in urine or in patients on methadone therapy.

With the latex agglutination type of test, only urine should be used if patient has rheumatoid arthritis.

Older techniques used animals (e.g., mouse, rat, frog, toad, rabbit) for injection of specimen (usually concentrated urine) followed by examination of the ovaries after specific periods of time. These methods are more cumbersome and more subject to false positive reactions (e.g., due to high titers of pituitary gonadotropin or high titers of follicle-stimulating hormone in menopause or primary ovarian failure; aspirin, chlorpromazine, phenothiazides within 48 hours) and false negative reactions due to toxic substances in urine (e.g., drugs, such as barbiturates and salicylates, excess electrolytes, such as potassium, and bacterial contamination).

Leukocyte alkaline phosphatase scoring may also be used as a test for pregnancy (see p. 114).

See also Urinary Chorionic Gonadotropins, p. 170.

HETEROPHIL AGGLUTINATION
(agglutination of sheep RBCs by serum of patients with infectious mononucleosis)

Titers ≦ 1:56 may occur in normal persons and in patients with other illnesses.

A titer of ≧ 1:224 is presumptive evidence of infectious mononucleosis but may also be caused by recent injection of horse serum or horse immune serum. Therefore a differential absorption test should be performed using guinea pig kidney and beef cell antigens.

Guinea pig absorption will not reduce the titer in infectious mononucleosis to < 25% of the original value; most commonly the titer is not reduced by more than 1 or 2 tube dilutions. If > 90% of the agglutination is removed by guinea pig adsorption, the test is considered negative.

Beef red cell absorption takes most (90%) or all of the sheep aggluti-

Table 13-13. Sample Titers in Heterophil Agglutination

Presumptive Test	After Guinea Pig Kidney Absorption	After Beef RBC Absorption	Interpretation of Diagnosis of Infectious Mononucleosis
1:224	1:112	0	+
1:224	1:56	0	+
1:224	1:28	0	+
1:224	1:14 or less	0	−
1:224	1:56	1:56	−
1:224	0	1:112	−
1:56	1:56–1:7	0	+
1:56	1:56	1:28	−
1:28	1:28–1:7	0	+

nations and does reduce the titer in infectious mononucleosis; failure to reduce the titer is evidence against a diagnosis of infectious mononucleosis.

Heterophil agglutination may be negative when positive hematologic and clinical findings are present; a second heterophil agglutination in 1–2 weeks may become positive later in the course of the disease. The heterophil agglutination may have become negative even though some residual hematologic findings are still present.

False positive tests are very rare and occur in relatively low titers.

SEROLOGIC TESTS FOR SYPHILIS

Nontreponemal Tests
(e.g., VDRL, RPR, ART)

Simple, convenient for routine screening at local level; frequent local requirement for premarital and prenatal serology

Does not become positive until 7–10 days after appearance of chancre.

High titer ($> 1:16$) usually indicates active disease.

Low titer ($\leq 1:8$) indicates biologic false positive (BFP) test or occasionally active disease.

Falling titer indicates response to treatment.

Rising titer indicates relapse or reinfection.

Serial titers should be done to differentiate congenital syphilis from passive transfer of maternal antibodies.

May be nonreactive in early primary, late latent, and late syphilis ($\cong 25\%$ of cases)

Prozone phenomenon in 1% of patients with secondary syphilis (VDRL negative in undiluted serum in presence of high titer)

Reactive and weakly reactive tests should be confirmed with FTA-ABS.

Quantitation of VDRL should always be performed before onset of treatment. Fourfold drop in titer indicates response to therapy. Titer response is unpredictable in late and latent syphilis. Treatment of primary syphilis usually causes progressive decline to negative VDRL within 2 years. In secondary syphilis, VDRL usually remains reactive 2 years after treatment despite fall in titer. In early congenital syphilis, treatment causes VDRL to become nonreactive, but after age 2 years, titer decreases slowly but may never become nonreactive.

Treponemal Tests

TPI (treponemal pallidum immobilization)

Very specific but less sensitive than FTA-ABS

Antibodies appear later so is less sensitive in early syphilis

Technical problems in performance

Is being replaced by MHA-TP

MHA-TP (microhemagglutination)

Confirmatory test for diagnosis of syphilis; not to be used for screening or to follow efficacy of treatment

Replacing TPI because it is

More easily performed

Can be automated and quantitated

Is more sensitive

Sensitized or unsensitized cells may occasionally be reactive with sera from patients with SLE, autoimmune diseases, viral infections, leprosy, drug addicts.

Compares well with FTA-ABS in sensitivity and specificity as a confirmatory test with fewer false positive reactions but is less sensitive in early primary syphilis

FTA-ABS-IgG (fluorescent treponemal antibody absorbed)

Most sensitive and specific test

More sensitive than MHA-TP in primary syphilis; parallels findings in other stages

Test of choice for confirmation of diagnosis (e.g., BFP)

Titers not correlated with clinical activity

Remains positive indefinitely in $\cong 95\%$ of patients reflecting previous infection

May be positive in late syphilis when VDRL is negative

Not used to document adequacy of treatment, as remains positive for 2 years after adequate therapy in 80% of cases of seropositive early syphilis; thus a positive test does not separate active from inactive disease.

Beaded pattern is common in collagen diseases (e.g., SLE) but is considered negative for syphilis.

Results of these tests are positive in presence of antibodies of related treponematoses (e.g., yaws, pinta, bejel). Once antibodies develop, the tests may thereafter remain positive despite therapy.

Table 13-14. % Reactive Patients within Different Stages

Test	Primary	Secondary	Late	Latent	Presumably Normal
VDRL	78	97	77	74	0
TPI	56	94	92	94	0
MHA-TP	72	100	77	73	< 1
FTA-ABS	85	99	95	95	< 1

Table 13-15. % Reactive Patients with BFP and Diseases Other than Syphilis

Test	BFP	Diseases Other than Syphilis	Presumably Normal
MHA-TP	13.1	15.3	0.6
FTA-ABS	23.1	22.7	0.8

(This is the mechanism for one type of BFP.) If therapy is given before antibodies develop, these tests may never be positive.

BFP should be confirmed with FTA-ABS.

$\leq$ 20% of reactive screening tests may be BFP. Two-thirds of these revert to normal within 6 months; patients have usually had recent infections or immunizations. The remaining third that do not become nonreactive in 6 months have serious underlying disease (e.g., SLE) in 25% or are shown to have syphilis in 50%. BFP occurs in 20–25% of narcotics addicts. $\leq$ 10% of patients over age 70 may show BFP. > 20% of patients with BFP also show positive tests for RA, antinuclear antibodies, antithyroid antibodies, cryoglobulins, elevated serum gamma globulins.

IgM-FTA-ABS for early detection of congenital syphilis in infants is no longer recommended.

See Syphilis, pp. 579–580.

ANTISTREPTOCOCCAL ANTIBODY TITERS (ASOT)

A high or rising titer is indicative only of current or recent streptococcal infection.

 Direct diagnostic value in
  Scarlet fever
  Erysipelas
  Streptococcal pharyngitis and tonsillitis
 Indirect diagnostic value in
  Rheumatic fever
  Glomerulonephritis

Antibody appears about 2 weeks after infection; titer rises for 4–6 weeks and may remain elevated for months.

Serial determinations are most desirable since individual determinations depend on various factors (e.g., duration and severity of infection, antigenicity). Even in severe streptococcal infection, there will be an elevated ASO titer in only 70–80% of patients.

Conditions	Usual ASO Titer (Todd Unit)
Normal persons	12–166
Active rheumatic fever	500–5000
Inactive rheumatic fever	12–250
Rheumatoid arthritis	12–250
Acute glomerulonephritis	500–5000
Streptococcal upper respiratory tract infections	100–333
Collagen diseases	12–250

Other streptococcal antigens may be tested:
> Antistreptococcal hyaluronidase (ASH) (significant titer > 128)
> Antideoxyribonuclease (ADNase) (significant titer > 10)

Useful In
Detecting subclinical streptococcal infection
Differential diagnosis of joint pains of rheumatic fever and rheumatoid arthritis

LUPUS ERYTHEMATOSUS (LE) CELL TEST
LE cells occur in
> 75% of patients with systemic lupus erythematosus (SLE)
> 10% of patients with rheumatoid arthritis (only half of these have multisystem disease)
> 10% of patients with scleroderma
> 100% of patients with lupoid hepatitis
> Patients with drug-induced lupuslike syndrome (e.g., due to procainamide, hydralazine, isoniazid, various anticonvulsants)
> Some infections

The test becomes negative in $\geq$ 4–6 weeks in 60% of patients treated successfully. It is not useful as a guide to therapy; it is not correlated with the clinical picture.

The test is positive when two typical LE cells are found; it may be repeated for verification. Because of gradual changes in LE cell factor, repetition in < 3 weeks is not useful; instead a more sensitive technique or a serologic test for antinuclear or anti-DNA antibodies should be used.

Rosettes (clusters of polynuclear leukocytes surrounding an extracellular hematoxylin body) are usually found in association with LE cells.

Hematoxylin bodies (homogeneous round extracellular material) may be found in SLE, rheumatoid arthritis, multiple myeloma, cirrhosis. In SLE they may be found without LE cells in the same sample.

See Systemic Lupus Erythematosus, pp. 633–635.

ANA PROFILE IN SLE*
Native DNA in 50–60% of patients at significant titers; very specific for SLE
DNP in up to 70% of patients usually > 1:10,000 by hemagglutination
Sm antigen in 30% of patients usually 1:40–1:640 by hemagglutination; very specific for SLE
Histones in up to 60% of patients; up to 95% of drug-induced lupus
SS-A in 30–40% of patients
SS-B in 15% of patients
RNP in 30–40% of patients
PCNA in < 5% of patients

---

*Data on ANA from E. M. Tan, Antinuclear antibodies in diagnosis and management. *Hosp. Pract.*, p. 79, Jan. 1983.

ANA PROFILE IN RHEUMATOID ARTHRITIS
RANA in 85–95% of patients at 1:16 titer by immunodiffusion and 1:32–1:64 by immunofluorescence
Histones in 20% of patients

ANA PROFILE IN SJÖGREN'S SYNDROME
SS-A in 70% of patients
SS-B in 60% of patients

ANA PROFILE IN MIXED CONNECTIVE TISSUE DISEASE (MCTD)
RNP in 95–100% of patients in high titer
Other ANAs are absent.

ANA PROFILE IN SCLERODERMA AND CREST
Sci-70 in 10–20% of patients
Nucleolar antigens in 40–50% of patients at 1:100–1:1000 titer by immunofluorescence
RNP, SS-A, SS-B at low titers
Centromere antigen is only antibody in 80–90% of CREST patients at 1:100–1:1000 titer by immunofluorescence.

ANA PROFILE IN POLYMYOSITIS AND DERMATOMYOSITIS
PM-1 antigen in 50% of polymyositis and 10% of dermatomyositis patients at 1:2–1:4 titer by immunodiffusion
Other nuclear antigens including Jo-1 may be present.

DISEASE ASSOCIATIONS OF ANAs

DNP (Deoxyribonucleoprotein)
SLE: 98% sensitivity
Connective tissue diseases (CT) and chronic active hepatitis (CAH): 15–40%

sDNA (Single-Stranded DNA)
SLE: > 90% sensitivity but low specificity
CT and CAH: 20–60%

nDNA (Native/Double-Stranded DNA)
SLE: 50–60%; very specific for SLE
Drug-induced SLE: negative
RA: 3–9%
Normal persons: 1%

Sm antigen (RNase-Resistant ENA)
SLE: 30%; low sensitivity but is the most specific test for SLE (< 1% in normal persons or in other diseases)

Histones
SLE: up to 60%
Drug-induced SLE: 95%
Rheumatoid arthritis: 20%

SS-A (Anti-Ro Antibodies)
Sjögren's syndrome: 70% of primary but < 10% of secondary Sjögren's syndrome

SLE: 30–40%
Scleroderma and MCTD: low frequency in low titer

SS-B (Anti-La Antibodies)
Sjögren's syndrome: 60% of primary but < 5% of secondary Sjögren's syndrome
SLE: 15%

RNP (Ribonucleoprotein: RNase-Sensitive Extractable Nuclear Antigen)
MCTD: 95–100% at > 1:10,000 titer
SLE: 30% at lower titers
Scleroderma: low frequency in low titer

PCNA
SLE: < 5%

Sci-70
Scleroderma: 10–20%

Nucleolar Antigens
Scleroderma: 40–50%

Centromere Antigens
CREST: 80–90%

RANA
Rheumatoid arthritis: 85–95% at 1:16 titer by immunodiffusion and 1:32–1:64 by immunofluorescence

PM-1
Polymyositis: 50% at titers 1:2–1:4
Dermatomyositis: 10% at titers 1:2–1:4

TEST FOR RHEUMATOID FACTOR (RA TEST)
The test is negative in one-third of patients with definite rheumatoid arthritis. It gives useful objective evidence of rheumatoid arthritis, but a negative RA test does not rule out rheumatoid arthritis.

It is positive in 5% of rheumatoid variants (arthritis associated with psoriasis, ulcerative colitis, regional enteritis, Reiter's syndrome, juvenile rheumatoid arthritis, rheumatoid spondylitis).

It is positive in ≤ 5% of normal persons; progressive increase with age ≤ 25% of persons over age 70.

It may be positive in up to one-third of patients with SLE.

It may be positive in syphilis, chronic infections, viral infections, scleroderma, sarcoidosis, chronic liver disease, subacute bacterial endocarditis, chronic pulmonary interstitial fibrosis, etc.

Use slide test only for screening; confirm positive test with tube dilution. Significant titer is ≥ 1:80. In rheumatoid arthritis, titers are often 1:640 to 1:5120 and sometimes ≤ 1:320,000. Titers in conditions other than rheumatoid arthritis are usually < 1:80.

See Rheumatoid Arthritis, p. 320.

Table 13-16. Immunologic Tests

Antibody Test	Interpretation
Acetylcholine receptor	Result < 1 unit makes the diagnosis of myasthenia gravis unlikely; result > 5 units confirms diagnosis of myasthenia gravis. Test may be negative in ocular myasthenia, Eaton-Lambert syndrome, and treated or inactive generalized myasthenia gravis.
Antiadrenal	High titers are characteristic of autoimmune hypoadrenalism (70%); not found in Addison's disease due to tuberculosis.
Antiglomerular basement membrane	High titer strongly suggests, but negative results do not rule out, Goodpasture's syndrome.
Anti-intrinsic factor	Antibodies indicate overt or latent pernicious anemia; present in 60% of cases.
Antimitochondrial	Absence is strong evidence against primary biliary cirrhosis (PBC). High titer strongly suggests PBC. Low titers are seen frequently in other liver diseases.
Antirheumatoid arthritis nuclear antigen	Found in 87% of patients with rheumatoid arthritis and in 15% of SLE cases.
Antireticulin	Presence supports the diagnosis of gluten-sensitive enteropathy. Especially useful in childhood where + in 80% of cases.
Anti-skin, interepithelial	+ test confirms diagnosis of pemphigus and is helpful in evaluating bullous diseases. + in > 90% of pemphigus cases; absence largely excludes that diagnosis. Rise and fall of titer may indicate impending relapse or effective control of disease. High sensitivity; lower specificity.
Anti-skin, dermal-epidermal	+ in > 80% of bullous pemphigus cases. Absence does not exclude that diagnosis. Some correlation of titer and severity. Low sensitivity; high specificity.
Antistriational	Absence is strong evidence against the presence of thymoma in myasthenia gravis. May be + in some patients with myasthenia gravis alone, thymoma alone, and in drug reactions, e.g., penicillamine.
Antithyroglobulin and antithyroid microsome	Absence of both antibodies is strong evidence against autoimmune thyroiditis. Persistent thyroid microsome antibodies may be predictive of elevated TSH (72%). + thyroid antibody titers and elevated TSH are associated with risk of hypothyroidism of 5% per year, even with initially normal T-4.

Antibody Test	Interpretation
C1 esterase inhibitor	Deficiency is characteristic of hereditary angioedema. In heterozygote, C1 inhibitor is substantially decreased. Patients have low CH100, C4, and C2 during attacks.
C1q	C1q can be very low in chronic urticaria and severe combined immunodeficiency and X-linked hypogammaglobulinemia.
TSI (thyroid-stimulating immunoglobulin)	Elevated TSI occurs in > 90% of Graves' disease. Failure of TSI to fall after antithyroid therapy predicts relapse. Elevated TSI in a patient who is HLA-DR3 positive predicts poor response to antithyroid therapy and suggests need for alternate mode of treatment.

Data from *The Use and Interpretation of Tests in Medical Laboratory Immunology.* Clinical Immunology Laboratories, Inc., 1981.

VARIOUS CAUSES OF DECREASED SERUM (C3 OR HEMOLYTIC) COMPLEMENT LEVELS IN ACUTE GLOMERULONEPHRITIS

	% of Cases in Which Occurs
Acute poststreptococcal GN	*Transient (3- to 8-week) decline in C3*
Membranoproliferative GN	
Type I ("classic" MPGN)	50–80%
Type II ("dense deposit disease")	80–90%; *C3 often remains depressed*
SLE	
Focal	75%
Diffuse	90%
Subacute bacterial endocarditis	90%
Cryoglobulinemia	85%
"Shunt" nephritis	90%

NORMAL SERUM COMPLEMENT LEVELS
Renal diseases
    IgG-IgA nephropathy (Berger's disease)
    Idiopathic rapidly progressive glomerulonephritis
    Anti–glomerular basement membrane disease
    Immune-complex disease
    Negative immunofluorescence findings
Systemic diseases
    Polyarteritis nodosa
    Hypersensitivity vasculitis
    Wegener's granulomatosis
    Schönlein-Henoch purpura
    Goodpasture's syndrome
    Visceral abscess

Table 13-17. Serologic Tests in Various Rheumatoid Diseases

Disease[a]	ANA[b]	LE Clot[c]	RF[d]	Serum Complement
SLE	100 (H)	70–80	30–40	D
Rheumatoid arthritis				
Adult	50 (L–M)	5–15	80–90	N or I
Juvenile	< 5 (L–M)	< 5	15	N
Mixed connective tissue disease	100 (M–H)	20	50	N or I
Dermatomyositis	25	< 5	10–15	N
Scleroderma	25–40	< 5	33	N
Periarteritis nodosa	< 5 (L)	< 5	5–10	N or D
Sjögren's syndrome	95 (M–H)	20	75	N or D
Ankylosing spondylitis	5–10	< 5	< 5	N

Numbers = % of cases positive for each test. D = decreased; N = normal; I = increased.

[a]Normal ESR in patients with nonspecific rheumatic symptoms suggests fibromyositis rather than any of the above disorders.

[b]ANA = fluorescent antinuclear antibody; H = titer > 1:200; M–H = titer 1:100–1:200; L–M = titer 1:20–1:100; ANA titer ≧ 1:160 with suggestive pattern and clinical setting is very helpful diagnostically, but when titer is negative, other laboratory tests are not productive. Anti-DNA antibodies correlate best with a diagnosis of SLE; they are positive in < 5% of patients with other immunologic diseases. Diagnosis of SLE is barely credible without a positive ANA test.

[c]LE cells in peripheral blood clot preparation.

[d]Positive RF (rheumatoid factor) test in rheumatoid arthritis shows a significantly higher titer than in other collagen diseases, but diagnosis is primarily clinical rather than serologic. Serial titers are not helpful to follow response to treatment since antiglobulins remain at constant levels despite clinical status. Frequently positive at low to moderate titers in polyclonal hypergammaglobulinemia (e.g., SLE, sarcoidosis, cirrhosis, active viral hepatitis, some acute viral infections).

COOMBS' (ANTIGLOBULIN) TEST

Positive Direct Antiglobulin Test (DAT) (Coombs' test)
(due to immunoglobulin antibodies and/or complement present on RBC membrane)

Erythroblastosis fetalis

Most cases of autoimmune hemolytic anemia, including ≦ 15% of certain systemic diseases, especially acute and chronic leukemias, malignant lymphomas, collagen diseases. Strength of reaction may be of prognostic value in patients with lymphoproliferative disorders.

Delayed hemolytic transfusion reaction

Drug induced

   Alpha methyldopa (in 30% of patients but < 1% show hemolysis)

   L-Dopa

   Mefenamic acid

   Penicillin

Cephalosporins
Quinidine
Digitalis
Insulin

Healthy blood donors (1:4,000–1:8,000 persons)

May be *weakly* positive in renal disease, epithelial malignancies, rheumatoid arthritis, inflammatory bowel diseases

Negative in hemolytic anemias due to intrinsic defect in RBC (e.g., glucose-6-PD deficiency, hemoglobinopathies)

Negative in 2–9% of patients with hemolytic anemia (due to smaller amount of IgG bound to RBC but similar response to splenectomy or steroid therapy or to IgM, IgA, or IgD rather than IgG). This is a diagnosis of exclusion.

Positive Indirect Coombs' Test
(using patient's serum which contains antibody)

Specific antibody—usually isoimmunization from previous transfusion

"Nonspecific" autoantibody in acquired hemolytic anemia

Incompatible crossmatched blood prior to transfusion

Beware of false positive and false negative results due to poor quality test serum, not using fresh blood (must have complement), etc.

FLUORESCENT ANTIBODY TESTS

Antimitochondrial antibodies are found in ≅ 85% of patients with primary biliary cirrhosis but almost never in diffuse extrahepatic biliary obstruction; therefore, antibodies are useful in differentiating these two conditions.

May also be found in two other liver disorders associated with autoimmune disease: active chronic hepatitis and cryptogenic cirrhosis.

Smooth muscle antibodies may be found in ≅ 80% of patients with chronic active hepatitis (lupoid hepatitis) and in patients with biliary cirrhosis.

Antibodies against the cross-striations of skeletal muscle are present in 30–40% of patients with myasthenia gravis; a changing titer may indicate response to treatment or thymectomy.

COLD AUTOHEMAGGLUTINATION

Increased In

Primary atypical (virus) pneumonia (30–90% of patients). Titer of ≥ 1:14–1:224. Negative titer does not rule out primary atypical pneumonia (see pp. 599–600).

Atypical hemolytic anemia
Paroxysmal hemoglobinuria
Raynaud's disease
Cirrhosis of the liver
Trypanosomiasis
Malaria
Infectious mononucleosis
Adenovirus infections
Influenza
Psittacosis
Mumps

Measles
Scarlet fever
Rheumatic fever

COUNTERCURRENT IMMUNOELECTROPHORESIS (CIE)

Provides rapid, specific, reliable detection of certain bacterial antigens in most body fluids. Is especially valuable when patient has received antibiotics before cultures and Gram stains are taken. In contrast to cultures, results can be obtained within several hours. Is most useful for identification of *Hemophilus influenzae* type B, *Streptococcus pneumoniae, Neisseria meningitidis* (groups A and C), group B streptococcus. Virtually any fluid obtained from the patient may be used (CSF, serum, urine, joint). A negative CIE does not, however, unequivocally exclude infection due to that organism. Larger amounts of antigen correlate with more complications and poorer prognosis.

Other Organisms Detected by CIE Include

Staphylococcus aureus in pleural fluid
Listeria monocytogenes in CSF
Klebsiella pneumoniae
Pseudomonas aeruginosa
Pneumocystis carinii pneumonitis
Entamoeba histolytica, especially in liver abscess material
Cryptococcus neoformans meningitis in CSF, urine, or serum
Candida precipitin titer = 1:8 or 4 times increase in titer indicates invasive candidiasis rather than *Candida* colonization.

Cross reaction and nonspecific precipitation may occur with some antisera.

Other sensitive immunologic tests for rapid identification of specific antigens include latex agglutination, coagglutination of *Staphylococcus aureus,* immunofluorescence, enzyme-linked immunosorbent assay (ELISA).

SEROLOGIC TESTS FOR VIRAL HEPATITIS A (HAV)

Anti-HAV IgM appears at the same time as symptoms and is detectable for 3–12 weeks after symptoms subside. Presence confirms the diagnosis of recent acute infection.
Anti-HAV IgG appears after the acute period and is usually detectable for life; found in 45% of adult population. Indicates previous exposure to HAV, recovery, and immunity to type A hepatitis. Usually order anti-HAV-Total and anti-HAV IgM tests simultaneously; positive anti-HAV-Total and negative anti-HAV IgM indicates anti-HAV IgG and immunity.
Serial testing is usually not indicated.

SEROLOGIC TESTS FOR VIRAL HEPATITIS B (HBV)

Hepatitis B Surface Antigen (HB$_s$Ag)

Earliest indicator of HBV infection. Usually appears in 27–41 days (as early as 14 days). Appears 7–26 days before biochemical abnormalities. Persists during the acute illness. Usually disappears 1–13 weeks after onset of laboratory abnormalities. Is the most

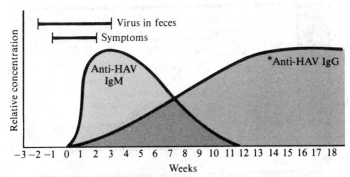

Fig. 3. Antibody markers in HAV. (Reproduced with permission of Abbott Laboratories, So. Pasadena, CA.)

reliable serologic marker of HBV infection. Titers are not of clinical value. May also be found in chronic infection.

Antibody to HB$_s$Ag

Indicates clinical recovery and immunity to HBV. May also occur after transfusion by passive transfer. Found in 80% of patients after clinical cure. Appearance may take several weeks or months after HB$_s$Ag has disappeared and after SGPT has returned to normal, causing a "serologic gap" during which time (usually 2–6 weeks) this system cannot identify patients who are recovering but may still be infectious.

In fulminant hepatitis—antibody is produced early and may coexist with low antigen titer. In chronic carriers—no antibody is present but antigen titers are very high.

Presence of antibody (without HB$_s$Ag detectable) indicates recovery from HBV infection, absence of infectivity, immunity from future HBV infection and does not need gamma globulin administration if exposed to infection; this blood can be transfused. Presence can be used to show efficiency of immunization program.

Hepatitis B "e" Antigen (HB$_e$Ag)

Indicates highly infectious state. Appears within 1 week after HB$_s$Ag; in acute cases disappears prior to disappearance of HB$_s$Ag; is found only when HB$_s$Ag is found. Occurs early in disease before biochemical changes. Usually lasts 3–6 weeks. Persistence > 10 weeks suggests progression to chronic carrier state and possible chronic hepatitis.

Antibody to HB$_e$ (Anti-HB$_e$)

Indicates decreasing infectivity, suggesting good prognosis for resolution of acute infection. Association with anti-HB$_c$ in absence of HB$_s$Ag and anti-HB$_s$ confirms recent acute infection (2–16 weeks).

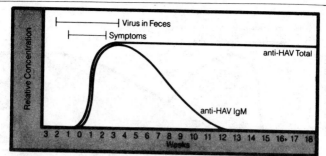

A

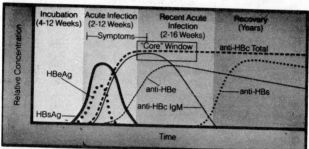

B

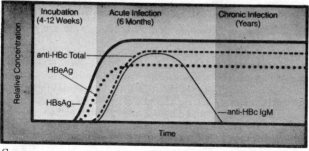

C

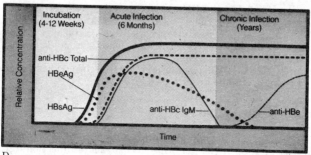

D

Table 13-18. Serologic Diagnosis of Acute Viral Hepatitis

Test			
HB$_s$Ag	Anti-HB$_c$IgM	Anti-HAV IgM	Interpretation
−	−	+	Recent HAV infection
+	+	−	Acute HBV infection
+	−	−	Early acute HBV infection or chronic HBV
−	+	−	Confirms recent HBV infection
−	−	−	Non-A, non-B hepatitis, or other causes of hepatitis (e.g., infectious mononucleosis, cytomegalovirus), or liver toxins
+	+	+	Recent HAV and simultaneous acute HBV (uncommon pattern)

If diagnosis is HBV, further testing should be done.

Antibody to Core Antigen-Total (Anti-HB$_c$-Total)

Occurs early in acute infection, 4–10 weeks after appearance of HB$_s$Ag, at same time as clinical illness; persists for years or for lifetime. With anti-HB$_c$IgM, may be the only serologic markers present after HB$_s$Ag and HB$_e$Ag have subsided but before these antibodies have appeared; this period is called the "serologic gap" or "window."

The earliest specific anti-HB$_c$ is IgM. This anti-HB$_c$IgM is found in high titer for a short time during the acute disease stage that covers the serologic window and then declines to low levels during recovery (see Fig. 13-7). Since this is the only test unique to recent infection, it can differentiate acute from chronic HBV. Is the only serologic test that can differentiate recent and remote infection with one specimen.

HEPATITIS B SURFACE ANTIGEN (HB$_s$Ag) AND BLOOD TRANSFUSIONS

Transfusion of blood containing HB$_s$Ag caused hepatitis or appearance of HB$_s$Ag in blood in > 70% of recipients; needle-stick from such blood causes hepatitis in 45% of cases. Transfusion of blood not containing HB$_s$Ag caused anicteric hepatitis in 16% of recipients and icteric hepatitis in 2%.

Screening out of blood donors with HB$_s$Ag will reduce posttransfusion hepatitis by 25–40%.

Fig. 13-7. Hepatitis serological profiles. A. Antibody response to hepatitis A. B. Hepatitis B core window identification. C, D. Hepatitis B chronic carrier profiles: no seroconversion (C); late seroconversion (D). (Reproduced with permission of Hepatitis Information Center, Abbott Laboratories, Abbott Park, IL.)

Table 13-19. Serologic Tests for Viral Hepatitis B (HBV)

	Test						
HBsAg	Anti-HBs	HBeAg	Anti-HBe	Anti-HBc-Total	Anti-HBc IgM		Interpretation
+	−	−	−	−	−		Late incubation or early acute HBV
+	−	+	−	−	−		Early acute HBV
+	−	+	−	+	+		Acute HBV
+	−	−	+	+	+		"Serologic window/gap" or acute HBV
+	−	−	−	+	+		Serologic gap
−	−	−	+	+	+		Convalescence
−	+	−	+	+	+		Early recovery
−	+	−	+	+	−		Recovery[a]
+	−	±	±	+	−		Chronic infection (chronic carrier)[a]
−	+	−	−	−	−		Old previous HBV with recovery and immunity or HBV vaccination or passive transfer antibody[b]
−	−	−	−	−	−		Not HBV infection

[a] Chronic carriers of HBV may have clinical hepatitis due to non-A, non-B hepatitis rather than HBV.
[b] Various serologic patterns may occur following blood transfusion or injection of immune (gamma) globulin by passive transfer. Anti-HBs can be found for up to 6–8 months after injection of high-titer HB immunoglobulin because of 25-day half-life.

When HB$_s$Ag carrier is discovered (e.g., in screening program), 60–80% show some evidence of hepatic damage.

Persons with a positive test for HB$_s$Ag should never be permitted to donate blood or plasma.

HB$_s$Ag is found in

Chronic persistent hepatitis	50%
Chronic active hepatitis	25%
Cirrhosis	3%
Prevalence in U.S.	0.25%
Multiple transfused patients	3.8%
Drug addicts	4.2%

NON-A, NON-B HEPATITIS

See pp. 249–250.

SEROLOGIC TESTS FOR VIRAL HEPATITIS D (HDV)

Hepatitis D (DELTA) is due to a transmissible virus that depends upon HBV for expression and replication. It consists of hepatitis D antigen (HDAg) within HB$_s$Ag. It may be found for 7–14 days in the serum during acute infection. Delta agent can cause acute or chronic hepatitis and is an important cause of severe progressive

Table 13-20. Serologic Diagnosis of HBV/HDV Hepatitis

Test				
HB$_s$Ag	Anti-HB$_c$ IgM	Anti-D IgM	Anti-D IgG	Interpretation
Transient +	+ High titer	Transient +	Transient low titer	Acute HBV and acute HDV[a]
Transient decrease due to inhibitory effect of HDV on HBV synthesis	Negative or low titers	High titer first, low titer later	Increasing titers	Acute HDV and chronic HBV[b]
May remain + in chronic HBV	Replaced by anti-HB$_c$ IgG in chronic HBV	+ correlates with HDAg in hepatocytes	High titers correlate with active infection; may remain + for years after infection resolves	Chronic HDV and chronic HBV[c]

[a]Clinically resembles acute viral hepatitis; fulminant hepatitis is rare, and progression to chronic hepatitis is unlikely. If HBV does not resolve, HDV can continue to replicate indefinitely.
[b]Clinically resembles exacerbation of chronic liver disease or of fulminant hepatitis with liver failure.
[c]Clinically resembles chronic liver disease progressing to cirrhosis.

liver disease. The course depends upon the presence of HBV infection. Simultaneous acute infection with HBV and HDV usually causes acute limited illness with additive liver damage due to each virus followed by recovery; HB_sAg and HDVAg are transient and followed by brief appearance of low titers of anti-HD. In contrast, when HDV is superimposed on chronic HBV carriers, severe chronic liver disease with persistent HDV infection often occurs; anti-HD is persistent in high titers, indicating continuing replication of HDV, and intrahepatic HDAg is present. In populations positive for HB_sAg, a high prevalence of HDV markers is found in drug addicts (43%) and hemophiliacs (25%) but not in homosexual men (< 1%); 8% of commercial blood donors and 4% of volunteer donors had such markers. Detection of HDAg is not a practical method; commercial testing for anti-HDV-total and anti-HDV-IgM will soon become available in kit form.

(ANTI-HTLV III) ANTIBODY TO HUMAN T-CELL LYMPHOTROPIC VIRUS

Antibody (anti-HTLV III) develops in all patients infected with this virus and is taken as evidence of past or present infection. Presence of antibody does not cause immunity, however, since virus can be cultured from antibody-positive individuals for years. Thus, antibody-positive persons can transmit the virus to others. Seroconversion can take up to 6 months.

Anti-HTLV III is used only for screening of blood donors and for epidemiologic studies. It is *not currently recommended for diagnosis of AIDS* (because of high false positive rate—see below) and because the medical significance of a positive test is unknown in terms of its predictive value in an asymptomatic person.

Incidence of HTLV-III antibody in donated blood is about 0.22% in the United States.

Recommended screening test uses ELISA technique, which has a sensitivity of 93–99% (assuming 100% prevalence in patients with AIDS) and a specificity of >99% (assuming 0% prevalence in random donors). Expected false positive rate is 68–89% when HTLV-III prevalence is 0.1% and 17–44% when HTLV-III prevalence is 1.0%.*

When ELISA test is positive or uncertain, the test is to be confirmed using Western blot technique, which is more specific but less sensitive and less standardized than ELISA. Second generation screening tests using viral proteins made by genetic engineering are not expected to be approved for at least another year.

A repeat positive test *requires* the donor facility to inform the donor.

Test may be positive in persons with subclinical infection who are asymptomatic, in active carriers of viral antigen, in persons with immunity, or due to false positive reactions.

Only 4–19% of people with a true positive test have developed AIDS so far.

ACQUIRED IMMUNODEFICIENCY SYNDROME (AIDS)

Due to a retrovirus, human T-cell lymphotropic virus (HTLV-III), also named lymphadenopathy-associated virus (LAV)

*Data from *J.A.M.A.* 254:1342, Sept. 13, 1985.

Criteria are diagnosed secondary disease that indicates underlying cellular immunodeficiency not due to known causes such as immunosuppressive therapy. These include:

  Kaposi's sarcoma in a patient < 60 years old

  Pneumocystis carinii pneumonia or other opportunistic infections including cytomegalovirus, herpes simplex and zoster, *Mycobacterium avium, M. intracellulare, Cryptococcus, Toxoplasma, Aspergillus,* Epstein-Barr virus, *Cryptosporidia*

In the absence of other opportunistic diseases, any of the following are considered indicative of AIDS if patient has a positive serologic or virologic test for HTLV-III:

  Disseminated histoplasmosis (not confined to lungs or lymph nodes) diagnosed by culture, histology, or antigen detection

  Isosporiasis causing diarrhea longer than 1 month diagnosed by histology or stool examination

  Bronchial or pulmonary candidiasis diagnosed by microscopy or characteristic gross plaques on bronchial mucosa but not by culture alone

  High grade pathologic type of non-Hodgkin's lymphoma (diffuse, undifferentiated) and of B-cell or unknown immunologic phenotype, diagnosed by biopsy

  Histologically confirmed Kaposi's sarcoma in patient > 60 years old

  Chronic lymphoid interstitial pneumonitis in child < 13 years old confirmed histologically

Anti-HTLV-III is positive (see p. 154).

Decreased number of T-helper lymphocytes and decreased ratio of OKT-4 (helper/inducer) to OKT-8 (suppressor-cytotoxic) T-lymphocytes

  Lymphopenia, leukopenia, anemia, and idiopathic thrombocytopenia are common.

Other immunologic abnormalities (many tests available only at special centers)

  Delayed hypersensitivity reaction

  Decreased lymphocyte blast transformation to antigens and mitogens

  Increased polyclonal B-cell activation

  Decreased monocyte/macrophage chemotaxis

Table 13-21. Distribution of Cases of AIDS by Sex and Risk Groups

	Men (%)	Women (%)	Total (%)
Homosexual/bisexual	78	0	73
IV drug user	15	56	17
Haitian	3	8	4
Hemophiliac	1	0	1
Transfusion associated	1	8	4
Heterosexual contact	0	11	1
None of these	3	17	4

Data from Centers for Disease Control. A. S. Fauci, et al., The acquired immunodeficiency syndrome: An update. *Ann. Intern. Med.* 102:800, 1985.

Diminished specific and nonspecific cytotoxicity
Production of soluble suppressor factors
Enhanced levels of an acid-labile form of alpha interferon
Increased alpha thymosin
Increased beta-2-microglobulin
Decreased free C3 receptors on RBCs
Positive Coombs' test

There is no laboratory test specific for AIDS.

CHRONIC LYMPHADENOPATHY SYNDROME

Found in homosexual men with lymphadenopathy for > 3 months
involving ≥ 2 extrainguinal sites without other illness or drug
use known to cause lymphadenopathy. If lymph node is biopsied,
shows reactive hyperplasia.

14

Urine

DETECTION OF BACTERIURIA

A colony count is significant if there are > 100,000 bacteria/cu mm under the following conditions: Periurethral area has first been thoroughly cleaned with soap; a midstream, clean-catch, first morning specimen is submitted in a sterilized container; and the specimen is refrigerated until the colony count is performed. When urine is allowed to remain at room temperature, the number of bacteria doubles every 3–45 minutes. Suprapubic sterile needle aspiration is the most reliable sampling technique, and the presence of any organisms on culture is virtually diagnostic of urinary tract infection; it is the only acceptable method in infants. A positive result in a single specimen containing gram-negative rods has an 85% chance of being the same in the next specimen (i.e., 15% error in a single specimen determination). Colony counts < 10,000/cu mm in the absence of therapy largely rule out bacteriuria. False low colony counts may occur with a high rate of urinary flow, low urine specific gravity, low urine pH, presence of antibacterial drugs, or inappropriate cultural techniques (e.g., tubercle bacilli, *Mycoplasma*, L-forms, anaerobes).

Direct microscopic examination of uncentrifuged urine unstained or gram-stained has 80–95% of the reliability of a colony count. It may show > 10% false positive results. Microscopic detection of pus cells is less sensitive and produces more false positive results than detection of bacteria. ≤50% of patients with bacteriuria may not show significant numbers of WBCs on urine microscopic examination; however, ≧10 WBCs/field is associated with bacteriuria in ≅ 90% of cases. Maximum sensitivity is obtained with microscopic detection of both bacteria and pus cells. "Sterile" pyuria (i.e., pyogenic infection is absent) may occur in renal tuberculosis, chemical inflammation, mechanical inflammation (e.g., calculi, instrumentation), early acute glomerulonephritis prior to appearance of hematuria or proteinuria, extreme dehydration, hyperchloremic renal acidosis, nonbacterial gastroenteritis and respiratory tract infections, and after administration of oral polio vaccine. Presence of both bacteria and WBCs has a higher predictive value than either alone.

Dye tests (bacterial reduction of nitrate to nitrite; tetrazolium reduction) do not detect 10–50% of infections. Bacteria show great variability in rate of dye reduction; some important bacteria do not reduce dye at all.

Decreased glucose in urine (< 2 mg/dl) in properly collected first morning urine (no food or fluid intake after 10 P.M., no urination during night) correlates well with colony count.

A culture should be performed for identification of the organism and determination of sensitivity when these screening tests are positive. If culture shows a common gram-positive saprophyte, it should be repeated because the second culture is often negative. Causative bacteria are usually enteric organisms; <10% are

Table 14-1. Sensitivity, Specificity, and Predictive Values of Tests in Predicting Bacteriuria (10^5 colonies/ml)

Test	Sensitivity (%)	Specificity (%)	Predictive Value (%) of Positive Test	Negative Test
>5 WBC/hpf	80	83	46	96
>10 WBC/hpf	63	90	53	93
Nitrite	69	90	57	94
Leukocyte esterase	71	85	47	94
Nitrite + leukocyte esterase (either positive)	86	86	54	97

gram-positive cocci (see Table 19-1, p. 192). If culture shows mixed flora, contamination should be suspected and culture should be repeated; but true mixed infections may occur after instrumentation or with chronic infection. *If* Pseudomonas *or* Proteus *is found, the patient may have an anatomic abnormality. If organism other than* Escherichia coli *is found, patient probably has chronic pyelonephritis even if this is the first clinical episode of infection.*

Bacteriuria may be found in
 10% of patients who are pregnant
 15% of patients with diabetes mellitus
 20% of patients with cystocele
 70% of patients with prostatic obstruction
 95% of patients (untreated) with an indwelling catheter for > 4 days

URINE SPECIFIC GRAVITY
Moderate increase of urine specific gravity results from
 Refrigeration of the urine
 Excretion of protein in urine
Marked increase of specific gravity results from
 Excretion of radiographic contrast medium (frequently ≦ 1.040–1.050)
 Sucrosuria (see p. 436)
None of these affect urinary osmolality.

See also urine concentration and dilution tests, pp. 103, 104.

DIFFERENTIATION OF URINARY PROTEINS
Precipitated by 5% Sulfosalicylic Acid
On boiling, precipitate remains	Albumin Globulin Pseudo–Bence Jones protein
On boiling, precipitate disappears	Bence Jones protein A "proteose"

Precipitated at 40–60°C

Resuspend precipitate in normal urine and an equal volume of 5% sulfosalicylic acid and boil:

Precipitate dissolves — Bence Jones protein
Precipitate does not dissolve — Pseudo–Bence Jones protein

CAUSES OF FALSE POSITIVE TESTS FOR PROTEINURIA
(see also p. 661)

	Dipstick	Sulfosalicylic Acid
Gross hematuria	+	+
Highly concentrated urine	+	+
Highly alkaline (pH > 8)	+	−
(e.g., urinary tract infection with urea-splitting bacteria)		
Antiseptic contamination (e.g., benzalkonium, chlorhexidine)	+	−
Phenazopyridine	+	−
Radiopaque contrast media	−	+
Tolbutamide metabolites	−	+
High levels of cephalosporin or penicillin analogs	−	+
Sulfonamide metabolites	−	+

BENCE JONES PROTEINURIA

About 20% of tests will be false positive (i.e., urine electrophoresis does not show a spike, and immunoelectrophoresis does not show a monoclonal light chain) due to
    Connective tissue disease (e.g., rheumatoid arthritis, SLE, scleroderma, polymyositis, Wegener's granulomatosis)
    Chronic renal insufficiency
    Lymphoma and leukemia
    Metastatic carcinoma of lung, GI, or GU tracts
    High doses of penicillin and aminosalicylic acid
    Presence of x-ray contrast media
80% of tests are true positive due to
    Myeloma (70% of all positive tests)
    Cryoglobulinemia
    Waldenström's macroglobulinemia
    Primary amyloidosis
    Adult Fanconi's syndrome
    Hyperparathyroidism
    Benign monoclonal gammopathy (see p. 370)

Positive test for Bence Jones proteinuria by heat test should always be confirmed by electrophoresis and immunoelectrophoresis of concentrated urine.

"Dipstick" test for albumin does not detect Bence Jones protein.

POSITIVE BENEDICT REACTIONS IN URINE

Glycosuria
  Hyperglycemia
    Endocrine (e.g., diabetes mellitus, pituitary, adrenal, thyroid disease)
    Nonendocrine (e.g., liver, CNS diseases)
    Due to administration of hormones (e.g., ACTH, corticosteroids, thyroid, epinephrine) or drugs (e.g., morphine, anesthetic drugs, tranquilizers)
  Renal tubular origin (low Tm_G)
    Renal diabetes
    Toxic renal tubular disease (e.g., due to lead, mercury, degraded tetracycline)
    Associated with defective amino acid transport
    Inflammatory renal disease (e.g., acute glomerulonephritis, nephrosis)
  Idiopathic
Melituria*
  Hereditary (e.g., galactose, fructose, pentose, lactose)
  Neonatal (e.g., physiologic lactosuria, sepsis, gastroenteritis, hepatitis)
  Lactosuria during lactation
Non-sugar-reducing substances (e.g., ascorbic acid, glucuronic acid, homogentisic acid, salicylates)

Galactosuria (in galactosemia) shows a positive urine reaction with Clinitest but negative with Clinistix and Tes-Tape.

False negative tests for glucose may occur in presence of ascorbic acid using glucose oxidase paper test (Labstix); found in > 1% of routine urine analyses in hospital.

KETONURIA

(ketone bodies—acetone, beta-hydroxybutyric acid, acetoacetic acid—appear in urine)

Occurs In
Metabolic conditions
    Diabetes mellitus
    Renal glycosuria
    Glycogen storage disease
Dietary conditions
    Starvation
    High-fat diets
Increased metabolic requirements
    Hyperthyroidism
    Fever
    Pregnancy and lactation
    Other

False positive results may occur after injection of Bromsulphalein (BSP test).

---

*5% of cases of melituria in the general population are due to renal glycosuria (incidence is 1:100,000), pentosuria (incidence is 1:50,000), essential fructosuria (incidence is 1:120,000).

SUBSTANCES AND CONDITIONS THAT MAY CAUSE ABNORMAL COLOR OF URINE

Porphyrins (see below)

Sickle cell crises produce a characteristic dark-brown color independent of volume or specific gravity that becomes darker on standing or on exposure to sunlight. Increase in total porphyrins, coproporphyrins, and uroporphyrins is routinely shown; increase in the porphyrin precursors (delta-aminolevulinic acid and porphobilinogen) is occasionally shown.

Hemoglobin (see p. 162)

Myoglobin (see pp. 162–163)

Melanin (see p. 163)

Red urine may be caused by ingestion of beets, blackberries, certain cold-drink and food dyes, certain drugs (e.g., phenolphthalein in laxatives); presence of urates and bile may also cause red urine.

Darkening of urine on standing, alkalinization, or oxygenation is nonspecific and may be due to melanogen, hemoglobin, indican, urobilinogen, porphyrins, phenols, salicylate metabolites (e.g., gentisic acid), homogentisic acid (due to alkaptonuria; *if acid pH, may not darken for hours*) and may appear in tyrosinosis. Darkened urine may follow administration of metronidazole (Flagyl).

Biliverdin: Blue or green color is due to oxidation of bilirubin in poorly preserved specimens. *Gives negative diazo tests for bilirubin (Ictotest), but oxidative tests (Harrison spot test) may still be positive.*

Methylene blue ingestion may cause a similar urine color. Blue urine occurs very rarely in *Pseudomonas* infection.

Blue diaper syndrome results from indigo blue in urine due to familial metabolic defect in tryptophan absorption associated with idiopathic hypercalcemia and nephrocalcinosis.

Red diaper syndrome is due to a nonpathogenic chromobacterium *(Serratia marcescens)* that produces a red pigment when grown aerobically at 25–30°C.

White cloud is due to excessive oxalic acid and glycolic acid in urine; occurs in oxalosis (primary hyperoxaluria).

Chyluria (see p. 163)

Lipuria (see p. 164)

URINE UROBILINOGEN

Increased In

Increased hemolysis (e.g., hemolytic anemias)

Hemorrhage into tissues (e.g., pulmonary infarction, severe bruises)

Hepatic parenchymal cell damage (e.g., cirrhosis, acute hepatitis in early and recovery stages)

Cholangitis

Decreased In

Complete biliary obstruction

PORPHYRINURIA

(due mainly to coproporphyrin)

Lead poisoning

Cirrhosis

Infectious hepatitis

Passive in newborn of mother with porphyria; lasts for several days
Porphyria

HEMATURIA

In one-third of children with gross hematuria, no cause is established.

In microscopic hematuria, number of RBCs is not related to the significance of the causative lesion.

Presence of blood clots virtually rules out glomerular origin of blood.

Phase microscopy of RBCs in urine sediment is said to show distortion of RBCs of glomerular origin but not of more distal origin.

RBC casts or hemoglobin casts indicate blood is of glomerular origin.

Some Causes of Hematuria*

	Gross	Microscopic
Kidney	15%	6%
Prostate	23%	27%
Urethra	4%	23%
Ureter	6%	1%
Bladder	40%	9%
General (e.g., GU tuberculosis, urinary tract infection)	2%	
Systemic (e.g., hemophilia, thrombocytopenia, dicumarol overdose)	1%	
Essential hematuria	8.5%	44%

HEMOGLOBINURIA

Renal threshold is 100–140 mg/dl plasma.

Infarction of kidney
Hematuria with hemolysis in urine
Intravascular hemolysis due to
>   Parasites (e.g., malaria, Oroya fever due to *Bartonella bacilliformis*)
>   Fava bean sensitivity
>   Antibodies (e.g., transfusion reactions, acquired hemolytic anemia, paroxysmal cold hemoglobinuria, paroxysmal nocturnal hemoglobinuria)
>   Hypotonicity (e.g., transurethral prostatectomy with irrigation of bladder with water)
>   Chemicals (e.g., naphthalene, sulfonamides)
>   Thermal burns injuring RBCs
>   Strenuous exercise and march hemoglobinuria

False positive (Occultest) results may occur in the presence of pus, iodides, bromides.

MYOGLOBINURIA

Renal threshold is 20 mg/dl plasma.

*Differing incidence of varying causes in the literature due to population groups studied (e.g., gross or microscopic hematuria, adult or child population, asymptomatic or symptomatic patient).

Hereditary
> Phosphorylase deficiency (McArdle syndrome)
> Metabolic defects (e.g., associated with muscular dystrophy)

Sporadic
> Ischemic (e.g., arterial occlusion) (in acute myocardial infarction, levels > 5 mg/ml occur within 1–2 hours and precede ECG and serum CK and CK-MB isoenzyme changes). Has 100% sensitivity but is less specific than CK-MB isoenzyme elevation.
> Crush syndrome
> Exertional (e.g., exercise, some cases of march hemoglobinuria, electric shock, convulsions, and seizures)
> Metabolic myoglobinuria (e.g., Haff disease, alcoholism, seasnake bite, carbon monoxide poisoning, diabetic acidosis, hypokalemia, fever and systemic infection, barbiturate poisoning)
> In ≦ 50% of patients with progressive muscle disease (e.g., dermatomyositis, polymyositis, SLE, others) in active stage

MELANOGENURIA

In some patients with malignant melanoma, when the urine is exposed to air for several hours, colorless melanogens are oxidized to melanin, and urine becomes deep brown and later black.

Is also said to occur in some patients with Addison's disease or hemochromatosis and in intestinal obstruction in blacks.

Confirmatory tests
> Ferric chloride test
> Thormählen's test
> Ehrlich's test

None of these is consistently more reliable or sensitive than observation of urine for darkening.

Melanogenuria occurs in 25% of patients with malignant melanoma; it is said to be more frequent with extensive liver metastasis. It is not useful for judging completeness of removal or early recurrence.

Beware of false positive red-brown or purple suspension due to salicylates.

CHYLURIA

Milky urine is due to chylomicrons recognized as fat globules by microscopy (this is almost entirely neutral fat). Protein is normal or low. Hematuria is common. Specific gravity is low, and reaction is acid.

A test meal of milk and cream may cause chyluria in 1–4 hours.

Chyluria is due to obstruction of the lymphochylous system, usually filariasis.

Microfilariae appear in the urine for 6 weeks after acute infection, then disappear unless endemic.

Laboratory findings are due to the pyelonephritis that is usually present.

LIPURIA
Lipids in the urine include all fractions. Double refractile (cholesterol) bodies can be seen. There is a high protein content.

May Occur In
Nephrotic syndrome
Severe diabetes mellitus
Severe eclampsia
Phosphorus poisoning
Carbon monoxide poisoning

URINE ELECTROLYTES
Usually of limited value because of the wide range of normal values (due to wide range of dietary intake of water and electrolytes), failure to obtain 24-hour excretion levels rather than random samples, or recent administration of diuretics; clinical problem may be more easily diagnosed if other tests are used.
Occasionally urinary electrolyte determination is useful in determining the cause of the problems listed in Table 14-2.

Table 14-2. Urine Electrolytes in Various Metabolic Conditions

Metabolic Problem	Cause	Urine Electrolytes*
Volume depletion	Extrarenal sodium loss	Sodium < 10 mEq/L
	Adrenal insufficiency or renal salt wasting	Sodium > 10 mEq/L
Acute oliguria	Prerenal azotemia	Sodium < 10 mEq/L
	Acute tubular necrosis	Sodium > 30 mEq/L
Hyponatremia	Severe volume depletion: edematous states	Sodium < 10 mEq/L
	Inappropriate antidiuretic hormone secretion; adrenal insufficiency; salt-wasting nephropathies	Sodium ≧ dietary intake
Hypokalemia	Extrarenal potassium loss	Potassium < 10 mEq/L
	Renal potassium loss (often associated with diuretic therapy)	Potassium > 10 mEq/L
Metabolic alkalosis	Chloride-responsive alkalosis	Chloride < 10 mEq/L
	Chloride-resistant alkalosis	Chloride parallels dietary intake

*Values based on patient not receiving diuretics.

URINE CALCIUM

Increased In

Hyperparathyroidism
Idiopathic hypercalciuria
High-calcium diet
    Excess milk intake
Immobilization (especially in children)
Lytic bone lesions
    Metastatic tumor
    Multiple myeloma
    Osteoporosis (primary or secondary to hyperthyroidism, Cushing's syndrome, acromegaly)
Excess vitamin D ingestion
Drug therapy
    Mercurial diuretics
    Ammonium chloride
Fanconi's syndrome
Renal tubular acidosis
Sarcoidosis
Glucocorticoid excess due to any cause
Rapidly progressive osteoporosis
Paget's disease

Decreased In

Hypoparathyroidism
Rickets, osteomalacia
Familial hypocalciuric (benign) hypercalcemia
Steatorrhea
Renal failure
Metastatic carcinoma of prostate

SOME CAUSES OF HYPERCALCIURIA WITHOUT HYPERCALCEMIA

Idiopathic hypercalciuria
Sarcoidosis
Glucocorticoid excess due to any cause
Hyperthyroidism
Rapidly progressive bone diseases, Paget's disease, immobilization, malignant tumors
Renal tubular acidosis
Medullary sponge kidney
Furosemide administration

URINE CREATINE

Increased In

Physiologic states
    Growing children
    Pregnancy
    Puerperium (2 weeks)
    Starvation
    Raw meat diet
Increased formation
    Myopathy
        Amyotonia congenita
        Muscular dystrophy

Poliomyelitis
Myasthenia gravis
Crush injury
Acute paroxysmal myoglobinuria
Endocrine diseases
Hyperthyroidism
Addison's disease
Cushing's syndrome
Acromegaly
Diabetes mellitus
Eunuchoidism
Therapy with ACTH, cortisone, or DOCA
Increased breakdown
Infections
Burns
Fractures
Leukemia
Disseminated lupus erythematosus

Decreased In
Hypothyroidism

FERRIC CHLORIDE TEST OF URINE
(to be used as screening test)

Positive In
Phenylketonuria (unreliable for diagnosis)
Tyrosinuria—transient elevation in newborns
Maple syrup urine disease
Alkaptonuria
Histidinemia
Tyrosinosis
Oasthouse urine disease

A positive test should always be followed by chromatography of blood and urine.

TYROSINE CRYSTALS IN URINE
Massive hepatic necrosis (acute yellow atrophy)

URINARY LACTIC DEHYDROGENASE (LDH) ACTIVITY

Increased In
Carcinoma of kidney, bladder, and prostate (high proportion of cases—useful for detection of asymptomatic lesions or screening of susceptible population groups and differential diagnosis of renal cysts)
Other renal diseases
Active glomerulonephritis, SLE with nephritis, nephrotic syndrome, acute tubular necrosis, diabetic nephrosclerosis, malignant nephrosclerosis, renal infarction
Active pyelonephritis (25% of patients), cystitis, and other inflammations
Instrumentation of the GU tract (especially cystoscopy with retrograde pyelography) (transient increase—<1 week)

Myocardial infarction and other conditions with considerably increased serum levels
Other

Normal In
Benign nephrosclerosis
Pyelonephritis (most patients)
Obstructive uropathy
Renal stones
Polycystic kidneys
Renal cysts

The test is not useful in routine screening for malignancy of kidney, renal pelvis, and bladder; increased values usually precede clinical symptoms. Increased levels suggest GU tract disease but do not indicate its nature.

Precautions: 8-hour overnight urine collection, clean voided to prevent bacterial and menstrual contamination. Refrigerate until analysis is begun. Specimen must be dialyzed to remove inhibitors in urine. Microscopic examination of urine should be performed first, since false positive LDH may occur if there are > 10 bacteria/hpf or if RBCs or hemolyzed blood is present.

URINARY EXCRETION OF FIGLU (FORMIMINOGLUTAMIC ACID)
Histidine loading is followed after 3 hours by a 5-hour urine collection.

Increased In
Folic acid deficiency occurring in
    Idiopathic steatorrhea ($\leqq 80$ mg/hour)
    Pregnancy, especially with toxemia and increased age, parity, and multiple pregnancy
    Administration of folic acid antagonists
    Malnutrition (some patients), chronic liver disease, use of anticonvulsant drugs, congenital hemolytic anemia

Normal is < 2 mg/hour or 3 mg/dl.

URINARY 5-HYDROXYINDOLEACETIC ACID (5-HIAA)
Increased in
Carcinoid syndrome
Ingestion of bananas, tomatoes, avocados, red plums, walnuts, eggplant, reserpine (Serpasil), mephenesin carbamate, phenothiazine derivatives, Lugol's solution, etc.

Normal is 2–9 mg/day; in carcinoid syndrome, 5-HIAA is > 40 mg/day, often 300–1000 mg/day.

URINARY ALDOSTERONE
Increased In
Primary and secondary aldosteronism (see pp. 488–490)

Decreased In
Hypoadrenalism
Panhypopituitarism

URINARY CATECHOLAMINES (NOREPINEPHRINE, NORMETANEPHRINE)*

Increased In
Pheochromocytoma
Neural crest tumors (neuroblastoma, ganglioneuroma, ganglioblastoma)
Progressive muscular dystrophy and myasthenia gravis (some patients)
May also be increased by vigorous exercise prior to urine collection (≤ 7 times)
False increase may be due to drugs that produce fluorescent urinary products (e.g., tetracyclines, Aldomet, epinephrine and epinephrine-like drugs, large doses of vitamin B complex; see p. 665). *Avoid such medications for 1 week before urine collection.*
Has also been reported in
    Guillain-Barré syndrome
    Acute intermittent porphyria
    Brain tumor
    Carcinoid syndrome
    Acute psychosis
    Clonidine withdrawal

URINE VANILLYLMANDELIC ACID (VMA)
VMA is the urinary metabolite of both epinephrine and norepinephrine.

Increased In
Pheochromocytoma
Neuroblastoma, ganglioneuroma, ganglioblastoma

Beware of false positive results due to certain foods (e.g., coffee, tea, chocolate, vanilla, some fruits and vegetables, especially bananas); certain drugs (e.g., vasopressor drugs); some antihypertensive drugs (e.g., methyldopa). Monoamine oxidase inhibitors may increase metanephrine and decrease VMA. See pp. 492, 665.

URINARY 17-KETOSTEROIDS (17-KS)

Increased In
Adrenocortical hyperplasia (causing Cushing's syndrome, adrenogenital syndrome)
Adrenocortical adenoma or carcinoma
Arrhenoblastoma and lutein cell tumor of ovary (if androgenic)
Interstitial cell tumor of testicle
Pituitary tumor or hyperplasia
ACTH administration
Severe stress
Third trimester of pregnancy
Testosterone administration
Nonspecific chromagens in urine

---

*Not all methods include dopamine in determination of total catecholamines.

Decreased In
Addison's disease
Panhypopituitarism
Hypothyroidism (myxedema)
Generalized wasting diseases
Nephrosis
Hypogonadism in men (castration)
Primary ovarian agenesis

Urinary 17-KS may have a daily variation of 100% in the same individual.

URINARY 17-KETOSTEROIDS BETA FRACTION

Increased In
Adrenal carcinoma

URINARY 17-KETOSTEROIDS BETA-ALPHA RATIO
Beta fraction is largely dehydroepiandrosterone; alpha fraction is
mostly androsterone and etiocholanolone.
Normal: Beta-alpha ratio is usually < 0.2.
Adrenocortical hyperplasia: Ratio is usually normal; even when it
is increased, it is rarely > 0.3.
Adrenal carcinoma: Ratio is usually 0.28–0.4. In adults, some patients may have a ratio > 0.2, but the ratio is increased in most
cases in children. The ratio is most helpful if it is > 0.4, when it is
most indicative of carcinoma.
Unless the total 17-KS is increased, the beta-alpha ratio is not
likely to be abnormal.

BLOOD AND URINARY CORTICOSTEROIDS
(17-KETOGENIC STEROIDS)

Increased In
Adrenal hyperplasia
Adrenal adenoma
Adrenal carcinoma
ACTH therapy
Stress

Decreased In
Addison's disease
Panhypopituitarism
Cessation of corticosteroid therapy
General wasting disease

URINARY PORTER-SILBER REACTION
This reaction measures only OH at C-17 and C-21 and O= at C-20;
does not measure pregnanetriol and other C-20 OH compounds.

Increased In
Cushing's syndrome (sometimes markedly)
Severe stress (e.g., eclampsia, pancreatitis [may be marked], infec-
tion, burns, surgery)
Third trimester of pregnancy (moderately)
Early pregnancy (slightly)

Severe hypertension (slightly)
Virilism (slightly)

Decreased or Normal In
Addison's disease
Hypopituitarism

Certain drugs (e.g., paraldehyde) interfere with determination.

URINARY DEHYDROISOANDROSTERONE (ALLEN BLUE TEST)

Increased In
Adrenal carcinoma

URINARY PREGNANEDIOL

Increased In
Luteal cysts of ovary
Arrhenoblastoma
Hyperadrenocorticism

Decreased In
Toxemia of pregnancy
Fetal death
Threatened abortion (some patients)
Amenorrhea

URINARY PREGNANETRIOL

Increased In
Adrenogenital syndrome (congenital adrenal hyperplasia)

URINARY ESTROGENS

Increased In
Granulosa cell tumor of ovary
Theca cell tumor of ovary
Luteoma of ovary
Interstitial cell tumor of testis
Pregnancy
Hyperadrenalism
Liver disease

Decreased In
Primary hypofunction of ovary
Secondary hypofunction of ovary

URINARY CHORIONIC GONADOTROPINS
(see also "Pregnancy" Test, p. 137)

Increased In
Normal pregnancy
Hydatidiform mole (sometimes markedly)
Chorionepithelioma (sometimes markedly)
    Of uterus
    Of testicle

Normal In
Nonpregnant state
Fetal death

URINARY PITUITARY GONADOTROPINS
This is a practical assay only for combined follicle-stimulating hormone and interstitial cell–stimulating hormone.

Increased In
Menopause
Male climacteric
Primary hypogonadism
Early hyperpituitarism

Decreased In
Secondary hypogonadism
Simmonds' disease
Late hyperpituitarism

OTHER PROCEDURES
Urine findings in various diseases (see Table 30-1, pp. 516–519)
Urine amylase (p. 271)
See also specific tests on urine in various chapters (e.g., Endocrine Diseases, Metabolic and Hereditary Diseases, Gastrointestinal Diseases, Hematologic Diseases).

Stool

OCCULT BLOOD IN STOOL
Chief usefulness is for screening for asymptomatic ulcerated lesions
of gastrointestinal tract, especially carcinoma of the colon that is
beyond the reach of routine sigmoidoscopy.

QUALITATIVE SCREENING TEST FOR STOOL FAT
Microscopic examination for neutral fat (ethyl alcohol + Sudan III)
and free fatty acids (acetic acid + Sudan III + heat) is made.
Random specimen is taken, on diet of > 60 gm of fat daily.
4 + fat in stool means excessive fecal fat loss.

Increased neutral fat
    Mineral and castor oil ingestion
    Dietetic low-calorie mayonnaise ingestion
    Rectal suppository use
    Steatorrhea

CHEMICAL DETERMINATION OF FECAL FAT
A 3-day stool sample is taken, on diet of 100 gm of fat daily.
Determination parallels but is more sensitive than triolein ^{131}I test
in chronic pancreatic disease.
Normal is < 6 gm/24 hours.
In chronic pancreatic disease, fecal fat is > 10 gm/24 hours.

UROBILINOGEN IN STOOL

Increased In
Hemolytic anemias

Decreased In
Complete biliary obstruction
Severe liver disease
Oral antibiotic therapy altering intestinal bacterial flora
Decreased hemoglobin turnover (e.g., aplastic anemia, cachexia)

MICROSCOPIC EXAMINATION OF DIARRHEAL STOOLS
FOR FECAL LEUKOCYTES
Primarily polynuclear leukocytes in
    Shigellosis
    Salmonellosis
    Invasive *Escherichia coli* colitis
    Yersinia infection
    Ulcerative colitis
Primarily mononuclear leukocytes in
    Typhoid
Leukocytes absent in
    Cholera
    Noninvasive *E. coli* diarrhea

Other bacterial toxins (e.g., *Staphylococcus, Clostridium perfringens*)

Viral diarrheas

Parasitic infestations (e.g., *Giardia lamblia, Entamoeba histolytica, Dientamoeba fragilis*)

FECAL ELECTROLYTES

	Sodium (mEq/24 hours)	Chloride (mEq/24 hours)	Potassium (mEq/24 hours)
Normal*	7.8 ± 2.0	3.2 ± 0.7	18.2 ± 2.5
Idiopathic proctocolitis	22.3	19.8	Normal
Ileostomy	30	19.0	4.1
Cholera	Increased	Increased	

*Average values for 8 healthy individuals.

OTHER PROCEDURES

Examination for ova and parasites

Trypsin digestion (see Cystic Fibrosis of Pancreas, pp. 273–274)

Microscopic examination (see Laboratory Diagnosis of Malabsorption, pp. 236–238)

Other

Gastric and Duodenal Fluids

GASTRIC ANALYSIS
1-hour basal acid

<2 mEq	Normal, gastric ulcer, or carcinoma
2–5 mEq	Normal, gastric or duodenal ulcer
>5 mEq	Duodenal ulcer
>20 mEq	Zollinger-Ellison syndrome

1-hour after stimulation (histamine or betazole hydrochloride)

0 mEq	Achlorhydria, gastritis, gastric carcinoma
1–20 mEq	Normal, gastric ulcer, or carcinoma
20–35 mEq	Duodenal ulcer
35–60 mEq	Duodenal ulcer, high normal, Zollinger-Ellison syndrome
>60 mEq	Zollinger-Ellison syndrome

Ratio of basal acid to poststimulation outputs

20%	Normal, gastric ulcer, or carcinoma
20–40%	Gastric or duodenal ulcer
40–60%	Duodenal ulcer, Zollinger-Ellison syndrome
>60%	Zollinger-Ellison syndrome

Serum gastrin levels are indicated with any of the following:
Basal acid secretion > 10 mEq/hour in patients with intact stomachs
Ratio of basal to poststimulation output > 40% in patients with intact stomachs
All patients with recurrent ulceration after surgery for duodenal ulcer
All patients with duodenal ulcer for whom elective gastric surgery is planned

When basal serum gastrin level is equivocal, serum gastrin level should be measured following stimulation with infusion of secretin or calcium.

Achlorhydria
Gastric carcinoma (50% of patients) even following histamine or betazole stimulation. Hypochlorhydria occurs in 25% of patients with gastric carcinoma; hydrochloric acid is normal in 25% of patients with gastric carcinoma; hyperchlorhydria is rare in gastric carcinoma.
Pernicious anemia (virtually all patients)

Adenomatous polyps of stomach (85% of patients)
Gastric atrophy
Achlorhydria occurs in normal persons: in 4% of children, increasing to 30% of adults over age 60.
True achlorhydria excludes duodenal ulcer.
Measure acid output after IV insulin to demonstrate adequacy of vagotomy (see below, Insulin Test Meal).
Hyperchlorhydria and hypersecretion
Duodenal ulcer
Zollinger-Ellison syndrome (see pp. 475–476). Twelve-hour night secretion shows acid of > 100 mEq/L and volume > 1500 ml. Basal secretion is > 60% of secretion caused by histamine or betazole stimulation.

Samples from upper GI tract should not be tested for blood using urine dipsticks or stool occult blood test kits (low pH may cause false negative and oral drugs false positive results).

INSULIN TEST MEAL
Aspirate gastric fluid every 15 minutes for 2 hours after IV administration of sufficient insulin (usually 15–20 units) to produce blood sugar of < 50 mg/dl.
Normal: Hypoglycemia increases free HCl.
Successful vagotomy produces achlorhydria.

PANCREOZYMIN-SECRETIN TEST
The test measures the effect of IV administration of pancreozymin and secretin on (1) volume, bicarbonate concentration, and amylase output of duodenal contents and (2) increase in serum lipase and amylase.

Normal duodenal contents
Volume: 95–235 ml/hour
Bicarbonate concentration: 74–121 mEq/L
Amylase output: 87,000–267,000 mg

This is the most sensitive and reliable test of chronic pancreatic disease; avoid gastric contamination.
Normally serum lipase and amylase do not rise above normal limits.

BENTIROMIDE
Bentiromide (Chymex), taken orally after overnight fast, is acted upon by pancreatic chymotrypsin, releasing PABA, which is readily absorbed and then excreted in urine, where it can be measured in a 6-hour sample that gauges pancreatic exocrine activity if there is normal kidney function, gastric emptying, and gut function. Is a useful initial test to rule out pancreatic disease in patients with chronic diarrhea, weight loss, or steatorrhea. Can be used in conjunction with D-xylose tolerance test for differentiation of pancreatic exocrine insufficiency from intestinal mucosal disease.

Serous Fluids (Pleural, Pericardial, and Ascitic)*

CHEMICAL TESTS

Glucose

Same value as serum in transudate

< 40 mg/dl may be found in empyema, tuberculosis, malignancy, SLE, rheumatoid arthritis. Therefore, only helpful if very low level (e.g., < 40). 0–10 mg/dl highly suspicious for rheumatoid arthritis.

Amylase

Increased in acute pancreatitis, perforated peptic ulcer, necrosis of small intestine (e.g., mesenteric vascular occlusion); sometimes in pancreatic pseudocyst; 10% of cases of metastatic cancer and esophageal rupture. Pleural fluid–serum ratio > 1 strongly favors pancreatitis. Isoenzyme studies show pancreatic type amylase in acute pancreatitis (often < 10,000 Somogyi units/dl) and pancreatic pseudocyst (often > 10,000 Somogyi units/dl); salivary type amylase is found in esophageal rupture (often > 10,000 Somogyi units/dl) and occasionally in carcinoma of ovary or salivary gland tumor (often < 10,000 Somogyi units/dl).

pH

Low pH (< 7.3) always means exudate, especially empyema, malignancy, rheumatoid pleurisy, SLE, tuberculosis, esophageal rupture. Esophageal rupture is only cause of pH close to 6.0; collagen vascular disease is only other cause of pH < 7.0.

Other Chemical Determinations

Carcinoembryonic antigen (CEA), beta$_2$-microglobulin, etc., have been suggested for diagnosis of cancer, but value not established. Also acid phosphatase in prostatic cancer, hyaluronic acid in mesothelioma, etc.

Gross Appearance

Clear, straw-colored—typical appearance of transudate

Cloudy, opaque—more cell components

Bloody—suggests malignancy, pulmonary infarct, trauma. Bloody fluid from traumatic thoracentesis should clot within several minutes, but blood present more than several hours has become defibrinated and does not form a good clot.

Chylous (milky)—usually due to trauma (e.g., auto accident, postoperative) but may be obstruction of duct (e.g., lymphoma). Pleural fluid triglyceride > 100 mg/dl or triglyceride pleural fluid > 2 times serum obtained at same time occurs only in chylous effusion (seen especially within a few hours after eating). After centrifugation, supernatant is white due to chylomicrons, which also stain with Sudan III.

Table 17-1. Comparison of "Typical"[a] Findings in Transudates and Exudates

Finding	Transudates (e.g., heart failure, nephrosis, cirrhosis)	Exudates (e.g., neoplasm, tuberculosis, infection)
Specific gravity[b]	<1.016	>1.016
Protein (gm/dl)[c]	<3.0	>3.0
Ratio pleural fluid–serum[d]	<0.5	>0.5
LDH ratio pleural fluid–serum[d] (if nonhemolyzed, nonbloody effusion)	<0.6	>0.6
Ratio pleural fluid–upper limit of normal serum LDH[d]	<2/3	>2/3
IU	<200	>200
LDH isoenzymes not shown to be useful in differentiating.		
WBC count	<1000/cu mm; mainly lymphocytes	>1000/cu mm; may be grossly purulent
RBCs	Few	Variable; few or may be grossly bloody
Glucose	Equivalent to serum	May be decreased because of bacteria or many WBCs
pH	Usually 7.4–7.5	Usually 7.35–7.45

[a] "Typical means 67–75% of patients.
[b] Long-standing transudates, however, can produce a high specific gravity.
[c] Protein level of 3.0 gm/dl misclassifies about 15% of effusions if used as only criterion.
[d] These three ratios are all found together and constitute the best differential of exudate and transudate. Any one of these three criteria has been used to define pleural fluid exudate and transudate. *All* three provide the best definition. Unequivocal criteria of transudate precludes the need for pleural biopsy in most cases unless two mechanisms are suspected (e.g., nephrotic syndrome with miliary tuberculosis, congestive heart failure with malignancy).

Purulent—infection

Foul odor—anaerobic empyema

Anchovy (dark red-brown) color—amebiasis

Turbid and greenish yellow—classic rheumatoid effusion. Turbidity may be due to lipids or increased WBCs; after centrifugation, a clear supernatant indicates WBCs as cause; white supernatant is due to chylomicrons.

Very viscous (clear or bloody)—characteristic of mesothelioma

Location

Typically left-sided—ruptured esophagus, acute pancreatitis. Pericardial disease is left-sided or bilateral; rarely exclusively right-sided. Typically right-sided or bilateral—congestive heart failure (if only on left, consider that right pleural space may be obliterated or patient has another process, e.g., pulmonary infarction).

Cell Count
(performed in counting chamber)

5000–6000 RBCs/cu mm needed to give red appearance to pleural fluid

Can be caused by needle trauma producing 2 ml of blood in 1000 ml of pleural fluid

> 100,000/cu mm is grossly hemorrhagic and suggests malignancy, pulmonary infarct, or trauma but occasionally seen in congestive heart failure alone

Empyema—WBCs usually > 50,000/cu mm

Smears

Wright's stain differentiates PMNs from mononuclear cells; cannot differentiate lymphocytes from monocytes.

Gram stain for early diagnosis

Acid-fast smears are positive in 20% of tuberculous pleurisy.

Mononuclear cells predominate in transudates and chronic exudates (lymphoma, carcinoma, tuberculosis, rheumatoid, uremia).

PMNs predominate in early inflammatory effusions (e.g., pneumonia, pulmonary infarct, pancreatitis, subphrenic abscess). After several days, mesothelial cells, macrophages, lymphocytes may predominate.

Large mesothelial cells > 5% are said to rule out tuberculosis (must differ from macrophages).

Eosinophilia in pleural fluid (>10% of total leukocytes) may mean blood or air in pleural space (e.g., repeated thoracenteses, pneumothorax, traumatic hemothorax) but is not diagnostically significant. It also said to be a sign of pulmonary infarction, polyarteritis nodosa, parasitic or fungal disease.

Cytology

Positive in 60% of malignancies on first tap, 80% by third tap. Therefore should repeat taps with cytologic examinations if cancer is suspected. Combined with needle biopsy, is positive in 90% of cases.

Needle Biopsy
(closed chest) (whenever cannot diagnose otherwise)

Positive for tumor in one-half of cases of malignancy

Positive for tubercles in two-thirds of cases on first biopsy with increased yield on second and third biopsies; therefore repeat biopsy if suspicious clinically. Can also culture biopsy material for tuberculosis.

Sputum

Smears and cultures for infections (e.g., pneumonias, tuberculosis, fungi)—must be adequate samples of sputum (i.e., not just saliva)
>   Cytology for carcinoma
>> Positive in 40% on first sample
>> Positive in 70% with 3 samples
>> Positive in 85% with 5 samples
>> False positive in < 1%
>   In bronchogenic carcinoma
>> Positive in 67–85% of squamous cell carcinoma
>> Positive in 64–70% of small-cell undifferentiated carcinoma
>> Positive in 55% of adenocarcinoma

Scalene Lymph Node Biopsy
(biopsy of scalene fat pad even without palpable lymph nodes)

Positive in 15% of bronchogenic carcinoma. May also be positive in various granulomatous diseases (e.g., tuberculosis, sarcoidosis, pneumoconiosis).

Bronchoscopy

For biopsy of endobronchial tumor in which obstruction may cause secondary pneumonia with effusion but still be resectable carcinoma

To obtain bronchial washings for malignant cells

To diagnose nonresectable tumors that should be treated with irradiation (e.g., oat cell carcinoma, Hodgkin's disease)

PLEURAL FLUID FINDINGS IN VARIOUS CLINICAL CONDITIONS

Tuberculous effusion—has high protein content and lymphocytes; acid-fast smears are positive in < 20%, and culture is positive in ≅ 67% of cases; culture combined with histologic examination establishes the diagnosis in 95% of cases. Needle biopsy can be done without hesitation. Tuberculosis often presents as effusion, especially in youth; pulmonary disease may be absent; risk of active pulmonary tuberculosis within 5 years is 60%.

Malignancy—can cause effusion by metastasis to pleura, causing exudate-type of fluid, or by metastasis to lymph nodes obstructing lymph drainage, giving transudate-type fluid. Low pH and glucose indicate a poor prognosis with short survival time. "Characteristic" effusion is moderate to massive, frequently hemorrhagic, moderate WBC count with predominance of mononuclear cells. Most common sources are lung, breast, stomach, ovary. Combined cytology and pleural biopsy give positive results in 90%. Pleural or ascitic effusion occurs in 20–30% of patients with malignant lymphoma; cytology establishes the diagnosis in approximately 50% of patients.

Rheumatoid effusion—"classic picture" is cloudy greenish fluid with 0 glucose level. Is < 30 mg/dl in 25% of patients. Rheumatoid arthritis cells may be found. Rheumatoid factor may also be found in other effusions (e.g., tuberculosis, cancer, bacterial pneumonia). Needle biopsy usually shows nonspecific chronic inflammation but may show characteristic rheumatoid nodule microscopically. *Nonpurulent, nonmalignant effusions not due to tuberculosis or rheumatoid arthritis almost always have glucose level > 70 mg/dl.*

Pulmonary infarct effusion—small volume, serous or bloody, predominance of PMNs, may show many mesothelial cells; this "typical pattern" seen in only 25% of patients. Effusion occurs in 50% of patients with pulmonary infarct; is bloody in one-third to two-thirds of patients; often no characteristic diagnostic findings occur.

Congestive heart failure—effusion is predominantly right-sided or bilateral. If unilateral or left-sided in patients with congestive heart failure, rule out pulmonary infarct.

Pneumonias—parapneumonic effusion is exudate type of effusion occurring in course of pneumonia.

Empyema—usually WBCs > 50,000/cu mm, low glucose, and low pH. Suspect clinically when effusion develops during adequate antibiotic therapy.

Aerobic gram-negative organisms *(Klebsiella, E. coli, Pseudomonas)* are associated with a high incidence of exudates (with 5000–40,000/cu mm, high protein, normal glucose, normal pH) and resolve with antibiotic therapy. Nonpurulent fluid with positive Gram stain or positive blood culture or low pH suggests that effusion will become or behave like empyema.

Streptococcus pneumoniae causes parapneumonic effusions in 50% of cases, especially with positive blood culture.

Staphylococcus aureus has effusion in 90% of infants, 50% of adults; usually widespread bronchopneumonia.

Streptococcus pyogenes usually has massive effusion, greenish color.

If pleural effusion occurs early in course of bacterial pneumonia, suspect Streptococcus *or* Staphylococcus, *since it takes 4–5 days to develop effusion in pneumococcus pneumonia.*

In parapneumonic effusions, pH < 7.0 and glucose < 40 mg/dl indicate need for closed chest tube drainage even without grossly purulent fluid. pH of 7.0–7.2 is questionable indication and should be repeated in 24 hours, but tube drainage is favored if pleural fluid LDH > 1000 IU/L. Tube drainage is also indicated if grossly purulent fluid or positive Gram stain or culture. Normal pH is alkaline and may approach 7.6. In *Proteus mirabilis* empyema, high ammonia level may cause a pH $\cong$ 8.0.

Viral or mycoplasma pneumonia—pleural effusions develop in 20% of cases

Legionnaires' disease—pleural effusion occurs in up to one-half of patients; may be bilateral.

Blood specimens should always be drawn at the same time as serous fluid for determination of glucose, protein, LDH, amylase, pH, etc. Pleural fluid for pH should be collected in the same way as arterial blood samples (i.e., heparinized syringe, maintained anaerobically on ice, analyzed promptly). Pleural fluid pH should be at least 0.15 greater than arterial blood pH.

SOME CAUSES OF PLEURAL EFFUSION

Transudate

Congestive heart failure (causes 15% of cases)
Cirrhosis with ascites (pleural effusion in $\cong$ 5% of these cases)
Nephrotic syndrome
Early (acute) atelectasis
Pulmonary embolism (some cases)
Superior vena cava obstruction
Hypoalbuminemia
Peritoneal dialysis
Early mediastinal malignancy
Misplaced subclavian catheter
Myxedema (rare cause)
Meigs' syndrome*

Exudate

Infection (causes 25% of cases)
    Parapneumonic effusion (empyema)
    Tuberculous empyema
    Fungal effusion (*Coccidioides, Cryptococcus, Histoplasma, Blastomyces, Aspergillus;* in immunocompromised host, *Aspergillus, Candida, Mucor*)
    Viral, mycoplasmal, rickettsial
    Parasitic (amoeba, hydatid cyst, filaria)
Pulmonary embolism/infarction
Neoplasms (metastatic carcinoma, lymphoma, leukemia, mesothelioma, pleural endometriosis) (causes 42% of cases)
Trauma (penetrating or blunt)
    Hemothorax
    Chylothorax
    Empyema
    Associated with rupture of diaphragm
Immunologic mechanisms
    Rheumatoid arthritis
    SLE
    Following myocardial infarction or cardiac surgery
    Vasculitis
    Hepatitis
    Sarcoidosis (rare cause)
    Familial recurrent polyserositis
    Drug reaction (e.g., nitrofurantoin hypersensitivity, methysergide)
Chemical mechanisms
    Uremic
    Pancreatic (pleural effusion occurs in $\cong$ 10% of these cases)
    Esophageal rupture
    Subphrenic abscess
Lymphatic abnormality
    Irradiation
    Milroy's disease
    Yellow nail syndrome
Injury
    Asbestosis

*Protein and specific gravity are often at the transudate-exudate border.

Table 17-2. Pleural Fluid Findings in Various Diseases

Disease	Appearance	Total WBC (1000/cu mm)	Predominant Type WBC	Total RBC (1000/cu mm)	pH	Glucose mg/dl	Glucose PF/S
Transudates							
Congestive heart failure	Clear, straw	<1	M	0–1	>7.4	>60	1
Cirrhosis	Clear, straw	<0.5	M	<1	>7.4	>60	1
Pulmonary embolus: atelectasis	Clear, straw	5–15	M	<5	>7.3	>60	1
Exudates							
Pulmonary embolus: infarction	Turbid to hemorrhagic	5–15	P	Bloody	>7.3	>60	1
Pneumonia	Turbid	5–40	P	<5	≧7.3	>60	1

Empyema	Turbid to purulent	25–100	P	<5	5.50–7.29	<60	<0.5
Tuberculosis	Straw; serosanguineous in 15%	5–10	M	<10	<7.3 in 20%	30–60 in 20%	1
Carcinoma	Straw to turbid to bloody	<10	M	1–>100	<7.3 in 30%	<60 in 30%	1
Rheumatoid arthritis effusion	Turbid or green or yellow	1–20	P in acute M in chronic	<1	<7.3; usually $\cong$ 7.0	<30 in 95%	
SLE	Straw to turbid		P in acute M in chronic		<7.3 in 30%	<60 in 30%	
Rupture of esophagus	Purulent		P		6.0	N or D	
Pancreatitis	Serous to turbid to serosanguineous	5–20	P	1–10	>7.3	>60	1

Table 17-2 (continued)

Disease	Protein PF/S	LDH PF/S	LDH IU/L	Amylase PF/S	Comment
Transudates					
Congestive heart failure	<0.5	<0.6	<200	≤1	
Cirrhosis	<0.5	<0.6	<200	≤1	Occurs in ≅ 5% of cirrhotics with clinical ascites.
Pulmonary embolus: atelectasis	<0.5	<0.6		≤1	
Exudates					
Pulmonary embolus: infarction	>0.5	>0.6		≤1	
Pneumonia	>0.5	>0.6		≤1	Occurs in 50% of bacterial pneumonias and Legionnaires' disease, 10% of viral and mycoplasma/pneumonias.

Empyema	>0.5	>0.6	May be >1000/L	≤1	Most commonly due to anaerobic bacteria, _S. aureus_, gram-negative aerobic bacteria.
Tuberculosis	>0.5	>0.6		≤1	AFB stain + in 15–20% & culture of fluid + in 30% of cases. Biopsy for histologic exam & culture of pleura are diagnostic in 75–85% of cases.
Carcinoma	>0.5	>0.6		≤1	Cytology of fluid plus biopsy are diagnostic in about 90% of cases.
Rheumatoid arthritis effusion	>0.5	>0.6	Often >1000/L	≤1	Biopsy is useful, especially in men with rheumatoid nodules & high RF titer.
SLE	>0.5	>0.6		>2	PF may show LE cells, antinuclear antibody titer, and low complement. Usually found only when lupus is active.
Rupture of esophagus	>0.5	>0.6		Salivary type	
Pancreatitis	>0.5	>0.6		>2	Occurs in 15% of acute cases. Left-sided in 70% of cases.

PF/S = ratio of pleural fluid to serum; M = mononuclear cells; P = polynuclear leukocytes; N = normal; D = decreased.

Altered pleural mechanics
    Late (chronic) atelectasis
    Trapped lung
Unknown ($\cong 15$ of all exudates)

*Cirrhosis, pulmonary infarct, trauma, and connective tissue diseases
compose $\cong 9\%$ of all cases.*

COMPARISON OF PLEURAL FLUID IN RHEUMATOID ARTHRITIS AND SLE

Test	Rheumatoid Arthritis	SLE
pH	$\leqq 7.2$	> 7.2
Glucose	< 30 mg/dl	Normal
LDH	> 700 IU/L	< 700 IU/L
Rheumatoid factor (RF)	Strongly +	− or weakly +
Pleural fluid–serum RF	> 1.0	< 1.0
Lupus cells	Absent	May be present
Rheumatoid arthritis cells (ragocytes)	May be present	Absent
Epithelioid cells	Present	Absent
C4	Markedly decreased ($< 10 \times 10^6$ gm/gm of protein)	Moderately decreased ($< 30 \times 10^6$ gm/gm of protein)
C1q-binding assay	Moderately +	Weakly +
Pleural fluid–serum C1q-binding	> 1.0	< 1.0

ASCITES

Chronic liver disease: Total protein is often not useful because of high protein content in 12–19% of these ascites as well as changes due to albumin infusion and diuretic therapies. Total WBCs are usually < 300/cu mm (one-half of cases) and neutrophils $< 25\%$ (two-thirds of cases).

Infected ascites: WBCs > 500/cu mm and neutrophils $> 50\%$ are presumptive of bacterial peritonitis. Gram stain is positive in 25% of cases. Acid-fast stains and culture establish the diagnosis of tuberculosis in only 25–50% of cases.

Pancreatic disease: Ascitic fluid amylase $>$ serum amylase is virtually specific for pancreatic disease, but both levels are normal in 10% of cases. Methemalbumin in serum or ascitic fluid and total protein > 4.5 gm/dl indicate poor prognosis.

Chylous ascites: 60% of cases are due to lymphoma or carcinoma. Ascitic fluid triglyceride is 2–8 times serum level. In pediatric patients, is often due to congenital lymphatic defects. (See also p. 243.)

Sweat

SWEAT ELECTROLYTES

Increased In
Cystic fibrosis of pancreas

Sweat Value (mEq/L)

	Chloride	Sodium	Potassium
Cystic fibrosis	50–120 (97)* 96% of cases are < 30	50–140 (103)	10–37 (15)
Normal	4–60 (18)	0–40 (24) Child 0–70 (40) Adult	6–25 (9)

Untreated adrenal insufficiency (Addison's disease)
Some unusual disease syndromes (e.g., glucose 6-PD deficiency, glycogen storage disease, vasopressin-resistant diabetes insipidus)

Sweat sodium is reduced by administration of mineralocorticoids (e.g., aldosterone) by ≅ 50% in normal subjects and 10–20% in cystic fibrosis patients whose final sodium concentration remains abnormally high.

Recommended sweat testing is pilocarpine iontophoresis performed in duplicate on separate days on samples of > 100 mg of sweat.

SWEAT COLOR
Brown—ochronosis
Red—rifampin overdose
Blue—occupational exposure to copper
Blue-black—idiopathic chromhidrosis (in black persons, axillary chromhidrosis may also be yellow, blue-green)

*Mean values are in parentheses.

Bacteria Commonly Cultured from Various Sites

Table 19-1. Most Common Bacteria Isolated in Cultures from Various Sites

Site	Normal Flora	Pathogens
External ear	*Staphylococcus epidermidis* Alpha-hemolytic streptococci Coliform bacilli Aerobic corynebacteria *Corynebacterium acnes* *Candida* species *Bacillus* species	*Pseudomonas* species *Staphylococcus aureus* Coliform bacilli Alpha-hemolytic streptococci *Proteus* species *Streptococcus (Diplococcus) pneumoniae* *Corynebacterium diphtheriae*
Middle ear	Sterile	<u>Acute Otitis Media</u> *Haemophilus influenzae* Beta-hemolytic streptococci Pneumococci <u>Chronic Otitis Media</u> *Staphylococcus aureus* *Proteus* species *Pseudomonas* species Other gram-negative bacilli Alpha-hemolytic streptococci Beta-hemolytic streptococci
Nasal passages	*Staphylococcus epidermidis* *Staphylococcus aureus* Diphtheroids Pneumococci Alpha-hemolytic streptococci Nonpathogenic *Neisseria* species Aerobic corynebacteria	<u>Acute Sinusitis</u> *Staphylococcus aureus* Pneumococci *Klebsiella-Enterobacter* species Alpha-hemolytic streptococci Beta-hemolytic streptococci <u>Chronic Sinusitis</u> *Staphylococcus aureus* Alpha-hemolytic streptococci Pneumococci

Table 19-1 (continued)

Site	Normal Flora	Pathogens
		Beta-hemolytic strep- tococci
		Mucor, Aspergillus species (especially in diabetics)
Pharynx and ton- sils	Alpha-hemolytic strep- tococci	Beta-hemolytic strep- tococci
	Neisseria species	*Corynebacterium diphtheriae*
	Staphylococcus epider- midis	*Bordetella pertussis*
	Staphylococcus aureus (small numbers)	*Neisseria meningitidis*
	Pneumococci	*Haemophilus influenzae* Group B
	Nonhemolytic (gamma) streptococci	*Staphylococcus aureus*
	Diphtheroids	*Candida albicans*
	Coliforms	
	Beta-hemolytic strep- tococci (not Group A)	
	Actinomyces israelii	
	Haemophilus species	
	Marked predominance of one organism may be clinically significant even if it is a normal inhabitant.	
Gastrointes- tinal tract		
Mouth	Alpha-hemolytic strep- tococci	*Candida albicans*
	Enterococci	*Borrelia vincentii* with *Fusobacterium fusiforme*
	Lactobacilli	
	Staphylococci	
	Fusobacteria	
	Bacteroides species	
	Diphtheroids	
Stomach	Sterile	
Small intes- tine	Sterile in one-third	
	Scant bacteria in others	
	Escherichia coli	
	Klebsiella-Enterobacter	
	Enterococci	
	Alpha-hemolytic strep- tococci	
	Staphylococcus epider- midis	
	Diphtheroids	

Table 19-1 (continued)

Site	Normal Flora	Pathogens
Colon	Abundant bacteria *Bacteroides* species *Escherichia coli* *Klebsiella-Enterobacter* Paracolons *Proteus* species Enterococci (Group D streptococci) Yeasts	Enteropathogenic *Escherichia coli* *Candida albicans* Various amebae and parasites *Aeromonas* species *Salmonella* species *Shigella* species *Campylobacter (Vibrio)* *fetus* *Yersinia enterocolitica* *Staphylococcus aureus* *Clostridium difficile* *Vibrio cholerae* *Vibrio parahaemolyticus* *Treponema pallidum* (anus) *Neisseria gonorrhoeae* (anus)
Gallbladder	Sterile	*Escherichia coli* Enterococci *Klebsiella-Enterobacter-* *Serratia* Occasionally Coliforms *Proteus* species *Pseudomonas* species *Salmonella* species
Blood	Sterile	Staphylococci (coagulase positive and negative) Coliform and related bacilli Alpha- and beta-hemo- lytic streptococci Pneumococci Enterococci *Haemophilus influenzae* *Clostridium perfringens* *Pseudomonas* species *Proteus* species *Bacteroides* and related anaerobes *Neisseria meningitidis* *Brucella* species *Pasteurella tularensis* *Listeria monocytogenes* *Achromobacter (Herellea)* species *Streptobacillus monilifor-* *mis* *Leptospira* species

Table 19-1 (continued)

Site	Normal Flora	Pathogens
		Vibrio fetus
		Opportunistic fungi
		Candida species
		Nocardia species
		Blastomyces dermatitidis
		Histoplasma capsulatum
		Salmonella species
Eye	Usually sterile Occasionally small numbers of diphtheroids and coagulase-negative staphylococci	*Staphylococcus aureus* *Haemophilus* species *Streptococcus (Diplococcus) pneumoniae* *Neisseria gonorrhoeae* Alpha- and beta-hemolytic streptococci *Achromobacter (Herellea)* species Coliform bacilli *Pseudomonas aeruginosa* Other enteric bacilli Morax-Axenfeld bacillus *Bacillus subtilis* (occasionally) *Chlamydia* species
Spinal fluid	Sterile	*Haemophilus influenzae* *Neisseria meningitidis* *Streptococcus pneumoniae* *Mycobacterium tuberculosis* Staphylococci, streptococci *Cryptococcus neoformans* Coliform bacilli *Pseudomonas* and *Proteus* species *Bacteroides* species
Urethra, male	*Staphylococcus aureus* *Staphylococcus epidermidis* Enterococci Diphtheroids *Achromobacter wolffi (Mima)* *Haemophilus vaginalis* *Bacillus subtilis*	*Neisseria gonorrhoeae* *Chlamydia* species Enterococci Beta-hemolytic streptococci (usually Group B) Anaerobic and microaerophilic streptococci *Bacteroides* species *Escherichia* and *Klebsiella-Enterobacter* *Staphylococcus aureus*

Table 19-1 (continued)

Site	Normal Flora	Pathogens
Urethra, female, and vagina	*Lactobacillus* (large numbers) Coli-aerogenes Staphylococci Streptococci (aerobic and anaerobic) *Candida albicans* *Bacteroides* species *Achromobacter wolffi (Mima)* *Haemophilus vaginalis*	Yeasts and *Candida albicans* *Clostridium perfringens* *Listeria monocytogenes* *Haemophilus vaginalis* *Trichomonas vaginalis* *Neisseria gonorrhoeae* (See also entries under Urethra, male) *Chlamydia* species
Prostate	Sterile	*Streptococcus faecalis* *Staphylococcus epidermidis* *Escherichia coli* *Proteus mirabilis* *Pseudomonas* species *Klebsiella* species
Uterus		Anaerobic and microanaerophilic streptococci (alpha, beta, and gamma types) *Bacteroides* species Enterococci Beta-hemolytic streptococci (usually Group B) Staphylococci *Proteus* species *Clostridium perfringens* *Escherichia coli* and *Klebsiella-Enterobacter-Serratia* *Listeria monocytogenes*
Urine	Staphylococci, coagulase-negative Diphtheroids Coliform bacilli Enterococci *Proteus* species Lactobacilli Alpha- and beta-hemolytic streptococci	*Escherichia coli* and *Klebsiella-Enterobacter-Serratia* *Proteus* species *Pseudomonas* species Enterococci Staphylococci, coagulase-positive and negative *Alcaligenes* species *Achromobacter (Herellea)* species *Candida albicans* Beta-hemolytic streptococci *Neisseria gonorrhoeae* *Mycobacterium tuberculosis* *Salmonella* and *Shigella* species

Table 19-1 (continued)

Site	Normal Flora	Pathogens
Wound		*Staphylococcus aureus* *Streptococcus pyogenes* Coliform bacilli *Bacteroides* species; other gram-negative rods *Proteus* species *Pseudomonas* species *Clostridium* species Enterococci *Achromobacter (Herellea)* species *Serratia* species
Pleura	Sterile	*Staphylococcus aureus* *Streptococcus pneumoniae* *Haemophilus influenzae* *Mycobacterium tuberculosis* Anaerobic streptococci *Streptococcus pyogenes* *Actinomyces* species *Nocardia* species Fungi
Peritoneum	Sterile	*Escherichia coli* Enterococci *Streptococcus pneumoniae* *Bacteroides* species; other gram-negative rods Anaerobic streptococci *Clostridium* species
Bones	Sterile	*Staphylococcus aureus* *Haemophilus influenzae* Beta-hemolytic streptococci *Neisseria gonorrhoeae* *Mycobacterium tuberculosis* *Salmonella* species in sickle cell disease
Joints (see also pp. 318–319	Sterile	*Staphylococcus aureus* Beta-hemolytic streptococci Pneumococci Gram-negative pathogens in newborns *Salmonella* species in sickle cell disease

Nuclear Sex Chromatin and Karyotyping

NUCLEAR SEXING

Epithelial cells from buccal smear (or vaginal smear, etc.) are stained with cresyl violet and examined microscopically.

A dense body (Barr body) on the nuclear membrane represents one of the X chromosomes and occurs in 30–60% of female somatic cells. The maximum number of Barr bodies is 1 less than the number of X chromosomes.

If there are < 10% of the cells containing Barr bodies in a patient with female genitalia, karyotyping should be done to delineate probable chromosomal abnormalities.

A normal count does not rule out chromosomal abnormalities.
  2 Barr bodies may be found in
     47 XXX female
     48 XXXY male (Klinefelter's syndrome)
     49 XXXYY male (Klinefelter's syndrome)
3 Barr bodies may be found in
     49 XXXXY male (Klinefelter's syndrome)

EVALUATION OF SEX CHROMOSOME IN LEUKOCYTES

Presence of a "drumstick" nuclear appendage in $\cong$ 3% of leukocytes in normal females indicates the presence of 2 X chromosomes in the karyotype. It is not found in males.

It is absent in the XO type of Turner's syndrome.

There is a lower incidence of drumsticks in Klinefelter's syndrome (XXY) as opposed to the extra Barr body. *(Mean lobe counts of neutrophils are also decreased.)*

Incidence of drumsticks is decreased and mean lobe counts are lower also in mongolism.

Double drumsticks are exceedingly rare and diagnostically impractical.

SOME INDICATIONS FOR CHROMOSOME ANALYSIS (KARYOTYPING)

Suspected Autosomal Syndromes
Down's (mongolism)
E_{18} trisomy
D_{13} trisomy
Cri du chat syndrome

Suspected Sex-Chromosome Syndromes
Klinefelter's XXY, XXXY
Turner's XO
"Superfemale" XXX, XXXX
"Supermale" XYY
"Funny-looking kid" syndromes, especially with multiple anomalies including mental retardation and low birth weight

Table 20-1. Chromosome Number and Karyotype in Various Clinical Conditions

Clinical Condition	Chromosome Number and Karyotype	Incidence
Normal male	46 XY	
Normal female	46 XX	
Turner's syndrome	45 XO	1 in 3000 live female births
	46 XX	Rare
	Mosaics	Infrequent
Klinefelter's syndrome	47 XXY	1 in 600 live male births
	48 XXXY	
	48 XXYY	
	49 XXXXY	Rare
	49 XXXYY	
	Mosaics	Infrequent
Superfemale	47 XXX	1 in 1000–2000 live female births
	48 XXXX	
	49 XXXXX	Rare
	Mosaics	
Supermale	47 XYY	1 in 1000 live male births
	48 XYYY	Rare
	Mosaics	Rare
Down's syndrome (mongolism; trisomy 21)	47 XX, G+ or 47 XY, G+	1 in 700 live births (2% are 46 count due to translocation and have 10% risk of Down's syndrome in subsequent pregnancies; 2% are 46/47 mosaics)
D_1 trisomy	47 XX, D+ or 47 XY, D+	1 in 5000 live births
	Translocations	Rare
	Mosaics	Rare
E_{18} trisomy	47 XX, E+ or 47 XY, E+	1 in 3000 live births
	Translocations	Rare
	Mosaics	Rare
Cri du chat syndrome	46 with partial B deletion	1 in 30,000 live births

Possible myelogenous leukemia to demonstrate Philadelphia chromosome (22)
Ambiguous genitalia
Infertility (some patients)
Repeated miscarriages
Primary amenorrhea or oligomenorrhea
Mental retardation with sex anomalies
Hypogonadism
Delayed puberty
Abnormal development at puberty
Disturbances of somatic growth

Diseases of Organ Systems

Diseases of Organ Systems

Cardiovascular Diseases

HYPERTENSION

(present in 18% of adults in the United States)

Laboratory findings due to the primary disease. *These conditions are often occult or unsuspected and should always be carefully ruled out, since many of them represent curable causes of hypertension.* (See Plasma Renin Activity, pp. 87–88.)

Systolic hypertension

Hyperthyroidism

Chronic anemia with hemoglobin < 7 gm/dl

Arteriovenous fistulas—advanced Paget's disease of bone; pulmonary arteriovenous varix

Beriberi

Systolic and diastolic hypertension

Essential (primary) hypertension (causes > 90% of cases of hypertension)

Secondary hypertension (causes < 10% of cases of hypertension)

Endocrine diseases

Adrenal

Pheochromocytoma (< 0.64% of cases of hypertension)

Aldosteronism (< 1% of cases of hypertension)

Cushing's syndrome

Pituitary disease

Signs of hyperadrenal function

Acromegaly

Hyperthyroidism

Hyperparathyroidism

Renal diseases

Vascular (4% of cases of hypertension)

Renal artery stenosis (usually due to atheromatous plaque in elderly patients and to fibromuscular hyperplasia in younger patients) (0.18% of cases of hypertension)

Nephrosclerosis

Embolism

Arteriovenous fistula

Aneurysm

Parenchymal

Glomerulonephritis

Pyelonephritis

Polycystic kidneys

Kimmelstiel-Wilson syndrome

Amyloidosis

Collagen diseases

Renin-producing renal tumor (Wilms' tumor; renal hemangiopericytoma)

Miscellaneous

Urinary tract obstructions

Central nervous system diseases
Cerebrovascular accident
Brain tumors
Poliomyelitis
Other
Toxemia of pregnancy
Polycythemia
Laboratory findings indicating the functional renal status (e.g., urinalysis, BUN, creatinine, uric acid, serum electrolytes, PSP, creatinine clearance, radioisotope scan of kidneys, renal biopsy)
Laboratory findings due to complications of hypertension (e.g., congestive heart failure, uremia, cerebral hemorrhage, myocardial infarction)
Laboratory findings due to administration of some antihypertensive drugs
Oral diuretics (e.g., benzothiadiazines)
Increased incidence of hyperuricemia (to 65–75% of hypertensive patients from incidence of 25–35% in untreated hypertensive patients)
Hypokalemia
Hyperglycemia or aggravation of preexisting diabetes mellitus
Less commonly, bone marrow depression, aggravation of renal or hepatic insufficiency by electrolyte imbalance, cholestatic hepatitis, toxic pancreatitis
Hydralazine
Long-term dosage of > 200 mg/day may produce syndrome not distinguishable from systemic lupus erythematosus (SLE). Usually regresses after drug is discontinued. Antinuclear antibody may be found in ≦ 50% of asymptomatic patients.
Methyldopa
≦ 20% of patients may have positive direct Coombs' test, but relatively few have hemolytic anemia. When drug is discontinued, Coombs' test may remain positive for months but anemia usually reverses promptly.
Abnormal liver function tests indicate hepatocellular damage without jaundice associated with febrile influenzalike syndrome.
Rheumatoid arthritis and LE tests may occasionally be positive.
Rarely, granulocytopenia or thrombocytopenia may occur.
Monoamine oxidase inhibitors (e.g., pargyline hydrochloride)
Wide range of toxic reactions, most serious of which are
Blood dyscrasias
Hepatocellular necrosis
Diazoxide
Sodium and fluid retention
Hyperglycemia (usually mild and manageable by insulin or oral hypoglycemic agents)
When hypertension is associated with decreased serum potassium, rule out
Primary aldosteronism
Pseudoaldosteronism (due to excessive ingestion of licorice)
Secondary aldosteronism (e.g., malignant hypertension)
Hypokalemia due to diuretic administration

Potassium loss due to renal disease
Cushing's syndrome

SOME CAUSES OF CARDIOMYOPATHY
Idiopathic
  Fibrotic (e.g., associated with mitral valve prolapse*)
  Hypertrophic*
  Löffler's fibroplastic endocarditis†
Infectious (e.g., viral, bacterial, rickettsial, protozoal)†
Endocrine
  Hyperthyroidism*
  Hypothyroidism*
  Hypoparathyroidism
  Hyperparathyroidism
  Acromegaly
  Diabetes mellitus
  Carcinoid†
Metabolic
  Electrolyte abnormalities (e.g., potassium, magnesium, phosphate)
  Nutritional (e.g., thiamine, protein)
Infiltrative
  Amyloidosis†
  Hemochromatosis†
  Glycogen storage disease†
Sarcoidosis†
Immunologic (e.g., cardiac allograft rejection†)
Toxic (e.g., doxorubicin administration,† methysergide administration*)
Physical agents (e.g., ionizing radiation†)
Associated with neuromuscular diseases (e.g., Friedreich's ataxia, progressive muscular dystrophies, myotonic dystrophy*)
Associated with collagen diseases (e.g., SLE, rheumatoid arthritis, polymyositis, progressive systemic sclerosis)
Associated with cardiovascular disease (e.g., ischemic, hypertensive, valvular)

CORONARY HEART DISEASE
Increased risk factors
  Increased serum triglyceride is not considered an independent risk factor
  Increased serum total cholesterol
  Increased serum LDL cholesterol
  Decreased serum HDL cholesterol
  HDL/LDL ratio > 5 indicates high risk, < 3 indicates low risk, intermediate ratio is a gray zone.
  Lipoprotein electrophoresis (see Table 28-5, pp. 424–427) shows a specific abnormal pattern in < 2% of Americans (usually Types II, IV). Only purpose of test now is to identify rare familial disorders (I, III, V) to anticipate problems in children.
  Also hyperglycemia, significant glycosuria, impaired glucose tolerance, increased serum uric acid (> 8.5 mg/dl), hypertension

*Endomyocardial biopsy documents myocardial changes.
†Endomyocardial biopsy confirms or clarifies myocardial diagnosis.

Laboratory workup for evaluation of hyperlipidemia (especially men age 20–35 years)
1. Serum cholesterol and fasting triglycerides
2. Determine serum HDL and HDL/LDL ratio if any of the following:
   Serum cholesterol > 225 mg/dl
   Serum triglycerides > 200 mg/dl
   Clinical evidence of coronary artery disease or atherosclerosis in patient < age 40
   Family history of premature coronary artery disease
3. Perform lipoprotein electrophoresis if any of the following:
   Serum cholesterol > 300 mg/dl
   Serum triglycerides > 300 mg/dl
   Fasting serum is lipemic
   Strong family history of premature coronary artery disease
Calculation of LDL cholesterol

LDL = total cholesterol − HDL − (triglycerides/5)

ACUTE MYOCARDIAL INFARCTION

Laboratory Determinations Required

Because ECG changes may be inconclusive (e.g., masked by bundle-branch block or Wolff-Parkinson-White syndrome or may not reveal intramural or diaphragmatic infarcts)

For differential diagnosis (e.g., angina pectoris, pulmonary infarction). Normal serum enzyme levels during 48 hours after onset of clinical symptoms indicate no myocardial infarction.

To follow the course of the patient with acute myocardial infarction

To estimate prognosis (e.g., marked elevation of serum enzyme [4–5 times normal] correlates with increased incidence of ventricular arrhythmia, shock, heart failure, and with higher mortality)

Blood should be drawn promptly after onset of symptoms. Repeat determinations should be performed at appropriate intervals (see Fig. 21-1, p. 207) and also if symptoms recur or new signs or symptoms develop. Changes may indicate extension or additional myocardial infarction or other complications (e.g., pulmonary infarction).

Specific Findings

Serum creatine kinase (CK) is particularly valuable for the following reasons:
   Increased levels occur in > 90% of the patients when blood is drawn at the appropriate time.
   It allows early diagnosis because increased levels appear within 3–6 hours after onset and peak levels in 24–36 hours.
   It is a more sensitive indicator than other enzymes because an increased CK level shows a larger amplitude of change (6–12 times normal).
   Less diagnostic confusion occurs because CK is not increased by many diseases that may be associated with myocardial infarction (e.g., liver damage due to congestion, drug therapy, etc., may increase SGOT) or that may be difficult to distinguish from myocardial infarction (e.g., pulmonary infarction may increase LDH).

It returns to normal by third day; a poorer prognosis is suggested if the increase lasts more than 3–4 days. Reinfarction is indicated by an elevated level after the fifth day that had previously returned to normal.

It is useful in differential diagnosis of diseases with normal enzyme level (e.g., angina pectoris) or from those with increased levels of other enzymes (e.g., increased LDH in pulmonary infarction).

Serum creatine kinase (CK) isoenzymes: MB isoenzyme is increased in acute myocardial infarction, cardiac surgery, and muscular dystrophy; it is not increased by cardiac catheterization or transvenous pacemakers even though total serum CK may be increased. In acute myocardial infarction, MB isoenzyme is evident at 4–8 hours, peaks at 24 hours, and is present in 100% of patients within the first 48 hours. By 72 hours, two-thirds of patients still show some increase in MB isoenzyme. CK isoenzyme studies provide the best laboratory discrimination between the presence or absence of myocardial necrosis.

Serum isoenzymes: In patients with suspected acute myocardial infarction, blood samples should be taken on admission and at 24 and 48 hours, and isoenzyme determinations should be performed when total CK or LDH is increased. *If increased CK-MB isoenzyme and flipped LDH both occur in any of the blood specimens (not necessarily at the same time), it is virtually certain that the patient has acute myocardial infarction and there is no need for further diagnostic testing; if these criteria are not met within 48 hours, the diagnosis is considered not to be acute myocardial necrosis and enzyme measurement can be terminated.*

Serum LDH is almost always increased, beginning in 10–12 hours and reaching a peak in 48–72 hours (of about 3 times normal). The prolonged elevation of 10–14 days is particularly useful for late diagnosis when the patient is first seen after sufficient time has elapsed for CK and SGOT to become normal. Levels > 2000 units suggest a poorer prognosis. Because many other diseases may increase the LDH, isoenzyme studies should be performed. Increased serum LDH with an LDH_1/LDH_2 ratio > 1 ("flipped" LDH) occurs in acute renal infarction and hemolysis associated with hemolytic anemia, pernicious anemia, or prosthetic heart valves, as well as in acute myocardial infarction. In acute myocardial infarction, flipped LDH usually appears in 12–24 hours and is present within 48 hours in 80% of patients; after 1 week, it is still present in < 50% of patients even though total serum LDH may still be elevated. Flipped LDH never appears before CK-MB isoenzyme. LDH_1 may remain elevated after total LDH has returned to normal; with small infarcts, LDH_1 may be increased while total LDH remains normal.

Serum SGOT is useful for the following reasons:

It is increased in > 95% of the patients when blood is drawn at the appropriate time.

It allows early diagnosis because increased levels appear within 6–8 hours and peak levels in 24 hours. Usually returns to normal in 4–6 days.

Peak level is usually $\cong$ 200 units (5 times normal). A higher level (> 300 units), along with a more prolonged increase, suggests a poorer prognosis.

Reinfarction is indicated by a rise following a return to normal.

Table 21-1. Summary of Increased Serum Enzyme Levels After Acute Myocardial Infarction[a]

Serum Enzymes	Earliest Increase (hours)	Maximum Level (hours)	Return to Normal by (days)	Amplitude of Increase × Normal	Comment[b]
CK	3–6	24–36	3	7	Recommended for early diagnosis
MDH	4–6	24–48	5	4	Early use parallels CK; no advantage over other enzymes; technically difficult to do
SGOT	6–8	24–48	4–6	5	
LDH	10–12	48–72	11	3	See α-HBD; isoenzyme determination to differentiate pulmonary infarction, congestive heart failure, etc.
α-HBD	10–12	48–72	13	3–4	Particularly useful for later diagnosis (in 2nd week) when other enzymes have returned to normal, because of longer duration of increased activity; more specific than LDH
ALD	6–8	24–48	4	4	
SGPT			Usually normal unless liver damage due to congestive heart failure, shock, drug therapy (e.g., Coumadin)		
ICD			Usually normal		

[a]The time periods all represent average values.
[b]Least number of false positive results occur with tests of CK, α-HBD, heat-stable LDH.

Table 21-2. Comparison of Sensitivity and Specificity of Various Tests for Myocardial Infarction*

Test	Sensitivity (%)	Specificity (%)
ECG	63–84	100
SGOT increased	89–97	48–88
CK increased	93–100	57–88
CK-MB increased	94–100	93–100
LDH increased	87	88
$LDH_1 > LDH_2$ (on third day after chest pain)	61–90	94–99

*Range of values because different studies used various methods, time periods after onset of symptoms, benchmarks for establishing the diagnosis, etc. Refers to levels in serum.

High sensitivity of CK-MB is combined with the high specificity of LDH isoenzymes by ordering both performed on same specimen where the diagnosis is uncertain.

Table 21-3. Triad of Laboratory Tests Suggested for Differential Diagnosis of Acute Myocardial Infarction[a]

	Serial Tests Done Within 2 Days of Onset		
	SGOT	LDH	Serum Bilirubin
Acute myocardial infarction	I	I	N
Angina pectoris	N	N	N
Pulmonary embolism or infarction[b]	Usually N	I	I ≅ 20% of patients
Pneumonia or atelectasis	N	N	N
Congestive heart failure	N	N	May be slightly I
Pulmonary embolism and myocardial infarction	I	I	I

I = increased; N = normal.

[a] Not useful in presence of severe liver disease.

[b] "Triad" of increased LDH and serum bilirubin associated with normal SGOT is found in only ≅ 15% of patients.

Serum SGPT is usually not increased unless there is liver damage due to congestive heart failure, drug therapy, etc.

Serum α-HBD parallels increase of fast-moving LDH with peak (3–4 times normal) in 48 hours and persistent elevation for up to 2 weeks.

Serum MDH is useful because an early increase (4–6 hours) parallels changes in CK.

Serum ICD is normal.

Leukocytosis is almost invariable; commonly detected by second day but may occur as early as 2 hours. Usually the WBC is 12,000–15,000; up to 20,000 is not rare; sometimes it is very high. Usually there are 75–90% neutrophilic leukocytes with only a slight shift to the left. Leukocytosis is likely to develop before fever.

Sedimentation rate (ESR) is increased, usually by second or third day (may begin within a few hours); peak rate is in 4–5 days, persists for 2–6 months. Increased ESR is sometimes more sensitive than WBC, as it may occur before fever and it persists after temperature and WBC have returned to normal. Degree of increase of ESR does not correlate with severity or prognosis.

Glycosuria and hyperglycemia occur in ≦ 50% of patients.

Glucose tolerance is decreased.

Myoglobinuria often occurs (see p. 163). Increased myoglobin in serum peaks and returns to normal earlier than CK; useful for diagnosis within 6 hours of onset of symptoms.

Differential Diagnosis

Serum enzymes not elevated in angina pectoris; increased levels mean myocardial infarction or another condition.

Serum enzymes usually show little or no increase in inflammatory myocardial lesions (e.g., rheumatic fever) unless disease is severe. (Salicylates may cause some increase of SGOT and SGPT due to liver damage.)

Little or no change occurs in chronic heart failure.

Some increase of SGOT and SGPT may occur in acute heart failure due to liver congestion; it is quickly reversed with appropriate therapy. There may be marked increase in cardiac tamponade due to pericardial effusion.

SGPT is higher than SGOT (which is only slightly increased) in pulmonary infarction and upper abdominal disease (e.g., liver injury).

CONGESTIVE HEART FAILURE

Renal changes: Urine—slight albuminuria (< 1 gm/day) is common. There are isolated RBCs and WBCs, hyaline, and (sometimes) granular casts. Urine is concentrated, with specific gravity > 1.02. Oliguria is a characteristic feature of right-sided failure. PSP excretion and urea clearance are usually depressed. Moderate azotemia (BUN usually < 60 mg/dl) is evident with severe oliguria; may increase with vigorous diuresis. *(Primary renal disease is indicated by proportionate increase in serum creatinine and low specific gravity of urine despite oliguria.)*

ESR may be decreased because of decreased serum fibrinogen.

Plasma volume is increased. Serum albumin and total protein are decreased, with increased gamma globulin. Hematocrit reading is slightly decreased, but red cell mass may be increased.

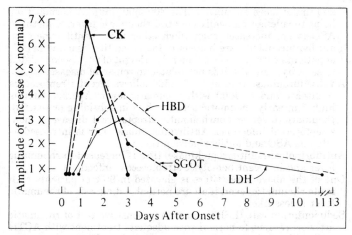

Fig. 21-1. Sequential changes in serum enzymes after acute myocardial infarction.

Liver function changes (see pp. 262–263).

Laboratory findings due to underlying disease (e.g., rheumatic fever, viral myocarditis, bacterial endocarditis, chronic severe anemia, hypertension, hyperthyroidism, Hurler's syndrome).

    Urine sodium is decreased. Plasma sodium and chloride tend to fall but may be normal before treatment. Total body sodium is markedly increased. Plasma potassium is usually normal or slightly increased (because of shift from intracellular location); may be somewhat reduced with hypochloremic alkalosis due to some diuretics. Total body potassium is decreased. Saliva sodium and chloride are decreased and potassium is increased.

    Acidosis (reduced blood pH) occurs when renal insufficiency is associated or there is CO_2 retention due to pulmonary insufficiency, low plasma sodium, or ammonium chloride toxicity.

    Alkalosis (increased blood pH) occurs in uncomplicated heart failure itself, in hyperventilation, in alveolar-capillary block due to associated pulmonary fibrosis, after mercurial diuresis that causes hypochloremic alkalosis, because of potassium depletion.

    Alkalosis (with normal or increased blood pH) showing increased plasma bicarbonate and moderately increased PCO_2 after acute correction of respiratory acidosis is due to CO_2 retention when there is chloride deficit and usually decreased potassium.

ACUTE RHEUMATIC FEVER

Antistreptolysin O (ASO) titer increase indicates recent hemolytic streptococcus infection and indirectly corroborates clinical findings of rheumatic fever. Increased titer develops only after the second week and reaches a peak in 4–6 weeks. Increasing titer is more significant than a single determination. Titer is usually >

250 units; more significant if > 400–500 units. A normal titer helps to rule out clinically doubtful rheumatic fever. Sometimes ASO is not increased even when other titers (antifibrinolysin. antihyaluronidase) are increased. Increased titer is found in 80% of patients within the first 2 months. Height of titer is not related to severity; rate of fall is not related to course of disease.

Antihyaluronidase titer of 1000–1500 follows recent streptococcus A disease and ≦ 4000 with rheumatic fever. Average titer is higher in early rheumatic activity than in subsiding or inactive rheumatic fever or nonrheumatic streptococcal disease or nonstreptococcal infections. Antihyaluronidase titer is increased as often as ASO and antifibrinolysin titers.

Antifibrinolysin (antistreptokinase) titer is increased in rheumatic fever and in recent hemolytic streptococcus infections.

One of the above three titers is elevated in 95% of patients with acute rheumatic fever; if all are normal, a diagnosis of rheumatic fever is less likely.

Sedimentation rate (ESR) increase is a sensitive test of rheumatic activity; returns to normal with adequate treatment with ACTH or salicylates. It may remain increased after WBC becomes normal. It is said to become normal with onset of congestive heart failure even in the presence of rheumatic activity. It is normal in uncomplicated chorea alone.

C-reactive protein (CRP) parallels ESR.

Serum proteins are altered, with decreased serum albumin and increased alpha$_2$ and gamma globulins. *(Streptococcus A infections do not increase alpha$_2$ globulin.)* Fibrinogen is increased.

WBC may be normal but usually is increased (10,000–16,000/cu mm) with shift to the left; increase may persist for weeks after fever subsides. Count may decrease with salicylate and ACTH therapy.

Anemia (hemoglobin usually 8–12 gm/dl) is common; gradually improves as activity subsides; microcytic type. Anemia may be related to increased plasma volume that occurs in early phase of acute rheumatic fever.

Urine: There is a slight febrile albuminuria. Often mild abnormality of Addis count (protein, casts, RBCs, WBCs) indicates mild focal nephritis. Concomitant glomerulonephritis appears in ≦ 2.5% of cases.

Blood cultures are usually negative. Occasional positive culture is found in 5% of patients (bacteria usually grow only in fluid media, not on solid media), in contrast to bacterial endocarditis.

SGOT may be increased, but SGPT is normal unless the patient has cardiac failure with liver damage.

Determine clinical activity—follow ESR, CRP, and WBC. Return to normal should be seen in 6–12 weeks in 80–90% of patients; it may take ≦ 6 months. Normal findings do not prove inactivity if patient is receiving hormone therapy. When therapy is stopped after findings have been suppressed for 6–8 weeks, there may be a mild rebound for 2–3 days and then a return to normal. Relapse after cessation of therapy occurs within 1–8 weeks.

CHRONIC RHEUMATIC VALVULAR HEART DISEASE

Laboratory findings due to complications
    Congestive heart failure
    Rheumatic activity

Bacterial endocarditis
Embolic phenomena

CHRONIC NONRHEUMATIC VALVULAR HEART DISEASE
Laboratory findings due to associated or underlying disease
Syphilis
Carcinoid syndrome
Marfan's syndrome
Genetic disease of mucopolysaccharide metabolism (Hurler's syndrome, Scheie's syndrome, Morquio-Ullrich syndrome)
Rheumatoid arthritis
Congenital defect (e.g., Ebstein's anomaly of tricuspid valve, bicuspid aortic valve)
Calcific aortic stenosis
Endocardial fibroelastosis
Nonbacterial thrombotic endocarditis (see below)
Laboratory findings due to complications
Heart failure
Bacterial endocarditis
Embolic phenomena

MITRAL VALVE PROLAPSE
Anatomically present in 4–7% of general population, but only a small proportion of these have the clinical syndrome.
Anatomic findings in connective tissue of valve are similar in Marfan's syndrome and Ehlers-Danlos syndrome.
Increased 24-hour urinary excretion of catecholamines (epinephrine and norepinephrine) in symptomatic patients, but not diagnostically useful
Normal thyroid function tests, diurnal cortisol secretion, 17-ketosteroid and 17-hydroxyketosteroid excretion, and oral glucose tolerance test
Laboratory findings due to complications (e.g., ruptured chordae tendineae, severe mitral regurgitation, embolization, bacterial endocarditis)

NONBACTERIAL THROMBOTIC ENDOCARDITIS
(TERMINAL ENDOCARDITIS; MARANTIC ENDOCARDITIS)
Laboratory findings due to underlying or predisposing conditions
Rheumatic valvular disease
Congenital valvular heart disease
Terminal systemic neoplasms
Other
Laboratory findings due to complications
Systemic emboli (e.g., cerebral, renal)
Bacterial endocarditis

BACTERIAL ENDOCARDITIS
Blood culture is positive in 80–90% of patients. *Streptococcus viridans* causes 40–50% of cases, *Staphylococcus aureus* 15–20%, *Streptococcus pneumoniae* 5%, and enterococcus 5–10%. Other causes may be gram-negative bacteria (about 10% of cases—e.g., *Escherichia coli, Pseudomonas aeruginosa, Klebsiella, Proteus*) and fungi (e.g., *Candida, Histoplasma, Cryptococcus*).
Progressive normochromic normocytic anemia is a characteristic feature; in 10% of patients, hemoglobin is < 7 gm/dl. Rarely there

is a hemolytic anemia with a positive Coombs' test. Serum iron is decreased. Bone marrow contains abundant hemosiderin. WBC is normal in $\cong$ 50% of patients and elevated $\leqq$ about 15,000/cu mm in the rest, with 65–86% neutrophils. Higher WBC indicates presence of a complication (e.g., cerebral, pulmonary). Occasionally there is leukopenia. Monocytosis may be pronounced. Large macrophages may occur in peripheral blood.

Platelet count is usually normal, but occasionally it is decreased; rarely purpura occurs.

Serum proteins are altered, with an increase in gamma globulin; therefore positive ESR, cryoglobulins, rheumatoid factor (RA test), etc., are found.

Hematuria (usually microscopic) occurs at some stage in many patients due to glomerulitis or renal infarct or focal embolic glomerulonephritis. Albuminuria is almost invariable even without these complications. Renal insufficiency with azotemia and fixed specific gravity is infrequent now. Nephrotic syndrome is rare.

Cerebrospinal fluid findings in various complications. See sections on meningitis (p. 289), brain abscess (p. 297).

Proper blood cultures require adequate volume of blood, at least 5 cultures taken during a period of several days with temperature 101°F or more (preferably when highest), anaerobic as well as aerobic growth, variety of enriched media, prompt incubation, prolonged observation (growth is usual in 1–4 days but may require 2–3 weeks). Beware of negative culture due to recent antibiotic therapy. Beware of transient bacteremia following dental procedures, tonsillectomy, etc., which does not represent bacterial endocarditis (in these cases, streptococci usually grow only in fluid media; in bacterial endocarditis, many colonies also occur on solid media). Blood culture is also negative in bacterial endocarditis due to *Rickettsia burnetii*, but Phase 1 complement fixation test is positive.

Positive blood cultures may be more difficult to obtain in prosthetic valve endocarditis (due to unusual and fastidious organisms), right-sided endocarditis, uremia, and long-standing endocarditis. A single positive culture must be interpreted with extreme caution. Aside from the exceptions noted in this paragraph, the diagnosis should be based on 2 or more cultures positive for the *same* organism.

Serum bactericidal test measures ability of serial dilutions of *patient's* serum to sterilize a standardized inoculum of *his* infecting organisms; it is sometimes useful to demonstrate inadequate antibiotic levels or to avoid unnecessary drug toxicity.

Laboratory findings due to underlying or predisposing diseases
    Rheumatic heart disease
    Congenital heart disease
    Infection of genitourinary system
    Other

MYXOMA OF LEFT ATRIUM OF HEART

Anemia that is hemolytic in type and mechanical in origin (due to local turbulence of blood) is to be looked for and may be severe. Bizarre poikilocytes may be seen in blood smear. Reticulocyte count may be increased. Other findings may reflect effects of hemolysis or compensatory erythroid hyperplasia. The anemia is recognized in $\cong$ 50% of patients with this tumor. Increased serum LDH reflects hemolysis.

Serum gamma globulin is increased in $\cong$ 50% of patients. IgG may be increased.

Increased ESR is a reflection of abnormal serum proteins.

Platelet count may be decreased (possibly the cause here also is mechanical) with resultant findings due to thrombocytopenia.

Negative blood cultures differentiate this tumor from bacterial endocarditis.

Occasionally WBC is increased, and CRP may be positive.

Laboratory findings due to complications
> Emboli to various organs *(increased SGOT may reflect many small emboli to striated muscle)* (see next section)
> Congestive heart failure

These findings are reported much less frequently in myxoma of the right atrium, which is more likely to be accompanied by secondary polycythemia than anemia.

EMBOLIC LESIONS

See separate sections for laboratory findings due to infarction of kidney, intestine, brain, etc.

Laboratory findings due to underlying causative disease
> Bacterial endocarditis
> Nonbacterial thrombotic vegetations on heart valves
> Chronic rheumatic mitral stenosis with mural thrombi
> Chronic atrial fibrillation *(rule out underlying hyperthyroidism)*
> Mural thrombus due to underlying myocardial infarction
> Myxoma of left atrium (see preceding section)

POSTCOMMISSUROTOMY SYNDROME

This condition occurs after cardiac surgery (e.g., commissurotomy, correction of pulmonary stenosis with atrial septal defect); it is the same as the postcardiac injury syndrome.

WBC is increased.

ESR is increased.

CRP is present by the second day.

SGOT is increased to 4–7 times normal by the second day.

COR PULMONALE

Secondary polycythemia

Increased blood CO_2 when cor pulmonale is secondary to chest deformities or pulmonary emphysema.

Laboratory findings of the primary lung disease (e.g, chronic bronchitis and emphysema, multiple small pulmonary emboli, pulmonary schistosomiasis)

TETRALOGY OF FALLOT

Secondary polycythemia is present. Mortality for complete surgical correction is higher in patients with Hb > 18 gm/dl than in those with Hb < 18 gm/dl. Surgical risk is decreased if polycythemia is first reduced by a preliminary systemic-pulmonary anastomosis.

Laboratory findings due to complications (see next section)

COMPLICATIONS OF CONGENITAL HEART DISEASE
Laboratory findings due to
    Congestive heart failure
    Bacterial endocarditis
    Pulmonary tuberculosis, especially with pulmonary stenosis
    Paradoxical embolism—with right-to-left communication, especially patent foramen ovale
    Brain abscess, especially with interventricular septal defect, particularly in tetralogy of Fallot; also in atrial septal defect
    Rupture of aorta
    Secondary polycythemia

COBALT-BEER CARDIOMYOPATHY
(bizarre syndrome of fulminating heart failure in drinkers of large amounts of beer of a brand that contains cobalt)
Polycythemia
Lactic acidosis and shock
Increased SGOT, CK, and LDH, often to extremely high levels; these may rise even further after recovery from shock.
Laboratory findings due to pericardial effusion and, less frequently, pleural effusion

ACUTE PERICARDITIS

Due To
Active rheumatic fever (40% of patients)
Bacterial infection (20% of patients)
Other infections (e.g., viral, rickettsial, parasites)
Uremia (11% of patients)
Benign nonspecific pericarditis (10% of patients)
Neoplasms (3.5% of patients)
Collagen disease (e.g., disseminated lupus erythematosus, polyarteritis nodosa) (2% of patients)
Acute myocardial infarction, postcardiac injury syndrome
Trauma
Myxedema
Others (e.g., hypersensitivity, unknown origin or in association with various syndromes)

Findings
See appropriate sections for laboratory findings of primary disease.
Radioisotope scan of cardiac pool
WBC—usually increased in proportion to fever; normal or low in viral disease and tuberculous pericarditis; markedly increased in suppurative bacterial pericarditis
Examination of aspirated pericardial fluid (see Table 17-1, p. 177)
    Smears and cultures for pyogenic bacteria and tubercle bacilli
    Cytologic examination for LE cells and neoplastic cells

CHRONIC PERICARDIAL EFFUSION
See appropriate sections for primary diseases and sections (Table 17-1, p. 177) on body fluids.

Due To
Tuberculosis
Myxedema

Metastatic tumor
Disseminated lupus erythematosus

Rarely Due To
Severe anemia
Scleroderma
Polyarteritis nodosa
Rheumatoid arthritis
Irradiation therapy
Mycotic infections
Endomyocardial fibrosis of Africa
Idiopathic causes

CHRONIC CONSTRICTIVE PERICARDITIS
Altered liver function tests
    Thymol turbidity increased (some patients)
    Other abnormalities as occur in congestive heart failure
Decreased serum albumin with normal total protein

AORTIC ARCH SYNDROME (TAKAYASU'S SYNDROME; PULSELESS DISEASE)
WBC usually normal
Serum proteins abnormal with increased gamma globulins (mostly
    composed of IgM)
Increased ESR

Women patients have a continuous high level of urinary total estro-
    gens (rather than the usual rise during luteal phase after a low
    excretion during follicular phase)

SYPHILITIC AORTITIS
Laboratory findings due to associated lesions
    Syphilitic aortic insufficiency, with congestive heart failure
    Myocardial infarction due to coronary ostial stenosis
Laboratory findings due to complications
    Hemorrhage (into pericardium, esophagus, bronchial tree, etc.)
    Pressure or erosion or obstruction of adjacent structures in
        mediastinum
Laboratory evidence of syphilis (see Serologic Tests for Syphilis, p.
    138–140)
Serologic tests for syphilis (e.g., VDRL, Kolmer complement-
    fixation) are negative in > 25% of patients with syphilitic aortitis
    at autopsy.

DISSECTING ANEURYSM OF AORTA
If patient survives the immediate episode
    Increased WBC
    Increased ESR
    Laboratory findings due to hemorrhage
    Normal serum CK, SGOT, SGPT, LDH, α-HBD, unless compli-
        cations occur
Laboratory findings due to complications
    Hemopericardium
    Interference with blood supply to heart, brain, kidney, intes-
        tine, etc.

Laboratory findings due to underlying disease
  Marfan's syndrome

ARTERIOSCLEROTIC ANEURYSM OF ABDOMINAL AORTA
Laboratory findings due to complications
  Hemorrhage, especially retroperitoneal; rarely into duodenum, etc.
  Obstruction of branches (e.g., renal arteries)

LÖFFLER'S PARIETAL FIBROPLASTIC ENDOCARDITIS
Eosinophilia $\leq 70\%$; may be absent at first but appears sooner or later
WBC frequently increased
Laboratory findings due to frequently occurring
  Mural thrombi in heart and embolization of spleen and lung
  Mitral and tricuspid regurgitation

MYOCARDIAL DISEASE ASSOCIATED WITH MARKED EOSINOPHILIA
Due To
Trichinosis
Polyarteritis nodosa
Eosinophilic leukemia with infiltration of heart
Loeffler's fibroplastic endocarditis

SHOCK
Leukocytosis is common, especially with hemorrhage. There may be leukopenia when shock is severe, as in gram-negative bacteremia. Circulating eosinophils are decreased.
Hemoconcentration (e.g., dehydration, burns) or hemodilution (e.g., hemorrhage, crush injuries, and skeletal trauma) takes place.
Hyperglycemia occurs early.
Acidosis appears when shock is well developed, with increased blood lactate, low serum sodium, low CO_2-combining power with decreased alkaline reserve. Serum potassium may be increased. Blood pH is usually relatively normal but may be decreased. BUN and creatinine may be increased.
Urine examination
  Volume: Normovolemic patients have output ≥ 50 ml/hour; should investigate cause if $< 25–30$ ml/hour. In hypovolemia, normal kidney may lower 24-hour urine output to 300–400 ml.
  Specific gravity: >1.02 with low urine output suggests patient is fluid-depleted. <1.01 with low urine output suggests renal insufficiency. Specific gravity depends on weight rather than concentration of solutes; therefore is more affected than osmolarity by high molecular weight substances such as urea, albumin, and glucose.
  Osmolarity: Hypovolemia is suggested by high urine osmolarity and urine-plasma osmolarity ratio $\geq 1:2$. Renal failure is suggested by low urine osmolarity with oliguria and urine-plasma osmolarity ratio $\leq 1:1$.

Table 21-4. Diagnosis of Acute Deep Vein Thrombosis Using Venography as Benchmark Test

	Impedance Plethysmography	Fibrin Degradation Products (Staphylococcal Clumping Test)	Both Tests Combined
Sensitivity	77%	88%	77%
Specificity	79%	66%	93%

Source: Data from M. E. G. Foti and V. Gurewich, Fibrin degradation products and impedance plethysmography. *Arch. Intern. Med.* 140:903–906, 1980.

PHLEBOTHROMBOSIS OF LEG VEINS

Staphylococcal clumping test measures breakdown products of fibrin in serum; these indicate the presence of a clot that has begun to dissolve.

Serial dilution protamine sulfate test measures the presence of a fibrin monomer that is one of the polymerization products of fibrinogen. It is less sensitive than the staphylococcal clumping test but indicates clotting earlier.

Tests indicate recent extensive clotting of any origin (e.g., postoperative surgical status).

Laboratory findings of pulmonary infarction (see pp. 224–225) should be sought as evidence of embolization.

RECURRENT THROMBOPHLEBITIS

Laboratory findings will be due to the underlying disease, which is often occult and may be without other manifestations.

Due To

Carcinoma, especially of pancreas; also bronchus, ovary, others

Kaposi's disease

Polycythemia

Vibrio fetus infection

SEPTIC THROMBOPHLEBITIS

Laboratory findings due to associated septicemia

    Increased WBC (often > 20,000/cu mm) with marked shift to left and toxic changes in neutrophils

    Disseminated intravascular coagulation may be present (see pp. 400, 402–404).

    Respiratory alkalosis due to ventilation-perfusion abnormalities with hypoxia. Significant acidosis indicates shock.

    Azotemia

    Positive blood culture

Laboratory findings due to complications (e.g., septic pulmonary infarction)

Laboratory findings due to underlying disease

CONGENITAL ANGIOMATOUS ARTERIOVENOUS FISTULAS

Platelet count may be decreased.

RAYNAUD'S PHENOMENON

May Occur With
High titer of cold agglutinins
Presence of cryoglobulins (e.g., in multiple myeloma, leukemia)
Scleroderma
Other diseases without specific laboratory findings

LABORATORY FINDINGS OF HEART TRANSPLANT REJECTION AS GUIDE TO IMMUNOSUPPRESSIVE TREATMENT

Increasing ESR
Increasing WBC
Increased isoenzyme LDH_1 as amount (>100 IU) and percent (35%) of total LDH during first 4 weeks after surgery

These findings are reversed with effective immunosuppressive therapy. Total LDH continues to be increased even when LDH_1 becomes normal.

Respiratory Diseases

CERVICAL LYMPHADENITIS
Diagnostic tests for specific causative agents (see appropriate separate sections)
>   Beta-hemolytic streptococci cause 75–90% of cases.
>   *Staphylococcus aureus*
>   *Mycobacterium tuberculosis*
>   Atypical mycobacteria
>   Cat-scratch fever
>   Infectious mononucleosis
>   Viruses (e.g., rubella, measles, herpes simplex, adenoviruses)

Occasionally biopsy may be indicated to rule out malignancy.

DISEASES OF LARYNX
Culture and smears for specific organisms (e.g., tubercle bacilli, fungi)
Biopsy for diagnosis of visible lesions (e.g., leukoplakia, carcinoma)

CROUP (EPIGLOTTITIS, LARYNGOTRACHEITIS)
Cultures, smears, and tests for specific causative agents
Group B *Hemophilus influenzae* causes > 90% of cases of epiglottitis; other bacteria include beta-hemolytic streptococci and pneumococci.
Clinical picture in infectious mononucleosis or diphtheria may resemble epiglottitis.
Laryngotracheitis is usually viral (especially parainfluenza) but rarely bacterial in origin.
Blood cultures should be taken at the same time as throat cultures.
Neutrophilic leukocytosis is present.

CHRONIC SINUSITIS
Laboratory findings due to infection
Laboratory findings of underlying disease that may be present
>   Cystic fibrosis of pancreas
>   Mucopolysaccharidosis
>   Allergy
>   Hypothyroidism

CHRONIC BRONCHITIS
WBC normal or increased
Eosinophil count increased if there is allergic basis or component
ESR normal or increased
Sputum bacterial smears and cultures (most common pathogens: pneumococcus, *Hemophilus influenzae;* occasionally *Staphylococcus aureus* or gram-negative rods)
Smears and cultures of bronchoscopic secretions
Laboratory findings due to associated or coexisting diseases (e.g., emphysema, bronchiectasis)

Table 22-1. Sample Arterial Blood Gas Values in Bronchial Asthma

	PO_2 (mmHg)	PCO_2 (mmHg)	pH	HCO_3^- (mEq/L)
Normal	90	40	7.40	24
Status asthma attack	55	30	7.48	22
Nasal O_2 therapy during asthma attack	75	35	7.42	22
Respiratory failure (severe alveolar hypo-ventilation with CO_2 retention, acidemia)	50	75	7.04	20

ACUTE BRONCHITIS (ASTHMATIC BRONCHITIS)
WBC may be increased.
ESR may be increased.

BRONCHIAL ASTHMA
Sputum is white and mucoid without blood or pus (unless infection is present). Eosinophils, crystals (Curschmann's spirals), and mucus casts of bronchioles may be found.

Eosinophilia may be present.

Blood CO_2 may be decreased in early stages and may be increased in later stages.

With severe respiratory distress, rapid deterioration of patient's condition may be associated with precipitous fall in arterial PO_2 and rise in PCO_2. When patient requires hospitalization, arterial blood gases should be measured frequently to assess his status.

Laboratory findings due to underlying diseases that may be primary and that should be ruled out, especially
  Polyarteritis nodosa
  Parasitic infestation
  Bronchial carcinoid
  Drug reaction (especially aspirin)
  Poisoning (especially cholinergic drugs and pesticides)
  Hypogammaglobulinemia

BRONCHIECTASIS
WBC usually normal unless pneumonitis is present

Mild to moderate normocytic normochromic anemia with chronic severe infection

Sputum abundant and mucopurulent (often contains blood); sweet-ish smell

Sputum bacterial smears and cultures

Laboratory findings due to complications (pneumonia, pulmonary hemorrhage, brain abscess, sepsis, cor pulmonale)

Rule out cystic fibrosis of the pancreas and hypogammaglobulinemia or agammaglobulinemia.

BRONCHIOLITIS
Due To
Usually virus, especially respiratory syncytial virus (see p. 600).

When recurrent especially in young infants, rule out cystic fibrosis (see pp. 273–274).

OBSTRUCTIVE PULMONARY EMPHYSEMA

Laboratory findings of underlying disease that may be primary (e.g., pneumoconiosis, tuberculosis, sarcoidosis, kyphoscoliosis, marked obesity, fibrocystic disease of pancreas, alpha$_1$ antitrypsin deficiency)

Laboratory findings of associated conditions, especially duodenal ulcer

Laboratory findings due to decreased lung ventilation
    Arterial blood oxygen decreased and CO_2 increased
    Ultimate development of respiratory acidosis
    Secondary polycythemia
    Cor pulmonale

ADULT RESPIRATORY DISTRESS SYNDROME

Laboratory findings due to preceding or associated acute events—trauma, shock, infections, drugs, aspiration of gastric contents, inhalational injury; gram-negative sepsis is most common cause.

Arterial blood gases show profound hypoxemia with hypocarbia; arterial PO_2 is often not raised by breathing 100% O_2 because of extensive right-to-left intrapulmonary shunting. As disease progresses, PCO_2 increases and pH decreases due to increased pulmonary congestion.

ATELECTASIS

No specific laboratory findings

Rule out underlying lesions (e.g., tumor, tuberculosis, cystic fibrosis of pancreas).

PNEUMONIA

Due To

Bacteria—pneumococcus, staphylococcus, *Klebsiella pneumoniae*, *Hemophilus influenzae*, streptococcus, enterobacteria, tularemia, plague, tubercle bacilli

Diplococcus pneumoniae causes 60–70% of bacterial pneumonia in patients requiring hospitalization. Blood culture positive in 25% of untreated cases during first 3–4 days.

Staphylococcus causes < 1% of all acute bacterial pneumonia with onset outside the hospital but more frequent after outbreaks of influenza; may be secondary to measles, mucoviscidosis, prolonged antibiotic therapy, debilitating diseases (e.g., leukemia, collagen diseases). Bacteremia in < 20% of patients.

H. influenzae is important in 6- to 24-month age group; rare in adults except for middle-aged men with chronic lung disease and/or alcoholism. Can mimic pneumococcal pneumonia; may be isolated with *Diplococcus pneumoniae*.

Gram-negative bacilli (e.g., *K. pneumoniae*, enterobacteria, *Escherichia coli*, *Proteus mirabilis*, *Pseudomonas aeruginosa*) are common causes of hospital-acquired pneumonia but unlikely outside the hospital. *K. pneumoniae* causes 1% of primary bacterial pneumonias, especially in alcoholics and upper lobe pneumonia; tenacious red-brown sputum is typical.

Anaerobic lung abscess—marked increase in sputum that is foul-smelling. Gram stain is diagnostic—sheets of polynuclear leukocytes with a bewildering variety of organisms.

Mycoplasma pneumoniae

Viruses—influenza, parainfluenza, adenoviruses, respiratory syncytial virus, echovirus, Coxsackievirus, reovirus, cytomegalic inclusion virus, viruses of exanthems, herpes simplex

Rickettsiae—Q fever, typhus

Fungi—*Histoplasma and Coccidioides* in particular

Protozoans—*Toxoplasma, Pneumocystis carinii*

Laboratory Findings

WBC is frequently normal or slightly increased in nonbacterial pneumonias; considerable increase in WBC is more common in bacterial pneumonia. *In severe bacterial pneumonia, WBC may be very high or low or normal. Since individual variation is considerable, there is limited value in distinguishing bacterial and nonbacterial pneumonia.*

In the urine, protein, WBCs, hyaline and granular casts in small amounts are common. Ketones may occur with severe infection. *Check for glucose to rule out underlying diabetes mellitus.*

Sputum reveals abundant WBCs in bacterial pneumonias. Gram's stain shows abundant organisms in bacterial pneumonias (e.g., pneumococcus, staphylococcus). Culture sputum for appropriate bacteria.

In all cases of pneumonia, blood culture and sputum culture and smear for Gram stain should be performed before antibiotic therapy is started. Optimum specimen of sputum shows > 25 polymorphonuclear leukocytes (PMNs) and < 10 squamous epithelial cells/lpf (10 ×), but > 10 PMNs and < 25 epithelial cells may be considered acceptable sputum specimen. < 10 PMNs and > 25 epithelial cells indicate unsatisfactory specimen of saliva.

Sputum that contains many organisms and WBCs on smear but no pathogens on aerobic culture may indicate aspiration pneumonia.

Sputum is not appropriate for anaerobic culture.

In *H. influenzae* pneumonia, sputum analysis is unreliable, since sputum culture is negative in > one-half of patients with positive cultures from blood, pleural fluid, or lung tissue, but organisms may be present in the sputum in the absence of disease.

SPUTUM COLOR IN VARIOUS CONDITIONS

Rusty	Lobar pneumonia
Anchovy-paste (dark brown)	Amebic liver abscess rupture into bronchus
Red-currant-jelly	*K. pneumoniae*
Red (pigment, not blood)	*Serratia marcescens;* rifampin overdose
Black	*Bacteroides melaninogenicus* pneumonia; anthracosilicosis
Green (with WBCs, sweet odor)	*Pseudomonas* infection
Milky	Bronchioalveolar carcinoma
Yellow (without WBCs)	Jaundice

Acute-phase serum should be stored at onset. If etiologic diagnosis is not established, a convalescent-phase serum should be taken. A fourfold increase in antibody titer establishes the etiologic diagnosis.

Serologic tests determine whether pneumonia is due to *Histoplasma, Coccidioides,* etc.

Diagnostic lung puncture to determine specific causative agent as a guide to antibiotic therapy may be indicated in critically ill children.

LEGIONNAIRES' DISEASE *(LEGIONELLA PNEUMOPHILA)*

Increased WBC is typical; leukopenia is a bad prognostic sign.

Gram stain of sputum shows few to moderate number of polymorphonuclear leukocytes; bacteria are not seen because the gram-negative *Legionella* stains poorly in clinical specimens.

Direct fluorescent antibody stain on sputum, pleural fluid, lung, or other tissue is extremely useful for rapid specific diagnosis.

Culture on special media of normally sterile material (pleural fluid, lung, transtracheal aspirate of lower respiratory secretions) may show growth in 2–3 days.

Indirect fluorescent antibody titer shows 4-fold increase to 1:128 in two-thirds of patients in 3 weeks and all patients in 6 weeks or single titer of 1:256; may be useful only for retrospective diagnosis.

Mild to moderate increase of SGOT, alkaline phosphatase, LDH, or bilirubin in serum is found in ≅ 50% of patients.

Hypoalbuminemia <2.5 gm/dl.

Decreased serum phosphorus and sodium occurs in ≅ 50% of patients.

Proteinuria occurs in ≅ 50% of patients; microscopic hematuria.

Renal failure and DIC are unusual complications.

Pleural effusions in up to 50% of patients may be bilateral; organism has been isolated from pleural fluid.

CSF is normal.

LIPID PNEUMONIA

Sputum shows fat-containing macrophages that stain with Sudan.

They may be present only intermittently; therefore, examine sputum more than once.

DIFFUSE INTERSTITIAL PNEUMONITIS

Serum LDH is increased.

LUNG ABSCESS

Sputum
    Abundant, foul
    Purulent; may be bloody; contains elastic fibers
    Bacterial cultures (including tubercle bacilli)—anaerobic as well as aerobic *(rule out amebas, parasites)*
    Cytologic examination for malignant cells
Blood culture—may be positive in acute stage
Increased WBC in acute stages (15,000–30,000/cu mm)
Increased ESR
Normochromic normocytic anemia in chronic stage
Albuminuria frequent

Findings of underlying disease—especially bronchogenic carcinoma; also drug addiction, postabortion state, coccidioidomycosis, amebic abscess, tuberculosis, alcoholism

BRONCHOGENIC CARCINOMA

Cytologic examination of sputum for malignant cells—positive in 40% of patients on first sample, 70% with three samples, 85% with five samples. False positive tests are < 1%.

Sputum cytology gives highest positive yield with squamous cell carcinoma (67–85%), intermediate with small cell undifferentiated carcinoma (64–70%), lowest with adenocarcinoma (55%).

Biopsy of scalene lymph nodes for metastases to indicate inoperable status—positive in 15% of patients

Findings of complicating conditions (e.g., pneumonitis, atelectasis, lung abscess)

Findings due to metastases (e.g., Addison's disease, diabetes insipidus, liver metastases with functional hepatic changes, malignant cells in pleural fluid)

Findings due to secretion of active hormone substances (e.g., Cushing's syndrome, hypercalcemia, serotonin production by carcinoid of bronchus) (see p. 513)

Biopsy of bronchus, pleura, lung, metastatic sites in appropriate cases

Transthoracic needle aspiration provides definitive cytologic diagnosis of cancer in 80–90% of cases; useful when other methods (e.g., sputum cytology, bronchoscopy) fail to provide a microscopic diagnosis.

Cancer cells in bone marrow and rarely in peripheral blood

PULMONARY ALVEOLAR PROTEINOSIS

Serum LDH increases when protein accumulates in lungs and drops to normal when infiltrate resolves.

PAS-positive material appears in sputum.

PSP dye injected intravenously is excreted in sputum for long periods of time.

Biopsy of lung for histologic examination is in order.

PULMONARY INFILTRATIONS ASSOCIATED WITH EOSINOPHILIA

Due To

Allergic conditions (e.g., asthma, serum sickness, drug reaction, farmer's lung, pulmonary aspergillosis)

Collagen disorders (e.g., polyarteritis nodosa, Wegener's granulomatosis, SLE)

Neoplasms (e.g., malignant lymphoma, eosinophilic leukemia)

Infections (e.g., fungus, tuberculosis, brucellosis)

Infestations (e.g., trichinosis, ascariasis, tropical eosinophilia due to *Dirofilaria immitis*)

Idiopathic causes, including Löffler's syndrome of recurrent transient pulmonary infiltration

PNEUMOCONIOSIS

Biopsy of lung, scalene lymph node—histologic, chemical, spectrographic, and x-ray diffraction studies (e.g., silicosis, berylliosis; also metastatic tumor, sarcoidosis, tuberculosis, fungus infection)

Increased WBC if associated infection

Secondary polycythemia or anemia
Bacterial smears and cultures of sputum (especially for tubercle bacilli)
Cytologic examination of sputum and bronchoscopic secretions for malignant cells

Additional Types of Pneumoconiosis
Asbestosis
    Asbestos bodies sometimes in sputum after exposure to asbestos dust even without clinical disease
    Associated malignancy, especially mesothelioma of pleura and squamous cell carcinoma of bronchus
Acute beryllium disease
    Occasional transient hypergammaglobulinemia
Chronic beryllium disease
    Secondary polycythemia
    Increased serum gamma globulin
    Increased urine calcium
    Increased beryllium in urine long after beryllium exposure has ended
Pneumoconiosis of coal workers
Diatomaceous earth pneumoconiosis
Talcosis
Bauxite fume fibrosis
Siderosis
Byssinosis (dust from carding and spinning of cotton contains fibers, mold, fungi, etc.)
Bagassosis (dust from sugar cane fibers)

FARMER'S LUNG
(bagassosis; thresher's lung; respiratory disease of mushroom workers; etc.)

Due To
Hypersensitivity to inhaled organic dusts (e.g., sugar cane, wheat, corn, oats, straw, hay, barley, tobacco)

Laboratory Findings
Normal WBC; increased in presence of infection
Eosinophilia $\leq 45\%$
Increased ESR
Sputum smear and culture nonspecific
Lung biopsy—acute granulomatous interstitial pneumonitis

IDIOPATHIC PULMONARY HEMOSIDEROSIS
Hemosiderin-laden macrophages in sputum and gastric washings
Hypochromic microcytic anemia due to pulmonary hemorrhages with decreased serum iron; sometimes findings of hemolytic type of anemia (increased indirect serum bilirubin and urine urobilinogen) (see pp. 344, 355–356)
Eosinophilia in $\leq 20\%$ of patients

GOODPASTURE'S SYNDROME
Malignant hypertension associated with pulmonary hemorrhages
Eosinophilia absent and iron deficiency anemia more marked than in idiopathic pulmonary hemosiderosis

Proteinuria and RBCs and RBC casts in urine
Renal function may deteriorate rapidly
Renal biopsy may show characteristic linear immunofluorescent deposits or focal or diffuse proliferative glomerulonephritis

IDIOPATHIC PULMONARY FIBROSIS (HAMMAN-RICH SYNDROME)

Morphologic changes in biopsy specimen are nonspecific.
ESR is usually increased.
WBC and differential are usually normal.
Polycythemia is unusual.
Occasional patients have positive tests for ANA, rheumatoid factor, cryoglobulins, or other autoimmune abnormalities, but these are probably nonspecific.
Bronchoalveolar lavage in untreated active disease usually shows increased number of cells, predominantly macrophages and neutrophils with smaller number of eosinophils and lymphocytes and few basophils. (Normal values are macrophages = 90%, lymphocytes = 10%, neutrophils < 1%; in this disease, macrophages = 68%, neutrophils = 20%, lymphocytes = 7%, eosinophils = 5%.)
^{67}Ga scan is positive in 70% of cases, usually showing diffuse pattern in lung parenchyma.
Mild decrease in PO_2 and PCO_2 at rest, which always fall with exercise

PULMONARY SARCOIDOSIS

Diagnosis requires demonstration of noncaseating granulomas in biopsy; method of choice for intrathoracic tissue is transbronchial biopsy.
See pp. 637–638 for laboratory test findings.
Bronchoalveolar lavage shows 3–5 times increase in cells; T-lymphocytes are increased to 36%; B-lymphocytes = 4%; macrophages decreased to 55%; if neutrophils and eosinophils are present, they are < 5%.
^{67}Ga scan is usually positive with a diffuse lung pattern and uptake in lymph nodes and other organs with active disease.
Gas exchange is usually normal early in disease; later PO_2 is decreased with marked fall after exercise.

HISTIOCYTOSIS X
(see also p. 448 for laboratory test findings [e.g., diabetes insipidus])
Pulmonary disorder is the major manifestation of this disease; bone involvement in minority of cases with lung disease.
Bronchoalveolar lavage shows increase in total number of cells; 2–20% are Langerhans' cells, small numbers of eosinophils, neutrophils, and lymphocytes and 70% macrophages.
Most adults do not have positive ^{67}Ga scans.
Mild decrease in PO_2, which falls with exercise

PULMONARY HEMOSIDEROSIS SECONDARY TO MITRAL STENOSIS
Hemosiderin-laden macrophages in sputum

PULMONARY EMBOLISM AND INFARCTION
Arterial blood gases (obtained when patient is breathing room air) is the most sensitive and specific laboratory test

$PO_2 < 80$ mm Hg in 88% of cases but normal PaO_2 does not rule out pulmonary embolus

Hypocapnia and slightly elevated pH

Increased WBC in 50% of patients is rarely > 15,000/cu mm (whereas in acute bacterial pneumonia is often > 20,000/cu mm)

Increased ESR

Increased serum LDH (due to isoenzymes 2 and 3) in 80% of patients rises on first day, peaks on second, normal by tenth day.

Serum SGOT is usually normal or only slightly increased. Serum enzymes differ from acute myocardial infarction.

Serum bilirubin is increased (as early as fourth day) to ≅ 5 mg/dl in 20% of cases.

"Triad" of increased LDH and bilirubin with normal SGOT is found in only 15% of cases.

Fibrin degradation products and soluble fibrin complexes are higher in blood of patients with thromboembolism.

Pleural effusion occurs in one half of patients; bloody in one-third to two-thirds of cases; typical pattern in only one-fourth of cases.

See Table 21-3, p. 205.

These laboratory findings depend on the size and duration of the infarction, and the tests must be performed at the appropriate time to detect abnormalities.

CAVERNOUS HEMANGIOMA (CONGENITAL ARTERIOVENOUS ANEURYSM OR VARIX) OF LUNG

Polycythemia

Table 22-2. Endocrine Syndromes That May Be Associated with Pulmonary Disease

Syndrome	Pulmonary Lesion
Hypokalemic alkalosis, edema, Cushing's syndrome	Oat cell carcinoma, adenoma
Hyponatremia (syndrome of inappropriate secretion of antidiuretic hormone)	Oat cell carcinoma, adenoma, tuberculosis, pneumonia, aspergillosis
Hypercalcemia	Squamous cell carcinoma
Gynecomastia (adults), precocious puberty (children)	Anaplastic, "large cell" carcinoma
Hypertrophic osteoarthropathy	Squamous cell carcinoma
"Carcinoid"	Bronchial adenoma, oat cell carcinoma
Hypoglycemia	Mesenchymal cell tumors
Diabetes	Fibrosarcoma
Galactorrhea (or no symptoms)	Anaplastic cell carcinoma
Multiple syndromes	Anaplastic cell carcinoma

Source: Adapted from H. H. Friedman and S. Papper, *Problem-Oriented Medical Diagnosis.* Boston: Little, Brown, 1975.

Table 22-3. Effect of Respiratory Abnormalities on Arterial Blood Gases[a]

Abnormality	Response to	Arterial PO_2	Arterial PCO_2	pH
Ventilation-perfusion abnormality	Resting	D	D–I	
	Oxygen[b]	Variably I	N–I	
	Exercise test[c]	Slightly I	D–I	
Generalized alveolar hypoventilation	Resting	D	I	If acute, pH is D; if chronic, pH is near N
	Oxygen	Markedly I	I	
	Exercise test	V	V	

Decreased pulmonary diffusing capacity	Resting	D	Usually D; may be N
	Oxygen	Markedly I	I
	Exercise test	Especially D	D
Right-to-left shunt or increased venous admixture	Resting	D	D–N	Oxygen effect measures extent of shunt
	Oxygen	Slightly I	I
	Exercise test	D	I
Hyperventilation	Resting	Slightly I	Always D	If acute, pH is I; if chronic, pH is N

N = normal; V = variable; I = high or increased; D = low or decreased.

[a] See also Hypoxemia; Hypercapnia; Hypocapnia, pp. 51–53, and Respiratory Acidosis; Respiratory Alkalosis, pp. 414–415.

[b] Oxygen = effect of breathing 100% O_2 for 15 minutes.

[c] Exercise test = effect of standard physical exercise test.

Source: Adapted from H. H. Friedman, Problem-Oriented Medical Diagnosis (3rd ed.) (Boston: Little, Brown, 1983), and G. L. Baum and E. Wolinsky, of Pulmonary Disease (3rd ed.) (Boston: Little, Brown, 1983).

PULMONARY SEQUESTRATION
The only laboratory findings are due to associated localized chronic
bronchitis and bronchiectasis

TUMORS (PRIMARY OR SECONDARY) OF PLEURA
Examination of pleural fluid (see Table 17-1, p. 177, Table 22-2, p.
225)
Biopsy of pleura

RHEUMATOID PLEURISY WITH EFFUSION
Decreased glucose level (< 30 mg/dl in 25% of patients) is the most
useful finding clinically. Nonpurulent nonmalignant effusions
other than those due to tuberculosis or rheumatoid arthritis almost always have glucose levels > 60 mg/dl.
Exudate is frequently turbid and may be milky.
Smears and cultures for bacteria, tubercle bacilli, and fungi are
negative.
Cytologic examination for malignant cells is negative. Rheumatoid
arthritis cells may be found.
Protein level is > 3 gm/dl.
Increased LDH (usually higher than in serum) is commonly found
in other chronic pleural effusions and is not useful in differential
diagnosis.
Rheumatoid factor may be present but may also be found in other
types of pleural effusion (e.g., with carcinoma, tuberculosis, bacterial pneumonia).
Needle biopsy of pleura usually shows nonspecific chronic inflammation, but characteristic changes of rheumatoid pleuritis may
be found histologically.
Other laboratory findings or rheumatoid arthritis are found (see pp.
320–321).

PNEUMOTHORAX
No abnormal laboratory findings
Laboratory findings *if* underlying disease is present (e.g., tuber-
culosis, sarcoidosis, lung abscess, silicosis, carcinoma)

PNEUMOMEDIASTINUM
Leukocytosis—variable, nonspecific

MEDIASTINAL NEOPLASMS
See
> Thymoma
> Malignant lymphoma
> Ganglioneuroma
> Neuroblastoma
> Pheochromocytoma
> Substernal goiter
> Parathyroid adenoma
> Metastatic tumors
> Sarcoidosis
> Tuberculosis
> Other

DERMOID CYST OF MEDIASTINUM
Hair in sputum may occur with rupture into bronchus.

DIAPHRAGMATIC HERNIA
Microcytic anemia (due to blood loss) may be present.
Stool may be positive for blood.

TIETZE'S SYNDROME
(costochondritis; costochondralgia; rib syndrome; etc.)
No abnormal laboratory findings

Gastrointestinal Diseases

LABORATORY FINDINGS IN ORAL MANIFESTATIONS OF SOME SYSTEMIC DISEASES

Infections
- Bacterial (e.g., diphtheria, scarlet fever, syphilis, Vincent's angina)
- Viral (e.g., herpes simplex, herpangina, measles, infectious mononucleosis)
- Fungal (e.g., actinomycosis, histoplasmosis, mucormycosis, moniliasis)

Hematologic diseases
- Pernicious anemia—glossitis
- Iron deficiency anemia—atrophy
- Polycythemia—erosions
- Granulocytopenia—ulceration and inflammation
- Acute leukemia—edema and hemorrhage

Vitamin deficiencies
- Pellagra
- Riboflavin deficiency
- Scurvy

Systemic diseases
- Systemic lupus erythematosus (SLE)
- Primary amyloidosis
- Hereditary hemorrhagic telangiectasia (Osler-Weber-Rendu disease)

GASTROINTESTINAL MANIFESTATIONS OF SOME SYSTEMIC DISEASES

Lymphoma and leukemia
Metastatic carcinoma
Collagen diseases (e.g., scleroderma, polyarteritis nodosa, SLE)
Amyloidosis
Parasitic infestation (schistosomiasis)
Bacterial infection (lymphogranuloma venereum)
Osler-Weber-Rendu disease
Henoch's purpura
Hemolytic crises (e.g., sickle cell disease)
Porphyria
Lead poisoning
Embolic accidents in rheumatic heart disease, bacterial endocarditis
Ischemic vascular disease
Uremia
Allergy
Cystic fibrosis of pancreas
Hirschsprung's disease
Cirrhosis (esophageal varices, hemorrhoids, peptic ulcer)
Zollinger-Ellison syndrome (peptic ulcer)
Peptic ulcer associated with other diseases (in 8–22% of patients

with hyperparathyroidism, 10% of patients with pituitary tumor, etc.)
Other

SYSTEMIC MANIFESTATIONS OCCURRING IN SOME GASTROINTESTINAL DISEASES
Carcinoid syndrome
Anemia (e.g., due to bleeding occult neoplasm)
Arthritis, uveitis, etc., in ulcerative colitis
Vitamin deficiency (e.g., sprue, malabsorption)
Endocrine manifestations due to replacement by metastatic tumors of GI tract

MALLORY-WEISS SYNDROME
(spontaneous cardioesophageal laceration following retching)
Laboratory findings due to hemorrhage from cardioesophageal laceration

SPONTANEOUS PERFORATION OF ESOPHAGUS
Gastric contents in thoracocentesis fluid

PLUMMER-VINSON SYNDROME
Hypochromic anemia associated with dysphagia and cardiospasm in women

CARCINOMA OF ESOPHAGUS
Cytologic examination of esophageal washings is positive for malignant cells in 75% of patients. It is false positive in < 2% of patients.

DIAPHRAGMATIC HERNIA
Microcytic anemia (due to blood loss) may be present.
Stool may be positive for blood.

ESOPHAGEAL INVOLVEMENT DUE TO PRIMARY DISEASES ELSEWHERE
Scleroderma (*esophageal involvement in > 50% of patients with scleroderma*)
Esophageal varices (see Cirrhosis of Liver, pp. 253–257)
Malignant lymphoma

SOME CONDITIONS OF GASTROINTESTINAL TRACT IN WHICH NO USEFUL ABNORMAL LABORATORY FINDINGS OCCUR
Acute esophagitis
Chronic esophagitis
Diverticula of esophagus and stomach
Esophageal spasm
Prolapse of gastric mucosa
Foreign bodies in stomach

PEPTIC ULCER OF STOMACH
Laboratory findings due to underlying conditions
    Administration of ACTH and adrenal steroids
    Acute burns (Curling's ulcer)

Cerebrovascular accidents and trauma and inflammation (Cushing's ulcer)
Various drugs (e.g., salicylates)
Uremia
Cirrhosis

Laboratory findings due to complications
Gastric retention—dehydration, hypokalemic alkalosis
Perforation—increased WBC with shift to the left, dehydration, increased serum amylase, increased amylase in peritoneal fluid
Hemorrhage

Curling's ulcer—hemorrhage 8–10 days and perforation 30 days after burn, causes death in 15% of fatal burn cases

See Chronic Duodenal Ulcer, p. 233.

CHRONIC GASTRITIS

Diagnosis depends on biopsy of gastric mucosa. (Other forms of chronic gastritis include hypertrophic [see below], eosinophilic, granulomatous.)

Anemia due to iron deficiency and malabsorption may occur.

Gastric acid studies are of limited value. Severe hypochlorhydria or achlorhydria after maximal stimulation usually denotes mucosal atrophy.

Fasting serum gastrin is greatly increased in chronic gastritis with achlorhydria and relative sparing of antral mucosa but may be normal with severe antral involvement even with achlorhydria.

Parietal cell antibodies and intrinsic factor antibodies help define the autoimmune type of chronic gastritis and those patients prone to pernicious anemia; absence does not rule out significant chronic gastritis.

Chronic antral gastritis is consistently present in patients with benign gastric ulcer.

BENIGN GIANT HYPERTROPHIC GASTRITIS (MENETRIER'S DISEASE)

Serum albumin decreased in 80% of cases.
Hypochlorhydria by gastric analysis in 75% of cases
See Protein-Losing Enteropathy, p. 238.

ADENOMATOUS POLYP OF STOMACH

Gastric analysis—achlorhydria in 85% of patients
Sometimes evidence of bleeding

Polyps occur in 5% of patients with pernicious anemia and 2% of patients with achlorhydria.

CARCINOMA OF STOMACH

Anemia due to chronic blood loss
Occult blood in stool
Gastric analysis
Achlorhydria following histamine or betazole in 50% of patients
Hypochlorhydria in 25% of patients
Normal in 25% of patients
Hyperchlorhydria rare

Exfoliative cytology positive in 80% of patients; false positive in less than 2%

Lymph node biopsy for metastases; needle biopsy of liver, bone marrow, etc.

Carcinoma of the stomach should always be searched for by periodic prophylactic screening in high-risk patients, especially those with pernicious anemia, gastric atrophy, gastric polyps.

LEIOMYOMA, LEIOMYOSARCOMA, MALIGNANT LYMPHOMA OF STOMACH
May show evidence of bleeding

CHRONIC DUODENAL ULCER
Laboratory findings due to associated conditions
    Zollinger-Ellison syndrome (ulcerogenic tumor of pancreas) (see pp. 475–476)
    Chronic pancreatitis
    Mucoviscidosis
    Rheumatoid arthritis
    Chronic pulmonary disease (e.g., pulmonary emphysema)
    Cirrhosis
    Certain drugs (e.g., ACTH)
    Hyperparathyroidism
    Polycythemia vera
Laboratory findings due to treatment
    Milk-alkali (Burnett's) syndrome—alkalosis, hypercalcemia, azotemia, renal calculi, or nephrocalcinosis
    Inadequate vagotomy—use insulin test meal (see p. 175)
        Gastric acidity shows late response >4.5 mEq total free acid in 30 minutes or any early response.

To obtain valid collection, Levin tube must be correctly placed fluoroscopically.

Dumping syndrome (occurs in ≦ 70% of post-subtotal gastrectomy patients)—during symptoms may have
        Rapid prolonged alimentary hyperglycemia
        Decreased plasma volume
        Decreased serum potassium
        Increased blood and urine serotonin
    Hypoglycemic syndrome (occurs in < 5% of post-subtotal gastrectomy patients)
        Prolonged alimentary hyperglycemia followed after 2 hours by precipitous hypoglycemia
        Late hypoglycemia shown by 6-hour oral GTT
    Stomal gastritis—anemia due to chronic bleeding
    Postgastrectomy malabsorption
    Postgastrectomy anemia (due to chronic blood loss, malabsorption, vitamin B_{12} deficiency, etc.)
    Afferent-loop obstruction—marked increase in serum amylase to > 1000 units
Laboratory findings due to complications of gastric or duodenal ulcer
    Hemorrhage
    Perforation

    Obstruction
    Other
Gastric analysis
    True achlorhydria following maximum stimulation rules out duodenal ulcer. Normal secretion or hypersecretion does not prove the presence of an ulcer.

Duodenal ulcer is absent in patients with ulcerative colitis (unless under steroid therapy), carcinoma of stomach, pernicious anemia, pregnancy.

REGIONAL ENTERITIS (CROHN'S DISEASE)

No pathognomonic findings for this disease or to distinguish from ulcerative colitis
Increased WBC, ESR, CRP, other acute phase reactants
Anemia due to iron deficiency or vitamin B_{12} or folate deficiency
Decreased serum albumin, increased gamma globulins
Diarrhea may cause hyperchloremic metabolic acidosis, dehydration, decreased sodium, potassium, magnesium.
Mild liver function test changes due to pericholangitis (especially increased alkaline phosphatase)
Serum carcinoembryonic antigen (CEA) may be increased.

ACUTE APPENDICITIS

Increased WBC (12,000–14,000/cu mm) with shift to the left in acute catarrhal stage; higher and more rapid rise with suppuration or perforation
ESR—may be normal during first 24 hours
Later—laboratory findings due to complications (e.g., dehydration, abscess formation, perforation with peritonitis)

ACUTE DIVERTICULITIS

Increased WBC and ESR
Hypochromic microcytic anemia (some patients)
Occult blood in stool
Cytologic examination of stool—negative for malignant cells
Laboratory findings due to complications
    Hemorrhage
    Perforation
    Obstruction

MOST COMMON AGENTS OF FOODBORNE DISEASE OUTBREAKS (GASTROENTERITIS)*

	% of Cases (known etiology)
Viral	5.5
Parasitic	0.8
Chemical (scromboid)	5.1
Bacterial†	88.6
Salmonella	31.9
Staphylococcus aureus	16.5
Clostridium botulinum	0.4

*Source: Data from H. L. Kazal, Laboratory diagnosis of foodborne diseases. *Ann. Clin. Lab. Sci.* 6:381, 1976.
†Confirm by culture of food, patient's stool, or food handler's stool.

Clostridium perfringens	18.5
Shigella	18.0
Vibrio parahaemolyticus	0.03
Bacillus cereus	0.03
Streptococcus, Group A	3.2
Brucella melitensis	0.1

ACUTE MEMBRANOUS ENTEROCOLITIS
Laboratory findings due to antecedent condition
    Disease for which antibiotics are administered
    Myocardial infarction
    Surgical procedure
    Other
Laboratory findings due to shock, dehydration
Culture of staphylococci from stool or rectal swab

WHIPPLE'S DISEASE (INTESTINAL LIPODYSTROPHY)
Characteristic biopsy of intestine and mesenteric lymph nodes
Malabsorption syndrome (see pp. 235–238)
Arthritis

CELIAC DISEASE (GLUTEN-SENSITIVE ENTEROPATHY, NONTROPICAL SPRUE, IDIOPATHIC STEATORRHEA)
Malabsorption syndrome (see pp. 235–238); return to normal on gluten-free diet
Biopsy of small intestine

TUMORS OF SMALL INTESTINE
Laboratory findings due to complications
    Hemorrhage
    Obstruction
    Intussusception
    Malabsorption
Laboratory findings due to underlying condition
    Peutz-Jeghers syndrome
    Malignant lymphoma
    Carcinoid syndrome

MULTIPLE DIVERTICULA OF JEJUNUM
Laboratory findings due to malabsorption syndrome

MECKEL'S DIVERTICULUM
Laboratory findings due only to complications
    Gastrointestinal hemorrhage
    Intestinal obstruction
    Perforation or intussusception ($\cong$ 20% of patients; the other 80% of patients are asymptomatic)

CLASSIFICATION OF MALABSORPTION
Inadequate mixing of food with bile salts and lipase (e.g., pyloroplasty, subtotal or total gastrectomy, gastrojejunostomy)
Inadequate lipolysis due to lack of lipase (e.g., cystic fibrosis of the pancreas, chronic pancreatitis, cancer of the pancreas or ampulla of Vater, pancreatic fistula, vagotomy)
Inadequate emulsification of fat due to lack of bile salts (e.g., obstructive jaundice, severe liver disease)

Primary absorptive defect in small bowel
  Inadequate absorptive surface due to extensive mucosal disease
  (e.g., regional enteritis, tumors, amyloid disease, scleroderma, irradiation)
Biochemical dysfunction of mucosal cells (e.g., celiac-sprue syndrome, severe starvation, intestinal infections, infestations, or administration of drugs such as neomycin sulfate, colchicine, or
  PAS)
Obstruction of mesenteric lymphatics (e.g., by lymphoma, carcinoma, Whipple's disease, intestinal tuberculosis)
Inadequate length of normal absorptive surface (e.g., surgical resection, fistula, shunt)
Miscellaneous (e.g., "blind loops" of intestine, diverticula, Zollinger-
  Ellison syndrome, agammaglobulinemia, endocrine and metabolic disorders)

LABORATORY DIAGNOSIS OF MALABSORPTION
Direct stool examination
  Gross—oil droplets, egg particles, buttery materials
  Sudan III stain—3 globules/microscopic hpf or globules > 75 μ
  Weight—much heavier than normal (normal weight is < 200
  gm/24 hours or normal fecal solids of 25–30 gm/24 hours)
Chemical analysis of fecal fat
  Normal—< 6 gm of fat/24 hours as average of 3-day collection
  when diet includes 100 gm of fat/day
  Chronic pancreatic disease—> 10 gm/24 hours
Indirect indices of fat absorption
  Serum cholesterol may be decreased.
  Prothrombin time may be prolonged due to malabsorption of
  vitamin K.
  Serum carotene (for screening purposes) is always abnormal in
  steatorrhea unless therapy is successful.
    Normal is 70–290 μg/ml.
    30–70 μg/dl indicates mild depletion; < 30 indicates severe
    depletion.
    May also be low in liver disease and diets low in carotene-
    containing foods
  Vitamin A tolerance test (for screening steatorrhea)
    Measure plasma vitamin A level 5 hours after ingestion.
    Normal rise is 9 times fasting level.
    Flat curve in liver disease
    Not useful after gastrectomy
    With vitamin A as ester of long-chain fatty acid, flat curve
    occurs, in both pancreatic disease and intestinal mucosal
    abnormalities; when water-soluble forms of vitamin A
    are used, the curve becomes normal in patients with pan-
    creatic disease but remains flat in intestinal mucosal ab-
    normalities.
  Triolein ^{131}I absorption with measurement of blood and fecal
    radioactivity (see p. 100)
  Oleic acid [131]I (see p. 100)
Carbohydrate absorption indices
  Oral glucose tolerance test—limited value
    Flat curve or delayed peak occurs in celiac disease and non-
    tropical sprue.
    Curve is normal in pancreatic insufficiency.

D-Xylose tolerance test—useful test of carbohydrate absorption
Measure total 5-hour urine excretion; perhaps also measure blood levels at ½, 1, and 2 hours (almost no absorption from ileum). Accuracy is 90% in distinguishing pancreatic disease from intestinal mucosal disease.

Absorption is normal, but urinary excretion is decreased in renal disease and myxedema; also decreased in the elderly.

Na_2CO_3 and Nile blue dye give blue color to stool proportional to the concentration of oleates.

Protein absorption indices
Normal fecal nitrogen is < 2 gm/day. There is marked increase in sprue and severe pancreatic deficiency.

Measure plasma glycine or urinary excretion of hydroxyproline after gelatin meal. Plasma glycine increases 5 times in 2½ hours in normal persons. In those with cystic fibrosis of the pancreas, the increase is < 2½ times.

Serum albumin may be decreased.

See Bentiromide, p. 175.

Schilling test (using ^{60}Co- or ^{57}Co-labeled vitamin B_{12}) shows poor absorption of vitamin B_{12} that is not improved by the addition of intrinsic factor.

Electrolyte absorption indices
Serum calcium, magnesium, potassium, and vitamin D may be decreased.

PVP-^{131}I test is indicated (see p. 100).

^{51}Cr albumin test (IV dose of 30–50 μCi) shows increased excretion in 4-day stool collection due to protein-losing enteropathy.

Biopsy of small intestine mucosa is excellent for verification of sprue, celiac disease, and Whipple's disease.

Anemia is due to deficiency of iron, folic acid, vitamin B_{12}, or various combinations, depending on their decreased absorption.

DISACCHARIDE MALABSORPTION

Due To

Primary malabsorption (congenital or acquired) due to absence of specific disaccharidase in brush border of small intestine mucosa
Sucrose-isomaltose malabsorption (inherited recessive defect)
Oral sucrose tolerance curve is flat, but glucose plus fructose tolerance test is normal. Occasionally there is an associated malabsorption with increased stool fat and abnormal D-xylose tolerance test although intestinal biopsy is normal.

Isolated lactase deficiency (most common defect; occurs in > 10% of whites and 60% of blacks; congenital or acquired)
Oral lactose tolerance curve is flat, but glucose plus galactose tolerance test is normal. Intestinal biopsy shows normal histology but decreased lactase activity.

After a lactose load, diarrheal stools typically show low pH, high osmolality, positive test for reducing substances (e.g., Clinitest tablets); unabsorbed lactose in stool can be demonstrated by chromatography.

Glucose-galactose malabsorption (inherited autosomal recessive defect that affects kidney and intestine)
Oral glucose or galactose tolerance curve is flat, but intra-

venous tolerance curves are normal. Glucosuria is common. Fructose tolerance test is normal.

Secondary malabsorption

Resection of > 50% of disaccharidase activity

Lactose is most marked, but there may also be sucrose.

Oral disaccharide tolerance (especially lactose) is abnormal, but intestinal histology and enzyme activity are normal.

Diffuse intestinal disease—especially celiac disease in which activity of all disaccharidases may be decreased, with later increase as intestine becomes normal on gluten-free diet; also cystic fibrosis of pancreas, severe malnutrition, ulcerative colitis, severe *Giardia* infestation, blind-loop syndrome, beta-lipoprotein deficiency, effect of drugs (e.g., colchicine, neomycin, birth control pills)

Oral tolerance tests (especially lactose) are frequently abnormal, with later return to normal with gluten-free diet. Tolerance tests with monosaccharides may also be abnormal because of defect in absorption as well as digestion.

Laboratory Findings

Oral carbohydrate (disaccharide) tolerance test is abnormal (blood glucose rises 0–21 mg/dl above fasting level).

Oral tolerance test using constituent monosaccharides. Normal result demonstrates normal absorption of monosaccharides.

Examine stool during disaccharide tolerance test.

pH of ≦ 5 is abnormal.

Measure disaccharide (Clinitest tablet).

>0.5% is abnormal.

0.25–0.5% is suspicious.

<0.25% is normal.

Biopsy of small intestine mucosa will reveal activity of specific disaccharidase.

PROTEIN-LOSING ENTEROPATHY

Secondary (i.e., disease states in which clinically significant protein-losing enteropathy may occur as a manifestation)

Giant hypertrophy of gastric rugae

Gastric neoplasms

Regional enteritis

Whipple's disease

Nontropical sprue

Inflammatory and neoplastic diseases of small and large intestine

Ulcerative colitis

Constrictive pericarditis

Primary (i.e., hypoproteinemia is the major clinical feature)

Intestinal lymphangiectasia

Nonspecific inflammatory or granulomatous disease of small intestine

Serum total protein, albumin, and gamma globulin decreased

Serum alpha and beta globulins normal

Serum cholesterol usually normal

Mild anemia

Eosinophilia (occasionally)

Serum calcium decreased

Steatorrhea with abnormal tests of lipid absorption
Increased permeability of GI tract to large molecular substances
shown by IV PVP-^{131}I test (see p. 100)
Proteinuria absent

PERORAL BIOPSY OF THE PROXIMAL SMALL INTESTINE
For differential diagnosis of malabsorption, diarrhea, and associ-
ated nutritional deficiencies
Biopsy is always useful in
    Celiac sprue
    Whipple's disease
    Agammaglobulinemia
    Abetalipoproteinemia (see p. 77: acanthotic RBCs, steatorrhea,
        failure of beta-lipoprotein manufacture, neurologic findings)
Biopsy may or may not be of specific diagnostic value in
    Amyloidosis
    Intestinal lymphangiectasia
    Malignant lymphoma of small bowel
    Eosinophilic gastroenteritis
    Regional enteritis
    Hypogammaglobulinemia and dysgammaglobulinemia
    Systemic mastocytosis
    Parasitic infestations (giardiasis, coccidiosis, strongyloidiasis,
        capillariasis)
Biopsy may be abnormal but not diagnostic in
    Tropical sprue
    Folate deficiency
    Vitamin B$_{12}$ deficiency
    Irradiation enteritis
    Zollinger-Ellison syndrome
    Stasis with intraluminal bacterial overgrowth
    Drug-induced lesions (neomycin, antimetabolites)
    Malnutrition
Biopsy is normal in
    Cirrhosis
    Pancreatic exocrine insufficiency
    Postgastrectomy malabsorption without intestinal mucosal dis-
        ease
    Functional bowel disease (irritable colon, nonspecific diarrhea)

*Biopsy taken at duodenojejunal junction by x-ray localization,
prompt fixation of tissue, proper orientation of tissue for histologic
sectioning, and serial sectioning of specimen are all necessary for
proper interpretation. Multiple biopsies may be necessary for
patchy lesions.*

RECTAL BIOPSY
Rectal biopsy is particularly useful in diagnosis of
    Cancer of rectosigmoid
    Polyps of rectosigmoid
    Secondary amyloidosis
    Amebic ulceration
    Schistosomiasis (even when no lesions are visible)
    Hirschsprung's disease

HIRSCHSPRUNG'S DISEASE (AGANGLIONIC MEGACOLON)
Rectal biopsy to include muscle layers shows absence of myenteric
  plexus ganglia in muscle layers.

CHRONIC NONSPECIFIC ULCERATIVE COLITIS
Laboratory findings parallel severity of the disease
    Anemia due to blood loss (frequently Hb = 6 gm/dl)
    WBC usually normal unless complication occurs (e.g., abscess)
    ESR often normal or only slightly increased
Stools
    Positive for blood (gross and/or occult)
    Negative for usual enteric bacterial pathogens and parasites;
      high total bacterial count
Changes in liver function
    Microscopic changes in needle biopsy of liver
    Serum alkaline phosphatase often increased slightly
    Other liver function tests usually normal
Changes in serum electrolytes due to diarrhea or to therapy with
  adrenal steroids or ACTH
Laboratory changes due to complications or sequelae
    Malabsorption due to involvement of small intestine
    Perforation
    Abscess formation
    Hemorrhage
    Carcinoma
    Arthritis
    Other
Rectal biopsy

ACUTE PROCTITIS
In homosexual men, specific etiology can be found in 80% of cases
  completely studied. The most common causes are *Neisseria gonorrhoeae,* herpes simplex virus type 2, *Chlamydia trachomatis,
  Treponema pallidum.*

Histopathology of rectal biopsy in acute proctocolitis due to C.
  trachomatis *is indistinguishable from Crohn's disease; culture for*
  C. trachomatis *and serologic tests for lymphogranuloma venereum
  should be performed in such cases. Primary or secondary syphilitic
  proctitis may be very severe and of variable appearance; serologic
  test for syphilis should be performed in such cases.*

HEREDITARY GASTROINTESTINAL POLYPOSIS
Laboratory findings due to intestinal polyps and due to associated
  lesions
    Familial polyposis of colon
    Occasional discrete polyps of colon and rectum
    Peutz-Jeghers syndrome
    Gardner's syndrome (see next section)
    Turcot syndrome (CNS tumors)
    Oldfield's syndrome (extensive sebaceous cysts)
    Zollinger-Ellison syndrome
    Generalized juvenile polyposis
Laboratory findings due to complications (e.g., bleeding, intussusception, obstruction, malignancy)

GARDNER'S SYNDROME
(multiple osteomas, fibrous and fatty tumors of skin and mesentery, epidermoid inclusion cysts of skin, multiple polyposis)
Polyposis of the colon and rectum may develop before puberty and show great tendency to become malignant.

CARCINOMA OF COLON
Blood in stool (occult or gross)
Evidence of inflammation
    Increased WBC and ESR
Anemia
    May be the only symptom of carcinoma of right side of colon (present in > 50% of these patients)
    Usually hypochromic
    Stools sometimes negative for occult blood
Evidence of metastases (see Metastatic or Infiltration Disease of Liver, p. 262)
Biopsy of colon lesion
Serum CEA (see pp. 92–93)

Villous tumor of rectum may cause potassium depletion with decreased serum potassium.
Carcinoid tumors may cause increased 5-HIAA in urine.

Laboratory findings due to complications
    Hemorrhage
    Perforation
    Obstruction
Laboratory findings due to underlying condition
    Hereditary polyposis (see above)
    Chronic nonspecific ulcerative colitis
    Granulomatous colitis (Crohn's disease)

VILLOUS ADENOMA OF RECTUM
Stool
    Large amount of mucus tinged with blood; frequent watery diarrhea
Serum potassium sometimes decreased
Biopsy of lesion

MESENTERIC VASCULAR OCCLUSION
Chronic (mesenteric arterial insufficiency)
    Laboratory findings due to malabsorption and starvation
Acute
    Marked increase in WBC ($\geq$ 15,000–25,000/cu mm) with shift to the left
    Laboratory findings due to intestinal hemorrhage, intestinal obstruction, metabolic acidosis, shock
    Infarction of intestine causes increased serum LDH; selective increase of intestinal isoenzyme of serum alkaline phosphatase is described.

INTESTINAL OBSTRUCTION
WBC is normal early. Later it tends to rise, with increase in polynuclear leukocytes; 15,000–25,000/cu mm suggests strangulation; >30,000/cu mm suggests mesenteric thrombosis.

Hemoglobin and hematocrit levels are normal early but later increase, with dehydration.

Urine

Specific gravity increases, with deficit of water and electrolytes unless preexisting renal disease is present. Urinalysis helps rule out renal colic, diabetic acidosis, etc.

Gastric contents

Positive guaiac test suggests strangulation; there may be gross blood if strangulated segment is high in jejunum.

Rectal contents

Gross rectal blood suggests carcinoma of colon or intussusception.

Decreased serum sodium, potassium, chloride, and pH and increased CO_2 are helpful indications for following the course of the patient and to guide therapy.

Increased BUN suggests blood in intestine or renal damage.

Serum amylase may be moderately increased in absence of pancreatitis.

Increased serum LDH may indicate strangulation (infarction) of small intestine.

GALLSTONE ILEUS

Laboratory findings due to preceding chronic cholecystitis and cholelithiasis

Laboratory findings due to acute obstruction of terminal ileum (*accounts for 1–2% of patients*)

GASTROINTESTINAL COMPLICATIONS OF ANTICOAGULANT THERAPY

Hemorrhage into gastrointestinal tract occurs in 3–4% of patients on anticoagulant therapy; may be spontaneous or secondary to unsuspected disease (e.g., peptic ulcer, carcinoma, diverticula, hemorrhoids). Occasionally there is hemorrhage into the wall of the intestine with secondary ileus. Prothrombin time may be in the therapeutic range or, more commonly, is increased. *Coumarin drug action is potentiated by administration of aspirin, antibiotics, phenylbutazone, and thyroxine and T-tube drainage of the common bile duct, especially if pancreatic disease is present.*

Hypersensitivity to phenindione may cause hepatitis or steatorrhea.

GASTROINTESTINAL HEMORRHAGE

Due To

Duodenal ulcer (25% of patients)

Esophageal varices (18% of patients)

Gastric ulcer (12% of patients)

Gastritis (12% of patients)

Esophagitis (6% of patients)

Mallory-Weiss syndrome (5% of patients)

Other (22% of patients)

With previously known GI tract lesions, 40% of patients bled from a different lesion.

Table 23-1. Rectal Bleeding in Children

Cause	Newborn	Ages 1 Week– 2 Years	Ages 2–13 Years
Swallowed blood	3+	–	–
Rectal trauma	1+	1+	–
Milk allergy	1+	1+	–
Bleeding diathesis	2+	1+	1+
Peptic ulcer	2+	2+	1+
Congenital anomalies	1+	2+	1+
Meckel's diverticulum	–	2+	1+
Intussusception	–	2+	1+
Anal fissure	–	4+	4+
Polyps	–	2+	3+
Portal hypertension	–	1+	2+
Ulcerative colitis	–	1+	3+

4+ = most frequent; 1+ = least frequent; – = rare or absent.
Source: Adapted from H. L. Barnett, *Pediatrics.* New York: Appleton-Century-Crofts, 1972.

In addition to the main cause of bleeding, 50% of patients have an additional lesion that could cause hemorrhage (especially duodenal ulcer, esophageal varices, hiatus hernia).

ACUTE PERITONITIS
Primary: Gram stain of direct smear of peritoneal fluid shows streptococci or pneumococci in absence of *Escherichia coli.*
  Marked increase in WBC ($\leq$ 50,000/cu mm) and PMN (80–90%)
Secondary: Laboratory findings due to underlying condition (e.g., appendicitis, perforated ulcer, volvulus)

CHYLOUS ASCITES
Fat content $\leq$ 5%; varies with diet
Protein content 2–3 gm/dl

Due To
Filariasis
Inflammation, tumor, or obstruction of small intestine
Trauma to chest or abdomen

See p. 186.

Hepatobiliary Diseases and Disorders of the Pancreas

HEPATIC INVOLVEMENT IN SYSTEMIC DISEASES

Infections (e.g., infectious mononucleosis, cytomegalic inclusion disease, Q fever, leptospirosis, lobar pneumonia, typhoid, granulomas, such as those with tuberculosis and brucellosis)

Infestations (e.g., schistosomiasis, echinococciasis, ascariasis, infection with *Toxocara canis*, amebiasis, toxoplasmosis)

Intoxications (e.g., alcohol)

Vascular diseases (e.g., congestive heart failure)

Hematologic diseases (e.g., leukemias, lymphomas, hemolytic anemias, polycythemia)

Endocrine diseases (e.g., hyperthyroidism, diabetes mellitus, pregnancy)

Hereditary and metabolic diseases (e.g., mucopolysaccharidoses, glycogen-storage diseases, sickle cell disease, histiocytoses, Wilson's disease, mucoviscidosis, fatty liver, ulcerative colitis)

Collagen diseases (e.g., systemic lupus erythematosus [SLE], polyarteritis)

ACUTE VIRAL HEPATITIS

In the U.S., about 60% of acute viral hepatitis is type B (HBV), about 20% is type A (HAV), about 20% is non-A, non-B (NANB).

Prodromal period

    Serologic markers appear in serum (see pp. 148–154).

    Bilirubinuria occurs before serum bilirubin increases.

    There is an increase in urinary urobilinogen and total serum bilirubin just before clinical jaundice occurs.

    Serum SGOT and SGPT both rise during the preicteric phase and show very high peaks (>500 units) by the time jaundice appears.

    ESR is normal.

    Leukopenia (lymphopenia and neutropenia) is noted with onset of fever, followed by relative lymphocytosis and monocytosis; may find plasma cells and <10% atypical lymphocytes (in infectious mononucleosis is > 10%).

Asymptomatic hepatitis

    Biochemical evidence of acute hepatitis is scant and often absent.

Acute icteric period (tests show parenchymal cell damage)

    Serum bilirubin is 50–75% direct in the early stage; later, indirect bilirubin is proportionately more.

    Serum SGOT and SGPT fall rapidly in the several days after jaundice appears and become normal 2–5 weeks later.

    In hepatitis associated with infectious mononucleosis, peak levels are usually < 200 units and peak occurs 2–3 weeks after onset, becoming normal by the fifth week. *In toxic hepatitis,* levels depend on severity; slight elevations may be associated with therapy with anticoagulants, anovulatory drugs, etc.; poisoning (e.g., carbon tetrachloride) may cause levels $\leq$ 300 units. *In severe toxic hepatitis (especially carbon tetrachloride poisoning),* serum enzymes may be 10–20 times higher than in acute hepatitis and show a different pattern, i.e., increase in LDH > SGOT > SGPT. *In acute hepatitis,* SGPT > SGOT > LDH.

Serum aldolase is increased in 90% of patients, $\leq$ 10 times normal. It parallels transaminase with a sharp rise before serum bilirubin and a return to normal 2–3 weeks after jaundice begins.

Serum isocitric dehydrogenase (ICD) is usually elevated in the early stage (5–10 times normal) but returns to normal in 2–3 weeks; increase persists in chronic hepatitis.

Other liver function tests are often abnormal, depending on severity of the disease—bilirubinuria, abnormal serum protein electrophoresis, alkaline phosphatase, etc.

Serum cholesterol–ester ratio is usually depressed early; total serum cholesterol is decreased only in severe disease. Serum phospholipids are increased in mild but decreased in severe hepatitis. Plasma vitamin A is decreased in severe hepatitis.

Urine urobilinogen is increased in the early icteric period; at peak of the disease it disappears for days or weeks; urobilinogen simultaneously disappears from stool.

ESR is increased; falls during convalescence.

Serum iron is often increased.

Urine: Cylindruria is common; albuminuria occurs occasionally; concentrating ability is sometimes decreased.

In acute viral hepatitis, very high SGOT and serum bilirubin are not reliable indicators of patient's clinical course, but prolonged prothrombin time, especially > 20 seconds, indicates the likely development of acute hepatic insufficiency; therefore the prothrombin time should be performed when patient is first seen. Triad of prolonged prothrombin time, increased PMN, and nonpalpable liver is omen of massive hepatic necrosis and likely development of coma.

Acute viral hepatitis completely resolves in 90% of patients within 12 weeks with disappearance of HB_sAg and development of anti-HB_s. Up to 10% of patients have disease for > 6 months (chronic hepatitis): 70% of these have benign chronic persistent hepatitis and 30% have chronic active hepatitis that can progress to cirrhosis and liver failure (see Table 24-1). Fulminant hepatitis occurs in 1–2% of patients with HBV, and 90% die within 2–4 weeks. Relapse, usually within 1 year, has been recognized in 20% of patients by some elevation of SGOT and changes in liver biopsy.

Defervescent period

Diuresis occurs at onset of convalescence.

Bilirubinuria disappears while serum bilirubin is still increased.

Urine urobilinogen increases.

Serum bilirubin becomes normal after 3–6 weeks.

ESR falls.

Table 24-1. Two Forms of Chronic Hepatitis

	Chronic Active Liver Disease	Benign Persistent Hepatitis
Synonyms	Lupoid hepatitis, subacute hepatitis, plasma cell hepatitis, chronic active hepatitis, chronic liver disease in young women, autoimmune hepatitis, juvenile cirrhosis, chronic aggressive hepatitis, active chronic hepatitis	Chronic persistent hepatitis, chronic lobular hepatitis, chronic portal hepatitis, triaditis, transaminitis, unresolved hepatitis
Criteria for diagnosis	After 12 weeks of hepatitis, tenfold increase in SGOT or fivefold increase in SGOT, with a twofold increase in gamma globulin	

	Chronic Active Liver Disease		Benign Persistent Hepatitis	
		% of Patients		*% of Patients*
Laboratory abnormalities in serum	Increase in SGOT	100	Increase in SGOT may be stable or fluctuate widely, from < 6 times normal to > 10 times normal	75
	Increase in gamma globulin	90		
	Increase in alkaline phosphatase	90	Other liver function tests are near normal	10
	Increase in bilirubin	90		
	Increase in immunoglobulin G	80		
	Smooth muscle antibody	80	Twofold increase in alkaline phosphatase	50

Prolonged prothrombin time	50	Increase in bilirubin $\leq$ 4 mg/dl	20
Increase in immunoglobulin M	50	Increase in gamma globulin twofold	50
Decrease in albumin	50		
Increase in immunoglobulin A	33		
Antinuclear antibody	33		
Antisalmonella antibody	33		
Antimitochondrial antibody	20		
HB_sAg	10–60	HB_sAg	$\leq$50
Laboratory findings of associated diseases (e.g., Hashimoto's thyroiditis, Sjögren's syndrome, primary biliary cirrhosis, pernicious anemia, idiopathic thrombocytopenic purpura)	25	No associated autoimmune diseases present	
Liver biopsy	Different histologic criteria for diagnosis of each condition		
Laboratory findings of sequelae	Cirrhosis, portal hypertension, or liver failure may occur; primary hepatocellular carcinoma is uncommon in U.S. but very important elsewhere	Do not occur	

Anicteric Hepatitis
Laboratory findings are the same as in the icteric type, but abnormalities are usually less marked and there is slight or no increase of serum bilirubin.

Acute Fulminant Hepatitis With Hepatic Failure
Develops in ≅ 1–3% of adults with acute icteric type B hepatitis with resultant death.

Findings are the same as in acute hepatitis but more severe.

There are findings of hepatic failure (see p. 263).

Serum bilirubin is very high unless death occurs in the prodromal period.

Serum cholesterol and esters are markedly decreased.

Aminoaciduria occurs.

Patient may show anemia, leukocytosis, thrombocytopenia, etc.

Serologic markers are similar in cases of typical acute hepatitis, but seroconversion from HB_eAg to anti-HB_e or from HB_sAg to anti-HB_s is uncommon. As patient deteriorates, titers of HB_sAg and HB_eAg may often fall and disappear.

Cholangiolitic Hepatitis
Same as acute hepatitis, but evidence of obstruction is more prominent (e.g., increased serum alkaline phosphatase and direct serum bilirubin), and tests of parenchymal damage are less marked (e.g., SGOT increase may be 3–6 times normal).

Chronic Hepatitis
(see Table 24-1, pp. 246–247)

Occurs in 5–10% of adults with acute HBV.

Is generally divided into three stages:

1. Stage of acute hepatitis: usually lasts 1–6 months with mild or no symptoms.
   SGOT and SGPT are increased > tenfold.
   Serum bilirubin is usually normal or only slightly increased.
   HB_sAg gradually arises to high titers and persists; HB_eAg also appears.
   Gradually merges with next stage.
2. Stage of chronic hepatitis: may last only 1 year or several decades with mild or severe symptoms; most cases resolve, but some develop cirrhosis and liver failure.
   SGOT and SGPT fall to 2–10 times normal range.
   HB_sAg usually remains high, and HB_eAg remains present.
3. Chronic carrier stage: are usually, but not always, healthy and asymptomatic.
   SGOT and SGPT fall to normal or < 2 times normal.
   HB_eAg disappears, and anti-HB_e appears.
   HB_sAg titer falls although may still be detectable; anti-HB_s subsequently develops, marking the end of carrier stage.
   Anti-HB_c is usually present in high titer (>1:512).

Serologic tests refer to HBV, but NANB may also cause chronic hepatitis (see pp. 249–250).

GENERALIZATIONS ON LIVER FUNCTION TEST INTERPRETATION

Patterns of abnormalities rather than single test changes are particularly useful despite sensitivities of only 65% in some cases.

Tests may be abnormal in many conditions that are not primarily hepatic (e.g., heart failure, sepsis, infections such as brucellosis, subacute bacterial endocarditis).

Individual tests are normal in high proportions of patients with proven specific liver diseases, and normal values may not rule out liver disease.

SOME PARTICULARLY USEFUL PATTERNS (TEST COMBINATIONS) OF LIVER FUNCTION CHANGES

Serum bilirubin (direct-total ratio)

<20%	Constitutional hyperbilirubinemias (e.g., Gilbert's disease, Crigler-Najjar syndrome)
	Hemolytic states
20–40%	Favors hepatocellular disease rather than extrahepatic obstruction
40–60%	Occurs in either hepatocellular or extrahepatic type
>50%	Favors extrahepatic obstruction rather than hepatocellular disease

Total serum bilirubin level is generally less markedly elevated (≤ 10 mg/dl) than in periampullary carcinomas (≤ 20 mg/dl) or intrahepatic cholestasis.

Increased serum bilirubin with normal alkaline phosphatase suggests constitutional hyperbilirubinemias or hemolytic states.

Normal serum bilirubin with increased alkaline phosphatase (of liver origin) suggests obstruction of one hepatic duct or metastatic or infiltrative disease of liver (see p. 262).

Mild increase of SGOT and SGPT (usually <500 IU) with alkaline phosphatase increased >3 times normal indicates cholestatic jaundice, but more marked increase of SGOT and SGPT (especially > 1000 IU) with alkaline phosphatase increased < 3 times normal indicates hepatocellular jaundice.

SGOT/SGPT ratio > 1 with SGOT > 300 mU/ml will identify 90% of cases of alcoholic liver disease. SGOT increased up to 300 IU with normal or slightly increased SGPT favors alcoholic hepatitis in cases of liver disease.

GGTP/alkaline phosphatase ratio > 5 favors alcoholic liver disease.

Serum 5'-nucleotidase and leucine aminopeptidase (LAP) parallel the increase in alkaline phosphatase in obstructive type of hepatobiliary disease, but the 5'-nucleotidase is increased only in the latter and normal in pregnancy and bone disease, whereas the LAP is increased in pregnancy but usually normal in bone disease. Therefore, these two enzymes are useful in determining the source of increased serum alkaline phosphatase.

NON-A, NON-B HEPATITIS

Causes up to 25% of sporadic cases of acute viral hepatitis in adults, 90% of posttransfusion hepatitis, and 35% of fulminant cases of hepatitis.

Should be considered in hepatitis in drug addicts, hemophilia, thalassemia, hemodialysis, and renal transplant patients. 3–7% of blood donors in U.S. are asymptomatic carriers.

No serologic, laboratory, or clinical findings establish the diagnosis, which is made by excluding other causes of acute hepatitis (e.g., HAV, HBV, infectious mononucleosis, Epstein-Barr virus, cytomegalovirus, herpes virus, Coxsackievirus B, drugs, toxins).

Typically is less severe than acute HBV. Is often asymptomatic and anicteric.

Biochemical abnormalities are usually mild; 50% of patients are anicteric. But may cause one-third of fulminant cases with mortality up to 90%.

Transaminase levels characteristically show waxing and waning pattern returning to almost normal levels (formerly called acute "relapsing" hepatitis); is highly suggestive but only occurs in 25% of cases; may be extreme, unpredictable course separated by weeks of almost normal enzyme levels. SGPT is usually < 800 IU.

Biochemical and histologic evidence of abnormality occurs in 7% of sporadic cases, up to 60% of posttransfusion cases, and up to 80% of immunosuppressed patients.

Anicteric patients with SGPT > 300 IU/L are at high risk for progressing to chronic hepatitis.

40–60% of posttransfusion cases and 10% of sporadic cases become chronic. Cirrhosis develops in 10–25% of cases.

In chronic disease, > 50% remit spontaneously within 3 years; death is rare due to chronic disease; hepatocellular carcinoma has not been recognized.

FATTY LIVER

Laboratory findings are due to underlying conditions (most commonly alcoholism; also diabetes mellitus, poor nutritional state, toxic chemicals, etc.).

Needle biopsy of liver establishes the diagnosis.

Liver function tests are normal in at least 50% of patients; others may show abnormalities of one or several tests, including clinical jaundice.

Mild anemia and increased WBC may occur.

Not infrequently, fatty liver is the only postmortem finding in cases of sudden, unexpected death.

ALCOHOLIC HEPATITIS

SGOT is increased (rarely > 300 IU), but SGPT is normal or only slightly elevated. SGOT and SGPT are more specific but less sensitive than GGTP. Levels of SGOT and SGPT do not correlate with severity of liver disease.

SGOT/SGPT ratio > 1 associated with SGOT > 300 mU/ml will identify 90% of patients with alcoholic liver disease; is particularly useful for differentiation from viral hepatitis, in which increase of SGOT and SGPT are about the same.

In acute alcoholic hepatitis, GGTP level is usually higher than SGOT level. GGTP is often abnormal in alcoholics even with normal liver histology. Is more useful as index of occult alcoholism or to indicate that elevated serum alkaline phosphatase is of bone or liver origin than to follow course of patient for which SGOT and SGPT are most useful.

Serum alkaline phosphatase may be normal or increased and is not useful as a diagnostic test.

Serum bilirubin is not useful as a diagnostic test. However, if bilirubin continues to increase during a week of therapy in the hospital, it indicates a poor prognosis (because of failure to respond to therapy or development of renal failure).

Decreased serum albumin means long-standing or relatively severe disease. Decreased serum albumin and increased serum globulin are frequent.

Increased serum IgA

Increased prothrombin time that is not corrected by parenteral administration of 10 mg/day of vitamin K for 3 days is best indicator of poor prognosis.

Increased WBC ($>15,000$) in up to one-third of patients with shift to left (*WBC is decreased in viral hepatitis*); normal WBC may indicate folic acid depletion.

Anemia in $> 50\%$ of patients may be macrocytic (folic acid or vitamin B_{12} deficiency), microcytic (iron or pyridoxine deficiency), mixed, or hemolytic. Increased MCV may be a valuable clue to alcoholism.

Metabolic alkalosis may occur due to K^+ loss with pH normal or increased, but pH < 7.2 often indicates disease is becoming terminal.

In terminal stage (last week before death) of chronic alcoholic liver disease, there is often decrease of serum sodium and albumin and increase of prothrombin time and serum bilirubin; SGOT and LDH decrease from previously elevated levels.

Indocyanine green (50 mg/kg) is abnormal in 90% of patients.

Liver biopsy should be done in any alcoholic with enlarged liver as the only way to make definite diagnosis of alcoholic hepatitis. Many have normal liver biopsy; others show characteristic alcoholic hyalin.

COMPARISON OF CHOLESTATIC AND HEPATOCELLULAR JAUNDICE

	Cholestatic	Hepatocellular
Serum bile acids	Very high	Moderately increased
Serum cholesterol	Increased	Decreased
SGOT, SGPT	May be slightly increased; rarely > 500 IU	More markedly increased; may be > 1000 IU
Serum alkaline phosphatase	>3 times normal	<3 times normal
Prothrombin time response to parenteral vitamin K	Yes	No
Steatorrhea	Common	Not common

Increased serum alkaline phosphatase < 3 times normal in 15% of patients with extrahepatic biliary obstruction, especially if incomplete or due to benign conditions.

Occasionally SGOT and LDH are markedly increased in biliary obstruction or liver cancer.

Table 24-2. Increased Serum Enzyme Levels in Liver Diseases

Serum Enzyme	Acute Viral Hepatitis		Complete Biliary Obstruction		Cirrhosis		Liver Metastases	
	Frequency	Amplitude	Frequency	Amplitude	Frequency	Amplitude	Frequency	Amplitude
SGOT	>95%	14	>95%	3	75%	2	50%	1–2
SGPT	>95%	17	>95%	4	50%	1	25%	1–2
Alkaline phosphatase	60%	1–2	>95%	4–14	55%	1–2	50%	1–10 (tuberculosis)
							40%	1–3 (sarcoidosis)
							80%	1–14 (carcinoma)
							Frequently	1–20 (amyloidosis)
LAP	80%	1–2	85%	3	30%	1	70%	2–3
ICD	>95%	6	10%	1	20%	1	40%	2
5'-Nucleotidase	70%	1–2	>95%	6	50%	1–2	65%	3–4
Aldolase	90%	10	>95%	Normal		Normal	20%	

Frequency = average % frequency of patients with increased serum enzyme level when blood taken at optimal time.
Amplitude = average number of times normal that serum level is increased.

SOME CAUSES OF CHOLESTASIS

Canalicular

Drugs (e.g., estrogens, anabolic steroids)—most common cause (see Table 24-5)
Normal pregnancy
Alcoholic hepatitis
Acute viral hepatitis
Sickle cell crisis
Postoperative state following long procedure and multiple transfusions
Benign recurrent familial intrahepatic cholestasis—rare condition
Hodgkin's disease (some cases)
Gram-negative sepsis

Interlobular Bile Ducts

Sclerosing pericholangitis (associated with inflammatory bowel disease)
Primary biliary cirrhosis
Postnecrotic cirrhosis (20% of cases)
Congenital intrahepatic biliary atresia

Interlobular and Larger Intrahepatic Bile Ducts

Multifocal lesions (e.g., metastases, lymphomas, granulomas)

Larger Intrahepatic Bile Ducts

Caroli's disease (congenital biliary ectasia)
Sclerosing cholangitis
Intraductal stones
Intraductal papillomatosis
Cholangiocarcinoma

Extrahepatic Ducts (Surgical or Extrahepatic Jaundice)

Carcinoma (e.g., pancreas, ampulla, bile ducts, gallbladder)
Stricture, stone, cyst, etc., of ducts
Pancreatitis (acute, chronic), pseudocysts

LABORATORY FINDINGS IN CHOLESTASIS

Increased serum alkaline phosphatase
Increased 5'-nucleotidase and LAP parallel alkaline phosphatase and confirm the hepatic source of alkaline phosphatase.
Increased GGTP (also increased in many other conditions; see pp. 60–61)
Increased serum cholesterol and phospholipids but not triglycerides
Increased fasting serum bile acid (>1.5 μg/ml) with ratio of cholic acid–chenodeoxycholic acid > 1 in primary biliary cirrhosis and many intrahepatic cholestatic conditions but <1 in most chronic hepatocellular conditions (e.g., Laennec's cirrhosis, chronic active hepatitis). *(There is relatively little experience with this test.)*

Cholestasis may occur without hyperbilirubinemia.

CIRRHOSIS OF LIVER

Serum bilirubin is often increased; may be present for years. Fluctuations may reflect liver status due to insults to the liver (e.g., alcoholic debauches). Most bilirubin is of the indirect type unless

Table 24-3. Serum Enzymes in Differential Diagnosis of Various Liver Diseases

Disease	Alkaline Phosphatase	SGOT	SGPT	ICD
Acute viral hepatitis	N to 3 × N (15–70 BU during obstructive phase)	Both rise during preicteric phase to peaks (up to 50 × N) by the time jaundice appears; then rapid fall in several days; become normal 2–5 weeks after onset of jaundice		500–2000 units in first week; <800 units after 2 weeks; slightly elevated in third week
Alcoholic hepatitis	Rarely > 5 × N	SGOT rarely > 10 × N; SGOT/SGPT > 2:1		
Portal cirrhosis	<2 × N (5–15 BU in 40–50% of cases)	≦ 300 units in 65–75% of patients	≦ 200 units in 50% of patients; wide fluctuation	<500 units; poor prognosis if higher
Primary biliary cirrhosis	3–20 × N	<5 × N (≦ 200 units) in 90% of cases		
Cholestasis (e.g., drugs)	2–10 × N	N to 5 × N (<300 units)	N to 5 × N (<300 units)	

Incomplete biliary obstruction (or obstruction of 1 duct)	Frequently 10–14 BU (≦70 BU in 100% of patients)	
Complete biliary obstruction		
Stones*	≦10 × N	May *abruptly* rise to 10 × N
Periampullary CA*	Many × > stones	Often N
Metastatic focal disease		
Metastatic CA	≦70 BU in 80% of cases	
Tuberculosis	≦50 BU in 50% of cases	
Sarcoidosis	≦18 BU in 40% of cases	
Amyloidosis	≦100 BU frequently	

BU = Bodansky units; N = normal; CA = carcinoma.
*Serum bilirubin ≧ 20 mg/dl (mostly direct) due to CA; < 10 mg/dl due to stones causing complete biliary obstruction.

cirrhosis is of the cholangiolitic type. Higher and more stable levels occur in postnecrotic cirrhosis; lower and more fluctuating levels occur in Laennec's cirrhosis. Terminal icterus may be constant and severe.

Serum SGOT is increased ($\leqq 300$ units) in 65–75% of patients. Serum SGPT is increased ($\leqq 200$ units) in 50% of patients. Transaminases vary widely and reflect activity or progression of the process (i.e., hepatic parenchymal cell necrosis).

Serum ICD is normal or only slightly increased (< 500 units) in 20% of patients. A large increase suggests a poorer prognosis.

Serum 5'-nucleotidase is increased in 50% of patients.

Serum alkaline phosphatase is increased ($\leqq 15$ Bodansky units) in 40–50% of patients. Serum LAP is slightly increased in 30% of patients.

Total serum protein is usually normal or decreased. Serum albumin parallels functional status of parenchymal cells and may be useful for following progress of liver disease; but it may be normal in the presence of considerable liver cell damage. Lowering of serum albumin may reflect development of ascites or hemorrhage. Serum globulin level is usually increased; it reflects inflammation and parallels the severity of the inflammation. Increased serum globulin may cause increased total protein, especially in chronic (viral) hepatitis and posthepatitic cirrhosis. Increased globulin is usually gamma. (See Table 13-3, pp. 70–73.)

Total serum cholesterol is normal or decreased. Decreased esters reflect more severe parenchymal cell damage.

Urine bilirubin is increased; urobilinogen is normal or increased.

Laboratory findings due to complications or sequelae
  Ascites
  Bleeding esophageal varices
  Hypersplenism
  Hepatoma
  Portal vein thrombosis
  Hepatic coma
  Other

BUN is often decreased (< 10 mg/dl); increased with gastrointestinal hemorrhage.

Serum uric acid is often increased.

Electrolytes and acid-base balance are often abnormal and reflect various combinations of circumstances at the time, such as malnutrition, dehydration, hemorrhage, metabolic acidosis, respiratory alkalosis. In cirrhosis with ascites, the kidney retains increased sodium and excessive water, causing dilutional hyponatremia.

Anemia reflects increased plasma volume and some increased destruction of RBCs. If more severe, rule out hemorrhage in gastrointestinal tract, folic acid deficiency, excessive hemolysis, etc.

WBC is usually normal with active cirrhosis; increased ($\leqq 50,000$/cu mm) with massive necrosis, hemorrhage, etc.; decreased with hypersplenism.

Blood ammonia level is increased in liver coma and cirrhosis and with portacaval shunting of blood.

Abnormalities of coagulation mechanisms
  Prolonged prothrombin time (does not respond to parenteral vitamin K as frequently as in patients with obstructive jaundice)

Abnormal TGT reflecting various abnormalities
Biopsy of liver is valuable.
Laboratory findings due to associated diseases or conditions (see appropriate separate sections)
  Alcoholism
  Wilson's disease
  Hemochromatosis
  Mucoviscidosis
  Glycogen-storage diseases
  Galactosemia
  Alpha$_1$ antitrypsin deficiency
  Porphyria
  Fanconi's syndrome
  Schistosomiasis
  Gaucher's disease
  Ulcerative colitis
  Osler-Weber-Rendu disease

PRIMARY BILIARY CIRRHOSIS (CHOLANGIOLITIC CIRRHOSIS, HANOT'S HYPERTROPHIC CIRRHOSIS, ETC.)

Laboratory findings of complete biliary obstruction are of long duration (may last for years) and often of fluctuating intensity.
Direct serum bilirubin is increased in 80% of patients; levels > 5 mg/dl in only 20% of patients; levels > 10 mg/dl in only 6% of patients. Serum bilirubin is normal in early phase but increases with progression of disease and is a reliable prognostic indicator. Indirect bilirubin is normal or slightly increased.
Serum alkaline phosphatase is markedly increased; in 50% of cases, > 70 King-Armstrong units (normal is $\leq$ 13). Be wary of making this diagnosis with values < 40. This is one of the few conditions that will elevate both serum alkaline phosphatase and GGPT to striking levels.
Serum IgM is increased in $\cong$ 75% of patients; levels may be very high (4–5 times normal). Other serum immunoglobulins are also increased.
The triad of increased serum bilirubin, alkaline phosphatase, and IgM should strongly suggest primary biliary cirrhosis.
Serum mitochondrial antibody titer is strongly positive in 90% of patients (1:40–1:80); similar titers occur in 5% of patients with chronic hepatitis; low titers occur in 10% of patients with other liver disease.
Biopsy of liver is often diagnostic or compatible with the diagnosis.
Marked increase in total cholesterol and phospholipids takes place, with normal triglycerides; serum is not lipemic; serum triglycerides become elevated in late stages. The increase is associated with xanthomas and xanthelasmas.
Serum globulins (especially beta and alpha$_2$) are increased. Albumin is normal or slightly decreased early; later decreased.
ESR is increased 1–5 times normal in 80% of patients.
Laboratory findings show relatively little evidence of parenchymal damage. SGOT and SGPT may be slightly increased (up to 1–5 times normal) in 90% of patients.
There are laboratory findings of steatorrhea, but prothrombin time is normal or restored to normal by parenteral vitamin K.
Urine contains urobilinogen and bilirubin.
Laboratory findings due to associated diseases (e.g., rheumatoid

arthritis, autoimmune thyroiditis, Sjögren's syndrome, scleroderma, breast cancer, cholelithiasis)
Laboratory findings due to complications (e.g., portal hypertension, treatment-resistant osteoporosis)
Liver copper level may be increased to 10–100 times normal.

HEMOCHROMATOSIS

Due To
Idiopathic hemochromatosis (rare inherited form)
Secondary
> Increased intake (e.g., excessive medicinal iron ingestion, Bantu siderosis, long-term frequent transfusions)
> Anemias with increased erythropoiesis (especially thalassemia major; also thalassemia minor, some other hemoglobinopathies, paroxysmal nocturnal hemoglobinuria, sideroblastic anemias, refractory anemias with hypercellular bone marrow, etc.)
> Porphyria cutanea tarda
> Following portal-systemic shunt
> Congenital atransferrinemia

Serum iron is increased (usually 200–300 μg/dl).
Total iron-binding capacity is decreased ($\cong$ 200 μg/dl; often approaches zero; generally higher in secondary than primary type).
Transferrin saturation is increased and frequently approaches 100%.
Serum ferritin is increased (usually > 1000 μg/L); elevated in $\cong$ two-thirds of patients with idiopathic type.
Increased stainable iron in bone marrow and liver biopsy; predominantly in parenchymal cells of liver in idiopathic type and predominantly in Kupffer's cells in secondary type
Liver iron is increased to 80–300 μmol/gm of dry liver (normal = 5–40 by atomic absorption methodology).
Urinary iron following deferoxamine (0.5 gm administered IM) is increased to 5–20 mg/24 hours (normal is < 2 mg/24 hours).
Liver function tests are same as in other types of cirrhosis.
Laboratory findings due to diabetes, underlying diseases (see above), associated alcoholism; hepatocellular carcinoma develops in $\cong$ 30% of cases.
One-third of heterozygotes for primary hemochromatosis have increased transferrin saturation or serum ferritin; more characteristic is hepatic iron concentration 6–10 times greater than normal.

WILSON'S DISEASE
Serum ceruloplasmin is decreased (< 20 mg/dl). (*It is normal in 5% of patients with overt Wilson's disease.*)
Total serum copper is decreased.
Nonceruloplasmin copper is increased.
Urinary copper is increased (> 100 μg/24 hours).
Liver biopsy shows high copper concentration (> 250 μg/gm of dry liver).
Liver biopsy may show no abnormalities, moderate to marked fatty changes with or without fibrosis, or active or inactive cirrhosis.

Table 24-4. Liver Function Tests in Differential Diagnosis of Jaundice

Disease	Urine		Stool		Serum Bilirubin		Serum Cholesterol	
	Bilirubin	Uro-bilinogen	Bilirubin	Uro-bilinogen	Direct	Indirect	Total	Esters
Viral hepatitis	I	N or I	D	D	I early	I predom.	N or D	Mildly to markedly D
Hepatitis due to drugs Hepatitic type	I	N or I	D	D	I early	I predom.	N	
Cholestatic type	I	N or D	D	D	I	Slightly I	I	
Cirrhosis	I	N or I			I < indirect	I > direct	N or D	Mildly to markedly D
Extrahepatic biliary obstruction	I	D	Markedly D	Markedly D	I	N or slightly I	Mildly to markedly I	

I = increased; D = decreased; N = normal.

Table 24-5. Comparison of Three Main Types of Liver Disease Due to Drugs

	Predominantly Cholestatic	Predominantly Hepatitic	Mixed Biochemical Pattern
Laboratory findings	Obstructive type of jaundice (see pp. 251–255) Average duration of jaundice = 2 weeks; may last for years Serum bilirubin may be > 30 mg/dl		Some aspects of each type, but one may be more marked
	Alkaline phosphatase and LAP are markedly increased; may remain increased for years after jaundice has disappeared	Less markedly increased	
	SGOT, SGPT, LDH show mild to moderate increase	More markedly increased	
Some causative drugs	Organic arsenicals Anabolic steroids* Estrogens*	Cinchophen Monoamine oxidase inhibitors (particularly iproniazid)	Phenytoin Phenylbutazone
	Sulfonylurea derivatives (including sulfonamides, phenothiazine tranquilizers, antidiabetic drugs, oral diuretics) Antithyroid drugs (e.g., methimazole) Chlorpromazine PAS (usually this type but may be mixed) Erythromycin	Isonicotinic acid hydrazide	PAS and other antituberculosis agents
Pathology	Centrilobular bile stasis Low incidence High mortality (20%)	Same as acute viral hepatitis	

*Alkaline phosphatase, SGOT, and SGPT are not increased as much compared with other drugs.

Findings of liver function tests may not be abnormal, depending on the type and severity of disease (e.g., transaminase).

Aminoaciduria (especially cystine and threonine) and decreased serum uric acid may occur due to renal tubular dysfunction.

Coombs-negative hemolytic anemia may occur.

Decreased serum ceruloplasmin (<20 mg/dl) with increased hepatic copper (> 250 µg/gm) occurs only in Wilson's disease or normal infants aged < 6 months.

Heterozygous gene for Wilson's disease occurs in 1 of 200 in the general population; 10% of these have decreased serum ceruloplasmin; liver copper is not increased (<250 µg/gm of dry liver).

Homozygous gene (clinical Wilson's disease) occurs in 1 of 200,000 in the general population.

Measure serum ceruloplasmin in any patient under age 30 with hepatitis, hemolysis, or neurologic symptoms to allow early diagnosis and treatment of Wilson's disease.

PORTAL HYPERTENSION (WITH SHUNT FROM PORTAL SYSTEM VIA COLLATERAL CIRCULATION)

Increased blood ammonia

Increased postprandial blood glucose

Increased urine urobilinogen

Laboratory findings due to underlying disease

> Posthepatic obstruction (e.g., constrictive pericarditis, obstruction of hepatic veins, obstruction of inferior vena cava, cirrhosis)
>
> Intrahepatic obstruction (e.g., sickle cell disease)
>
> Prehepatic obstruction (e.g., occlusion of portal vein by thrombus or tumor, tumors, scars—as from schistosomiasis)
>
> Shunts (e.g., arteriovenous fistulas, hamartomas of liver)

Laboratory findings due to complications and sequelae

> Hypersplenism
>
> Intestinal malabsorption or protein loss
>
> Bleeding from esophageal varices

SURGICAL PORTACAVAL ANASTOMOSIS

In cirrhosis

> Operative mortality is < 5% if
>
>> Serum bilirubin is < 3.0 mg/dl.
>>
>> Serum albumin is at least 3.5 gm/dl.
>
> Operative mortality is ≅ 50% if
>
>> Serum bilirubin is > 8.0 mg/dl.
>>
>> Serum albumin is ≅ 2.5 gm/dl.

Following surgery

> Serum indirect bilirubin is slightly increased.
>
> Blood ammonia is increased.
>
> Laboratory findings of hypersplenism decrease.

PORTAL VEIN THROMBOSIS

Laboratory findings due to underlying conditions (e.g., polycythemia, cirrhosis, neoplastic invasion of portal vein)

Laboratory findings due to infarction of intestine

HEPATOMA
Serum alpha-fetoprotein present in 50% of white and 75–90% of nonwhite patients

Laboratory findings associated with metastatic lesions of liver

Laboratory findings associated with underlying disease (>60% occur with preexisting cirrhosis)

>   Hemochromatosis (≦ 20% of patients die of hepatoma)

>   More frequent in postnecrotic than in alcoholic cirrhosis

Sudden progressive worsening of laboratory findings of underlying disease

Hemoperitoneum—ascites in ≅ 50% of patients but tumor cells found irregularly

Laboratory findings due to obstruction of hepatic or portal veins or inferior vena cava

Occasional marked hypoglycemia unresponsive to epinephrine injection

ESR and WBC sometimes increased

Anemia uncommon unless hemorrhage occurs

Serologic marker of HBV frequently present

METASTATIC OR INFILTRATIVE DISEASE OF LIVER
Increased serum alkaline phosphatase is the most useful index of *partial obstruction of the biliary tree* when serum bilirubin is usually normal and urine bilirubin is increased.

>   Increased in 80% of patients with metastatic carcinoma (≦70 Bodansky units)

>   Increased in 50% of patients with tuberculosis (≦50 Bodansky units)

>   Increased in 40% of patients with sarcoidosis (≦18 Bodansky units)

>   Increased frequently in patients with amyloidosis (≦100 Bodansky units)

Increased serum LAP parallels alkaline phosphatase but is not affected by bone disease.

Whenever the alkaline phosphatase is increased, a simultaneous increase of 5′-nucleotidase establishes biliary disease as the cause of the elevated alkaline phosphatase.

SGOT is increased in 50% of patients (≦300 units).

SGPT is increased less frequently (≦150 units).

ICD may show a moderate increase.

Detection of metastatic carcinoma by panel of blood tests (alkaline phosphatase, LDH, transaminase, bilirubin) has sensitivity of 85%.

Radioactive scanning of the liver has 65% sensitivity.

Blind needle biopsy of the liver is positive in 65–75% of patients.

Laboratory findings due to primary disease are noted. See also

>   Carcinoid syndrome

>   Pyogenic liver abscess

>   Other

LIVER FUNCTION ABNORMALITIES IN CONGESTIVE HEART FAILURE
Serum bilirubin is frequently increased (indirect more than direct); usually 1–5 mg/dl. It usually represents combined right- and left-sided failure with hepatic engorgement and pulmonary infarcts.

Serum bilirubin may suddenly rise rapidly if superimposed myocardial infarction occurs.

Urine urobilinogen is increased. Urine bilirubin is increased in the presence of jaundice.

SGOT and SGPT are increased in $\cong$ 12% of patients. They are disproportionately increased compared with other liver function tests in left-sided heart failure.

Serum LDH is increased in $\cong$ 40% of patients.

Serum alkaline phosphatase shows mild to moderate increase (6–25 Bodansky units) in 45% of cases.

Hypoalbuminemia is common with cardiac fibrosis of liver.

Prothrombin time may be slightly increased, with increased sensitivity to anticoagulant drugs.

Serum cholesterol and esters may be decreased.

Pattern of abnormal liver function tests is variable. All will return to normal when heart failure responds to treatment. Serum alkaline phosphatase is usually the last to become normal, and this may be weeks to months later.

These findings may occur with marked liver congestion due to other conditions (e.g., Chiari's syndrome [occlusion of hepatic veins] and constrictive pericarditis).

HEPATIC FAILURE

Serum bilirubin progressively increases; may become very high.

Decreased albumin and also total protein

Previously elevated SGOT and SGPT that fall abruptly with onset of hepatic failure

Decreased blood glucose

Prolonged prothrombin time; is never normal in acute hepatic failure.

Blood ammonia level usually increased

Laboratory findings of hemorrhage, especially in GI tract

HEPATIC ENCEPHALOPATHY
(neurologic and mental abnormalities in some patients with liver failure)

Respiratory alkalosis due to hyperventilation is frequent.

Hypokalemic metabolic alkalosis may occur due to diuretic excess.

Arterial ammonia is increased in 90% of patients but does not reflect the degree of coma. Normal level in comatose patient suggests another cause of coma.

Serum amino acid profile is abnormal. All serum amino acids are markedly increased in coma due to acute liver failure.

CSF is normal except for increased glutamine level.

Diagnosis is clinical; characteristic laboratory findings are supportive but not specific.

COMPLETE BILIARY OBSTRUCTION (INTRAHEPATIC OR EXTRAHEPATIC)

Direct serum bilirubin is increased; indirect serum bilirubin is normal or slightly increased.

Urine bilirubin is increased; urine urobilinogen decreased.

There is decreased stool bilirubin and urobilinogen (clay-colored stools).

Serum alkaline phosphatase is markedly increased (15–70 Bodansky units). In extrahepatic type, the increase is related to the completeness of obstruction.

Serum LAP parallels alkaline phosphatase.

SGOT is increased ($\leqq 300$ units), and SGPT is increased $\leqq 200$ units); they usually return to normal in 1 week after relief of obstruction.

Serum cholesterol is increased (acute, 300–400 mg/dl; chronic, $\leqq 1000$ mg/dl).

Serum phospholipids are increased.

Prothrombin time is prolonged, with response to parenteral vitamin K more frequent than in hepatic parenchymal cell disease.

Laboratory findings due to underlying causative disease are noted (e.g., stone, carcinoma of duct, metastatic carcinoma to periductal lymph nodes).

OBSTRUCTION OF ONE HEPATIC BILE DUCT

Serum bilirubin remains normal in the presence of serum alkaline phosphatase that is markedly increased.

DUBIN-JOHNSON SYNDROME (SPRINZ NELSON SYNDROME)

Inherited familial disease may resemble mild viral hepatitis. It is characterized by mild recurrent jaundice with hepatomegaly and right upper quadrant abdominal pain. It is due to inability to transport bilirubin glucuronide through the parenchymal hepatic cell into the canaliculi; however, conjugation of bilirubin glucuronide is normal. Usually it is compensated, except in periods of stress. Jaundice (innocuous and reversible) may be produced by estrogens, last trimester of pregnancy, or birth control pills.

Serum direct bilirubin is increased (3–10 mg/dl).

Urine contains bile and urobilinogen.

Other liver function tests are normal.

Serum alkaline phosphatase is normal.

Liver biopsy shows large amounts of yellow-brown or slate-black pigment in hepatic cells in centrilobular location; small amounts of Kupffer's cells.

ROTOR'S SYNDROME

Inherited condition of defective transfer of bilirubin from liver to bile; usually detected in adolescents or adults. Jaundice may be produced or accentuated by pregnancy, birth control pills, alcohol, infection, surgery.

Mild chronic conjugated hyperbilirubinemia

Other liver function tests normal

GILBERT'S DISEASE (UNCONJUGATED HYPERBILIRUBINEMIA WITHOUT OVERT HEMOLYSIS)

Mild symptomatic benign condition with an evanescent increase of indirect serum bilirubin, which is usually discovered on routine laboratory examinations. The disease may be due to inadequacy of glucuronyl-transferase or bilirubin transfer from plasma to liver and probably represents a heterogeneous group (e.g., late infectious hepatitis, mild familial congenital disease), or it may be an inherited defect that is aggravated by other medical conditions. Jaundice is usually accentuated by pregnancy, fever, exercise, and various drugs, including alcohol and birth control pills.

Indirect serum bilirubin is increased. It may rise to 18 mg/dl but usually is < 4 mg/dl. Fasting (<400 calories/day) for 72 hours causes elevated indirect bilirubin to increase > 100% in Gilbert's disease but not in normal persons or those with liver disease or hemolytic anemia.

Fecal urobilinogen may be decreased.

Urine shows no increased bilirubin.

Liver function tests are usually normal.

HEREDITARY GLUCURONYL-TRANSFERASE DEFICIENCY, GROUP I (CRIGLER-NAJJAR SYNDROME)

This rare familial autosomal recessive disease is due to marked congenital deficiency or absence of glucuronyl-transferase, which conjugates bilirubin to bilirubin glucuronide in hepatic cells (counterpart is the homozygous Gunn rat).

Indirect serum bilirubin is increased; it appears on first or second day of life, rises to 12–45 mg/dl, and persists for life.

Fecal urobilinogen is very low.

Liver function tests are normal.

Liver biopsy is normal.

There is no evidence of hemolysis.

Nonjaundiced parents have diminished capacity to form glucuronide conjugates with menthol, salicylates, and tetrahydrocortisone.

This syndrome has been divided into two groups:

	Group I	Group II
Transmission	Autosomal recessive	Autosomal dominant
Hyperbilirubinemia	More severe (usually > 20 mg/dl)	Less severe and more variable (usually < 20 mg/dl)
Kernicterus	Frequent	Absent
Bile	Essentially colorless	Normal color
	Only traces of unconjugated bilirubin	Contains bilirubin-glucuronide
Phenobarbital administration	Hyperbilirubinemia unaffected	Jaundice disappears
Bile	Very low bilirubin concentration (<10 mg/dl)	Nearly normal bilirubin concentration (50–100 mg/dl)
	Total absence of bilirubin glucuronide	Contains bilirubin glucuronide
	Essentially colorless	Normal color
Stool color	Pale yellow	Normal
Parents	Normal serum bilirubin in both parents	One parent usually shows minimal to severe icterus
	Partial defect (about 50%) in glucuronide conjugation in both parents	Defect in glucuronide conjugation may be present only in one parent.
		Level of conjugation cannot be distinguished from Group I.

Table 24-6. Differential Diagnosis of Adult Jaundice When Other Liver Chemistries Are Normal and There Are No Signs or Symptoms of Liver Disease

	When Increased Bilirubin Is Conjugated (direct)		When Increased Bilirubin Is Unconjugated (indirect)		
	Dubin-Johnson Syndrome	Rotor's Syndrome	Gilbert's Disease	Crigler-Najjar Syndrome	Hemolytic Jaundice
Serum Bilirubin					
Direct	I	I			
Indirect			I	I	I
Urine					
Bilirubin	I	N or I	N	N	Absent
Urobilinogen	I	N or I	N or D	N or D	I
Stool					
Bilirubin			D	D	I
Urobilinogen			N or D	N or D	I
Impaired excretion of dyes (e.g., BSP) requiring conjugation	Present	Present	May be slightly impaired		
Liver biopsy	Characteristic pigment	No pigment	N	N	N

N = normal; D = decreased; I = increased.

HEPATIC CHOLESTEROL ESTER STORAGE DISEASE

In this inherited familial disorder, an enlarged liver contains excessive deposition of cholesterol esters, and serum bile acid levels are increased.

Serum bilirubin is usually 3–7 mg/dl (mostly direct).

Liver chemical function tests are normal.

Other blood chemistries are normal (including carotene, vitamin A, ceruloplasmin).

Serum lipid profiles may show a moderate increase in esterified cholesterol, phospholipid, triglyceride.

Lipoprotein electrophoresis may show a slight decrease in alpha-lipoproteins or a slight increase in beta- and pre-beta-lipoproteins.

Biopsy of liver reveals brilliant orange-yellow color. Polarized light shows crystalline material in parenchymal cells. There is chemical and histochemical confirmation of cholesterol esters. Septate cirrhosis may be present histologically.

RECURRENT FAMILIAL CHOLESTASIS

Rare familial condition with early onset of multiple episodes of conjugated hyperbilirubinemia with spontaneous complete remissions and exacerbations.

LIVER TRAUMA

Serum LDH is frequently increased (> 1400 units) 8–12 hours after major injury. *Shock due to any injury may also increase LDH.*

Other serum enzymes and liver function tests are not generally helpful.

Findings of abdominal paracentesis

    Bloody fluid (in ≅ 75% of patients) confirming traumatic hemoperitoneum and indicating exploratory laparotomy

    Nonbloody fluid (especially if injury occurred > 24 hours earlier)

        Microscopic—some red and white blood cells

        Determine amylase, protein, pH, presence of bile.

PRIMARY SCLEROSING CHOLANGITIS

Chronic fibrosing inflammation of intra- and extrahepatic bile ducts predominantly in men under age 45, usually associated with inflammatory bowel disease especially ulcerative colitis, characteristic cholangiography image; slow, relentless, progressive course of chronic cholestasis to death. Diagnosis should not be made if previous bile duct surgery or gallstones.

Cholestatic biochemical profile

    Serum alkaline phosphatase may fluctuate but is always increased.

    SGOT is mildly increased in > 90%.

    Bilirubin is increased in one-half of patients; occasionally is very high; may fluctuate markedly.

No serologic markers in serum; antimitochondrial antibody, smooth-muscle antibody, rheumatoid factor, ANA are negative in > 90% of patients. HB$_s$Ag is negative.

Copper metabolism tests are abnormal; have diagnostic and prognostic value.

    Serum ceruloplasmin is increased in 75% of cases.

Hepatic copper is increased to levels seen in Wilson's disease and primary biliary cirrhosis.

Urine copper level is increased.

Liver biopsy provides only confirmatory evidence in patients with compatible history, laboratory and x-ray findings.

Adenocarcinoma of bile ducts develops in some patients.

SUPPURATIVE CHOLANGITIS

Marked increase in WBC ($\leqq$ 30,000/cu mm) with increase in granulocytes

Blood culture often positive

Laboratory findings of incomplete duct obstruction due to inflammation or of preceding complete duct obstruction that caused the cholangitis (e.g., stone, tumor, scar)

Laboratory findings of parenchymal cell necrosis and malfunction
Increased serum SGOT, SGPT, etc.
Increased urine urobilinogen

SEPTIC PYLEPHLEBITIS

Polynuclear leukocytosis in > 90% of patients; usually > 20,000/cu mm

Anemia of varying severity

Moderate increase in serum bilirubin in $\cong$ 33% of patients

Other liver function tests positive in $\cong$ 25% of patients

Needle biopsy of liver not helpful; contraindicated

Blood culture sometimes positive

Laboratory findings due to preceding disease (e.g., acute appendicitis, diverticulitis, ulcerative colitis)

Laboratory findings due to complications (e.g., portal vein occlusion)

PYOGENIC LIVER ABSCESS

Increase in WBC due to increase in granulocytes

Abnormalities of liver function tests
Decreased serum albumin, increased serum globulin
Increased serum alkaline phosphatase
Increased serum bilirubin (> 10 mg/dl usually indicates pyogenic rather than amebic and suggests poorer prognosis because of more tissue destruction)
Other laboratory findings (see Metastatic or Infiltrative Disease of Liver, p. 262)

Anemia frequent

Laboratory findings due to complications (e.g., subphrenic abscess, pneumonia, empyema, bronchopleural fistula)

Patients with amebic abscess of liver due to *Entamoeba histolytica* also show positive serologic tests for ameba (see pp. 623–624).
Stools may be negative for cysts and trophozoites.
Needle aspiration of abscess may show *Entamoeba histolytica* in 50% of patients. (*Characteristic brown or anchovy-sauce color may be absent; secondary bacterial infection may be superimposed.*)

ACUTE CHOLECYSTITIS

Increased ESR, WBC (average 12,000/cu mm; if > 15,000 suspect empyema or perforation) and other evidence of acute inflammatory process

Increased serum bilirubin in 20% of patients (usually >4 mg/dl; if higher, suspect associated choledocholithiasis)

Increased serum alkaline phosphatase (some patients) even if serum bilirubin is normal

Increased serum amylase and lipase in some patients

Laboratory findings of associated biliary obstruction if such obstruction is present

Laboratory findings of preexisting cholelithiasis (some patients)

Laboratory findings of complications (e.g., empyema of gallbladder, perforation, cholangitis, liver abscess, pylephlebitis, pancreatitis, gallstone ileus)

Serum SGOT is increased in 75% of patients.

CHRONIC CHOLECYSTITIS

May be mild laboratory findings of acute cholecystitis or no abnormal laboratory findings

May be laboratory findings of associated cholelithiasis

CHOLELITHIASIS

Laboratory findings of underlying conditions causing hypercholesterolemia (e.g., diabetes mellitus)

Laboratory findings of causative chronic hemolytic disease (e.g., hereditary spherocytosis)

Laboratory findings of resultant cholecystitis or choledocholithiasis, etc.

CHOLEDOCHOLITHIASIS

During or soon after an attack of biliary colic
    Increased WBC
    Increased serum bilirubin in ≅ one-third of patients
    Increased urine bilirubin in ≅ one-third of patients
    Increased serum and urine amylase

Fluctuating laboratory evidence of biliary obstruction (see p. 251)

Laboratory findings due to secondary cholangitis

In duodenal drainage, crystals of both calcium bilirubinate and cholesterin (some patients); 50% accurate (only useful in nonicteric patients)

BILIARY DYSKINESIA

Normal laboratory tests of biliary, hepatic, and pancreatic function

Normal WBC

CANCER OF GALLBLADDER AND BILE DUCTS

Laboratory findings reflect varying location and extent of tumor infiltration that may cause partial intrahepatic duct obstruction or obstruction of hepatic or common bile duct, metastases in liver or associated cholangitis (see pp. 251–255, 262, 268); 50% of patients have jaundice at the time of hospitalization.

Laboratory findings of duct obstruction are of progressively increasing severity in contrast to the intermittent or fluctuating changes due to duct obstruction caused by stones. A papillary intraluminal duct carcinoma may undergo periods of sloughing, producing the findings of intermittent duct obstruction.

Stool is frequently positive for occult blood.

Anemia is present.

Cytologic examination of aspirated duodenal fluid may demonstrate malignant cells.

Laboratory findings of the preceding cholelithiasis are present (gallbladder cancer occurs in ≅ 3% of patients with gallstones).

PARASITIC INFESTATION OF BILIARY SYSTEM
Laboratory findings due to biliary obstruction and to cholangitis
Infestation due to *Echinococcus, Ascaris,* liver flukes

POSTOPERATIVE JAUNDICE
This is usually due to a combination of factors.
Overproduction of bilirubin
Resorption of blood (e.g., hematoma, hemoperitoneum)
Glucose-6-PD deficiency (see p. 353)
Sickle cell disease (see p. 345)
Hemolysis of transfused RBCs. The amount of hemoglobin produced is insufficient to cause jaundice unless other conditions (e.g., sepsis, hypoxemia, anesthesia) are present.
Impaired hepatocellular function
Halothane toxicity: Occurs 1:10,000 cases. WBC is increased in 2 days. Jaundice may not appear for several weeks but may occur earlier if there has been previous exposure. Laboratory findings of severe liver necrosis are present (e.g., marked increase of SGOT, prolonged prothrombin time), and there is 20% fatality.
Shock: Severe jaundice in 2% of patients is due to trauma. *(Multiple factors are usually present, e.g., drugs, infection, transfusions.)* Serum bilirubin reaches 5–20 mg/dl 2–10 days after surgery; SGOT is 100–500 units; serum alkaline phosphatase is 2–3 times normal. *Clinical jaundice is found in only 20% of patients with massive liver necrosis.*
Syndrome of benign postoperative intrahepatic cholestasis: Occurs in patients with difficult prolonged surgery, multiple transfusions, postoperative complications (e.g., hemorrhage, sepsis, kidney failure, heart failure). Serum bilirubin reaches 15–40 mg/dl 2–10 days after surgery; SGOT is usually < 200 units; serum alkaline phosphatase shows marked but variable increase. Liver biopsy reveals dilated bile canaliculi with bile casts, and minimal necrosis or infiltration of lymphocytes.
Bacterial infections, especially gram-negative septicemia and pneumococcal pneumonia: Occurs 5–12 days after onset of infection. Increased serum bilirubin is mild; there is variable increase in SGOT and serum alkaline phosphatase. Liver biopsy reveals intrahepatic cholestasis with mild periportal infiltration of leukocytes; there is little or no hepatic cell necrosis.
Preexisting anicteric hepatitis or cirrhosis
Drugs (see Table 24-5, p. 260)
Extrahepatic bile duct obstruction
Injury to bile duct. Jaundice usually occurs within 1 week. See also Primary Sclerosing Cholangitis, p. 267; Suppurative Cholangitis, p. 268.
See also Cholecystitis, p. 269; Choledocholithiasis, p. 269.

ACUTE PANCREATITIS

Serum amylase increase begins in 3–6 hours, rises to >250 Somogyi units within 8 hours in 75% of patients, reaches maximum in 20–30 hours, and may persist for 48–72 hours. The increase may be ≦ 40 times normal, but the height of the increase and rate of fall do not correlate with the severity of the disease, prognosis, or rate of resolution; however, a prolonged increase suggests an associated cancer of pancreas or a complication (e.g., pseudocyst). The level should be ≧ 500 Somogyi units/dl to be significant of acute pancreatitis. *Similar high values may occur in obstruction of pancreatic duct; they tend to fall after several days. >10% of patients with acute pancreatitis may have normal values, even when dying of acute pancreatitis.*

Serum lipase increases in 50% of patients and may remain elevated for as long as 14 days after amylase returns to normal. *(Lipase should always be determined whenever amylase is determined, since the amylase may have already returned to normal values.)* Urinary lipase is not clinically useful.

Serum calcium is decreased in severe cases 1–9 days after onset (due to binding to soaps in fat necrosis). The decrease usually occurs after amylase and lipase levels have become normal. Tetany may occur. *(Rule out hyperparathyroidism if serum calcium is high or fails to fall in hyperamylasemia of acute pancreatitis.)*

Increased urinary amylase tends to reflect serum changes by a time lag of 6–10 hours, but sometimes increased urine levels are higher and of longer duration than serum levels. The 24-hour level may be normal even when some of the 1-hour specimens show increased values. Amylase levels in hourly samples of urine may be useful (>40 Somogyi units/hour). Ratio of amylase clearance to creatinine clearance is increased (>5%) and avoids the problem of timed urine specimens.

Serum bilirubin may be increased when pancreatitis is of biliary tract origin but is usually normal in alcoholic pancreatitis. SGOT may correlate with serum bilirubin rather than with amylase, lipase, or calcium levels. Serum alkaline phosphatase is increased when serum bilirubin is elevated and parallels serum bilirubin.

Serum trypsin is increased.

WBC is slightly to moderately increased (10,000–20,000/cu mm).

Hemoconcentration occurs (increased hematocrit). Hematocrit may be decreased in severe hemorrhagic pancreatitis.

Glycosuria appears in 25% of patients.

Ascites may develop, cloudy or bloody or "prune juice" fluid, 0.5–2.0 L in volume, containing increased amylase with a level higher than that of serum amylase. No bile is evident (unlike in perforated ulcer). Gram stain shows no bacteria (unlike in infarct of intestine).

Adult respiratory distress syndrome (with pleural effusion, alveolar exudate, or both) may occur in ≅ 40% of patients; arterial hypoxemia is present.

Hypokalemia, metabolic alkalosis, or lactic acidosis may occur.

Laboratory findings due to predisposing conditions

    Alcoholism and biliary tract disease account for 65–90% of cases.

    Idiopathic (up to 25% of cases)

Infections (especially viral)
Trauma and postoperative
Drugs (e.g., steroids, thiazides, azathioprine)
Tumors (pancreas, ampulla)
Hereditary
Miscellaneous (collagen vascular disease, pregnancy, ischemia)

Poorer prognosis is indicated when $\geq$ 3 of the following laboratory findings are present:

Initial WBC > 16,000/cu mm
Initial blood glucose > 200 mg/dl
Initial serum LDH > 350 IU/L
Initial SGOT > 2500 Sigma units/L
Decreased serum calcium < 8.0 mg/dl
Fall in hematocrit > 10%
Rise in BUN > 5 mg/dl
Arterial PO_2 < 60 mmHg
Metabolic acidosis with base deficit > 4 mEq/L

Diagnostic Efficiency of Amylase and Lipase in Acute Pancreatitis

	Sensitivity (%)	Specificity (%)
Serum amylase	70–98	70–76
Urine amylase	80–98	80–90
Amylase-creatinine clearance ratio	93–100	80–97
Amylase isoenzymes	100	92
Serum lipase	75–100	70–86
Serum amylase and lipase	Up to 90–97	

CHRONIC PANCREATIC DISEASE (CHRONIC PANCREATITIS; CARCINOMA OF PANCREAS)

Examine duodenal contents (volume, bicarbonate concentration, amylase output) after IV administration of pancreozymin and secretin. Some abnormality occurs in > 85% of patients with chronic pancreatitis. Amylase output is the most frequent abnormality. When all three are abnormal, there is a greater frequency of abnormality in the tests listed below.

Serum amylase and lipase increase after administration of pancreozymin and secretin in $\cong$ 20% of patients with chronic pancreatitis. They are more often abnormal when duodenal contents are normal.

Fasting serum amylase and lipase increase in 10% of patients with chronic pancreatitis.

There will be a diabetic oral glucose tolerance test (GTT) in 65% of patients with chronic pancreatitis and frank diabetes in >10% of patients with chronic relapsing pancreatitis. When GTT is normal in the presence of steatorrhea, the cause should be sought elsewhere than in the pancreas.

Chemical determination of fecal fat demonstrates steatorrhea. It is more sensitive than tests using triolein [131]I.

Triolein ^{131}I is abnormal in one-third of patients with chronic pancreatitis.

Starch tolerance test is abnormal in 25% of patients with chronic pancreatitis.

Radioactive scanning of pancreas (selenium) yields variable findings in different clinics.

See Laboratory Diagnosis of Malabsorption, p. 236.

Laboratory findings due to underlying conditions are noted (e.g., alcoholism, trauma, duodenal ulcer, cholelithiasis).

PSEUDOCYST OF PANCREAS

Serum direct bilirubin is increased (>2 mg/dl) in 10% of patients.

Serum alkaline phosphatase is increased (>5 Bodansky units) in 10% of patients.

Fasting blood sugar is increased in $<10\%$ of patients.

Laboratory findings of preceding acute pancreatitis are present (this is mild and unrecognized in one-third of patients). Persistent increase of serum amylase and lipase after an acute episode may indicate formation of a pseudocyst.

Duodenal contents after secretin-pancreozymin stimulation usually show decreased bicarbonate content (<70 mEq/L) but normal volume and normal content of amylase, lipase, and trypsin.

Laboratory findings due to conditions preceding acute pancreatitis are noted (e.g., alcoholism, trauma, duodenal ulcer, cholelithiasis).

CYSTIC FIBROSIS OF PANCREAS (MUCOVISCIDOSIS)

Striking increase in sweat sodium and chloride (>60 mEq/L) and, to a lesser extent, potassium is present in virtually all homozygous patients. It is present throughout life from time of birth and is not related to severity of disease or organ involvement. There is a broad range of values in this disease and in normal but minimal overlap (see Sweat Electrolytes, p. 187). *(Sweat chloride is somewhat more reliable than sodium for diagnostic purposes.)* Sweat sodium and chloride increase is not useful for determination of heterozygosity or genetic counseling.

Serum chloride, sodium, potassium, calcium, and phosphorus are normal unless complications occur (e.g., chronic pulmonary disease with accumulation of CO_2, massive salt loss due to sweating).

Urine electrolytes are normal.

Submaxillary saliva has slightly increased chloride and sodium but not potassium; however, considerable overlap with normal persons prevents diagnostic use. Submaxillary saliva also is more turbid, with increased calcium, total protein, and amylase. These changes are not generally found in parotid saliva.

Serum protein electrophoresis shows increasing gamma globulin with progressive pulmonary disease, mainly due to immunoglobulins G and A; M and D are not appreciably increased.

Glucose intolerance in $\cong 40\%$ of patients with glycosuria and hyperglycemia in 8%

Serum albumin is often decreased (because of hemodilution due to cor pulmonale; may be found before cardiac involvement is clinically apparent). In late stages of chronic lung disease, decreased serum electrolytes, hemoglobin, hematocrit level, etc., may also reflect hemodilution.

Bacteriology: Hemolytic *Staphylococcus aureus* is the most frequent and important organism in the respiratory tract; *Pseudomonas aeruginosa* has recently been found increasingly often.

Adrenal and pituitary function tests are normal.

Laboratory changes secondary to complications (e.g., pancreatic deficiency, chronic pulmonary disease, sinusitis, nasal polyps, excessive loss of electrolytes in sweat, biliary cirrhosis, cholelithiasis, aspermia, intestinal obstruction)

> Pancreas (see Laboratory Diagnosis of Malabsorption, p. 236
>> 80% of patients show loss of all pancreatic enzyme activity.
>> 10% of patients show decrease of pancreatic enzyme activity.
>> 10% of patients show normal pancreatic enzyme activity.
> Cirrhosis (in > 25% of patients at autopsy)
> Chronic lung disease (especially upper lobes) with laboratory changes due to accumulation of CO_2, severe recurrent infection, secondary cor pulmonale, etc.
> Meconium ileus during early infancy

Stool and duodenal fluid show lack of trypsin digestion of x-ray film gelatin; this is a useful screening test up to age 4; decreased chymotrypsin production gauged by bentiromide (Chymex) test (see p. 175).

CARCINOMA OF BODY OR TAIL OF PANCREAS

Laboratory tests are often normal.

Serum amylase and lipase may be slightly increased in early stages (< 10% of cases); with later destruction of pancreas, they are normal or decreased. They may increase following secretin-pancreozymin stimulation before destruction is extensive; therefore, the increase is less marked with a diabetic glucose tolerance curve. Serum amylase response is less reliable.

Glucose tolerance curve is of the diabetic type with overt diabetes in 20% of patients with pancreatic cancer. Flat blood sugar curve with IV tolbutamide tolerance test indicates destruction of islet cell tissue. Unstable, insulin-sensitive diabetes that develops in an older man should arouse suspicion of carcinoma of the pancreas.

Secretin-pancreozymin stimulation evidences duct obstruction when duodenal intubation shows decreased volume of duodenal contents (< 10 ml/10-minute collection period) with usually normal bicarbonate and enzyme levels in duodenal contents. Acinar destruction (as in pancreatitis) shows normal volume (20–30 ml/10-minute collection period), but bicarbonate and enzyme levels may be decreased. Abnormal volume, bicarbonate, or both is found in 60–80% of patients with pancreatitis or cancer. In carcinoma, the test result depends on the relative extent and combination of acinar destruction and of duct obstruction. Cytologic examination of duodenal contents shows malignant cells in 40% of patients. Malignant cells may be found in up to 80% of patients with periampullary cancer.

Serum leucine aminopeptidase (LAP) is increased (> 300 units) in 60% of patients with carcinoma of pancreas due to liver metastases or biliary tract obstruction. *It may also be increased in chronic liver disease.*

Triolein ^{131}I test demonstrates pancreatic duct obstruction with absence of lipase in the intestine causing flat blood curves and increased stool excretion.

Radioisotope scanning of pancreas may be done (^{75}Se) for lesions > 2 cm.

CARCINOMA OF HEAD OF PANCREAS

The abnormal pancreatic function tests that occur with carcinoma of the body of the pancreas (see p. 274) may be evident.

Laboratory findings due to complete obstruction of common bile duct

    Serum bilirubin increased (12–25 mg/dl), mostly direct (increase persistent and nonfluctuating)

    Serum alkaline phosphatase increased (usually 12–30 Bodansky units)

    Urine and stool urobilinogen absent

    Increased prothrombin time; normal after IV vitamin K administration

    Increased serum cholesterol (usually > 300 mg/dl) with esters not decreased

    Other liver function tests are usually normal.

The most useful diagnostic tests are ultrasound or CAT scanning followed by endoscopic retrograde cholangiopancreatography (ERCP) (at which time fluid is also obtained for cytologic and pancreatic function studies). This combination will correctly diagnose or rule out cancer of pancreas in ≧ 90% of cases.

CEA level in bile (obtained by percutaneous transhepatic drainage) was reported elevated in 76% of a small group of cases.

Needle biopsy (with radiologic guidance) may be positive.

See tests listed in sections on other diseases of pancreas, pp. 271–275.

MACROAMYLASEMIA

Serum amylase persistently increased

Urine amylase normal or low

Amylase-creatinine clearance ratio < 1% with normal renal function

Macroamylase is identified in serum by special gel filtration technique.

May be found in ≅ 1% of randomly selected patients and 2.5% of persons with increased serum amylase.

Diseases of the Central and Peripheral Nervous System

METABOLIC CAUSES OF COMA
Hypoglycemia (due to insulin, liver diseases, etc.)
Metabolic deficiencies (e.g., vitamin B_{12}, thiamine, niacin, pyridoxine)
Diseases of other organs
    Hepatic coma
    Uremia
    Lung (CO_2 narcosis)
    Pancreas (diabetic coma, hypoglycemia)
    Thyroid (myxedema, thyrotoxicosis)
    Parathyroid (hypoparathyroidism, hyperparathyroidism)
    Adrenal (Addison's disease, pheochromocytoma, Cushing's syndrome)
    Pituitary
    Porphyria
    Aminoacidurias
    Also leukodystrophies, lipid storage diseases, Bassen-Kornzweig syndrome, etc.
Abnormalities of electrolytes and acid-base balance
    Acidosis (metabolic, respiratory)
    Alkalosis (metabolic, respiratory)
    Water and sodium (hypernatremia, hyponatremia)
    Serum potassium (increased, decreased)
    Serum calcium (increased, decreased)
    Serum magnesium (increased, decreased)
Poisons
    Sedatives (especially alcohol, barbiturates)
    Enzyme inhibitors (especially salicylates, heavy metals, organic phosphates, cyanide)
    Other (e.g., methyl alcohol, paraldehyde, ethylene glycol)
Cerebral hypoxia
    Decreased blood O_2 content with normal tension (e.g., anemia, carbon monoxide poisoning, methemoglobinemia)
    Decreased blood O_2 content and tension (e.g., decreased atmospheric PO_2 [high altitude] lung disease, alveolar hypoventilation)
Cerebral ischemia
    Decreased cardiac output (e.g., cardiac arrhythmias and Adams-Stokes disease, congestive heart failure, myocardial infarction, aortic stenosis)
    Decreased peripheral resistance in systemic circulation (e.g., low blood volume, syncope, carotid sinus hypersensitivity)
    Increased cerebral vascular resistance (e.g., increased blood viscosity as in polycythemia, hypertensive encephalopathy, hyperventilation syndrome)

SOME CONDITIONS ASSOCIATED WITH EPILEPSY THAT MAY HAVE ASSOCIATED LABORATORY ABNORMALITIES

Metabolic
>   Carbohydrate (e.g., glycogen storage disease, hypoglycemia)
>   Protein (e.g., phenylketonuria, maple syrup urine disease)
>   Fat (e.g., leukodystrophies, lipidoses)
>   Electrolytes (e.g., hypocalcemia, hypomagnesemia, hyponatremia, hypernatremia)
>   Other (e.g., porphyria)

Malformations (e.g., vascular malformations and shunts)

Infections
>   Fetal (e.g., rubella, cytomegalic inclusion disease, toxoplasmosis)
>   Encephalitis, meningitis
>   Postinfectious encephalitis (e.g., measles, mumps)

Allergic (e.g., postvaccinal encephalitis, drug reaction)

Circulatory (e.g., thrombosis, embolism, hemorrhage, hypertensive encephalopathy)

Neoplasms

Degenerative diseases of the brain

Hematologic (e.g., sickle cell anemia, leukemia)

Normal CSF

Found in
>   Korsakoff's syndrome
>   Wernicke's encephalopathy
>   Alzheimer's disease (diffuse cerebral atrophy)
>   Jakob-Creutzfeldt disease
>   Tuberous sclerosis (protein rarely increased)
>   Idiopathic epilepsy (*If protein is increased, rule out neoplasms; if cell count is increased, rule out neoplasm or inflammation.*)
>   Narcolepsy, cataplexy, etc.
>   Parkinson's disease
>   Hereditary cerebellar degenerations
>   Huntington's disease
>   Migraine
>   Ménière's syndrome
>   Psychiatric conditions (e.g., neurocirculatory asthenia, hysteria, depression, anxiety, schizophrenia) (*Rule out psychiatric condition as a manifestation of primary disease, e.g., drugs, porphyria, primary endocrine diseases.*)
>   Transient cerebral ischemia
>   Amyotrophic lateral sclerosis
>   Muscular dystrophy
>   Progressive muscular atrophy
>   Syringomyelia
>   Vitamin B_{12} deficiency with subacute combined degeneration of spinal cord
>   Pellagra
>   Beriberi
>   Subacute myelo-opticoneuropathy (SMON)
>   Minimal brain dysfunction of childhood
>   Cerebral palsies
>   Febrile convulsions of childhood

See Chapter 31 for metabolic and hereditary diseases that affect the nervous system (e.g., gangliosidosis, mucopolysaccharidoses, glycogen storage disease).

Table 25-1 Cerebrospinal Fluid Findings in Various Diseases

Disease	Appearance	Initial Pressure (mm of water)	Protein (mg/dl)	Fasting Sugar (mg/dl)	WBC/cu mm
Normal					
Ventricular	Clear, colorless, no clot	70–180	5–15	45–80	0–10
Cisternal			10–25		
Lumbar			15–45		
Tuberculous meningitis	O, slightly yellow, delicate clot	Usually I	45–500	10–45	25–1000, chiefly L
Acute pyogenic meningitis	O–Pu, slightly yellow, coarse clot	Usually I	50–1500	0–45	25–10,000, chiefly P
Aseptic meningeal reaction	C or T or X	Often N	20–200+	N	≦ 500, occasionally 2000
Syphilis Tabes dorsalis	N	N	25–100	N	10–80
General paresis	N	N	50–300	N	10–150
Meningovascular syphilis	N	N	45–150, N in 30% of patients	N	10–100, N in 45%

Acute anterior poliomyelitis	C or slightly O, may be slightly yellow, may be delicate clot	Usually N, may be I	20–350	N	10–500+, L > P
Other virus Mumps	N or O	N or slightly I	20–125	N	0–2000+
Measles	N or O	N or slightly I	Slightly I	N	≤500
Herpes zoster	N	N	20–110	N	≤300, 40% of patients
Equine, St. Louis encephalitis, choriomeningitis	N or slightly T	N or I	20–200+	N	10–200, occasionally to 3000
Postinfectious encephalitis	N	May be slightly I	15–75	N	5–200, rarely to 1000
Toxoplasmosis (congenital)	X	I	≤2000		50–500, chiefly monocytes
Cryptococcal meningitis	N	I	≤500 in 90%	Moderately decreased in 55%	≤800 (L > P)
Coccidioidomycosis		I	I	N early, then D	≤200 early; may be higher later

Table 25-1 (continued)

Disease	Appearance	Initial Pressure (mm of water)	Protein (mg/dl)	Fasting Sugar (mg/dl)	WBC/cu mm
Primary amebic meningoencephalitis (due to free-living *Naegleria*)	Sanguino-purulent, may be T or Pu	I	I	Usually D	400–21,000 (predominantly P). Usually RBCs are also found. Amebas seen on Wright's stain
Tumor Cord	C, occasionally X	N or D	≦3500 in 85%, N in 15%	N	≦100, chiefly L; N in 60%
Brain	C, occasionally X	I	≦500	N	≦150, N in 75%
Pseudotumor cerebri	N	I	N	N	N
Cerebral thrombosis	N	25% I, 75% N	≦100+, N in 60%	N	≦50, N in 75%
Cerebral hemorrhage	N in 15%, X in 10%, B in 75%	80% I, 20% N	≦2000, usually I	N	Same as in blood, N in 10%
Subarachnoid hemorrhage (ruptured berry aneurysm)	B, X in 24 hours, no clot	Usually I	≦1000+, usually I	N	Same as in blood

	B	N or D	I by blood	N	Same as in blood
Bloody tap (traumatic)			I by blood	N	Same as in blood
Head trauma	N, B, or X	Often I	I if bloody	N	Same as in blood
Subdural hematoma	N, B only with contusion	80% I, 20% N	N or slightly I	N	Same as in blood
Multiple sclerosis (see pp. 295–296)	N	N	≦130, N in 75%; IgG I in 75%	N	≦40, N in 70%
Polyneuritis Polyarteritis	N; X if protein is very I	N	Usually N	N	N, but albuminocytologic dissociation in Guillain-Barré syndrome that may occur in heavy metal poisoning, infection, etc.
Porphyria		N	Usually N	N	
Beriberi		N	Usually N	N	
Alcohol		N	Usually N	N	
Arsenic		N	Usually N	N	
Diabetes mellitus		N	Often ≦300	N	
Acute infections		N	≦1500	N	
Lead encephalopathy	N or slightly yellow	I	≦100	N	0–100

Table 25-1 (continued)

Disease	Appearance	Initial Pressure (mm of water)	Protein (mg/dl)	Fasting Sugar (mg/dl)	WBC/cu mm
Alcoholism	N	May be I	N	N	Usually N
Diabetic coma	N	D	N	I	Usually N
Uremia	N	Usually I	N or I	N or I	Usually N
Epilepsy	N	N	N	N	N

C = clear; O = opalescent; T = turbid; N = normal; X = xanthochromic; B = bloody; Pu = purulent; I = increased; D = decreased; P = polynuclear neutrophilic leukocyte; L = lymphocyte.

CEREBROSPINAL FLUID (CSF)

Viscous CSF may occur with metastatic mucinous adenocarcinoma (e.g., colon), large numbers of cryptococci, or rarely, injury to annulus fibrosus with release of nucleus pulposus fluid.

Turbidity may be due to presence of microorganisms (bacteria, fungi, amebae), contrast media, epidural fat aspirated during lumbar puncture, as well as increased WBC or RBC.

WBC of 200–300/cu mm causes cloudiness of CSF.

Protein > 100 mg/dl usually causes CSF to look faintly yellow.

CSF with RBC > 6000/cu mm appears grossly bloody; with RBC = 500–6000/cu mm appears cloudy, xanthochromic, or pink-tinged (in bright light in clear glass tubes containing > 1 ml of CSF).

Xanthochromia may be due to prior (at least 2–4 hours) bleeding, or markedly elevated protein (>150 mg/dl), or serum bilirubin > 6 mg/dl.

CSF WBC may be corrected for presence of blood (e.g., traumatic tap, subarachnoid hemorrhage) by subtracting 1 WBC for each 700 RBCs/cu mm counted in CSF if the CBC is normal. If there is significant anemia or leukocytosis,

$$\text{Corrected WBC} = \text{WBC in bloody CSF} - \frac{\text{WBC (blood)} \times \text{RBC (CSF)}}{\text{RBC (blood)}}$$

(all values are cells per cu mm)

CSF total protein may be corrected for presence of blood by subtracting 1 mg/dl of protein for each 1000 RBCs/cu mm (if serum protein and CBC are normal and CSF protein and cell count are performed on same tube of CSF).

WBCs are usually polynuclear leukocytes in early stages of all types of meningitis; mononuclear cells only appear later. Similarly, protein may not be increased in early stages of many types of meningitis.

CSF glucose is decreased by utilization by bacteria (pyogens or tubercle bacilli) or occasionally cancer cells in CSF. Normally is about 60–80% of blood glucose, which should be drawn simultaneously. CSF glucose lags behind blood glucose by about 1 hour. In pyogenic meningitis, is usually < 50% of blood level; may rapidly become normal after onset of antibiotic therapy; is decreased in only ≅ 50% of cases of bacterial meningitis. May be decreased in 10–20% of cases of lymphocytic choriomeningitis, encephalitis due to mumps or herpes simplex. May also be decreased in rheumatoid meningitis, lupus myelopathy, chemical meningitis, meningeal parasites, hypoglycemia, granulomatous meningitis (e.g., sarcoid), some cases of subarachnoid hemorrhage. 40–45 mg/dl is almost always abnormal. CSF glucose < 40 mg/dl is always abnormal.

CSF lactic acid is increased (>35 mg/dl) in both bacterial and fungal meningitis but not in viral meningitis. Level is still high after 1–2 days of antibiotic therapy in bacterial meningitis. Is increased whenever CSF glucose is very low or CSF WBC is elevated.

CSF protein, glucose, and WBC levels may not return to normal in ≅ 50% of cases clinically cured of bacterial meningitis and therefore are not recommended as a test of cure.

CSF protein is normal in 10% of patients with bacterial meningitis (20% of meningococcal meningitis).

CSF protein > 500 mg/dl is infrequent and occurs chiefly in meningitis, bloody CSF, or cord tumor with spinal block and occasionally in polyneuritis and brain tumor. With complete spinal block, the lower the level of cord tumor, the higher the protein concentration.

CSF protein may show mild to moderate elevation in myxedema (25% of cases), uremia, connective tissue disorders, Cushing's syndrome.

Decreased CSF protein (3–20 mg/dl) may occur in hyperthyroidism, one-third of patients with benign intracranial hypertension, after removal of large volumes of CSF (e.g., during pneumoencephalography), in children 6–24 months old.

CSF chloride reflects only blood chloride level, although in tuberculous meningitis a decrease of 25% may exceed the decrease of serum chloride due to dehydration and electrolyte loss. Is not useful in diagnosis of tuberculous meningitis.

CSF glutamine > 35 mg/dl is associated with hepatic encephalopathy (due to conversion from ammonia).

Blood and CSF serology is positive in CNS syphilis (see p. 138); positive in 7–10% of active cases of infectious mononucleosis

Colloidal gold test is no longer used and replaced by protein electrophoresis of CSF. IgG in CSF is increased 14–35% in two-thirds of patients with neurosyphilis. IgG oligoclonal bands are seen in neurosyphilis as well as in multiple sclerosis.

Smears for Gram and acid-fast stains must be made routinely, since the other findings may be normal in meningitis. Occasionally animal inoculations may be required. Gram stain of CSF sediment is positive in ≅ 80% of cases of meningitis and negative in 20% because at least 10^5 bacteria/ml CSF must be present to demonstrate 1–2 bacteria/100 × microscopic field.

Positive CSF culture has sensitivity of 92%, specificity of 95%, false negative rate of 8%, false positive rate of 5%.

Limulus amebocyte lysate is a rapid specific indicator of endotoxin produced by gram-negative bacteria (*Neisseria meningitidis, Hemophilus influenzae* type B, *Escherichia coli, Pseudomonas*). Is not affected by prior antibiotic therapy; is more rapid and sensitive than counterimmunoelectrophoresis (CIE).

CIE detects bacterial antigens in CSF; identifies *H. influenzae* and meningococci but does not recognize *N. meningitidis* group B.

In eclampsia, CSF shows gross or microscopic blood and increased protein (up to 200 mg/dl) in most cases. Glucose is normal. Uric acid is increased (to 3 times normal level) in all cases reflecting the marked increase in serum level. (In normal pregnancy, CSF values have same reference range as in nonpregnant women.)

The presence of leukemic cells in CSF in children with myelogenous leukemia indicates need for intrathecal chemotherapy.

DIFFERENTIATION OF BLOODY CSF DUE TO SUBARACHNOID HEMORRHAGE AND TRAUMATIC LUMBAR PUNCTURE

CSF Findings	Subarachnoid Hemorrhage	Traumatic Lumbar Puncture
CSF pressure	Often increased	Low
Blood in tubes for collecting CSF	Mixture with blood is uniform in all tubes	Earlier tubes more bloody than later tubes

CSF clotting	Does not clot	Often clots
Xanthochromia	Present if more than 8–12 hours since cerebral hemorrhage	Absent unless patient is icteric
Immediate repeat of lumbar puncture at higher level	CSF same as initial puncture	CSF clear

TRANSAMINASE (GOT) IN CEREBROSPINAL FLUID

Normal CSF is not permeable to serum enzymes. Changes in GOT are irregular and generally of limited diagnostic value.

Increased In

Large infarcts of brain during first 10 days. (In severe cases, serum GOT may also be increased; occurs in ≅ 40% of patients.)

≅ 40% of CNS tumors (various benign, malignant, and metastatic), depending on location, growth rate, etc.; chiefly useful as indicator of organic neurologic disease

Some other conditions (e.g., head injury, subarachnoid hemorrhage)

LACTIC DEHYDROGENASE (LDH) IN CEREBROSPINAL FLUID

Changes are of limited diagnostic value.

Increased In

Cerebrovascular accidents—increase occurs frequently, reaches maximum level in 1–3 days, and is apparently not related to xanthochromia, RBC, WBC, protein, sugar, or chloride levels.

CNS tumors (primary and metastatic), depending on location, growth rate, etc.

Meningitis—mild increase in viral meningitis due to LDH_1 and LDH_2; more marked increase in bacterial meningitis due to LDH_4 and LDH_5

CREATINE KINASE (CK) IN SPINAL FLUID

Test not useful because

It does not consistently increase in various CNS diseases

No relationship to CSF protein, WBC, or RBC values

No pattern of relationship of LDH and GOT in CSF

No correlation of serum CK and cerebrospinal fluid CK

See Serum Creatine Kinase, p. 67.

HEAD TRAUMA

Laboratory findings due to single or various combinations of brain injuries

Contusion

Laceration

Subdural hemorrhage

Extradural hemorrhage

Subarachnoid hemorrhage

Laboratory findings due to complications (e.g., pneumonia, meningitis)

In possible skull fractures, it has been recommended that nasal secretions may be differentiated from CSF by absence of glucose (using test tapes or tablets) in latter, but this is not reliable since nasal secretions may normally contain glucose. If enough fluid can be obtained to perform immunoelectrophoresis, CSF transferrin shows a double arc (gull wing), but serum transferrin has a single arc.

ACUTE EPIDURAL HEMORRHAGE
CSF is usually under increased pressure; clear unless there is associated cerebral contusion, laceration, or subarachnoid hemorrhage.

SUBDURAL HEMATOMA
CSF findings are variable—clear, bloody, or xanthochromic, depending on recent or old associated injuries (e.g., contusion, laceration).

Chronic subdural hematoma fluid is usually xanthochromic; protein content is 300–2000 mg/dl.

Anemia is often present in infants.

CEREBROVASCULAR ACCIDENT (NONTRAUMATIC)

Due to

Occlusion (thrombosis, embolism, etc.) in 80% of patients
Hemorrhage
    Ruptured berry aneurysm (45% of patients)
    Hypertension (15% of patients)
    Angiomatous malformations (8% of patients)
    Miscellaneous (e.g., brain tumor, blood dyscrasia)—infrequent
    Undetermined (rest of patients)
CSF
    In early subarachnoid hemorrhage (< 8 hours after onset of symptoms), the test for occult blood may be positive before xanthochromia develops. After bloody spinal fluid occurs, WBC/RBC ratio may be higher in CSF than in peripheral blood.
    Bloody CSF clears by tenth day in 40% of patients. CSF is persistently abnormal after 21 days in 15% of patients. ≅ 5% of cerebrovascular episodes due to hemorrhage are wholly within the parenchyma with normal CSF.

See Serum Creatine Kinase, pp. 67–68.
See Serum Transaminase, p. 64.

CEREBRAL THROMBOSIS
Laboratory findings due to some diseases that may be causative
    Hematologic (e.g., polycythemia, sickle cell disease, thrombotic thrombopenia, macroglobulinemia)
    Arterial (e.g., polyarteritis nodosa, Takayasu's syndrome, dissecting aneurysm of aorta, syphilis, meningitis)
    Hypotension (e.g., myocardial infarction, shock)

CSF
> Protein normal or may be increased ≦ 100 mg/dl
> Cell count normal or ≧ 10 leukocytes/cu mm during first 48 hours and rarely ≧ 2000 leukocytes/cu mm transiently on third day

See Serum Creatine Kinase, p. 67.
See Serum Transaminase, p. 64, and Table 25-1, pp. 278–282.

CEREBRAL EMBOLISM

Laboratory findings due to underlying causative disease
> Bacterial endocarditis
> Nonbacterial thrombotic vegetations on heart valves
> Chronic rheumatic mitral stenosis. (*Rule out underlying hypothyroidism.*)
> Mural thrombus due to underlying myocardial infarctions
> Myxoma of left atrium
> Myocardial infarction
> Fracture of long bones in fat embolism
> Neck, chest, or cardiac surgery in air embolism

CSF
> Usually findings are the same as in cerebral thrombosis. One-third of patients develop hemorrhagic infarction, usually producing slight xanthochromia several days later; some of these patients may have grossly bloody CSF (10,000 RBCs/cu mm). Septic embolism (e.g., bacterial endocarditis) may cause increased WBC (≦200/cu mm with variable lymphocytes and polynuclear leukocytes), increased RBC (≦1000/cu mm), slight xanthochromia, increased protein, normal sugar, negative culture.

INTRACEREBRAL HEMORRHAGE

Increased WBC (15,000–20,000/cu mm) (*higher than in cerebral occlusion, e.g., embolism, thrombosis*)
Increased ESR
Urine
> Transient glycosuria
> Laboratory findings of concomitant renal disease

Laboratory findings due to other causes of intracerebral hemorrhage (e.g., leukemia, aplastic anemia, purpuras, hemophilias, anticoagulant therapy, SLE, polyarteritis nodosa)

CSF
> See Table 25-1, pp. 278–282.
> See Differentiation of Bloody CSF, pp. 284–285.
> See Cerebrovascular Accident (Nontraumatic), p. 286.

Especially if blood pressure is normal, always rule out ruptured berry aneurysm, hemorrhage into tumor, angioma.

Laboratory findings due to other diseases that occur with increased frequency in association with berry aneurysm
> Coarctation of the aorta
> Polycystic kidneys
> Hypertension

RUPTURED BERRY ANEURYSM OF CEREBRAL VESSELS
See preceding section and Cerebrovascular Accident (Nontraumatic), p. 286.

ANGIOMAS OF BRAIN (ARTERIAL-VENOUS COMMUNICATIONS)
Laboratory findings due to complications
    Subarachnoid hemorrhage (20% of patients)
    Intracerebral hemorrhage (20% of patients)
    Convulsion (50% of patients)
Oxygen tension in jugular venous blood may be increased.

HYPERTENSIVE ENCEPHALOPATHY
Laboratory findings due to changes in other organ systems
    Cardiac
    Renal
    Endocrine
    Toxemia of pregnancy
Laboratory findings due to progressive changes that may occur (e.g., focal intracerebral hemorrhage)
CSF frequently shows increased pressure and protein $\leqq$ 100 mg/dl.

PSEUDOTUMOR CEREBRI
CSF normal except for increased pressure
Laboratory findings due to underlying causative condition
    Corticosteroid administration, usually after reduction of dosage or change to different preparation
    Sex hormone administration
    Addison's disease
    Lateral sinus thrombosis (most commonly after otitis media)
    Acute hypocalcemia
    Vitamin A intoxication

BRAIN TUMOR
CSF findings
    CSF is clear, occasionally xanthochromic or bloody if there is hemorrhage into the tumor.
    WBC may be increased $\leqq$ 150 cells/cu mm in 75% of patients; normal in others.
    Protein is usually increased.
    Tumor cells may be demonstrable in 20–40% of patients with all types of solid tumors, but failure to find malignant cells does not exclude meningeal neoplasm.
    Glucose may be decreased if cells are present.

    CSF protein is particularly increased with meningioma of the olfactory groove and with acoustic neurinoma.

    Brain stem gliomas, which are characteristically found in childhood, usually show normal CSF.
    "Diencephalic syndrome" of infants due to glioma of hypothalamus usually show normal CSF.

Laboratory findings due to underlying causative disease
    Primary brain tumors
    Metastatic tumors, especially of bronchus, breast, kidney, GI

tract (*hemorrhagic tumor particularly with choriocarcinoma and some bronchogenic carcinomas*)

Leukemias and lymphoma: Acute lymphocytic leukemia involves CNS more frequently than myeloblastic type. Meninges may be involved in 50% of patients with acute lymphocytic type.

Infections (e.g., tuberculoma, schistosomiasis, torulosis, hydatid cyst, cysticercosis)

Pituitary adenomas—CSF protein and pressure usually normal

LEUKEMIC INVOLVEMENT OF CNS

Intracranial hemorrhage—principal cause of death in leukemia (may be intracerebral, subarachnoid, subdural)

> More frequent when WBC is > 100,000/cu mm and with rapid increase in WBC, especially in blastic crises
>
> Platelet count frequently decreased
>
> Evidence of bleeding elsewhere
>
> Cerebrospinal fluid findings of intracranial hemorrhage (see p. 280)

Meningeal infiltration of leukemic cells: Meninges are involved in less than 5% of patients with malignant lymphoma, but malignant cells are found in CSF in 60–80% of cases with meningeal involvement.

> CSF may show
>> Increased pressure
>>
>> Increased cells that are not usually recognized as blast cells because of poor preservation
>>
>> Increased protein
>>
>> Glucose decreased to < 50% of blood level

Complicating meningeal infection (see next two sections)
> Various bacteria
>
> Opportunistic fungi (see pp. 630–631)

BACTERIAL MENINGITIS

CSF

See Table 25-1, pp. 278–282.

75% of cases are due to *N. meningitidis,* pneumococcus, *H. influenzae. Bacteria can be identified in only 90% of cases; culture is more reliable than Gram stain, although the stain offers a more immediate guide to therapy.*

Laboratory findings due to preceding diseases
> Pneumonia, otitis media, sinusitis, skull fracture prior to pneumococcal meningitis
>
> *Neisseria* epidemics prior to this meningitis
>
> Bacterial endocarditis, septicemia, etc.

Laboratory findings due to complications (e.g., Waterhouse-Friderichsen syndrome, subdural effusion)

ASEPTIC MENINGITIS

CSF

> Protein is normal or slightly increased.
>
> Increased cell count shows predominantly leukocytes at first, mononuclear cells later.
>
> Glucose is normal.
>
> Bacterial cultures are negative.

Table 25-2 Etiology of Bacterial Meningitis by Age

	Newborns	Less Than 1 Year	1–5 Years	5–14 Years	More Than 15 Years
Most frequent	*Escherichia coli*	*Hemophilus influenzae*		*Neisseria meningitidis*	*Pneumococcus*
Common	*Klebsiella-Aerobacter* Beta-hemolytic streptococcus *Staphylococcus aureus*	*Neisseria meningitidis* Pneumococcus		*Hemophilus influenzae* Pneumococcus	*Neisseria meningitidis* *Staphylococcus aureus*
Uncommon	Paracolon bacilli *Pseudomonas* species *Hemophilus influenzae*	*Pseudomonas* species *Staphylococcus aureus* Beta-hemolytic streptococcus *Escherichia coli*	Beta-hemolytic streptococcus		Beta-hemolytic streptococcus *Escherichia coli* *Pseudomonas* species
Rare	*Neisseria meningitidis*		*Klebsiella-Aerobacter*, paracolons, various other gram-negative organisms		*Hemophilus influenzae*

The frequency of different organisms may vary from year to year, in presence of epidemics, or by geographic location. Occasionally more than one organism is recovered.

Hemophilus influenzae (almost always type B) causes most cases between age 6 months and 3 years but is unusual before age 2 months. Enteric bacteria are so rarely found in older children that in their presence immunologic defect or congenital dermal sinus should be ruled out. If surgery has not been performed, congenital dermal sinus should be ruled out if *Staphylococcus aureus* is present.

A Gram stain of CSF should always be done in addition to a culture because it provides a more immediate clue to the causative agent and the proper therapy and because the culture may be negative if the patient received antibiotics soon before the lumbar puncture. Cultures should also be obtained from blood and petechial skin lesions if present. Gram stain of buffy coat of blood is often useful.

CSF glucose is very useful in differentiating bacterial and viral meningitis and is a good index to the severity of the infection, with a lower level in more severe infections. *Newborns with overwhelming pneumococcal infections may have no decrease in glucose or increase of cells.*

CSF should be reexamined in 24 hours as a guide to therapeutic response; a good response shows negative gram-stained smear and culture, increased glucose level, and a changing cell count from predominance of polymorphonuclear cells to predominance of mononuclear cells; total cell count and protein may show an initial rise. CSF should be reexamined when therapy is to be stopped; treatment should not be stopped unless CSF is normal except for slight increase of cells ($\leq$ about 20 lymphocytes).

If glucose levels are decreased, rule out tuberculosis, cryptococcosis, leukemia, lymphoma, metastatic carcinoma, sarcoidosis.

Due To (clinically most important types)
Viral infections (especially poliomyelitis, Coxsackievirus, echovirus, lymphocytic choriomeningitis, infectious mononucleosis, and many others)
Leptospirosis, syphilis
Tuberculosis, cryptococcosis (*CSF glucose levels may not be decreased until later stages.*)
Brain abscess, incompletely treated bacterial meningitis
Neoplasm (leukemia, carcinoma)

RECURRENT MENINGITIS

May Be Associated With
Bacterial infections
    Anatomic defects (traumatic or congenital)
    Adjacent foci of infection (e.g., paranasal sinusitis, mastoiditis, brain abscess, epidural abscess, subdural empyema)
    Immunologic deficiencies (e.g., sickle cell anemia, lymphoma, decreased immunoglobulins)
    Various infections (brucellosis, leptospirosis, tuberculosis, idiopathic)
Fungal infections
    Cryptococcosis
    Treatment failure in cases of blastomycosis, coccidioidomycosis, and histoplasmosis
Other infections
    Viral
    Cerebral hydatid cyst
Neoplasms of brain and spinal cord (e.g., hemangioma of third ventricle, ependymoma, craniopharyngioma)
Unknown etiology
    Sarcoidosis
    Mollaret's meningitis
    Behçet's syndrome
    Vogt-Koyanagi syndrome
    Harada's syndrome

PRIMARY AMEBIC MENINGOENCEPHALITIS
(due to free-living amebas—*Naegleria*)
Increased WBC, predominantly neutrophils
CSF findings (see Table 25-1, p. 280)
    Fluid may be cloudy, purulent, or sanguinopurulent.
    Protein is increased.
    Glucose is usually decreased; may be normal.
    Increased WBCs are chiefly polynuclear neutrophilic leukocytes. RBCs are frequently present also. Motile amebas are seen in hemocytometer chamber.
    Amebas are seen on Wright's stain. Gram's stain and cultures are negative for bacteria and fungi.

VON ECONOMO'S ENCEPHALITIS LETHARGICA
CSF changes appear in 50% of patients—increase in lymphocytes and variable increase in protein.

ACUTE ENCEPHALOMYELITIS
(postvaccinal, postexanthematous, postinfectious)
CSF shows increased protein and lymphocytes.
Laboratory findings due to preceding condition (e.g., measles) are
noted.

SUBACUTE SCLEROSING PANENCEPHALITIS
Chronic encephalitis associated with measles virus in children and
adolescents; insidious onset, slow progress of 3–4 years, usually
fatal.
CSF shows normal pressure and cell count; protein is normal or
slightly increased. Striking elevation of gamma globulins with
presence of oligoclonal bands on agarose gel electrophoresis (see
Multiple Sclerosis, pp. 295–296).

REYE'S SYNDROME
Childhood syndrome of pernicious vomiting without clinical jaun-
dice, beginning one week after an infection, with acute alter-
ations of consciousness or coma, not due to CNS infection, intoxi-
cation (e.g., salicylates, lead), or brain trauma.
SGOT and SGPT are increased to > 100 units.
Blood ammonia is increased (often > 200 µg/dl).
Prothrombin time is prolonged by 2 seconds or more.
Blood amino acids are increased (alanine, glutamine, lysine, alpha-
amino-n-butyrate), which distinguishes condition from severe
salicylism.
Liver biopsy shows marked fatty changes.
Serum LDH and CK (isoenzyme MM) may be increased due to mus-
cle damage.
Plasma free fatty acids are increased with pyruvic and lactic
acidosis (severe metabolic acidosis).
Hypoglycemia is often present.
Serum bilirubin and GGT are usually normal.
Serum uric acid and BUN may be increased.
CSF shows normal cell count; glucose is decreased proportional to
decreased serum level.

MOLLARET'S MENINGITIS
Numerous recurrent episodes (2–7 days each) of aseptic meningitis
occur over a period of several years with symptom-free intervals
showing mild leukopenia and eosinophilia. Other organ systems
are not involved. There is frequently a history of previous severe
trauma with fractures and concussions.
CSF during first 12–24 hours may contain ≦ several thousand cells/
cu mm, predominantly polynuclear neutrophils and 66% of a
large type of mononuclear cell. The mononuclear cells (sometimes
called "endothelial" cells) are of unknown origin and significance
and are characterized by vague nuclear and cytoplasmic outline
with rapid lysis even while being counted in the hemocytometer
chamber; they may be seen only as "ghosts" and are usually not
detectable after the first day of illness. After the first 24 hours,
the polynuclear neutrophils disappear and are replaced by lymphocytes, which, in turn, rapidly disappear when the attack subsides.
CSF protein may be increased ≦ 100 mg/dl. CSF glucose is normal
or may be slightly decreased.

CHEMICAL MENINGITIS
(due to injection of anesthetic, antibiotic, radiopaque dye, etc.)
CSF
Pleocytosis is mild to moderate, largely lymphocytic.
Protein shows variable increase.
Glucose is usually normal.

GUILLAIN-BARRÉ SYNDROME
CSF shows albuminocytologic dissociation with normal cell count and increased protein (average 50–100 mg/dl). Protein increase parallels increasing clinical severity; increase may be prolonged.
Laboratory findings due to underlying disease are noted (e.g., infectious mononucleosis, Refsum's disease).

MENTAL RETARDATION
Laboratory findings due to underlying causative condition (see appropriate separate sections)

Prenatal
Infections (e.g., syphilis, rubella, toxoplasmosis, cytomegalic inclusion disease)
Metabolic (e.g., diabetes mellitus, toxemia, placental dysfunction)
Chromosomal (e.g., Down's syndrome, E_{18} trisomy, cri du chat syndrome, Klinefelter's syndrome)
Metabolic abnormalities
Amino acid metabolism (e.g., phenylketonuria, maple syrup urine disease, hemocystinuria, cystathioninuria, hyperglycemia, arginosuccinicaciduria, citrullinemia, histidinemia, hyperprolinemia, oasthouse urine disease, Hartnup disease, Joseph's syndrome, familial iminoglycinuria)
Lipid metabolism (e.g., Batten's disease, Tay-Sachs disease, Niemann-Pick disease, abetalipoproteinemia, Refsum's disease, metachromatic leukodystrophy)
Carbohydrate metabolism (e.g., galactosemia, mucopolysaccharidoses)
Purine metabolism (e.g., Lesch-Nyhan syndrome, hereditary orotic aciduria)
Mineral metabolism (e.g., idiopathic hypercalcemia, pseudo- and pseudopseudohypoparathyroidism)
Other syndromes (e.g., tuberous sclerosis, Louis-Bar syndrome)

Perinatal
Kernicterus
Prematurity
Anoxia
Trauma

Postnatal
Poisoning (e.g., lead, arsenic, carbon monoxide)
Infections (e.g., meningitis, encephalitis)
Metabolic (e.g., hypoglycemia)
Postvaccinal encephalitis
Cerebrovascular accidents
Trauma

SENILE DEMENTIA (ALZHEIMER-PICK DISEASE; CEREBRAL ATROPHY)

There are no abnormal laboratory findings, but laboratory findings are useful to rule out other diseases that may resemble these syndromes but are amenable to therapy.

Metabolic: uremia, Wilson's disease

Endocrine: Cushing's syndrome, Addison's disease, hypo- or hyperthyroidism, hypo- or hyperparathyroidism, hyper- or hypoglycemia, hypopituitarism, SIADH

Deficiency: pellagra, pernicious anemia, folate deficiency

Toxic: bromism, drug abuse, lead and other heavy metal poisoning, alcohol abuse

Infectious: CNS lues, bacterial endocarditis, cerebral abscess, residua of viral encephalitis

Trauma: cerebral injury, subdural hematoma

Vascular: multiple infarcts

Collagen disease

Neoplastic: primary or metastatic intracranial tumor

Hereditary: Huntington's disease

Other (see conditions listed under Metabolic Causes of Coma, p. 276)

REFSUM'S DISEASE

This is a rare hereditary recessive lipidosis of the nervous system with retinitis pigmentosa, peripheral neuropathy, cerebellar ataxia, nerve deafness, and ichthyosis.

CSF shows albuminocytologic dissociation (normal cell count with protein usually increased to 100–700 mg/dl).

METACHROMATIC LEUKODYSTROPHY

Urine sediment may contain metachromatic lipids (from breakdown of myelin products).

CSF protein may be normal or elevated $\leq$ 200 mg/dl.

Biopsy of dental or sural nerve with demonstration of accumulated metachromatic sulfatide is diagnostic.

PROGRESSIVE CEREBELLAR ATAXIA WITH SKIN TELANGIECTASIAS (LOUIS-BAR SYNDROME)

This is an autosomal recessive multisystem disease with cerebellar ataxia and oculocutaneous telangiectasia.

Some patients have

Glucose intolerance

Abnormal liver function tests

Decreased or absent serum IgA and IgE causing recurrent pulmonary infections; IgM present

Increased serum alpha-fetoprotein

See also Table 27-15, p. 383.

TUBEROUS SCLEROSIS

This is a hereditary, familial, congenital anomaly of adenoma sebaceum, epilepsy, and mental retardation associated with sclerotic areas in the brain.

There are no abnormal laboratory findings.
Rarely, CSF protein is increased.

BASSEN-KORNZWEIG SYNDROME

Abnormal RBCs (acanthocytes) are present in the peripheral blood smear.

There may be
>Marked deficiency of serum beta-lipoprotein and cholesterol
>Abnormal pattern of RBC phospholipids
>Marked impairment of GI fat absorption
>Low serum carotene levels (see p. 77)

LINDAU-VON HIPPEL DISEASE (HEMANGIOBLASTOMAS OF RETINA AND CEREBELLUM)

Laboratory findings due to associated conditions
>Polycythemia
>Pheochromocytomas
>Various tumors (e.g., kidney)

MULTIPLE SCLEROSIS (MS)

No changes of diagnostic value in peripheral blood.

CSF WBC is slightly elevated in about 25% of patients but usually < 20 mononuclear cells/cu mm. > 50 cells/cu mm should be interpreted with extreme caution.

CSF total protein may be mildly elevated in about 25% of cases. Levels > 100 mg/dl should cast doubt on diagnosis.

CSF IgG is increased in about 70% of cases, often when total protein is normal. Increase of IgG is expressed as ratio of CSF total protein or albumin to rule out increased IgG due to disruption of blood-brain barrier. CSF IgG does not correlate with duration, activity, or course of MS. Increase may also be found in neurosyphilis, acute Guillain-Barré syndrome, 5–15% of miscellaneous neurologic diseases, and a few normal persons; recent myelogram is said to invalidate the test.

CSF IgM and IgA may also be elevated but are not useful for diagnosis.

Agar or agarose gel electrophoresis of CSF shows discrete bands of oligoclonal proteins (due to abnormal gamma globulins) in 85–95% of MS patients; is the most sensitive marker of MS. Positive results also occur in 2–10% of noninflammatory neurologic disease and 40% of acute aseptic CNS inflammation (e.g., neurosyphilis, viral encephalitis, subacute sclerosing panencephalitis). Not known to correlate with severity, duration, or course of MS. During steroid treatment, prevalence of oligoclonal bands and other gamma globulin abnormalities may be reduced by 30–50%.

A few patients with definite MS may have normal CSF immunoglobulins and lack oligoclonal bands.

Myelin basic protein is elevated in 70–90% of MS patients during an acute exacerbation and usually returns to normal within 2 weeks. Is frequently elevated in other causes of demyelination and tissue destruction (e.g., encephalitis, leukodystrophies, metabolic encephalopathies, CNS lupus, cranial irradiation and intrathecal chemotherapy, 45% of patients with recent stroke).

Increased association with certain histocompatibility antigens (e.g., whites with B7 and Dw2 antigen).

Abnormal CSF IgG Values in MS*

$$\text{CSF IgG index} = \frac{\text{CSF IgG} \times \text{serum albumin}}{\text{CSF albumin} \times \text{serum IgG}}$$

$$(\text{normal} = <0.77 \text{ mg/dl})$$

CSF IgG: normal = <7.1 mg/dl

CSF albumin: normal = <26.0 mg/dl

CNS IgG synthesis (mg/day)

$$= 5 \times \text{CSF IgG} - \frac{\text{Serum IgG}}{68.2}$$

$$- 2.15 \times \left(\text{CSF albumin} - \frac{\text{Serum albumin}}{169}\right)\left(\frac{\text{Serum IgG}}{\text{Serum albumin}}\right)$$

$$(\text{normal} = <8.0 \text{ mg/day})$$

CSF IgG index > 0.77 mg/dl in 58% of definite MS, 42% of probable MS, 33% of inflammatory neurologic diseases, 12% of other neurologic disorders.

CSF IgG index has sensitivity of 88%, specificity of 95%.

Oligoclonal bands have sensitivity of 88%, specificity of 79%.

Diagnosis should not be made on CSF findings unless there are multiple clinical lesions in time and anatomic location.

CRANIAL ARTERITIS
ESR is markedly increased.

CAVERNOUS SINUS THROMBOPHLEBITIS
CSF is usually normal unless there is associated subdural empyema or meningitis, or it may show increased protein and WBC with normal glucose, or it may be hemorrhagic. *In the diabetic patient, mucormycosis may cause this clinical appearance.*

Laboratory findings due to preceding infections of paranasal sinuses, mastoid, etc., are noted.

Laboratory findings due to complications (e.g., meningitis, brain abscess) are noted.

Laboratory findings due to other causes of venous thromboses (e.g., sickle cell disease, polycythemia, dehydration) in patients with sinus thrombosis rather than thrombophlebitis

INTRACRANIAL EXTRADURAL ABSCESS
CSF shows increased neutrophils (20–1000/cu mm) and a slight increase in protein; glucose is normal.

Laboratory findings due to underlying osteomyelitis of middle ear or paranasal sinus are noted.

ACUTE SUBDURAL EMPYEMA
CSF

Cell count is increased to a few hundred, with predominance of polynuclear leukocytes.

---

*Data from H. Markowitz and E. Kokmen, Neurologic diseases and the cerebrospinal fluid immunoglobulin profile. *Proc. Mayo Clin.* 58:273–274, 1983.

Protein is increased.
Glucose is normal.
Bacterial smears and cultures are negative.
WBC is usually increased ($\leq 25,000$/cu mm).
Laboratory findings due to preceding diseases
> ENT infections, especially acute sinusitis
> Intracranial surgery

Streptococci are the most common organisms when preceding condition is sinusitis. Staphylococcus aureus *or gram-negative organisms are the most common organisms following trauma or surgery.*

BRAIN ABSCESS
CSF shows increased neutrophils, lymphocytes, RBCs, and WBC $\cong$ 25–300/cu mm. There may be increased protein level (75–300 mg/dl). The sugar level is normal. Bacterial cultures are negative. Findings depend on stage and duration of abscess.
Associated primary disease
> Ear, nose, and throat diseases (e.g., frontal sinusitis, middle ear infections, mastoiditis)
> Primary septic lung disease (e.g., lung abscess, bronchiectasis, empyema)
> Congenital heart disease with septal defects and pulmonary arteriovenous shunts

Due To
Usually mixed anaerobic (e.g., streptococci or *Bacteroides*) and aerobic organisms (e.g., streptococci, staphylococci, or pneumococci).
May be caused by almost any organism, including fungi, *Nocardia.*

TUBERCULOMA OF BRAIN
CSF shows increased protein with small number of cells. The tuberculoma may be transformed into tuberculous meningitis with increased protein and cells (50–300/cu mm), decreased sugar and chloride.
Laboratory findings due to tuberculosis elsewhere are noted.

SPINAL CORD TUMOR
CSF protein is increased. It may be very high and associated with xanthochromia when there is a block of the subarachnoid space. With complete block, lower levels of cord tumor are associated with higher protein concentration.
See Table 25-1, p. 280.

EPIDURAL ABSCESS OF SPINAL CORD
CSF protein is increased (usually 100–400 mg/dl), and WBCs (lymphocytes and neutrophils) are relatively few in number.
Most common organism is *Staphylococcus aureus,* followed by streptococci and gram-negative bacilli.
Laboratory findings due to preceding condition
> Vertebral osteomyelitis
> Bacteremia due to dental, respiratory, or skin infections
> Postoperative state

MYELITIS

CSF may be normal or may show increased protein and cells (20–1000/cu mm—lymphocytes and mononuclear cells).
See primary disease
 Poliomyelitis
 Herpes zoster
 Tuberculosis, syphilis, parasites, abscess
 Postvaccinal myelitis
 Multiple sclerosis
 Other

INFARCTION OF SPINAL CORD

CSF changes same as in cerebral hemorrhage or infarction
Laboratory findings due to causative condition
 Polyarteritis nodosa
 Dissecting aneurysm of aorta
 Arteriosclerosis of aorta with thrombus formation
 Iatrogenic (e.g., aortic arteriography, clamping of aorta during
  cardiac surgery)

CHRONIC ADHESIVE ARACHNOIDITIS
(due to spinal anesthesia, syphilis, etc.)
CSF protein may be normal or increased.

CERVICAL SPONDYLOSIS

CSF shows increased protein in some cases.

POLYNEURITIS OR POLYNEUROPATHY

Due To

Infectious mononucleosis—CSF shows increased protein and ≦ several hundred mononuclear cells.
Diphtheria—CSF protein is 50–200 mg/dl.
Leprosy
Metabolic condition (e.g., pellagra, beriberi, combined system disease, pregnancy, porphyria)—CSF usually normal. In about 70% of patients with diabetic neuropathy, CSF protein is increased to >200 mg/dl.
Uremia—CSF protein is 50–200 mg/dl, occurs in a few chronic cases of uremia.
Neoplasm (leukemia, multiple myeloma, carcinoma)—CSF protein often increased; may be associated with an occult primary neoplastic lesion outside CNS
Amyloidosis—CSF protein often increased
Sarcoidosis
Polyarteritis nodosa—CSF usually normal; nerve involvement in 10% of patients
Systemic lupus erythematosus
Toxic condition caused by drugs and chemicals (especially lead, arsenic, etc.)
Alcoholism—CSF usually normal
Bassen-Kornzweig syndrome
Refsum's disease
Chédiak-Higashi syndrome

DISEASES CAUSING NEURITIS OF ONE NERVE OR PLEXUS

Due To
Diphtheria
Herpes zoster
Sarcoidosis
Leprosy
Tumor (leukemias, lymphomas, carcinomas)—may find tumor cells in spinal fluid
Serum sickness
Bell's palsy
Idiopathic cause

MULTIPLE CRANIAL NERVE PALSIES

Laboratory findings due to causative condition
    Trauma
    Aneurysms
    Tumors (e.g., meningioma, neurofibroma, carcinoma, cholesteatoma, chordoma)
    Herpes zoster
Benign polyneuritis associated with cervical lymph node tuberculosis or sarcoidosis

FACIAL PALSY

Laboratory findings due to causative disease
    Bell's palsy—occasional slight increase in cells in CSF
    Herpes zoster
    Pontine lesions (tumor or vascular)
    Tumors invading the temporal bone
    Acoustic neuromas
    Sarcoidosis (uveoparotid fever or Heerfordt's syndrome)
    Leprosy
    Acute infectious polyneuritis

TRIGEMINAL NEURALGIA (TIC DOULOUREUX)

Laboratory findings due to causative disease
    Usually idiopathic
    May also stem from multiple sclerosis, herpes zoster

OPHTHALMOPLEGIA

Laboratory findings due to causative disease
    Diabetes mellitus
    Myasthenia gravis
    Hyperthyroid exophthalmos

VON RECKLINGHAUSEN'S DISEASE (MULTIPLE NEUROFIBROMAS)

CSF findings of brain tumor if acoustic neurinoma occurs

BITEMPORAL HEMIANOPSIA

Laboratory findings due to causative disease
    Usually pituitary adenoma
    Also metastatic tumor, sarcoidosis, Hand-Schüller-Christian disease, meningioma of sella, aneurysm of circle of Willis

RETROBULBAR NEUROPATHY

CSF is normal or may show increased protein and ≦ 200 lymphocytes.

75% of these patients ultimately develop multiple sclerosis.

GLOMUS JUGULARE TUMOR

CSF protein may be increased.

DEXAMETHASONE SUPPRESSION TEST (DST)

Blood is drawn at 11 P.M., 8 A.M., 12 noon, 4 P.M., and 11 P.M. for plasma cortisol levels. 1 mg of dexamethasone is given immediately after the first sample is taken. An abnormal test result is failure of suppression of plasma cortisol to level ≦ 5 μg/dl in any sample after the first.

A positive DST will "rule in" the diagnosis of melancholia (endogenous depression), but a negative DST will not rule it out, since it may be positive in only 40–50% of such patients.

In the presence of a positive DST, appropriate drug treatment (e.g., tricyclic antidepressants) that results in normalization of DST with clinical recovery is a good prognostic sign whereas failure of normalization of DST suggests a poor prognosis and the need for continued antidepressant therapy. Despite clinical improvement, treatment should be continued until DST becomes negative. With relapse, DST may become abnormal when symptoms are still mild, before fully developed syndrome develops. The need to continue treatment is indicated if a positive DST that became negative with therapy reverts to positive after discontinuation of drug treatment or lowering drug dosage.

Interference with DST may be caused by

Certain drugs that cause nonsuppression, especially phenytoin, barbiturates, meprobamate, carbamazepine, alcohol (chronic high doses or withdrawal within 3 weeks)

Enhanced suppression may be caused by benzodiazepines (high doses), corticosteroids (spironolactone, cortisone, artificial glucocorticoids such as prednisone, topical and nasal forms), dextroamphetamine.

Other drugs that are said to interfere include estrogens (not birth control pills), reserpine, narcotics, and indomethacin.

Medical conditions including weight loss to 20% below ideal body weight, pregnancy or abortion within 1 month, endocrine diseases, systemic infections, serious liver disease, cancer, other severe physical illnesses may also cause false positive test results.

Lithium maintenance therapy will not interfere with DST.

With a 50% prevalence of melancholia in the population studied and fulfillment of certain medical criteria, DST has sensitivity of 67%, specificity of 96%, and confidence level of 94% in diagnosis. Using only the 4 P.M. blood, the sensitivity ≅ 50%. However, there are still no clear indications for routine use of DST in clinical psychiatry, and many of the routine methods are not accurate at the decision level.

Response of thyroid-stimulating hormone (TSH) to administration of thyrotropin-releasing hormone (TRH) has also been suggested as useful in the diagnosis of unipolar depression and prediction of relapse. These patients have a maximum rise in serum TSH level of $< 7 \, \mu U/ml$ (normal = 17 ± 9). Use of this test with DST is said to add confidence to diagnosis of major unipolar depression; abnormal response to either test before treatment suggests that patient is particularly liable to early relapse unless there is laboratory as well as clinical recovery after treatment.

Musculoskeletal Diseases

MYASTHENIA GRAVIS

Serum enzymes are normal.

CBC and ESR are normal (occasional cases of associated macrocytic anemia).

Serum electrolytes are normal.

Thyroid function tests are normal (disease may be associated with, but independent of, hyperthyroidism or hypothyroidism).

Fluorescent antibodies to skeletal muscle cross-striations have been reported in 30–40% of patients.

Antibodies to acetylcholine receptor (AChR) occur in > 85% of cases, but normal levels do not rule out myasthenia gravis. False positive results have been seen in some patients with amyotrophic lateral sclerosis, especially those treated with cobra venom, and in a small percentage of patients treated with penicillamine who develop myasthenia-like symptoms. Titers only correspond roughly to clinical status of patients as a group but correlate better with the course of an individual patient and is particularly useful for monitoring during plasmapheresis therapy. Approximately 9% of patients with clinical myasthenia gravis lack detectable anti-AChR antibodies; these are of recent onset or mild and only involve extraocular muscles.

High frequency of associated diabetes mellitus is seen, especially in older patients; therefore GTT should be performed with or without cortisone.

Other immunologic abnormalities are frequent.

> Anti-DNA antibodies in 40% of cases
> ANA (antinuclear antibody), anti-parietal cell, anti–smooth-muscle, antimitochondrial, antithyroid antibodies, rheumatoid factor, etc., may be found.

Always rule out cancer of lung.

Thymic tumor is present in up to 10% of patients; 70% of patients have thymic hyperplasia with germinal centers in medulla. See p. 380.

POLYMYOSITIS

Total eosinophil count is frequently increased. WBC may be increased in fulminant disease.

Mild anemia may occur.

ESR is moderately to markedly increased; may be normal; not clinically useful.

Thyroid function tests are normal.

Serum enzymes are increased; occasionally they remain normal. The degree of increase reflects the activity of the disease; usually decrease occurs 3–4 weeks before improvement in muscle strength and increase 5–6 weeks before clinical relapse; the level

Table 26-1. Laboratory Findings in the Differential Diagnosis of Some Muscle Diseases

Disease	Complete Blood Count	ESR	Thyroid Function Tests	Percent of Patients with Increase in Various Serum Enzyme Levels	Muscle Biopsy	Comment
Myasthenia gravis	N	N	N	N	Lymphorrhages	Cancer of lung should always be ruled out; high frequency of associated diabetes mellitus, especially in older patients Serum electrolytes N
Polymyositis	Total eosinophil count frequently I	Moderately to markedly I; occasionally N	N	CK in 65%; levels may vary greatly and become N with steroid therapy; markedly I may occur in children ALD in 75%, LDH in 25%, SGOT in 25%; α-HBD parallels LDH; MDH offers no additional diagnostic value	Necrosis of muscle with phagocytosis of muscle fibers, infiltration of inflammatory cells	Associated cancer in $\leqq$ 17% of cases (especially lung; also breast) LE preparation and latex fixations occasionally positive; serum alpha$_2$ and gamma globulin may be increased.
Muscular dystrophy	N	N	N	In active phase; CK in 50%, ALD in 20%, LDH in 10%, SGOT in 15%	Various degenerative changes in muscle; late muscle atrophy; no cellular infiltration	

N = normal; I = increased.

frequently becomes normal with steroid therapy or in chronic myositis. It is important to measure more than one enzyme and to repeat the tests.

Serum CK is increased in two-thirds of patients. Levels may vary greatly. In childhood very high levels may occur.

Serum aldolase is increased in 75% of patients.

Serume LDH is increased in 25% of patients.

Serum SGOT is increased in ≅ 25% of the patients.

Serum alpha-hydroxybutyric dehydrogenase (α-HBD) may be increased, paralleling the increased LDH.

Serum MDH may be increased but offers no additional diagnostic value.

Urine shows a moderate increase in creatine and a decrease in creatinine. Myoglobinuria occurs occasionally in severe cases.

Increased ANA titers are found in 20% of cases. Rheumatoid factor (RA) tests may be positive in 50% of patients.

Serum gamma globulins may be increased.

Muscle biopsy shows necrosis of muscle, with phagocytosis of muscle fibers and infiltration of inflammatory cells.

Associated carcinoma is present in ≦ 20% of the patients and in ≦ 5% of patients over age 40 (especially cancer of lung and cancer of breast). The polymyositis may antedate the neoplasm by up to 2 years.

MUSCULAR DYSTROPHY
ESR is usually normal.

Thyroid function tests are normal.

Serum enzymes are increased, especially in

Young patients. Highest levels (≦ 50 times normal) are found at onset of infancy and childhood, with gradual return to normal.

The more rapidly progressive dystrophies (such as the Duchenne type) and may be slightly or inconsistently increased in the limb-girdle and facioscapulohumeral types

The active early phase. Increased levels are not constant and are affected by patient's age and duration of disease. Enzymes may be increased before disease is clinically evident.

Serum CK is increased in ≅ 50% of patients.

Serum aldolase is increased in ≅ 20% of patients.

Serum LDH is increased in ≅ 10% of patients.

Serum SGOT is increased in ≅ 15% of patients.

Serum CK is increased in ≅ 75% of female *carriers*. It is thus possible to identify carrier state and detect clinically unaffected male infants with Duchenne type.

Elevated serum enzyme levels are not affected by steroid therapy.

Muscle biopsy shows muscle atrophy but no cellular infiltration.

Urine creatine is increased; urine creatinine is decreased. These changes are less marked in limb-girdle and facioscapulohumeral types than in the Duchenne type.

MYOTONIC DYSTROPHY
Increased creatine in urine may occur irregularly.

Findings due to atrophy of testicle and androgenic deficiency are noted.

Urine 17-ketosteroids are decreased.
Thyroid function may be decreased.
Serum enzyme increases are slight and inconsistent. Female carriers may have higher levels of aldolase (ALD) and CK than control females.

SERUM ENZYMES IN SOME DISEASES OF THE MUSCULOSKELETAL SYSTEM

CK is the measurement of choice. It is more specific and sensitive than SGOT and LDH and more discriminating than ALD.

Increased In
Dermatomyositis
Progressive muscular dystrophy (see Muscular Dystrophy, p. 304)
Myotonic dystrophy (see p. 304)

Normal In
Rheumatoid arthritis
Scleroderma
Acrosclerosis
Discoid lupus erythematosus
Muscle atrophy of neurologic origin (e.g., old poliomyelitis, polyneuritis)
Hyperthyroid myopathy

CREATINE AND CREATININE
Decreased creatinine excretion
Increased creatine excretion
Increased blood creatinine

Occurs In
Progressive muscular dystrophy
Decreased muscle mass in
     Neurogenic atrophy
     Polymyositis
     Addison's disease
     Hyperthyroidism
     Male eunuchoidism

MYALGIAS—DIFFERENTIAL DIAGNOSIS
Rheumatoid arthritis
Rheumatic fever
Hyperparathyroidism
Hyperthyroidism and hypothyroidism
Hypoglycemia
Renal tubular acidosis
Myoglobinuria
McArdle syndrome
Brucellosis
Other infections (bacterial, viral, rickettsial, etc.)

METABOLIC DISEASES OF MUSCLE
Hyperthyroidism
     Increased urine creatine
     Decreased creatine tolerance

Normal serum enzyme levels
Normal muscle biopsy

Causes some cases of hypokalemic periodic paralysis.

Hypothyroidism (rarely associated with myotonia)
Decreased urine creatine
Increased creatine tolerance
Increased serum CK
Other serum enzyme levels normal
Associated with administration of adrenal corticosteroids and with Cushing's syndrome
Increased urine creatine
Increased serum enzymes (SGOT, ALD)—uncommon, and may be due to the primary disease
Muscle biopsy—degenerative and regenerative changes in scattered muscle fibers; no inflammatory cell infiltration

CONGENITAL MYOTONIA (THOMSEN'S DISEASE)
Mild creatine intolerance is found.
Urine creatine may be increased in some patients.
Muscle biopsy shows few changes that are not specific.
Serum enzymes are normal.

STIFF-MAN SYNDROME
Other laboratory examinations are normal.
CSF is normal.
Biopsy of muscle is normal or shows minimal nonspecific changes (e.g., slight atrophy).
Occasionally other alterations are present (e.g., persistent leukopenia with eosinophilia).

MYOTUBULAR MYOPATHY
Routine laboratory studies including measurement of serum enzymes are normal; occasionally serum CK is slightly increased.
Biopsy of muscle establishes the diagnosis.

MITOCHONDRIAL MYOPATHY
Routine laboratory studies including measurement of serum enzymes are normal.
Biopsy of muscle with histochemical staining reaction demonstrates hyperactivity of certain mitochondrial enzymes (e.g., DPNH diaphorase, succinate dehydrogenase, cytochrome oxidase).

NEMALINE (ROD) MYOPATHY
Routine laboratory tests are normal.
Serum enzymes are normal; occasionally serum CK is slightly increased.
Endocrine studies (including measurements of urine 17-ketosteroids and 11-oxysteroids) are normal.
Biopsy of muscle with appropriate special stains establishes the diagnosis.

MYOPATHY ASSOCIATED WITH ALCOHOLISM
Acute
Increased serum CK, SGOT, and other enzymes. Serum CK

Table 26-2. Increased Serum Enzyme Levels in Muscle Diseases

| | Muscular Dystrophy | | | | | | Myotonic Dystrophy | Polymyositis |
| | Duchenne | | Limb-Girdle | | Facioscapulohumeral | | | |
Enzyme	Frequency	Amplitude	Frequency	Amplitude	Frequency	Amplitude	Frequency	Frequency
CK	>95%	65	75%	25	80%	5	50%	70%
ALD	90%	9	25%	3	30%	2	20%	75%
SGOT	90%	4	25%	2	25%	1½	15%	25%
LDH	90%	4	15%	1½	10%	1	10%	25%

Frequency = average % frequency of patients with increased serum enzyme level when blood is taken at optimal time.
Amplitude = average number of times normal that serum level is increased.

Table 26-3. Types of Periodic Paralysis

	Hypokalemic (familial, sporadic, associated with hyperthyroidism)	Hyperkalemic (adynamia episodica hereditaria)	Normokalemic
Induced by	Glucose and insulin, ACTH, DOCA, epinephrine	KCl	KCl
Serum potassium during attack	Decreased	Increased	Normal or slightly decreased
Urine potassium excretion	Decreased	Normal	Decreased

    increases in 1–2 days; reaches peak in 4–5 days. CK in CSF is normal, even when serum level is elevated.
    Gross myoglobinuria
    Acute renal failure (some patients)
Chronic—may show some or all of the following changes
    Increased urine creatine
    Increased serum CK and SGOT
    Diminished ability to increase blood lactic acid with ischemic exercise
    Abnormalities on muscle biopsy (support the diagnosis)
    Myoglobinuria

FAMILIAL PERIODIC PARALYSIS
Serum potassium is decreased during the attack.
Urine potassium excretion decreases at the same time.
Serum enzymes are normal.

ADYNAMIA EPISODICA HEREDITARIA (GAMSTORP'S DISEASE)
Transient increase in serum potassium occurs during the attack; attack is induced by administration of potassium.
Urine potassium excretion is unchanged during or before the attack.

MALIGNANT HYPERTHERMIA
(autosomal dominant syndrome triggered by potent inhalational anesthetic agents, local anesthetic agents in large doses [e.g., lidocaine], muscle relaxants [e.g., succinylcholine, tubocurarine], various types of stress)
Combined metabolic and respiratory acidosis is the most consistent abnormality and is diagnostic in the presence of muscle rigidity or rising temperature. pH is often < 7.2, base excess [BE] > -10, and $PaCO_2$ 70–120 mmHg. *Immediate* arterial blood gas analysis should be performed.
Increased serum potassium and calcium initially with below-normal values later.

Serum CK, LDH, and SGOT are markedly increased with peak in 24–48 hours following surgery; CK levels are often 20,000–100,000 units/L.

Myoglobinemia and myoglobinuria may be present early.

Oliguria with acute renal shutdown may occur later.

Coagulopathy, including DIC, may occur later but is infrequent.

OSTEOMYELITIS

WBC may be increased, especially in acute case.

ESR is increased in < 50% of patients but may be important clue in occult cases (e.g., intervertebral disk space infection).

Bacteriology
  Staphylococcus aureus causes almost all infections of hip and two-thirds of infections of skull, vertebrae, and long bones. Other bacteria may simultaneously be present and contribute to infection.

  Gram-negative bacteria cause most infections of mandible, pelvis, and small bones.

  Salmonella is more commonly found in patients with sickle hemoglobinopathy.

Laboratory findings due to underlying conditions
  Postoperative status
  Irradiation therapy
  Foreign body, tissue gangrene, contiguous infection, etc.

SKELETAL INVOLVEMENT ASSOCIATED WITH SOME METABOLIC ABNORMALITIES

Primary hypophosphatemia
Hypophosphatasia
Rickets
Gaucher's disease
Gargoylism (mucopolysaccharides in urine; sometimes Riley bodies in white cells)
Gout
Alkaptonuria
Phenylketonuria
Familial hyperparathyroidism
Idiopathic hypercalcemia
Osteogenesis imperfecta
Marfan's syndrome
Other

SKELETAL INVOLVEMENT ASSOCIATED WITH SOME HEMATOLOGIC DISEASES

Anemia
  Hereditary hemolytic (e.g., sickle cell disease, thalassemia, hereditary spherocytosis)
  Iron deficiency anemia of childhood
  Congenital aplastic anemia (Fanconi's syndrome)
Coagulation defects (e.g., deficiency of AHG, PTC, or PTA)
Malignant lymphoma (e.g., leukemia, lymphosarcoma, Hodgkin's disease, multiple myeloma)
Primary reticulum cell sarcoma of bone
Reticuloendothelioses (e.g., Niemann-Pick disease, Gaucher's disease, Hand-Schüller-Christian disease, Letterer-Siwe disease, eosinophilic granuloma)
Myelosclerosis
Osteopetrosis (marble bone disease)
Other

RICKETS

Serum alkaline phosphatase is increased. This is the earliest and most reliable biochemical abnormality; parallels severity of the rickets. It may remain elevated until bone healing is complete.

Serum calcium is usually normal or slightly decreased.

Serum phosphorus is usually decreased. In some persons, serum calcium and phosphorus may be normal.

Generalized renal aminoaciduria is present; it disappears when adequate vitamin D is given.

Serum calcium and phosphorus rapidly become normal after institution of vitamin D therapy.

Vitamin D deficient state is suggested by
> Low serum phosphorus
> Severe liver disease
> Malabsorption
> Anticonvulsant therapy

OSTEOPENIA

(generic term for decreased mineralized bone on x-ray, but x-ray cannot distinguish osteomalacia from osteoporosis in most patients unless pseudofractures are seen)

Due To

Osteoporosis (total bone mass is decreased, but ratio of bone mineral to matrix is normal)

20% of patients with osteoporosis also have osteomalacia.

> Primary
> > Postmenopausal or senile
> > Idiopathic
> > Juvenile
> Secondary
> > Diabetes mellitus
> > Immobilization
> > Chronic liver disease
> > Alcoholism
> > Chronic renal disease
> > Cushing's syndrome
> > Turner's syndrome

Osteomalacia (failure of normal mineralization causes decreased ratio of bone mineral to matrix; usually due to vitamin D deficiency)

> Dietary
> GI tract malabsorption
> Pancreatic disease
> Anticonvulsant drug therapy
> Hepatobiliary disease
> Chronic renal disease
> Renal tubular acidosis
> Primary hypophosphatemia
> Vitamin D–dependent osteomalacia (1-α-hydroxylase deficiency)
> Tumor osteomalacia
> Others (e.g., hyperthyroidism)

Table 26-4. Serum Chemistries in Different Types of Osteopenia

	Serum Calcium	Serum Phosphorus	Serum Alkaline Phosphatase	Urine Calcium
Osteoporosis	N	N	N	N or I
Osteomalacia	N or D	Marked D*	I	D
Osteitis fibrosis	I	D	I	I

N = normal; D = decreased; I = increased.
*Is increased in chronic renal failure.

Malignancy
    Multiple myeloma
    Metastatic tumor
Osteitis fibrosa
    Hyperparathyroidism

All serum chemistries may be normal in any form of osteopenia.
All chemistries are commonly normal in osteomalacia, especially with coexisting osteoporosis.
Serum vitamin D that is below normal (e.g., 15 ng/ml of 25-hydroxy vitamin D) suggests osteomalacia
Diagnosis is established with bone biopsy that may be combined with tetracycline labeling.
During therapeutic trial of calcium and vitamin D, serum and urine calcium should be monitored monthly to avoid toxicity. Urine calcium is maintained < 300 mg/gm of creatinine and serum calcium < 10.2 mg/dl by reducing dose of vitamin D.

AXIAL OSTEOMALACIA
Axial skeleton shows x-ray changes resembling those in Paget's disease and metastatic tumor.
Bone biopsy is characteristic of osteomalacia.
Blood chemistries are normal.
There is no recognizable cause for axial osteomalacia.

RENAL TUBULAR HYPOPHOSPHATEMIA WITH ASSOCIATED RICKETS
Due To
Toxic injury or intrinsic metabolic defect of renal tubule cell

PRIMARY HYPOPHOSPHATEMIA (FAMILIAL VITAMIN D–RESISTANT RICKETS)
(hereditary metabolic defect in phosphate transport in renal tubules and possibly intestine)

Serum phosphorus is markedly decreased.
Serum calcium is relatively normal.
Serum alkaline phosphatase is moderately increased.
Stool calcium is increased, and urine calcium is decreased.
Administration of vitamin D does not cause serum phosphorus to

rise (in contrast to ordinary rickets), but urine and serum calcium
may be increased with sufficiently large dose.

Renal aminoaciduria is absent, in contrast to ordinary rickets.

Treatment is monitored by choosing dose of vitamin D that will not
increase serum calcium > 11 mg/dl or urine calcium > 200 mg/
day. Serum phosphorus usually remains low; increase > 4 mg/dl
may indicate renal injury due to vitamin D toxicity.

RENAL TUBULAR ACIDOSIS WITH RICKETS AND OSTEOMALACIA
(inborn error of renal tubular metabolism)

See pp. 521–522.

FANCONI'S SYNDROME

See pp. 521–522.

VITAMIN D–DEPENDENT RICKETS

Serum calcium is frequently decreased, sometimes causing tetany.

Serum phosphorus is decreased but not as markedly or as consistently as in hypophosphatemic rickets.

Serum alkaline phosphatase is increased.

Urine calcium is decreased.

Generalized renal aminoaciduria is present; it disappears when
adequate vitamin D is given.

Serum chemistries return to normal after adequate vitamin D is
given (may require very large doses).

May be due to familial genetic pattern.

METAPHYSEAL DYSOSTOSIS

Rare congenital disorder with progressive long bone deformities
that mimic chronic rickets.

Serum calcium, phosphorus, and alkaline phosphatase are normal.

VITAMIN D INTOXICATION

Serum calcium may be increased.

Serum phosphorus is usually also increased but sometimes is decreased, with increased urinary phosphorus.

FAMILIAL OSTEOECTASIA
**(uncommon inherited disorder of membranous bone showing painful
swelling of the periosteal soft tissue and spontaneous fractures)**

Serum alkaline phosphatase is increased.

Serum acid phosphatase and aminopeptidase are also increased.

OSTEOSCLEROSIS

Due To

Osteopetrosis (see next section)

Heavy-metal poisoning (e.g., lead, bismuth)

Hypoparathyroidism

Hypothyroidism

OSTEOPETROSIS (ALBERS-SCHÖNBERG DISEASE; MARBLE BONE DISEASE)

Normal serum calcium, phosphorus, alkaline phosphatase

Serum acid phosphatase increased (some patients)

Table 26-5. Usual Laboratory Findings in Different Types of Rickets

	Serum Calcium	Serum Phosphorus	Serum Alkaline Phosphatase	Serum Parathyroid Hormone	Urine Cyclic AMP	Tubular Reabsorption of Phosphate	Urine Amino Acids	Response to Vitamin D
Vitamin D resistant	N	D	I	N	N	D	N	Poor
Vitamin D dependent	D	D	I	I	I	D	I	Good with high dose
Vitamin D deficient	D	D	I	I	I	D	I	Good

N = normal; D = decreased; I = increased.
Source: Adapted from R. A. DeFronzo and S. O. Thier, Inherited tubule disorders. *Hosp. Pract.* Feb., 1982, pp. 111–128.

Myelophthisic anemia (some patients)
Laboratory findings due to complications
    Osteomyelitis
    Other infections

PAGET'S DISEASE OF BONE (OSTEITIS DEFORMANS)

Marked increase in serum alkaline phosphatase directly related to severity and extent of disease; sudden additional increase with development of osteogenic sarcoma

Normal serum calcium increased during immobilization (e.g., due to intercurrent illness or fracture)

Normal or slightly increased serum phosphorus

Frequently increased urine calcium; renal calculi common

Increase in hydroxyproline in urine may be marked.

OSTEOGENIC SARCOMA

Marked increase in serum alkaline phosphatase (≤ 40 times normal); reflects new bone formation and parallels clinical course (development of metastases, response to therapy, etc.); is said to occur in only 50% of patients.

Laboratory findings due to metastases—80% of patients have lung metastases at time of diagnosis.

Laboratory findings due to preexisting Paget's disease, if present.

OSTEOLYTIC TUMORS OF BONE
(e.g., Ewing's sarcoma)

Usually normal serum calcium, phosphorus, alkaline phosphatase

METASTATIC CARCINOMA OF BONE

Osteolytic metastases (especially from primary tumor of bronchus, breast, kidney, thyroid)
    Urine calcium is often increased; marked increase may reflect increased rate of tumor growth.
    Serum calcium and phosphorus may be normal or increased.
    Serum alkaline phosphatase is usually normal or slightly to moderately increased.
    Serum acid phosphatase is often slightly increased, especially in prostatic metastases.

Osteoblastic metastases (especially from primary tumor in prostate)
    Serum calcium is normal; it is rarely increased.
    Urine calcium is low.
    Serum alkaline phosphatase is usually increased.
    Serum acid phosphatase is increased in prostatic carcinoma.
    Serum phosphorus is variable.

FAT EMBOLISM

This occurs after trauma (e.g., fractures, insertion of femoral head prosthesis).

Unexplained fall in hemoglobin in 30–60% of patients

Decreased platelet count in 80% of patients

Free fat in urine in 50% of patients

Fat globules in sputum (some patients)

Decreased arterial PO_2 with normal or decreased PCO_2

Increased serum lipase in 30–50% of patients; increased free fatty acids; not of diagnostic value

Increased serum triglycerides

Fat globulinemia in 42–67% of patients and in 17–33% of controls
Normal cerebrospinal fluid
Hypocalcemia is a common nonspecific finding (due to binding to free fatty acids).
Arterial blood gas values are always abnormal in clinically significant fat embolism syndrome; are the most useful and important laboratory data. Show decreased lung compliance, abnormal ventilation-perfusion ratios, increased shunt effect.

Laboratory findings alone are inadequate for diagnosis.

CONDITIONS ASSOCIATED WITH THE DEVELOPMENT OF AVASCULAR (ASEPTIC) NECROSIS OF THE HEAD OF THE FEMUR

Due To
Traumatic interruption of blood supply
>25% of patients with fracture of neck of femur
Dislocation of hip
Slipped femoral capital epiphysis
Nontraumatic interference with blood supply
Caisson disease
Sickle cell disease and trait and sickle cell–hemoglobin C disease
Infection
Gout
Rheumatoid arthritis
Systemic lupus erythematosus (SLE)
Fabry's disease
Scleroderma
Gaucher's disease
Cushing's syndrome
Corticosteroid treatment
Alcoholism
Pancreatitis
X-ray irradiation
Idiopathic (Chandler's disease)

CLASSIFICATION OF ARTHRITIS*

Polyarthritis of unknown etiology
Rheumatoid arthritis
Juvenile rheumatoid arthritis (Still's disease)
Ankylosing spondylitis (Marie-Strümpell disease)
Psoriatic arthritis
Reiter's syndrome
Other
Collagen diseases (acquired connective tissue disorders)
SLE
Scleroderma (progressive systemic sclerosis)
Polymyositis and dermatomyositis
Necrotizing arteritis and other forms of vasculitis (e.g., polyarteritis nodosa, hypersensitivity angiitis, Wegener's granulo-

*Adapted from American Rheumatism Association, Primer on the rheumatic diseases, *J.A.M.A.* 224:662, 1973.

matosis, Takayasu's disease, Cogan's syndrome, giant cell arteritis)

Amyloidosis

Other

Rheumatic fever

Degenerative joint disease (osteoarthritis)

Primary

Secondary

Diseases with frequently associated arthritis

Sarcoidosis

Relapsing polychondritis

Schönlein-Henoch purpura

Ulcerative colitis

Regional ileitis

Whipple's disease

Sjögren's syndrome

Familial Mediterranean fever

Psoriatic arthritis

Other

Associated with infectious agents

Bacterial (e.g., *Brucella,* gonococcus, tubercle bacillus, *Salmonella,* pneumococcus, *Staphylococcus, Streptococcus moniliformis,* syphilis, yaws)

Rickettsial

Viral (especially rubella; also mumps, viral hepatitis)

Fungal (especially coccidioidomycosis; also histoplasmosis, blastomycosis, cryptococcosis, sporotrichosis)

Parasitic

Traumatic and/or neurogenic causes

Direct trauma

Tertiary syphilis (tabes dorsalis)

Diabetes mellitus with neurologic complications

Syringomyelia

Shoulder-hand syndrome

Mechanical derangement of joints

Endocrine diseases

Hyperparathyroidism

Acromegaly

Hypothyroidism

Biochemical and metabolic diseases

Gout

Pseudogout (chondrocalcinosis articularis)

Ochronosis

Hemophilias

Hemoglobinopathies

Agammaglobulinemia

Scurvy

Gaucher's disease

Hemochromatosis

Hyperlipoproteinemia Type II (xanthoma tuberosum and tendinosum)

Other

Inherited and congenital diseases

Mucopolysaccharidoses (e.g., Hurler's syndrome, Morquio's disease)

Homocystinuria

    Ehlers-Danlos syndrome
    Marfan's syndrome
    Osteogenesis imperfecta
    Congenital hip dysplasia
Tumors
    Multiple myeloma
    Leukemia
    Metastatic tumors
    Primary juxta-articular bone
    Synovioma
    Other
Allergy and drug reactions (e.g., serum sickness)
Miscellaneous
    Aseptic necrosis of bone
    Stevens-Johnson syndrome
    Erythema nodosum
    Hypertrophic osteoarthropathy
    Juvenile osteochondritis
    Osteochondritis dissecans
    Pigmented villonodular synovitis
    Tietze's syndrome
    Other
Nonarticular rheumatism
    Intervertebral disk and low back syndromes
    Fibrositis, myositis, tendinitis, bursitis, tenosynovitis, fasciitis
    Carpal tunnel syndrome
    Neuritis
    Panniculitis

NEEDLE BIOPSY OF JOINT (HISTOLOGIC EXAMINATION OF SYNOVIA)

May Be Useful In

Gout
Pseudogout
Ochronosis
Tuberculosis
Coccidioidomycosis
Pyogenic arthritis
Rheumatoid arthritis
Osteoarthritis
Reiter's syndrome
SLE

Provides major diagnostic assistance in about one-third of patients with early or difficult diagnosis.

OSTEOARTHRITIS

ESR may be slightly increased (possibly because of soft-tissue changes secondary to mechanical alterations in joints).

CBC, ESR, serum protein electrophoresis, rheumatoid factor, serum uric acid, calcium, phosphorus, alkaline phosphatase, VDRL tests, etc., are normal.

Laboratory tests are not helpful.

Table 26-6. Synovial Fluid Findings in Various Diseases of Joints

Property	Normal	Noninflammatory[a]	Hemorrhagic[b]	Acute Inflammatory[c]			Septic		
				Acute Gouty Arthritis	Rheumatic Fever	Rheumatoid Arthritis	Tuberculous Arthritis	Gonorrheal Arthritis	Septic Arthritis[e]
Volume	3.5 ml								
Appearance	Clear, colorless	Clear, straw	Bloody or xanthochromic	Turbid yellow			Turbid yellow		
Viscosity	High	High	V	D			D		
Fibrin clot	0	Usually 0	Usually 0	+			+		
Mucin clot	Good	Good	V	Fair to poor			Poor		
WBC (no./cu mm)[f]	<200	<5000	<10,000	Range 750–45,000 Average 13,500	300–98,000 17,800	300–75,000 15,500	2500–105,000 23,500	1500–108,000 14,000	15,600–213,000 65,400

				Range / Average					
Neutrophils (%)	<25	<25	<50	48–94 / 83	8–98 / 46	5–96 / 65	29–96 / 67	2–96 / 64	75–100 / 95
Blood-synovia glucose difference (mg/dl)[g]	<10	<10	<25	0–41 / 12	6	0–88 / 31	0–108 / 57	0–97 / 26	40–122 / 71
Culture[h]	0	0	0	0	0	0		See p. 326.	

I = increased; D = decreased; 0 = absent; + = positive; V = variable.

a For example, degenerative joint disease, traumatic arthritis, some cases of pigmented villonodular synovitis.

b For example, tumor, hemophilia, neuroarthropathy, trauma, some cases of pigmented villonodular synovitis.

c For example, rheumatoid arthritis, Reiter's syndrome, acute gouty arthritis, acute pseudogout, systemic lupus erythematosus, etc.

d For example, pneumococcal.

e In purulent arthropathy of undetermined cause, very high synovial fluid lactate (>2000 mg/dl) indicates a nongonococcal septic arthritis (gram-negative bacilli, gram-positive cocci, fungi). Lactate is <100 mg/dl in gonococcal infection, gout, rheumatoid arthritis, osteoarthritis, trauma.

f Use saline instead of acetic acid, which clumps the joint fluid.

g Joint tap should be performed preferably after patient has been fasting for >4 hours, and a blood glucose determination should be performed simultaneously.

h Material should be cultured aerobically and anaerobically. Culture for tubercle bacilli and guinea pig inoculation should be performed.

Synovial fluid analysis is primarily useful to diagnose or rule out infectious arthritis, gout, or pseudogout.

RHEUMATOID ARTHRITIS

Serologic tests for rheumatoid factor (e.g., using latex, bentonite, or sheep or human RBCs): Tests become positive after disease is active for 6 months. Positive in 75% of "typical" cases; positive in 95% of patients with subcutaneous nodules; high titers in patients with splenomegaly, vasculitis, or neuropathy. Positive in only 10–20% of patients with juvenile rheumatoid arthritis. May diminish or disappear during remission. Positive in 5% of normal population. False positive in other diseases (e.g., SLE, sarcoidosis, liver diseases, subacute bacterial endocarditis, syphilis, leprosy, tuberculosis). Negative in osteoarthritis, gout, ankylosing spondylitis, rheumatic fever, suppurative arthritis, arthritis associated with ulcerative colitis (see p. 240).

Anemia is moderate in degree, of the normocytic hypochromic type, and not responsive to administration of iron, folic acid, or vitamin B_{12} or to splenectomy.

Serum iron is decreased.

WBC is usually normal; there may be a slight increase early in the active disease.

Increased ESR and positive C-reactive protein (CRP) test are rough guides to activity and to therapy.

Serum protein electrophoresis shows increase in globulins, especially in gamma and alpha$_2$ globulins, and decreased albumin.

Positive LE test in $\leq$ 20% of patients is usually weakly reactive. Antinuclear factors are present in $\leq$ 65% of patients, depending on sensitivity of test.

Serum calcium, phosphorus, alkaline phosphatase, uric acid, and ASOT are normal.

Synovial biopsy is especially useful in monoarticular form to rule out tuberculosis, gout, etc.

For synovial fluid examination, see Table 26-6, pp. 318–319.
See Amyloidosis, pp. 639–640.

JUVENILE RHEUMATOID ARTHRITIS (STILL'S DISEASE)

Serologic tests for rheumatoid factor RA are positive in only 10–20% of patients.

WBC is usually increased with increased PMNs in 55% of cases.

Hypochromic anemia is frequent; varies from mild to severe.

Other findings are similar to those in adult rheumatoid arthritis.

Table 26-7. Comparison of Rheumatoid Arthritis and Osteoarthritis

Rheumatoid Arthritis	Osteoarthritis
Synovial fluid has high WBC and low viscosity	Effusions infrequent
	Synovial fluid has low WBC and high viscosity
ESR more markedly increased	ESR may be mildly to moderately increased
Rheumatoid factor usually present	RF usually absent
Positive biopsy of subcutaneous rheumatoid nodule and synovia	Rheumatoid changes in tissue absent

Table 26-8. ESR in Differential Diagnosis of Juvenile Rheumatoid Arthritis

Disease	ESR Falls to Normal
Untreated acute rheumatic fever	9–12 weeks
Salicylate-treated acute rheumatic fever	5 weeks
Steroid-treated acute rheumatic fever	2 weeks
Chronic rheumatic fever	Occasionally shows persistent elevation
Juvenile rheumatoid arthritis	May remain elevated for months or years despite therapy

Increased ESR and CRP parallels degree of inflammation.

Serum protein electrophoresis shows increased IgG, IgA, and IgM in 20–50% of cases.

Secondary amyloidosis appears in long-standing active disease (see Amyloidosis, pp. 639–640).

FELTY'S SYNDROME

The syndrome occurs in 5–10% of patients with rheumatoid arthritis associated with splenomegaly and leukopenia.

Rheumatoid arthritis is far advanced.

Serologic tests for rheumatoid factor are positive; RF may be present in high titers.

Positive LE test is more frequent than in rheumatoid arthritis.

Leukopenia is present. Anemia and thrombocytopenia may occur; they respond to splenectomy.

SJÖGREN'S SYNDROME*

May be secondary to connective tissue disease in one-half to two-thirds of cases or primary; immunologic abnormality associated with decreased secretion of salivary and lacrimal glands. 90% of patients are female.

Diagnosis is established by biopsy of gland (minor salivary gland of lower lip is easiest).

Autoantibodies: Anti-SS-A is present in 70–88% of primary and <10% of secondary type. Anti-SS-B is present in 48–73% of primary and <5% of secondary type. Anti-salivary duct antibody is present in <30% of primary and 76–83% of secondary type.

Rheumatoid factor is present in 52% of primary and 98% of secondary type.

Mild normochromic, normocytic anemia in 50% of patients

Leukopenia in up to one-third of cases

ESR is usually increased.

Serum protein electrophoresis shows increased globulins, largely due to IgG.

*Data from R. D. Collins and G. V. Ball, *J. Musculoskeletal Med.*, April 1984, pp. 42–51.

Table 26-9. Synovial Fluid Findings in Acute Inflammatory Arthritis of Various Etiologies

Disease	WBC	Complement Activity	Rheumatoid Factor (RF)	Crystals*	Other Findings
Acute gouty arthritis	I	I	0	Monosodium urate; within PMNs during acute stage	
Acute chondrocalcinosis (pseudogout)	I	I	0	Calcium pyrophosphate	
Reiter's syndrome	Markedly I	Markedly I	0		Macrophages with ingested leukocytes
Rheumatoid arthritis	I	Low	Usually +		
Juvenile rheumatoid arthritis	I	Low	0		Abundant lymphocytes (sometimes > 50%); immature lymphocytes and monocytes present
Systemic lupus erythematosus	Usually very low	Low or 0	V	0	LE cells may be present
Arthritis associated with psoriasis, ulcerative colitis, ankylosing spondylitis	I	I			

I = increased; 0 = absent; V = variable; PMN = polynuclear leukocyte; + = positive.
*Crystals should be identified using polarized light microscopy. Finding of characteristic crystals is diagnostic of gout and of chondrocalcinosis.

Laboratory findings due to primary disease
> Rheumatoid arthritis is found in 30–55% of patients with Sjögren's syndrome; SS is found in 20–100% of patients with RA.
> SLE is found in 4–5% of patients with SS; SS is found in 50–98% of patients with SLE.
> Primary biliary cirrhosis is found in 3% of patients with SS; SS is found in 50–100% of patients with primary biliary cirrhosis.
> Other associated diseases include generalized scleroderma, mixed connective tissue disease, chronic active hepatitis, thyroiditis.

Laboratory findings due to frequent concomitant diseases (e.g., lymphoma, pseudolymphoma, Waldenström's macroglobulinemia)

Immune complex glomerulonephritis may occur, but chronic tubulointerstitial nephritis is more characteristic.

ANKYLOSING RHEUMATOID SPONDYLITIS (MARIE-STRÜMPELL DISEASE)

ESR is increased in ≤ 80% of cases.

Mild to moderate hypochromic anemia appears in ≤ 30% of cases.

Serologic tests for rheumatoid factor are positive in <15% of patients with arthritis of only the vertebral region.

CSF protein is moderately increased in ≤ 50% of patients.

Secondary amyloidosis appears in 6% of patients.

Laboratory findings of carditis and aortitis with aortic insufficiency, which occur in 1–4% of patients, are noted.

Laboratory findings of frequently associated diseases
> Chronic ulcerative colitis
> Regional ileitis
> Psoriasis

Histocompatibility antigen HLA-B27 is found in about 95% of these white patients and in lesser numbers with variants of this condition. About 20% of persons carrying HLA-B27 have ankylosing spondylitis. Not helpful in establishing the diagnosis.

ARTHRITIS ASSOCIATED WITH PSORIASIS

Arthritis occurs in 2% of patients with psoriasis. There is no correlation between activity of skin and joint manifestations; either one may precede the other.

Increased serum uric acid is due to increased turnover of skin cells in psoriasis.

Serologic tests for rheumatoid factor are negative.

ARTHRITIS ASSOCIATED WITH ULCERATIVE COLITIS OR REGIONAL ENTERITIS

There may be rheumatoid arthritis, ankylosing spondylitis, or acute synovitis (monarticular or polyarticular—absent rheumatoid factor).

Joint fluid is sterile bacteriologically and microscopically. It is similar to fluid of rheumatoid arthritis and Whipple's disease (cell count, differential count, specific gravity, viscosity, protein, sugar, poor mucin clot formation). Joint fluid examination is principally useful in monarticular involvement to rule out suppurative arthritis.

Synovial biopsy is similar to rheumatoid arthritis biopsy.

ARTHRITIS ASSOCIATED WITH WHIPPLE'S DISEASE
This is a nonspecific synovitis.

HEMOCHROMATOSIS-ASSOCIATED ARTHRITIS
Laboratory findings of hemochromatosis
Negative RA factor
No subcutaneous nodules
Biopsy of synovia—iron deposits in synovia lining but not in cartilage, little iron in deep macrophages
> Hemarthrosis—iron diffusely distributed in macrophages (e.g., in hemophilia, trauma, and pigmented villonodular synovitis)
> Osteoarthritis—small amount of iron that is limited to deep macrophages
> Rheumatoid arthritis—iron in both deep macrophages and lining cells
Chondrocalcinosis frequently associated.

REITER'S SYNDROME
This triad of arthritis, urethritis, and conjunctivitis has additional features: dermatitis, buccal ulcerations, circinate balanitis, and keratosis blennorrhagica.
Increased ESR parallels the clinical course.
WBC is increased (10,000–20,000/cu mm), as are granulocytes.
Serum globulins are increased in long-standing disease.
Nonbacterial cystitis, prostatitis, or seminal vesiculitis is found (significance of culturing pleuropneumonia-like organisms is not determined).
HLA-B27 is found in up to 90% of white patients; not diagnostically useful.

GOUT
Serum uric acid is increased. Several determinations may be required to establish elevated values; beware of serum levels reduced to normal range by recent aspirin ingestion.
Serum uric acid levels are increased in $\cong$ 25% of asymptomatic relatives.
About 10% of adult males have elevated serum uric acid levels.
Only 1–3% of patients with hyperuricemia have gout.
$\cong$ 1% of patients with attacks of gout have serum uric acid < 6 mg/dl.
Uric acid stones occur 100 times more frequently in gouty patients than in the general population even though 75% of gouty patients have normal 24-hour excretion of uric acid.
Secondary hyperuricemia usually produces much higher uric acid level than primary type. If serum uric acid is > 10 mg/dl, underlying malignancy should be considered after renal failure has been ruled out.
24-hour urine for uric acid should be performed; if elevated (>600 mg/24 hours), it should be repeated after 3–5 days on purine-free diet. (If excretion < 600 mg/day and no history of kidney or GU tract disease, treatment is with probenecid; if > 600 mg/day or there is history of GU tract or kidney disease, allopurinol is drug of choice.) > 1100 mg/24 hours in asymptomatic hyperuricemia is indication for treatment.

Drug-induced gout may cause up to 50% of all new cases of gouty arthritis; these occur later in life and are more common in women than primary gout.

20% of patients with untreated hypertension have hyperuricemia. Other frequently associated conditions are diabetes mellitus, cardiovascular disease, myxedema, obesity, alcohol ingestion. Serum triglycerides are frequently increased, resulting in a high frequency of types IIb and IV liproprotein patterns; HDL-cholesterol level is frequently decreased.

10–25% of primary gout patients develop uric acid stones; in 40% of these, the stones appear > 5 years before an episode of gout.

Moderate leukocytosis and increased ESR occur during acute attacks; normal at other times.

Presence of crystals of monosodium urate from tophi and joint fluid (viewed microscopically under polarized light) establishes the diagnosis.

Uric acid crystals and amorphous urates are normal findings in urinary sediment.

Low-grade proteinuria occurs in 20–80% of gouty persons for many years before further evidence of renal disease appears.

Histologic examination of gouty nodule should be made.

See Tables 26-6, pp. 318–319, and 26-9, p. 322.
See also sections on renal diseases and serum uric acid.

DISEASES ASSOCIATED WITH GOUT
Hypertension in one-third of patients with gout
Diabetes mellitus
Familial hypercholesterolemia
Acute intermittent porphyria
von Gierke's disease
Sarcoidosis
Other

SECONDARY GOUT

Occurs In
Lead intoxication
Hematologic diseases (e.g., leukemia, polycythemia vera, secondary polycythemia, malignant lymphomas). *Blood dyscrasias are found in ≅ 10% of patients with clinical gout.*
Psoriasis

CHONDROCALCINOSIS ("PSEUDOGOUT")
Joint fluid contains crystals of calcium pyrophosphate dihydrate, inside and outside of WBCs; differentiated from urate crystals under polarized light.
Blood and urine findings are normal.

See Tables 26-6, pp. 318–319, and 26-9, p. 322.

CONDITIONS THAT MAY PRESENT AS ACUTE ARTHRITIS
Beware of conditions that may present as acute arthritis.
Acute leukemia in children
Hypertrophic pulmonary osteoarthropathy (clubbing) in lung tumors—may have acute onset and be painful

Drug reaction causing lupus erythematosus–like syndrome (e.g., procainamide)

Aortic insufficiency starting with back pain and symptoms of spondylitis

SEPTIC ARTHRITIS (SUPPURATIVE OR PURULENT ARTHRITIS)

Laboratory findings due to preexisting infections (e.g., subacute bacterial endocarditis, meningococcic meningitis, pneumococcal pneumonia, typhoid, gonorrhea, tuberculosis) are noted.

See Table 26-6, pp. 318–319.

Joint fluid
    In purulent arthritis
        Gram stain is particularly useful for establishing diagnosis promptly and in cases in which cultures are negative.
        Culture may be negative because of prior administration of antibiotics.
    In tuberculous arthritis
        Gram stain and bacterial cultures are negative, but acid-fast stain, culture for tubercle bacilli, guinea pig inoculation, and biopsy of synovia confirm the diagnosis.

PIGMENTED VILLONODULAR SYNOVITIS

CBC, ESR, blood cholesterol, and urinalysis are normal.

See Table 26-6, pp. 318–319.

POLYMYALGIA RHEUMATICA

ESR is usually markedly increased.

Mild hypochromic or normochromic anemia is commonly found.

WBC is usually normal.

Abnormalities of serum proteins are frequent, although there is no consistent or diagnostic pattern. Most frequently the albumin is decreased with an increase in alpha$_1$ and alpha$_2$ globulins and fibrinogen. Cryoglobulins are sometimes present.

Rheumatoid factor is present in serum in 7.5% of patients.

LE test is negative.

Serum enzymes (e.g., SGOT, CK, aldolase) are normal.

Muscle biopsy is usually normal or may show mild nonspecific changes.

Temporal artery biopsy is often positive because of the high incidence of associated cranial arteritis.

HYPERTROPHIC OSTEOARTHROPATHY (CLUBBING; HYPERTROPHIC "PULMONARY" OSTEOARTHROPATHY)

Due To

Pulmonary diseases (especially bronchogenic carcinoma, bronchiectasis, lung abscess)

Pleural disease (especially tumors, empyema)

Mediastinal lesions (e.g., malignant lymphoma, aortic aneurysm)

Cardiac diseases (especially subacute bacterial endocarditis, cyanotic congenital heart disease)

Hepatic disease (especially cholangiolitic cirrhosis)

Intestinal diseases (especially tuberculosis, amebic infection, regional enteritis, ulcerative colitis, neoplasms)
Rare hereditary and idiopathic causes

CARPAL TUNNEL SYNDROME

Rule out underlying conditions.
> Amyloidosis
> Pregnancy
> Acromegaly
> Rheumatoid inflammation
> Many others (e.g., fibrosis, trauma)

NORMAL LABORATORY FINDINGS IN DISEASES OF BONE
Polyostotic fibrous dysplasia (Albright's syndrome) (occasionally increased serum alkaline phosphatase)
Giant-cell tumor of bone
Achondroplasia
Dyschondroplasias
Tietze's syndrome
Osteitis pubis
Osteogenesis imperfecta

NORMAL LABORATORY FINDINGS IN DISEASES OF JOINTS
Slipped femoral epiphysis
Aseptic (avascular) necrosis of bone
Juvenile osteochondritis
Osteochondritis dissecans
Hypertrophic osteoarthropathy
Congenital dysplasia of hip
Joint mice
Intervertebral disk syndrome

NORMAL LABORATORY FINDINGS IN DISEASES OF MUSCULOSKELETAL SYSTEM
Fibrositis
Fasciitis
Bursitis
Capsulitis
Tenosynovitis
Tendinitis
Dupuytren's contracture

Hematologic Diseases

CLASSIFICATION OF ANEMIAS ACCORDING TO PATHOGENESIS

Marrow hypofunction with decreased RBC production

    Marrow replacement (myelophthisic anemias due to tumor or granulomas [e.g., tuberculosis])

In absence of severe anemia or leukemoid reaction, nucleated RBCs in blood smear suggest miliary tuberculosis or marrow metastases.

    Marrow injury (hypoplastic and aplastic anemias)

    Nutritional deficiency (e.g., megaloblastic anemias due to lack of vitamin B_{12} or folic acid)

    Endocrine hypofunction (e.g., pituitary, adrenal, thyroid)

Marrow hypofunction due to decreased hemoglobin production (hypochromic microcytic anemias)

    Deficient heme synthesis (iron deficiency anemia, pyridoxine-responsive anemias)

    Deficient globin synthesis (thalassemias, hemoglobinopathies)

Excessive loss of RBCs (hemolytic anemias due to genetically defective RBCs)

    Abnormal shape (hereditary spherocytosis, hereditary elliptocytosis)

    Abnormal hemoglobins (sickle cell anemia, thalassemias, hemoglobin C disease)

    Abnormal RBC enzymes (glucose-6-PD deficiency, congenital nonspherocytic hemolytic anemias)

Excessive loss of RBCs

    Hemolytic anemias with acquired defects of RBC and positive Coombs' test (autoantibodies, as in systemic lupus erythematosis [SLE], malignant lymphoma; or exogenous allergens, as in penicillin allergy)

Excessive loss of normal RBCs

    Hemorrhage

    Hypersplenism

    Chemical agents (e.g., lead)

    Infectious agents (e.g., *Clostridium welchii, Bartonella,* malaria)

    Miscellaneous diseases (e.g., uremia, liver disease, cancers)

    Physical agents (e.g., burns)

    Mechanical trauma (e.g., artificial heart valves, tumor microemboli)

Blood smear shows fragmented bizarre-shaped RBCs in patients with artificial heart valves.

Anemias are often multifactorial; the resultant characteristics depend on which factor predominates. The diagnosis must be reevaluated after the apparent causes have been treated.

Table 27-1. Red Blood Cell Indices

Type of Anemia	Mean Corpuscular Volume (MCV)[a] (fl)	Mean Corpuscular Hemoglobin (MCH)[b] (pg)	Mean Corpuscular Hemoglobin Concentration (MCHC)[c] (gm/dl)
Normal	82–92	27–31	32–36
Normocytic anemias	82–92	25–30	32–36
Macrocytic anemias	95–150	30–50	32–36
Microcytic (usually hypochromic) anemias	50–80	12–25	25–30

[a] Mean corpuscular volume (MCV) (fl) = hematocrit/RBC.
[b] Mean corpuscular hemoglobin (MCH) (pg) = hemoglobin/RBC; represents weight of hemoglobin in average RBC. Not as useful as MCHC.
[c] Mean corpuscular hemoglobin concentration (MCHC) (gm/dl) = hemoglobin/hematocrit; represents concentration of hemoglobin in average RBC.

MCHC is increased only in hereditary spherocytosis. MCHC is not increased in pernicious anemia.

RED BLOOD CELL INDICES IN VARIOUS ANEMIAS
Macrocytic (MCV > 95 fl; MCHC > 30 gm/dl)
   Megaloblastic anemia
      Pernicious anemia
      Sprue (e.g., steatorrhea, celiac disease, intestinal resection or fistula)
      Macrocytic anemia of pregnancy
      Megaloblastic anemia of infancy
      Fish tapeworm infestation
      Carcinoma of stomach, following total gastrectomy
      Drug therapy (e.g., estrogens, antimetabolites, phenytoin)
      Orotic aciduria
      Di Guglielmo's disease
      Liver disease
      Alcohol intoxication
   Miscellaneous macrocytic nonmegaloblastic anemias that are usually normocytic
      Anemia of hypothyroidism
      Hemolytic anemia
      Aplastic anemia
Normocytic (MCV = 80–94 fl; MCHC > 30 gm/dl)
   Following acute hemorrhage
   Hemolytic anemias
   Anemias due to inadequate blood formation
      Myelophthisic
      Hypoplastic
      Aplastic
   Endocrinopathies (hypopituitarism, hypothyroidism, hypoadrenalism, hypogonadism)

Anemia of chronic disease (chronic infections, neoplasms, uremia, etc.)

Microcytic (usually hypochromic) (MCV < 80 fl; MCHC < 30 gm/dl)
　　Iron deficiency
　　　　Inadequate intake
　　　　Poor absorption
　　　　Excessive iron requirements
　　　　Chronic blood loss
　　　　Other
　　Pyridoxine-responsive anemia
　　Thalassemia (major or combined with hemoglobinopathy)
　　Sideroblastic anemia (hereditary)
　　Lead poisoning
　　Chronic inflammation

Microcytic (usually normocytic)
　　Anemia of chronic diseases
　　Hemoglobinopathies

RED CELL DISTRIBUTION WIDTH (RDW)

Is coefficient of variation (CV) of the RBC size as determined by automated blood cell counting instruments.

$$CV = \frac{\text{standard deviation of RBC size}}{\text{mean corpuscular volume (MCV)}}$$

Normal = 11.5–14.5. No subnormal values have been reported.

MYELOPHTHISIC ANEMIA

Anemia is usually mild; not more than moderate.

Increased nucleated RBCs and normoblasts in peripheral smear, often without reticulocytosis, are out of proportion to the degree of anemia and may be found even in the absence of anemia. Polychromatophilia, basophilic stippling, and increased reticulocyte count may also occur.

WBC may be normal or decreased; occasionally it is increased up to a leukemoid picture; immature WBC may be found in peripheral smear.

Table 27-2. Classification of RBC Disorders by RDW and MCV

RDW	MCV	Disorder
N	D	Thalassemia minor; anemia of chronic disease
I	D	Iron deficiency; RBC fragmentation; Hb H disease; S beta thalassemia
N	N	Normal; anemia of chronic disease; hereditary spherocytosis; hemoglobinopathy traits (e.g., AS)
I	N	Early vitamin B_{12} or folate deficiency; sickle cell anemia; Hb SC disease
N	I	Aplastic anemia; myelodysplastic syndrome
I	I	Vitamin B_{12} or folate deficiency; immune hemolytic anemia; cold agglutinins

N = normal; D = decreased; I = increased.

Platelets may be normal or decreased, and abnormal forms may occur. Abnormalities may occur even when WBC is normal.
Bone marrow demonstrates primary disease.
> Metastatic carcinoma of bone marrow (especially breast, lung, prostate, thyroid)
> Hodgkin's disease, leukemia
> Multiple myeloma (5% of patients)
> Gaucher's, Niemann-Pick, and Hand-Schüller-Christian diseases
> Osteopetrosis
> Myelofibrosis

Mild anemia with normoblastemia should arouse suspicion of infiltrative disease of marrow.

Nonhemolytic normocytic anemias with no obvious cause characterized by marked RBC changes on blood smear should arouse suspicion of malignancy or marrow fibrosis.

IDIOPATHIC MYELOFIBROSIS (AGNOGENIC MYELOID METAPLASIA)
Normocytic anemia is usual.
Peripheral smear shows anisocytosis; teardrop poikilocytosis is striking; polychromatophilia and occasional nucleated RBCs are found.
Reticulocyte count is increased ($\leqq 10\%$).
WBC may be normal (50% of patients), increased or decreased, and abnormal forms may occur. Immature cells ($\leqq 15\%$) are usual. Basophils and eosinophils may be increased.
Platelets may be normal or decreased, and abnormal forms may occur.
Repeated bone marrow aspiration often produces no marrow elements. Surgical biopsy of bone for histologic examination shows fibrosis of marrow that is usually hypocellular.
Needle puncture of spleen and a lymph node shows extramedullary hematopoiesis.
Hypersplenism causes thrombocytopenia in 30% and leukopenia in 15% of these patients.
Leukocyte alkaline phosphatase is increased; may be marked.
Serum uric acid is often increased.
Prolonged prothrombin time is found in 75% of patients.
Laboratory findings due to complications
> Hemorrhage
> Hemolytic anemia
> Infection
> DIC occurs in 20% of patients.

Rule out other myeloproliferative diseases, underlying poisoning (e.g., phosphorus, fluorine, estrogens).

PURE RED CELL ANEMIA (AREGENERATIVE ANEMIA; IDIOPATHIC HYPOPLASTIC ANEMIA; PRIMARY RED CELL APLASIA, ETC.)
Severe normochromic normocytic anemia is present that is refractory to all treatment except transfusion and sometimes ACTH or corticosteroids.

Reticulocytes are decreased or absent.

WBC and differential blood count are normal.

There is no evidence of hemolysis.

Bone marrow usually shows marked decrease in erythroid series but sometimes is normal. Myeloid cells and megakaryocytes are normal.

Plasma iron (^{59}Fe) clearance is markedly reduced.

RBC uptake of ^{59}Fe is markedly decreased.

Increased erythropoietin level

The disease may be related to thymus tumors (see p. 380), leukemia, which develops in 10% of patients, chemicals, bronchogenic carcinoma (rarely), kwashiorkor, etc.

PANCYTOPENIA

Anemia

Leukopenia—absolute myeloid decrease may be associated with relative lymphocytosis or with lymphocytopenia.

Thrombocytopenia

Laboratory findings due to causative disease

Due To

Hypersplenism
>   Congestive splenomegaly
>   Malignant lymphomas
>   Histiocytoses
>   Infectious diseases (tuberculosis, kala-azar, sarcoidosis)
>   Primary splenic pancytopenia

Diseases of marrow
>   Metastatic carcinoma
>   Multiple myeloma
>   Aleukemic leukemia
>   Osteopetrosis
>   Myelosclerosis, myelofibrosis, etc.
>   Systemic mastocytosis (requires Giemsa or toluidine stain of bone marrow)

Aplastic anemias
>   Physical and chemical causes (e.g., ionizing irradiation, benzol compounds)
>   Idiopathic causes (familial or isolated; *"isolated" accounts for 50% of all cases of pancytopenia*)

Megaloblastic macrocytic anemias (e.g., pernicious anemia)

Paroxysmal nocturnal hemoglobinuria (rare)

APLASTIC ANEMIA

Peripheral blood pancytopenia associated with variable bone marrow hypocellularity in the absence of underlying myeloproliferative or malignant disease.

Anemia is usually normochromic, normocytic but may be slightly macrocytic.

Reticulocyte count corrected for hematocrit is decreased.

No poikilocytes are seen on peripheral blood smear.

Serum iron is increased.

Both bone marrow aspiration and biopsy should be performed.

Criteria for diagnosis (International Aplastic Anemia Study Group)
    Peripheral blood
        Neutrophils < 500/cu mm
        Platelets < 20,000/cu mm
        Reticulocyte count corrected for hematocrit < 1%
    Marrow
        Severe hypocellularity
        Moderate hypocellularity with < 30% of residual cells being hematopoietic
    At least any two peripheral blood criteria plus either of marrow criteria

    Following treatment with marrow transplantation
        Acute graft-versus-host disease develops in 25–30% of recipients and is fatal in 8%.
        Chronic graft-versus-host disease develops in 20–30% of patients who survive > 6 months.
        Most infections occur within 6 months. Interstitial pneumonia occurs in 16% of those conditioned by cyclophosphamide and up to 50% of those conditioned with whole body irradiation: mortality is 40–50%; one-half of cases are due to CMV and one-half are of unknown cause.
Laboratory findings represent the whole spectrum, from the most severe condition of the classic type with marked leukopenia, thrombocytopenia, anemia, and acellular bone marrow, to cases with involvement only of erythroid elements. In some cases, the marrow may be cellular or hyperplastic.

Due To
Idiopathic in 50% of cases
Ionizing irradiation (x-ray, radioisotopes)
Chemicals (e.g., benzene family)
Cytotoxic (e.g., nitrogen mustards, busulfan) and antimetabolite (e.g., antifolates, 6-mercaptopurine) drugs
Other drugs (e.g., chloramphenicol, antibiotics, anticonvulsants, phenylbutazone, gold)
Immunologic disorders (graft-versus-host reaction)
Malnutrition (e.g., kwashiorkor)
Infections (especially non-A, non-B hepatitis)
Constitutional, inherited (e.g., Fanconi's anemia)
Leukemia is the underlying disease in 1–5% of patients who present with aplastic anemia.
Paroxysmal nocturnal hemoglobinuria (PNH) develops in 5–10% of patients with aplastic anemia, and aplastic anemia develops in 25% of patients with PNH.

HEMATOLOGIC EFFECTS OF CHEMICALS THAT INJURE BONE MARROW
(especially benzene; also trinitrotoluene and others)
In order of decreasing frequency
    Anemia
    Macrocytosis
    Thrombocytopenia
    Leukopenia
    Other (e.g., decreased lymphocytes, increased reticulocytes, increased eosinophils)

Varying degrees of severity up to aplastic anemia
Hemolytic anemia is sometimes produced.

HEMATOLOGIC EFFECTS OF IRRADIATION
(depends on amount of irradiation received)
Severe
> Severe leukopenia with infection
> Thrombocytopenia and increased vascular fragility, causing hemorrhage; begins in 4–7 days, peak severity in 16–22 days
> Aplastic anemia if patient survives 3–6 weeks; laboratory findings due to complications, such as hemorrhage, infection, dehydration

Mild (< 300 R)
> Increased neutrophils within a few hours with onset of irradiation sickness
> Decreased lymphocytes after 24 hours, causing decrease in total WBC
> No anemia unless dose of radiation is greater; may appear in 4–8 weeks (*Early appearance of anemia with greater irradiation is due to hemorrhage and changes in fluid homeostasis rather than marrow injury.*)
> Platelets slightly decreased (some patients)

Chronic (occupational)
> Decreased granulocytes
> Increased lymphocytes, relative or absolute
> Varying degrees of leukocytosis and leukemoid reactions
> Varying degrees of anemia, normocytic or macrocytic; erythrocytosis
> Thrombocytopenia

Late
> Increased incidence of leukemia (e.g., in survivors of atomic bomb explosions)
> Increased incidence of visceral malignancy (e.g., liver cancer due to Thorotrast, bone cancer due to radium)

PERNICIOUS ANEMIA
Anemia sometimes shows RBC as low as 500,000/cu mm.

MCV is increased (95–110 fl with mild to moderate anemia; 110–150 fl with more severe anemia.

Macrocytosis may be absent in a substantial number of black patients, possibly due to an associated alpha thalassemia or iron deficiency.

MCH is increased (33–38 pg with moderate anemia; up to 56 pg with severe anemia).

MCHC is normal.

Poikilocytosis is moderate to marked; it is always present in relapse.

Anisocytosis is moderate to marked; it is always present in relapse.

Reticulocyte count is decreased or normal.

Blood smear may show polychromatophilia, stippled RBCs, Howell-Jolly bodies, Cabot's rings, etc. Large hypersegmented leukocytes (shift to the right) are usually present and may precede RBC abnormalities. Occasionally there is moderate eosinophilia.

Thrombocytopenia is present; abnormal and giant forms may be seen.

Leukopenia is usually < 4000/cu mm.

RBC survival is decreased.

Marrow shows megaloblastic and erythroid hyperplasia and abnormalities of myeloid and megakaryocytic elements.

Achlorhydria occurs even after administration of histamine—this is virtually essential for diagnosis. Decreased volume of gastric juice, high pH, and decreased or absent pepsin and rennin are also shown. Achlorhydria and gastric changes are rarely found in children.

Schilling test is diagnostic.

Serum vitamin B_{12} is decreased.

Serum intrinsic factor blocking antibody is present in 50–60% of patients with pernicious anemia. Positive test strongly supports diagnosis of pernicious anemia and therefore should be performed in patients with low serum B_{12}; however, a negative test does not rule out pernicious anemia since almost one-half of such patients are negative for this antibody. False positive results are rare.

Serum LDH (principally LDH_1 and LDH_2) is markedly increased.

Serum iron is almost always increased during relapse unless there is complicating iron deficiency. Total iron-binding capacity (TIBC) is normal or slightly decreased.

Serum indirect bilirubin is increased (< 4 mg/dl).

Urine urobilinogen and coproporphyrin I are increased.

Stool urobilinogen is increased.

Serum alkaline phosphatase is decreased; increases after treatment.

Serum cholesterol is moderately decreased.

Cholinesterase activity in RBC, plasma, and whole blood is decreased.

There is a characteristic therapeutic response to vitamin B_{12} administration.

RESPONSE OF LABORATORY TESTS TO SPECIFIC TREATMENT OF PERNICIOUS ANEMIA

Increased urinary urobilinogen and coproporphyrin I immediately revert to normal, preceding reticulocyte response.

Serum folate decreases at the same time reticulocytosis takes place.

Serum iron decreases to normal or less than normal at the same time reticulocytosis takes place.

Serum uric acid increases; peak precedes maximum reticulocyte count by about 24 hours; remains increased as long as rapid RBC regeneration goes on.

Serum LDH falls but is not yet normal by eighth day.

Serum cholesterol rises to greater than normal levels; most marked at peak of reticulocyte response.

RBC count reaches normal between 8th and 12th week regardless of severity of anemia; hemoglobin concentration may rise at a slower rate, producing hypochromia with microcytosis.

Reticulocyte response is proportional to severity of anemia. This response is characteristic: reticulocyte count begins to rise by fourth day after treatment and reaches maximum on eighth to ninth day; returns to normal by 14th day.

Megaloblasts disappear from marrow in 24–48 hours.

Achlorhydria persists.

RBC cholinesterase activity increases.

Serum alkaline phosphatase increases to normal.

MACROCYTIC ANEMIA OF LIVER DISEASE

Increased MCV (100–125 fl) in one-third to two-thirds of patients. Indices resemble those in other megaloblastic anemias. Low MCHC may indicate associated iron deficiency.

Uniform round macrocytosis is the cardinal finding. Target cells and stomatocytes may be present.

Hemolytic anemia or true folate deficiency is frequent in alcoholic liver disease.

WBC and platelet count may be decreased or normal.

MACROCYTIC ANEMIA OF SPRUE, CELIAC DISEASE, STEATORRHEA

See p. 235.

MEGALOBLASTIC ANEMIA OF PREGNANCY AND PUERPERIUM

Anemia may have been present during previous pregnancy with spontaneous remission after delivery.

Hematologic abnormalities are less marked than in pernicious anemia (see pp. 334-335).

If achlorhydria is present, it often disappears after delivery.

Therapeutic response to folic acid but usually not to vitamin B_{12}.

Urinary excretion of formiminoglutamic acid (FIGLU) is increased.

HEREDITARY OROTIC ACIDURIA

This disorder of pyrimidine metabolism is due to a defect in the conversion of orotic acid to uridylic acid.

The severe megaloblastic anemia is refractory to vitamin B_{12} and folic acid but responsive to oral prednisone and yeast extract containing uridylic and cytidylic acids.

Anemia is hypochromic or normocytic; there is marked anisocytosis.

Leukopenia is present with increased susceptibility to infection.

Table 27-3. Laboratory Tests in Differential Diagnosis of Causes of Vitamin B_{12} Deficiencies

| | Gastric Juice | | Schilling Test | |
Condition	HCl	Intrinsic Factor Assay	Without Intrinsic Factor	With Intrinsic Factor
Lack of intrinsic factor (usually pernicious anemia)	O	O	D	N
Intestinal lesion	P or O	P	D	D
Nutritional	P or O	P	N	N

O = absent; P = present; N = normal; D = decreased.

Presence of free HCl in gastric juice always rules out pernicious anemia (except for very rare cases); absence of HCl is not helpful.

Table 27-4. Laboratory Tests in Differential Diagnosis of Vitamin B_{12} and Folic Acid Deficiencies

	Serum Vitamin B_{12}	Serum Folate	RBC Folate
Normal	N	N or D	N
Vitamin B_{12} deficiency	D	N or I	D
Folic acid deficiency	N	D	D
Vitamin B_{12} and folic acid deficiencies	D	D	D

N = normal; D = decreased; I = increased.

Folate deficiency is reflected in RBC folate levels. Low serum folate indicates only negative folate balance, not folate deficiency. Serum folate serves to distinguish combined deficiency from vitamin B_{12} deficiency alone. Thus all three parameters should be measured simultaneously in suspected cases of megaloblastic anemia.

Iron deficiency is present in one-half of patients with folate deficiency and one-third with vitamin B_{12} deficiency. If iron deficiency is more severe than folate deficiency, results of serum and RBC folate tests are normal, and diagnosis cannot be made from these tests; hypersegmentation of leukocytes in blood smear is the only clue.

Orotic acid in urine is increased; crystals precipitate when urine stands at room temperature.
RBC orotidylic decarboxylase activity is decreased (<5.5 units).
Iatrogenic orotic aciduria occurs during cancer chemotherapy with 6-azauridine.

ANEMIA IN HYPOTHYROIDISM
Occurs in one-third to two-thirds of patients with hypothyroidism; usually mild (hematocrit > 35%)
Normochromic normocytic or macrocytic *(If hypochromic, rule out associated iron deficiency.)*
No anisocytosis or poikilocytosis
Decreased total blood volume and plasma volume
Normal RBC survival
Responds only to treatment of hypothyroidism

IRON DEFICIENCY ANEMIA

Due To (usually a combination of these factors)
Chronic blood loss (e.g., menometrorrhagia, bleeding from GI tract, especially from carcinoma of colon, hiatus hernia, peptic ulcer, parasites in intestine)
Decreased food intake (e.g., poverty, emotional factors)
Decreased absorption (e.g., steatorrhea, gastrectomy, achlorhydria)
Increased requirements (e.g., pregnancy, lactation)

Laboratory Findings
Hemoglobin is decreased (usually 6–10 gm/dl) out of proportion to decrease in RBC (3.5–5.0 million/cu mm); thus MCV is decreased (<80 fl), MCHC is decreased (25–30 gm/dl), and MCH is decreased (<30 pg). Hypochromia and microcytosis parallel severity

Table 27-5. Laboratory Tests in Differential Diagnosis of Microcytic (MCV < 80 fl) and Hypochromic (MCHC < 30 gm/dl) Anemias

1. Determine serum iron and TIBC (and also perhaps do iron stain on bone marrow smear—the most reliable index of iron deficiency).
2. If serum iron and TIBC are both normal, hemoglobin electrophoresis will establish the diagnosis of thalassemia.

If serum iron is abnormal, the cause may be iron deficiency (e.g., blood loss, dietary deficiency) or normochromic microcytic anemia of chronic disease.

Type of Anemia	Serum Iron	TIBC	Transferrin Saturation	Serum Ferritin	FEP*	Marrow Hemosiderin	Sideroblasts	Type of Hemoglobin	Anemia
Normal values	80–160 µg/dl in men 50–150 µg/dl in women	250–410 µg/dl	20–55%	20–150 ng/dl			30–50%	AA	
Iron deficiency	D	I	D	D	I	O	D	AA	Hypochromic, normocytic, or microcytic
Normochromic, normocytic or microcytic, of chronic disease	D	D or N	D or N	N or slightly I	I	N or I	D	AA	Normochromic, normocytic, or microcytic

								RBC Morphology
Thalassemia								
Major	I	D	I	I	I	N	20–90% F	Hypochromic Microcytic
Minor	N or I	N	N or I	I	N	N	2–8% F, A2 is I	
Sideroblastic	N or I	D or N	I	I	D	I	AA	Hypochromic and/or microcytic with normocytic or macrocytic changes; dimorphic RBC population

O = absent; D = decreased; I = increased; N = normal.

*FEP = free erythrocyte protoporphyrin is useful to distinguish between iron deficiency and beta thalassemia.

Iron depletion: Early—serum iron is normal; TIBC may be increased. Later—serum iron decreases; anemia is often normocytic when mild or of rapid onset; anemia first becomes microcytic, then hypochromic.

Iron deficiency may occur without anemia (transferrin saturation < 15%; decreased marrow iron and sideroblasts).

Table 27-6. Comparison of Sample Values in Iron Deficient States

	Normal	Iron Depletion	Iron Deficiency Erythropoiesis	Iron Deficiency Anemia
RBC morphology	N	N	N	Microcytic hypo-chromic
Sideroblasts (%)	40–60	40–60	<10	<10
RBC protoporphyrin (μg/dl RBC)	30	30	100	200
Transferrin saturation (%)	20–50	30	<15	<10
Plasma iron (μg/dl)	65–165	115	<60	<40
Plasma ferritin (ng/ml)	40–160	20	10	<10
Transferrin IBC (μg/dl)	300–360	360	390	410
RE marrow iron	2–3+	0–1+	0	0

of anemia. Polychromatophilia and nucleated RBCs are less common than in pernicious anemia or thalassemia. Diagnosis from peripheral blood smear is difficult and unreliable.

Serum iron is decreased (usually 40 μg/dl), total iron-binding capacity increased (usually 350–460 μg/dl), and transferrin saturation decreased (<15%). TIBC may be normal or moderately decreased in many patients with uncomplicated iron deficiency.

Decreased serum ferritin is sensitive index of iron deficiency but may be increased when there is coexisting liver disease or an inflammatory condition. Thus iron deficiency is suggested by serum ferritin <25 μg/L in a patient with inflammation, <50 μg/L in a hemodialysis patient, and <100 μg/L in liver disease.

Bone marrow shows normoblastic hyperplasia with decreased hemosiderin, later absent, and decreased percentage of sideroblasts.

Reticulocytes are normal or decreased, unless there is recent hemorrhage or administration of iron.

WBC is normal or may be slightly decreased; may be increased with fresh hemorrhage.

Serum bilirubin and LDH are not increased.

Platelet count is normal or may be slightly increased.

Coagulation studies are normal.

RBC fragility is normal or (often) increased to 0.21%.

RBC life span is normal.

Laboratory findings may disclose causative factors (e.g., GI bleeding).

Response to oral iron therapy

    Increased reticulocytes with peak of 8–10% on fifth to tenth day; proportional to degree of anemia

    Followed by rising hemoglobin (average 0.25–0.4 gm/dl/day) and rising hematocrit (average = 1%/day) during first 7–10

Table 27-7. Differential Diagnosis of Iron Deficiency and Thalassemia Minor Microcytic Anemias

	Iron Deficiency	No Differentiation	Thalassemia Minor
Hemoglobin	<9.3 M or F	9.3–13.5 M 9.3–12.5 F	>13.5 M >12.5 F
MCV when Hb in indeterminate zone (fl)		>68	<68
MCHC (gm/dl)	<30	>30	
RBC (per cu mm)	<4.2	4.2–5.5	>5.5
Mentzer formula* $\left(\dfrac{MCV}{RBC}\right)$	>13		<13
England-Fraser* formula (MCV − [5 × HB + RBC + K]) if K = 3.4)		Positive number	Negative number
Shine-Lal formula* (MCV^2 × MCH)			<1530

M = males; F = females.
*These formulas are not applicable if patient has been treated with iron and sometimes with blood transfusion or if both conditions coexist (e.g., England-Fraser formula produces a positive number). Furthermore, in patients with polycythemia vera who develop iron deficiency with resultant microcytosis, a negative number results. These formulas do not account for the indeterminate zone of no differentiation.
Patients with thalassemia minor must have at least one parent with the disorder. A trial of iron therapy for 1 month will correct the anemia and microcytosis of iron deficiency.

days; thereafter hemoglobin increases 0.1 gm/dl/day to level ≧ 11 gm/dl in 3–4 weeks. In elderly, increase of 1 gm/dl may take 1 month when younger patients increase hemoglobin 3 gm/dl and hematocrit 10%.

Failure to respond suggests incorrect diagnosis, coexistent deficiencies (folic acid, vitamin B_{12}, thyroid), associated conditions (e.g., lead poisoning, bleeding, malabsorption, liver or kidney disease).

ATRANSFERRINEMIA
(isolated absence of transferrin)
Iron deficiency anemia is unresponsive to therapy.
Hemosiderosis follows transfusions with involvement of adrenals, heart, etc.
Serum protein electrophoresis shows marked decrease in beta globulins.
Absence of transferrin is demonstrated with immunoelectrophoresis.

ANEMIAS OF CHRONIC DISEASES
Due To
Subacute or chronic infections (especially tuberculosis, bronchiectasis, lung abscess, empyema, bacterial endocarditis, brucellosis)
Neoplasms
Rheumatoid arthritis (*anemia parallels activity of arthritis*)
Rheumatic fever, SLE
Uremia (BUN > 70 mg/dl)
Chronic liver diseases

Laboratory Findings
Anemia is usually mild (hemoglobin > 9 gm/dl) but may be as low as 5 gm/dl in uremia.
Anemia is usually normocytic, normochromic. In one-fourth to one-third of these patients, is hypochromic and/or microcytic, in which case it is always less marked than in iron deficiency anemia.
Moderate anisocytosis and slight poikilocytosis are present.
Reticulocytosis, polychromatophilia, and nucleated RBCs are absent (*may be present with severe anemia or uremia*).
Serum iron is decreased. TIBC and transferrin saturation are decreased or normal. If TIBC is elevated, presence of iron deficiency must be ruled out. Transferrin saturation < 10% implies iron deficiency.
Serum ferritin is high, normal, or increased in contrast to iron deficiency.

In rheumatoid arthritis, liver disease, or neoplasms, normal serum ferritin does not exclude concomitant iron deficiency.

Marrow hemosiderin is increased or normal; sideroblasts are decreased.
RBC survival is slightly decreased in patient but not in normal recipient.
Platelet count is normal.
WBC count is consistent with infection.

See Table 27-5, pp. 338–339.

SIDEROBLASTIC ANEMIAS
(Miscellaneous group of diseases characterized by increased sideroblasts [erythroblasts containing iron inclusions] in marrow) (see Table 27-5, p. 338)

Due To
Drugs (e.g., isoniazid, chloramphenicol, alcohol, lead, cytotoxic drugs such as nitrogen mustard and azathioprine)
Diseases
    Hematologic (e.g., leukemia, polycythemia vera, megaloblastic anemia, hemolytic anemia)
    Neoplastic (e.g., lymphoma, carcinoma)
    Inflammatory (e.g., infection, RA, polyarteritis nodosa)
    Miscellaneous (uremia, myxedema, thyrotoxicosis, porphyria)

Hereditary (pyridoxine-responsive or -refractory)
Idiopathic (pyridoxine-responsive or -refractory)

Hereditary
Usual onset in young adults but may be in children or infants
Anemia is usually severe, hypochromic, microcytic with anisocytosis, poikilocytosis, target cells, basophilic stippling; dimorphic RBC population.
WBC and platelets are usually normal.
Bone marrow shows erythroid hyperplasia with normoblastic maturation; 10–40% of normoblasts are ringed sideroblasts; excessive hemosiderin. Megaloblastic changes indicate complicating folate deficiency.
Transferrin saturation is increased.
Less than 50% of patients respond to pyridoxine therapy.

Idiopathic Refractory
Usual onset in older adults (rarely < 50 years)
Anemia is usually moderate, normocytic, or macrocytic with a small population of hypochromic RBCs on blood smear, some of which show marked stippling.
WBC and platelet counts are variable but usually normal.
Bone marrow shows erythroid hyperplasia; 45–95% of normoblasts are ringed sideroblasts; excessive hemosiderin. Megaloblastic changes due to complicating folate deficiency are found in 20% of patients.
Transferrin saturation is increased (>90% in 33% of patients)
Serum ferritin is increased.
Acute leukemia develops in ≅ 10% of patients.

Secondary
Due to drugs and toxic agents (e.g., chloramphenicol, antituberculosis drugs, lead poisoning, alcoholism) or associated with other diseases such as neoplasms (e.g., lymphomas, myeloma), hematologic diseases (e.g., leukemia, polycythemia vera), inflammatory diseases (e.g., SLE, rheumatoid arthritis, polyarteritis nodosa), miscellaneous diseases (e.g., thyroid dysfunction, porphyrias, uremia)

PYRIDOXINE-RESPONSIVE ANEMIA
Severe hypochromic microcytic anemia is present.
Blood smear shows anisocytosis, poikilocytosis with many bizarre forms, target cells, hypochromia. Polychromatophilia and reticulocytosis are not increased.
Serum iron is increased; TIBC is somewhat decreased; transferrin saturation is markedly increased. Marrow sideroblasts and blood siderocytes are increased. Marrow and liver biopsy show increased hemosiderin.
Bone marrow usually shows normoblastic hyperplasia; occasionally it is megaloblastic.
Response to pyridoxine is always incomplete. Even when hemoglobin becomes normal, morphologic changes in RBCs persist.

CLASSIFICATION OF HEMOLYTIC ANEMIAS*

Membrane Disorders
Intrinsic
    Congenital or familial (usually autosomal dominant)

Hereditary spherocytosis	Common
Hereditary elliptocytosis	Rare
Hereditary stomatocytosis	Very rare
Other	Very rare
Acquired—paroxysmal nocturnal hemo-	Rare
globinuria	

Extrinsic
    Congenital or familial

Abetalipoproteinemia	Very rare

    Acquired

Autoimmune (Coombs' test usually positive;	Common
spherocytes may be found)	

        Idiopathic
        Secondary to
            Lymphoproliferative disease (e.g., Hodgkin's
                disease, chronic lymphocytic leukemia)
            Autoimmune diseases (e.g., infectious mononucle-
                osis, *Mycoplasma*)
            Drug induced (e.g., penicillin, methyldopa)

Isoimmune	
Blood transfusion reaction	Rare
Nonimmune (Coombs' test usually negative;	Rare
morphologic changes in blood smears are	
usually found)	

        Physical or mechanical
            Prosthetic heart valves
            Severe burns
            March hemoglobinuria
            Microangiopathic hemolytic disease, including
                DIC, thrombotic thrombocytopenic purpura, he-
                molytic uremic syndrome, etc.
        Infectious
            Protozoan (e.g., malaria, toxoplasmosis, leish-
                maniasis)
            Bacterial (e.g., clostridial toxins, bartonellosis)

Hemoglobin Disorders
Intrinsic
    Autosomal

Sickle cell (SS) disease	Common
Hemoglobin C, D, E diseases	Common
Thalassemias	Common
Unstable hemoglobins	Very rare

Metabolic Disorders
Intrinsic

Glucose-6-PD deficiency	Common
Others (e.g., pyruvate kinase deficiency)	Rare or
	very rare

*Source: Adapted from M. C. Brain, Hemolytic anemia. *Postgrad. Med.* 64:127, Oct. 1978.

Extrinsic
    Drugs
        In normal RBC (e.g., dapsone)
        In glucose-6-PD deficiency
    Others (e.g., lead poisoning, Wilson's disease)

LABORATORY SCREENING FOR HEMOGLOBINOPATHIES
Normocytic normochromic RBC except in
    Thalassemia syndromes—microcytic hypochromic
    Hemoglobin (Hb) C, D, E diseases—microcytic normochromic
Osmotic fragility—normal or decreased (especially in thalassemia)
    Symmetric shift in Hb C, D, E, diseases
    Asymmetric shift in other hemoglobin diseases
Target cells—in many of hemolytic diseases due to hemoglo-
    binopathies; 50% of RBCs in Hb C, D, E diseases
Sickle cell test—proves presence of Hb S
Inclusion bodies—in Hb H and C disorders
Hemoglobin electrophoresis
Alkali denaturation for Hb F

SICKLE CELL DISEASE
Sickle cell trait (heterozygous sickle cell or Hb AS disease—occurs
    in ≅ 10% of American blacks)
    Hemoglobin electrophoresis: Hb S is 20–40%, and Hb A is 60–
        80%; small amount of Hb F (≦2%) may be present.
    Sickle cell preparation is positive.
    Blood smear shows only a few target cells.
    No anemia or hemolysis or jaundice is present.
    Anoxia may cause systemic sickling (see below, Sickle cell
        anemia).
        Beware anesthesia, airplane flights, etc.
    Hematuria without any other demonstrable cause may be
        found.
    Hyposthenuria may occur.
Sickle cell anemia (homozygous Hb SS disease); (occurs in 1:625
    American blacks)
    Hemoglobin electrophoresis: Hb S is 80–100%, and Hb F com-
        prises the rest (see Fetal Hemoglobin, p. 129); Hb A is absent.
    The anemia is normocytic normochromic (hemoglobin 5–10 gm/
        dl).
    Sickle cell preparation is positive.
    Blood smear shows a variable number of RBCs with abnormal
        shapes, nucleated RBCs, Howell-Jolly bodies, target cells,
        spherical cells.
    Reticulocyte count is increased (5–30%).
    WBC is increased (10,000–30,000/cu mm) during a crisis, with
        normal differential or shift to the left.
    Platelet count is increased (300,000–500,000/cu mm), with ab-
        normal forms.
    Bone marrow shows hyperplasia of all elements.
    Decreased ESR becomes normal after blood is aerated.
    Osmotic fragility is decreased (more resistant RBCs).
    Mechanical fragility of RBCs is increased.
    RBC survival time is decreased.
    Indirect serum bilirubin is increased (≦6 mg/dl).
    Urine contains increased urobilinogen but is negative for bile.

Table 27-8. Comparison of Sickle Cell Anemia and Hemoglobin SC Disease in Adults

Feature	Sickle Cell Anemia	Hb SC Disease
RBC, Hb, Hct	Lower	Higher
MCV	Higher	Lower, mildly microcytic
MCH	Higher	Lower
MCHC	Lower	Higher in females
Peripheral smear		
Irreversible sickled cells	Up to 16%	None, fat sickle (boat-shaped) cells
Target cells	Less abundant	More abundant
Nucleated RBCs, Howell-Jolly bodies	More abundant	Less abundant
Changes due to hemolysis	More marked	Less marked
Reticulocyte count, WBC, platelet count, serum/ LDH, uric acid, total bilirubin	Higher	Lower
Changes probably due to more frequent transfusion— serum/Fe, ferritin, % transferrin saturation	Higher	Lower
TIBC	Same	Same
Leukocyte alkaline phosphatase decreased	Less often	More often
Serum alkaline phosphatase, SGOT	Higher (elevated)	Lower (normal)
Serum creatinine (within normal range)	Lower	Higher
Clinical		
Severity	More	Less
Frequency of crises	More	Less
Frequency of leg ulcers, cholelithiasis	More	Less
Frequency of papillary necrosis, eye lesions, thromboembolic complications	Less	More

Source: Adapted from S. K. Ballas, et al. Clinical, hematological, and biochemical features of Hb SC disease. *Am. J. Hematol.* 13:37–51, 1982.

Urobilinogen in stool is increased.

Hemosiderin appears in urine sediment.

Hematuria is frequent.

Renal concentrating ability is decreased, leading to a fixed specific gravity in virtually all patients after the first few years of life.

Serum uric acid may be increased.

Serum alkaline phosphatase is increased during crisis, representing vaso-occlusive bone injury as well as liver damage.

Leukocyte alkaline phosphatase activity is decreased.

Laboratory findings due to complications

Infarction of lungs, spleen, brain, bowel, etc.

Stasis and necrosis of liver—increased bile in urine, increased direct serum bilirubin ≤ 40 mg/dl, other findings of obstructive type of jaundice. Chronic cholecystitis and cholelithiasis in one-third of adults.

Salmonella osteomyelitis (see p. 571).

Anemia and hemolytic jaundice are present throughout life after age 3–6 months; hemolysis and anemia are not increased during crises.

Hb SC disease (occurs in 1:833 American blacks)

Hemoglobin electrophoresis: Hb A is absent; Hb S predominates (30–60%) with Hb C present; Hb F is 2–15%.

Blood smear shows tetragonal crystals within RBC in 70% of patients.

Other findings are the same as for sickle cell anemia, but there is less marked destruction of RBCs, anemia, etc., and the disease is less severe clinically. *Crises may cause a more marked fall in RBC than occurs in Hb SS disease.*

Sickle cell–thalassemia disease (occurs in 1:1667 American blacks)

Hemoglobin electrophoresis: Hb S is 20–80%; Hb F is 2–20%; Hb A is 0–50%.

Anemia is hypochromic microcytic; target cells are prominent; serum iron is normal.

Other findings resemble those of sickle cell anemia.

Sickle cell–persistent high fetal hemoglobin (occurs in 1:25,000 American blacks)

Hemoglobin electrophoresis: Hb F is 20–40%; absent, Hb A and A_2; Hb S is present.

Findings are intermediate between those of sickle cell anemia and of sickle cell trait.

Sickle cell–hemoglobin D disease (occurs in 1:20,000 American blacks)

Findings are intermediate between those of sickle cell anemia and of sickle sickle cell trait.

THALASSEMIAS
(see Tables 27-5 and 27-6, pp. 338 and 340)

Thalassemia trait

In uncomplicated cases, hemoglobin is normal or only slightly decreased (11–12 gm/dl), while the RBC is increased (5–7 million/cu mm). Most nonanemic patients with microcytosis have thalassemia minor. Microcytic anemia with anemia <

Table 27-9. Some Laboratory Findings in Hemoglobinopathies and Thalassemia

Condition	Hb Type	Hb F (fetal hemoglobin) % of Total	Sickling (stained blood smear)	% Target Cells	Microcytosis	Hypochromia	Severity of Anemia	Splenomegaly
Normal adult	AA	0–2	0	0	0	0	0	0
Normal newborn	AF	60–90	0	0	0	0	0	0
Sickle cell trait	AS	0–2	+	4	0	0	0	0
Sickle cell anemia	SS	2–30	++	5–30	0	0–1+	4+	0
Sickle cell–thalassemia	SF	2–20	+	20–40	3+	3+	3–4+	2+
Sickle cell–Hb C	SC	2–8	+	20–85	0	1–2+	2–3+	2+
Sickle cell–Hb D	SD	0–2	+	1+	0–1+	1–2+	3–4+	2+
Sickle cell–Hb G	SG	0–2	+	0	0	0	0	0
Sickle cell–hereditary spherocytosis	SA	0–2	+	1+	1+	0	1–4+	2+
Thalassemia minor	AA_2	0–8	0	1+	2–3+	2–3+	1+	±

Thalassemia major	AF	10–100	0	10–35	2–4+	2–4+	2–4+	3–4+	4+
Hb C–thalassemia	CA	0–2	0	3+	1+	1+	1+	0–1+	0
Hb E–thalassemia	EF	20–40	0	10–40	2+	2+	2+	1+	3+
Hb G–thalassemia	EG	0–2	0	1+	1+	1+	1+	1+	0
Hb H–thalassemia	AH	0–2	0	2+	1+	2+	1+	2+	±
Hb C trait	AC	0–2	0	1–100	0	1+	0	0	0
Hb C disease	CC	0–5	0	30–100	0–1+	3+	0–1+	1+	2+
Hb C–elliptocytosis	AC	0–2	0	1+	1+	2+	1+	0–1+	
Hb D trait	AD	0–2	0	0	0	0	0	0	0
Hb E trait	AE	0–2	0	0	0	0	0	0	0
Hb E disease	EE	0–9	0	25–60	2+	0	2+	0–1+	±
Hb G trait	AG	0–2	0	0	0	0	0	0	0
Hb G disease	GG	0–2	0	0	0	0	0	0	0
Hb I trait	AI	0–2	0	0–2	0	0	0	0	0

1+ to 4+ = degree present on a scale of 1–4.

9.3 gm/dl is unlikely to be thalassemia minor. MCV < 75 fl may be as low as 55 fl. MCHC > 31%.

Blood smear changes are less than in thalassemia major. Anisocytosis is less marked than in iron deficiency anemia. Microcytosis may be difficult to detect morphologically. Poikilocytosis is mild to moderate; more striking than iron deficiency anemia with Hb = 10–12 gm/dl. Target cells and oval forms may be numerous. Occasional RBCs show basophilic stippling in beta thalassemia minor (rare in blacks but common in Mediterranean patients).

Reticulocyte count is increased (2–10%).

Serum iron is normal or slightly increased; transferrin saturation may be increased. TIBC is normal.

Cellular marrow contains stainable iron.

Osmotic fragility is decreased.

Beta type of thalassemia minor has increased Hb A_2 (3–6%) on starch or agar electrophoresis and a slight increase in Hb F (2–10%). Hb A_2 is often decreased in iron deficiency; thus A_2 level may be normal in concomitant iron deficiency and beta thalassemia minor. Hb A_2 and F are absent in the alpha type of thalassemia. No specific laboratory identification of alpha thalassemia trait (carrier). Thus, normal hemoglobin electrophoresis and England-Fraser < −6 in the absence of iron deficiency implies alpha thalassemia minor; mild alpha thalassemia is a clinical diagnosis.

Alpha thalassemia coincident with sickle cell or Hb C trait reduces the proportion of Hb S or Hb C below the usual 35–40%; thus < 35% variant hemoglobin is good evidence for coexisting alpha thalassemia in such patients.

Thalassemia major

Fetal hemoglobin is 10–90%; Hb A is decreased; Hb A_2 is not increased.

There is marked hypochromic microcytic regenerative hemolytic anemia.

Blood smear shows marked anisocytosis, poikilocytosis, target cells, spherocytes, and hypochromic, fragmented, and bizarre RBCs; also many nucleated RBCs—basophilic stippling, Cabot's rings, siderocytes.

Reticulocyte count is increased.

WBCs are often increased, with normal differential or marked shift to the left.

Platelets are normal.

Bone marrow is cellular and shows erythroid hyperplasia and contains stainable iron.

Serum iron and TIBC are increased.

Serum LDH and indirect bilirubin are increased (1–3 mg/dl).

Urine urobilinogen is increased without bile.

Stool urobilinogen is increased.

RBC survival time is decreased.

Osmotic fragility is decreased.

Mechanical fragility is increased.

Laboratory findings due to secondary hypersplenism are present.

Hemoglobin E–thalassemia

The laboratory findings resemble those in thalassemia major.

HEMOGLOBIN C DISEASE

Hb C trait (occurs in 2% of American blacks, less frequently in other Americans)

Hemoglobin electrophoresis demonstrates the abnormal hemoglobin.

Blood smear shows variable number of target cells.

No other abnormalities are seen.

Hb C disease

Hemoglobin electrophoresis demonstrates the abnormal hemoglobin.

Mild hypochromic hemolytic anemia is present.

Blood smear shows many target cells, variable number of microspherocytes, occasional nucleated RBCs, a few tetragonal crystals within RBCs that increase following splenectomy.

Reticulocyte count is increased (2–10%).

Osmotic fragility is decreased.

Mechanical fragility is increased.

RBC survival time is decreased.

Hb F is slightly increased.

Increase in serum bilirubin is minimal.

Normoblastic hyperplasia of bone marrow is present.

HEMOGLOBIN D DISEASE

Homozygous Hb D disease

Hemoglobin electrophoresis demonstrates the abnormal hemoglobin at acid pH.

Mild microcytic anemia.

Target cells and spherocytes.

Decreased RBC survival time.

Heterozygous Hb D trait

Hemoglobin electrophoresis demonstrates the abnormal hemoglobin at acid pH.

There are no other laboratory findings.

Sickle cell–Hb D disease

Hemoglobin electrophoresis demonstrates the abnormal hemoglobin at acid pH.

Findings are intermediate between those of sickle cell anemia and sickle cell trait.

HEMOGLOBIN E DISEASE

Homozygous Hb E disease

Mild hypochromic hemolytic anemia

Target cells (25–60%)

Decreased osmotic fragility

Hb F sometimes slightly increased

Heterozygous Hb E trait

There are no laboratory findings.

Hb E–thalassemia

The laboratory findings resemble those in thalassemia major.

METHEMOGLOBINEMIA

Due To

Drugs and chemicals, especially aniline derivatives (e.g., acetanilid, phenacetin, certain sulfonamides, various clothing dyes)

Abnormal Hb M (several different Ms)
Inherited enzyme deficiency (e.g., methemoglobin reductase)

Laboratory Findings
Freshly drawn blood is chocolate-brown; does not become red after exposure to air.
Starch block electrophoresis identifies the Hb M.
Spectroscopic absorption analysis—band at 630 mμ disappears on addition of 5% KCN.
RBC is slightly increased; no other hematologic abnormalities are found; there is no jaundice.

Patient is cyanotic clinically but in apparent good health.

SULFHEMOGLOBINEMIA
Due To
Drugs, especially phenacetin (including Bromo-Seltzer) and acetanilid

Laboratory Findings
Spectroscopic absorption analysis—band at 618 mμ does not disappear on addition of 5% KCN.
Laboratory findings due to associated bromide intoxication. Bromide intoxication and sulfhemoglobinemia may be due to excessive intake of Bromo-Seltzer.

HEREDITARY ELLIPTOCYTOSIS (OVALOCYTOSIS)
Autosomal Mendelian dominant trait affecting 1:2500 persons in U.S.
Blood smear shows 25–90% of RBCs are oval. In normal individuals, up to 10–15% of RBCs may be oval or elliptical. Also seen frequently in thalassemias, hemoglobinopathies, iron deficiency, myelophthisic anemias. Only few ovalocytes are present at birth with gradual increase to stable value at 3–4 months old. Splenectomy does not affect ovalocytosis.
No other hematologic abnormalities are seen in most patients; about 12% of patients show a chronic congenital hemolytic anemia with decreased RBC survival time, moderate anemia, increased serum bilirubin, and increased reticulocyte count, increased osmotic fragility, and autohemolysis.
Hemoglobin electrophoresis is normal.
Osmotic fragility and autohemolysis are normal in patients without hemolytic anemia.
Mechanical fragility is increased.

HEREDITARY SPHEROCYTOSIS
Defective RBC membrane is abnormally permeable to sodium, causing water inflow and rupture.
Anemia (hemolytic type) is moderate (RBC = 3–4 million/cu mm), microcytic (MCV = 70–80 fl), and hyperchromic (MCHC = 36–40 gm/dl). MCHC $\geq$ 36% means congenital spherocytic anemia if cold agglutinins and hypertriglyceridemia have been excluded.
Anisocytosis is marked; poikilocytosis is slight.
Spherocytes are present.
Osmotic fragility is increased; when normal in some patients, the incubated fragility test shows increased hemolysis.

Autohemolysis (sterile defibrinated blood incubated for 48 hours) is increased (10–20% compared to normal of <4% of cells).

Abnormal osmotic fragility and autohemolysis are reduced by 10% glucose.

Mechanical fragility is increased.

Reticulocytes are increased.

WBC and platelet counts are usually normal; they may be increased during hemolysis.

Bone marrow shows marked erythroid hyperplasia; moderate hemosiderin is present.

Indirect serum bilirubin is increased.

Stool urobilinogen is usually increased.

Haptoglobins are decreased or absent.

Coombs' test is negative.

RBCs show Howell-Jolly bodies, Pappenheimer bodies, Heinz bodies.

Laboratory findings due to gallstones.

Diagnosis should be questioned if splenectomy does not cause a complete response.

HEREDITARY NONSPHEROCYTIC HEMOLYTIC ANEMIAS

This is a heterogeneous group. Some are due to deficiency of glucose-6-PD; others to unknown cause or to other rare congenital enzyme defects (e.g., glutathione).

Anemia is of the hemolytic type; may be severe; may begin in newborn; may be precipitated by certain drugs.

RBCs show Howell-Jolly bodies, Pappenheimer bodies, Heinz bodies, basophilic stippling; there may be slight macrocytosis.

Increase in reticulocyte count is marked, even with mild anemia.

Bone marrow shows marked erythroid hyperplasia; normal hemosiderin is present.

WBC, platelet count, hemoglobin electrophoresis, osmotic fragility, and mechanical fragility are normal.

Autohemolysis is present in some cases but not in others; reduction by glucose is less than in normal blood.

CONGENITAL STOMATOCYTOSIS

Rare condition of morphologic abnormality of RBCs in which one or more slitlike areas of central pallor produce a mouthlike appearance.

Findings resemble hereditary spherocytosis with variable degree of hemolytic anemia but *not* cured by splenectomy.

GLUCOSE 6-PHOSPHATE DEHYDROGENASE (GLUCOSE-6-PD) IN RBCS

After standard dose of primaquine in adult

Hematocrit usually begins to fall in 2–4 days; reaches nadir by 8–12 days.

Heinz bodies and increased serum bilirubin occur during first few days of hemolysis.

Reticulocytosis begins at about fifth day; reaches maximum in 10–20 days.

Recovery occurs in 10–40 days.

Decreased In
American black males (13%)
American black females (3%; 20% are carriers)
Some other ethnic groups (e.g., Greeks, Sardinians, Sephardic Jews)

May be associated with at least 4 clinical syndromes
> Some drug-induced acute hemolytic anemias (e.g., primaquine, sulfonamides, antipyretics)
> Favism
> Nonimmunologic hemolytic disease of the newborn
> Some cases of congenital nonspherocytic hemolytic anemia

Other Findings
Higher frequency of coronary heart disease and of cholelithiasis
Higher risk in presence of some other diseases (e.g., diabetes mellitus, viral hepatitis, pneumonia)

Increased In
Pernicious anemia to 3 times normal level; remains elevated for several months, even after administration of vitamin B_{12}
ITP (Werlhof's disease); becomes normal soon after splenectomy

Also reported in hepatic coma, hyperthyroidism, myocardial infarction (first week after), other megaloblastic anemias, and chronic blood loss.

ERYTHROCYTE PYRUVATE KINASE DEFICIENCY
Congenital inherited nonspherocytic hemolytic anemia showing
> Icterus
> Anemia that varies from mild to profound
> \> 5% and may be > 50%.
> Reticulocytosis
> Macrocytosis
> Few or no spherocytes
> Occasional "tailed poikilocytes"
> Varying abnormalities of incubated RBC osmotic fragility
> Deficiency of erythrocyte pyruvate kinase (10-25% of normal). If an infant has been transfused, the assay should be performed 3–4 months later. Assay will demonstrate heterozygous carrier state in parents who are hematologically normal.

Acquired type may be due to
> Drug ingestion
> Metabolic diseases of liver

PAROXYSMAL NOCTURNAL HEMOGLOBINURIA (MARCHIAFAVA-MICHELI SYNDROME)
Hemoglobinemia is present; increases during sleep.
Hemoglobinuria is evident on arising.
Serum haptoglobin is absent during an episode.
Chronic hemolytic anemia is well developed.
Urine contains hemoglobin, hemosiderin (in WBCs and epithelial cells of sediment), and increased urobilinogen.
Osmotic fragility is normal.
Serum iron may be decreased.
WBC is usually decreased.

Leukocyte alkaline phosphatase activity is decreased.
Platelet count is usually decreased but shows thrombotic rather than hemorrhagic complications.
Autohemolysis is increased.
RBC fragility is increased in acid medium (Ham test) and in hydrogen peroxide; amount of change is related to clinical severity.
RBC acetylcholinesterase activity is decreased.
Develops in 5–10% of patients with aplastic anemia, and aplastic anemia develops in 25% of patients with paroxysmal nocturnal hemoglobinuria.

PAROXYSMAL COLD HEMOGLOBINURIA
Sudden hemoglobinuria follows exposure to cold environment.
Findings are of acute hemolytic anemia.
Cold autohemolysin is present in blood.
Positive direct Coombs' test is present only during the attack.
There may be a biologic false positive test for syphilis, or the attack may be due to congenital syphilis.

ACQUIRED HEMOLYTIC ANEMIA
Laboratory findings due to increased destruction of RBCs
  RBC survival time differentiates intrinsic RBC defect from factor outside RBC.
  Blood smear often shows marked spherocytosis. Anisocytosis, poikilocytosis, and polychromasia are seen.
  Slight abnormality of osmotic fragility is shown.
  There is increased indirect serum bilirubin (less than 6 mg/dl because of compensatory excretory capacity of liver).
  Urine urobilinogen is increased (may vary with liver function; may be obscured by antibiotic therapy altering intestinal flora). Bile is absent from urine.
  Stool urobilinogen is increased.
  Hemoglobinemia and hemoglobinuria are present when hemolysis is very rapid.
  Haptoglobins are decreased or absent in chronic hemolytic diseases (removed following combination with free hemoglobin in serum).
  WBC is usually elevated.
Laboratory findings due to compensatory increased production of RBCs
  There is normochromic, normocytic anemia. MCV reflects immaturity of circulating RBCs. Polychromatophilia is present.
  Reticulocyte count is increased.
  Erythroid hyperplasia of bone marrow is evident.
Laboratory findings due to mechanism of RBC destruction
  Coombs' tests are positive.
  Warm antibodies are found.
  Cold agglutinins are found.
  There is a biologic false positive test for syphilis.
Laboratory findings due to underlying conditions
  Malignant lymphoma
  Collagen diseases (e.g., disseminated lupus erythematosus)
  Disseminated intravascular coagulation (see pp. 400, 402)
  Idiopathic pulmonary hemosiderosis (see p. 223)
  Infections, especially viral pneumonia

Drug-induced hemolytic anemia associated with a positive
Coombs' test

Other

MICROANGIOPATHIC HEMOLYTIC ANEMIA

Peripheral blood smear establishes the diagnosis by characteristic
burr cells, schistocytes, helmet cells, microspherocytes.

Nonimmune hemolytic anemia varies in severity depending on
underlying condition (see previous section).

Laboratory findings due to causative disease

Due To

Renal disease with uremia

Cardiac valvular disease (e.g., intracardiac valve prostheses, bacterial endocarditis, severe valvular heart disease)

Severe liver disease (e.g., cirrhosis)

Disseminated intravascular coagulation (see pp. 400, 402)

Snakebite (see p. 655)

LABORATORY FINDINGS DUE TO INTRAVASCULAR HEMOLYSIS

Plasma hemoglobin increases transiently with return to normal in
8 hours. Determinations lack accuracy and precision.

Plasma haptoglobin level decreases about 100 mg/dl in 6–10 hours
and lasts for 2–3 days after lysis of 20–30 ml blood. Determination is relatively reliable and very sensitive.

Urine hemosiderin occurs 3–5 days after hemolysis with positive
Prussian blue staining of renal tubular epithelial cells. It may be
difficult to detect a single episode. Urine hemosiderin is commonly found in paroxysmal nocturnal hemoglobinuria.

Hemoglobinuria occurs 1–2 hours after severe hemolysis and lasts
≤ 24 hours. It is a transient finding and is relatively insensitive.
False positive is due to myoglobinuria or to lysis of RBCs in urine.

Schumm's test for methemalbuminemia becomes positive 1–6 hours
after hemolysis of 100 ml blood and lasts 1–3 days. Methemalbuminemia also occurs in hemorrhagic pancreatitis.

Serum bilirubin increase depends on liver function and amount of
hemolysis. With normal liver function, it is increased 1 mg/dl in
1–6 hours to maximum in 3–12 hours following hemolysis of 100
ml blood.

Fecal urobilinogen may be increased but not useful because of wide
normal range and variability.

Urine urobilinogen is similarly insensitive and unreliable as an
index of hemolysis.

Extravascular hemolysis may cause increases in serum bilirubin
and urine and fecal urobilinogen and a decrease in serum haptoglobin.

ANEMIA DUE TO ACUTE BLOOD LOSS

RBC, hemoglobin, and hematocrit level are not reliable initially
because of compensatory vasoconstriction and hemodilution.
They decrease for several days after hemorrhage ceases. RBC
returns to normal in 4–6 weeks. Hemoglobin returns to normal in
6–8 weeks.

Anemia is normochromic, normocytic. *(If hypochromic or microcytic, rule out iron deficiency due to prior hemorrhages.)*

Reticulocyte count is increased after 1–2 days, reaches peak in 4–7 days ($\leq 15\%$). Persistent increase suggests continuing hemorrhage.

Blood smear shows no poikilocytes. Polychromasia and increased number of nucleated RBCs (up to 5:100 WBCs) may be found.

Increased WBC (usually $\leq$ 20,000/cu mm) reaches peak in 2–5 hours, becomes normal in 3–4 days. Persistent increase suggests continuing hemorrhage, bleeding into a body cavity, or infection. Differential count shows shift to the left.

Platelets are increased (≤ 1 million/cu mm) within a few hours; coagulation time is decreased.

BUN is increased if hemorrhage into lumen of GI tract occurs.

Serum indirect bilirubin is increased if hemorrhage into a body cavity or cystic structure occurs.

Laboratory findings due to causative disease (e.g., peptic ulcer, esophageal varices, leukemia) are noted.

ANEMIAS IN PARASITIC INFESTATIONS
Anemia due to blood loss, malnutrition, specific organ damage
Malaria
Hemolytic anemia
Diphyllobothrium latum (fish tapeworm)
Macrocytic anemia
Hookworm
Hypochromic microcytic anemia due to chronic blood loss
Schistosoma mansoni
Hypochromic microcytic anemia due to blood loss from intestine
Macrocytic anemia due to cirrhosis of schistosomiasis
Amebiasis
Due to blood loss and malnutrition

"ANEMIA" IN PREGNANCY
This is a normal physiologic change due to hemodilution—total blood volume and plasma volume increase more than red cell mass.

Onset is at eighth week; full development by 16–22 weeks; rapid return to normal in puerperium.

Hemoglobin averages 11 gm/dl; hematocrit value averages 33.

RBC morphology is normal.

RBC indices are normal.

If hemoglobin is < 10 gm/dl or there are hypochromic microcytic indices, rule out iron deficiency anemia, which may occur frequently during pregnancy.

See Megaloblastic Anemia of Pregnancy and Puerperium, p. 336.

POLYCYTHEMIA VERA
RBC is 7–12 million; may increase to > 15 million/cu mm.

Hemoglobin is 18–24 gm/dl.

Hematocrit value is increased.

MCV, MCH, and MCHC are normal or decreased.

Blood volume and red cell mass are increased; plasma volume is variable.

ESR is decreased.

Blood viscosity is increased.

Table 27-10. Laboratory Tests in Differential Diagnosis of Polycythemia Vera, Secondary Polycythemia, and Relative Polycythemia

Test	Polycythemia Vera	Secondary Polycythemia	Relative Polycythemia
Hematocrit	I	I	I
Blood volume	I	I	D or N
Red cell mass	I	I	D or N
Plasma volume	I or N	N or I	D or N
Platelet count	I	N	N
WBC with shift to left	I	N	N
Nucleated RBC, abnormal RBC	I	N	N
Serum uric acid	I	I	N
Serum vitamin B_{12}	I	N	N
Leukocyte alkaline phosphatase	I	N	N
Oxygen saturation of arterial blood	N	D	N
Bone marrow	Hyperplasia of all elements	Erythroid hyperplasia	N

I = increased; D = decreased; N = normal.

Osmotic fragility is decreased (increased resistance).

Platelet count is increased (often >1 million).

Moderate polynuclear leukocytosis is present (usually >15,000/cu mm; sometimes there is a leukemoid reaction).

Peripheral blood smear may show macrocytes, microcytes, polychromatophilic RBCs, normoblasts, large masses of platelets, neutrophilic shift to the left.

Reticulocyte count is normal unless there has been some recent hemorrhage.

Bone marrow shows general hyperplasia of all elements.

Serum uric acid may be increased.

Leukocyte alkaline phosphatase may be greatly increased.

Serum vitamin B_{12} is increased.

Oxygen saturation of arterial blood is normal.

Bleeding time and coagulation time are normal, but clot retraction may be poor.

Urine may contain increased urobilinogen, and occasionally albumin is present.

Laboratory findings of associated diseases
    Gout
    Duodenal ulcer
    Cirrhosis
    Hypertension

Laboratory findings due to complications
    Thromboses (e.g., cerebral, portal vein)

Intercurrent infection
Hemorrhage
Myelofibrosis
Chronic myelogenous leukemia (develops in 20% of patients)

SECONDARY POLYCYTHEMIA
Results from hypoxia with decreased oxygen saturation of arterial blood due to
    Decreased atmospheric pressure (e.g., high altitudes)
    Chronic heart disease
        Congenital (e.g., pulmonary stenosis, septal defect, patent ductus arteriosus)
        Acquired (e.g., chronic rheumatic mitral disease)
    Arteriovenous aneurysm
    Impaired pulmonary ventilation
        Alveolar-capillary block (e.g., Hamman-Rich syndrome, sarcoidosis, lymphangitic cancer)
        Alveolar hypoventilation (e.g., bronchial asthma, kyphoscoliosis)
        Restriction of pulmonary vascular bed (e.g., primary pulmonary hypertension, mitral stenosis, chronic pulmonary emboli, emphysema)
    Abnormal hemoglobin pigments (methemoglobinemia or sulfhemoglobinemia due to chemicals, such as aniline and coal tar derivatives)
Associated with tumors and miscellaneous conditions
    Renal disease (hypernephroma, benign tumors, hydronephrosis, polycystic kidneys)
    Pheochromocytoma
    Cushing's syndrome
    Hemangioblastoma of cerebellum
    Uterine fibromyoma
    Other

The polycythemia may be relative.

See Table 27-10, p. 358.

RELATIVE POLYCYTHEMIA
Relative polycythemia is not secondary to hypoxia but results from a decrease in plasma volume due to decreased fluid intake (e.g., dehydration) and/or excess loss of body fluids (e.g., burns, shock).

PRELEUKEMIA
(poorly defined hematologic syndrome that sometimes precedes acute nonlymphocytic leukemia; overt leukemia seen in one-third of these patients by 6 months, 50% by 12 months, and 74% by 24 months)
Anemia, leukopenia, and thrombocytopenia in various combinations are most common findings.
Leukocytosis, monocytosis, and immature granulocytes may occur.
Anisocytosis, poikilocytosis, oval macrocytes, nucleated RBCs, and normochromia are most common changes in RBC morphology.
Atypical and bizarre platelets are seen in most cases.
Bone marrow is usually hypercellular, and erythroid hyperplasia occurs in 50% of patients.

Erythroid maturation defects with bizarre (e.g., multinucleated) forms and megaloblastic features unresponsive to folic acid, vitamin B_{12}, and iron.

Megakaryocytes are often atypical or bizarre.

Variable increase in mature granulocyte precursors (usually myelocytes) and monocytosis occur frequently.

Leukocyte alkaline phosphatase is decreased in about 20% of cases.

Fetal hemoglobin is increased in about 80% of cases.

ACUTE LEUKEMIA

Peripheral blood

WBC is rarely > 100,000/cu mm. It may be normal and is commonly less than normal. Peripheral smear shows many cells that resemble lymphocytes; it may not be possible to differentiate the very young forms as lymphoblasts or myeloblasts, and special cytochemical stains may be used. Special immunologic markers distinguish T-cell, B-cell, and non-T, non-B cell types of acute lymphocytic leukemia, which is important because of different prognosis and relapse patterns in the three types. Prognosis is better when initial WBC is < 10,000/cu mm and worse when > 100,000/cu mm.

Anemia is almost always present at clinical onset. Usually normocytic and sometimes macrocytic, it is progressive and may become severe. Normoblasts and polychromatophilia are common.

Platelet count is usually decreased at clinical onset and becomes progressively severe. May show poor clot retraction, increased bleeding time, positive tourniquet test, etc.

Bone marrow smear

Blast cells are present even when none are found in peripheral blood. *(This finding is useful to differentiate from other causes of pancytopenia.)*

There is progressively increasing infiltration with earlier cell types (e.g., blasts, myelocytes).

The myeloid-erythroid ratio is increased.

Erythroid and megakaryocyte elements are replaced.

In acute myelogenous leukemia, serum LDH and MDH are frequently but inconstantly increased; there is normal to slight increase in SGOT, SGPT, aldolase.

Laboratory findings due to complications

Meningeal leukemia occurs in 25–50% of children with acute leukemia; CSF shows pleocytosis and increased pressure and LDH (see p. 289).

Urate nephropathy (see Chronic Myelogenous Leukemia, p. 361).

Infection causes 90% of deaths. Most important pathogens are gram-negative rods (especially *Pseudomonas aeruginosa*) and fungi (especially *Candida albicans*).

Hemolytic anemia (see pp. 355–356).

Complete remission is possible with drug therapy (e.g., prednisone in acute lymphoblastic leukemia).

WBC falls (or rises) to normal in 1–2 weeks with replacement of lymphoblasts by normal polynuclear leukocytes and return of RBC and platelet counts to normal; bone marrow may become normal. Maximum improvement in 6–8 weeks.

Amethopterin toxicity causes a macrocytic type of anemia with megaloblasts in marrow compared to leukemic normocytic anemia with blast cells in marrow.

CHRONIC MYELOGENOUS LEUKEMIA

Increased WBC due to increase in myeloid series is earliest change. In earlier stages the more mature forms predominate with sequentially fewer cells of the younger forms; in the later, more advanced stages the younger cells become predominant.

> Eosinophilic, basophilic leukocytes may increase. Monocytes are normal or only slightly increased.

> Lymphocytes are normal in absolute number but relatively decreased.

> WBC is usually 100,000–500,000/cu mm when disease is discovered.

> Decreased number of leukocytes show positive alkaline phosphatase staining reaction. Leukocyte alkaline phosphatase (LAP) score can rise to normal or high levels with infection, inflammation, secondary malignant disease, remission due to chemotherapy or onset of blast crisis.

Anemia is usually normocytic; absent in early stage and severe in late stage. Blood smear shows few normoblasts, slight polychromatophilia, occasional stippling. Reticulocyte count is usually < 3%. Anemia is due to myelophthisis; also due to bleeding (skin and GI tract), hemolysis (autoimmune hemolytic anemia is rare), and insufficient compensatory hematopoiesis. Degree of anemia is a good index of extent of leukemic process and therefore of prognosis. Anemia improves with appropriate therapy or becomes more marked as the disease progresses.

Platelet count is normal or, commonly, increased; decreased in terminal stages with findings of thrombocytopenic purpura. Low count may increase with therapy. Bleeding manifestations are usually due to thrombocytopenia.

Bone marrow

> Hyperplasia of granulocytic elements occurs, with increase in myeloid-erythroid ratio.

> Granulocytes are more immature than in the peripheral blood.

> The number of eosinophils and basophils is increased.

> Megakaryocytic hyperplasia is often present.

> Hemosiderin deposits are increased.

Needle aspiration of spleen

> The number of immature leukocytes is increased.

> Normoblastosis is present.

> Megakaryopoiesis is increased.

Serum and urine uric acid is increased, especially with high WBC and antileukemic therapy. Urinary obstruction may develop on account of intrarenal and extrarenal uric acid crystallization.

Serum LDH is increased; rises several weeks prior to relapse and falls several weeks prior to remission.

> Increased serum LDH, MDH, SGOT, SGPT, and aldolase show less elevation than in acute leukemia. SGOT, SGPT, and aldolase are normal in half the patients. LDH is useful for following course of therapy.

Serum protein electrophoresis shows decreased albumin with increased alpha and gamma globulins.

Thyroid uptake of radioactive iodine is normal.

Table 27-11. Differential Diagnosis of Chronic Myelogenous Leukemia

	Chronic Myelogenous Leukemia	Acute Myeloblastic Leukemia	Granulocytic Leukemoid Reaction	Myelofibrosis
WBC >100,000/cu mm	Yes	Rare	No	No
Whole spectrum of immature granulocytes	Yes	No (leukemic hiatus)	No	Yes
Myeloblasts and promyelocytes in blood or marrow	>30%	>30%	0	<30%
Leukocyte alkaline phosphatase	Usually <10	30–150	>150	Variable
Bone marrow	Granulocytic hyperplasia	>30% myeloblasts	Granulocytic hyperplasia	Fibrosis
Philadelphia chromosome	Yes	No	No	No

Coombs' test is positive in one-third of patients.

Serum vitamin B_{12} level is increased (often >1000 μg/ml).

Philadelphia chromosome (small satellite of one long arm of chromosome 22 is translocated usually to one long arm of chromosome 9: 9q+;22q−) is found in 90% of patients. Ph^1-negative patients are older, have lower WBC and platelet counts at presentation and poorer response to therapy with shorter survival.

Laboratory findings due to leukemic infiltration of organs (e.g., kidney [hematuria common; uremia rare], heart, liver). With increasing survival in blast crisis, meningeal leukemia has become more frequent (up to 40%) with leukemic cells in CSF indicative of need for intrathecal chemotherapy.

Many patients experience an accelerated phase before a blast crisis: progressive anemia, leukocytosis without an increased percentage of blast cells in blood or marrow, basophilia (may be >20%), increased LAP, thrombocytosis, new karyotypic abnormalities, and myelofibrosis associated with clinical manifestations of blast crisis (e.g., fever, malaise, increasing splenomegaly).

Approximately one-third of patients with CML in blast crisis have leukemic cells with morphologic, antigenic, enzymatic (TdT), and other *lymphoid* characteristics.

Peripheral blood remission due to drugs—decreased WBC to nearly normal levels (decrease in spleen size is usually parallel) with only rare immature cells, correction of anemia, control of thrombocytosis, and LAP may occasionally rise to normal; marrow continues to show granulocytic hyperplasia and Philadelphia chromosome.

CHRONIC LYMPHOCYTIC LEUKEMIA

Peripheral blood

> WBC is increased (usually 50,000–250,000/cu mm) with 90% lymphocytes. These are uniformly similar, producing a monotonous blood picture of small lymphocytes with minimal cytoplasm. Blast cells are uncommon. Neutropenia is a late occurrence.

> Anemia—see Chronic Myelogenous Leukemia, pp. 361–363. Autoimmune hemolytic anemia occurs in 25% of patients. Anemia and/or thrombocytopenia correlate with marked change in survival time.

> Platelet count is less likely to increase with therapy than in myelogenous leukemia.

Bone marrow

> Infiltration with earlier cell types is progressively increased.

> There is replacement of erythroid, myeloid, and megakaryocyte series.

Lymph node aspirate or imprint. The number of immature leukocytes, predominantly blast cells, is increased.

Uric acid levels are not increased.

Philadelphia chromosome is not found.

Serum enzyme levels are less frequently elevated and show a lesser increase than in chronic myelogenous leukemia. Even serum LDH is frequently normal.

Direct Coombs' test is positive in up to one-third of patients.

Hypogammaglobulinemia occurs in most cases depending on duration of disease; monoclonal gammopathy (most often IgM) is found in some cases.

INFECTIOUS MONONUCLEOSIS

Mononucleosis syndrome, characterized hematologically by $\geq 50\%$ lymphocytes and monocytes and $\geq 10\%$ characteristically atypical lymphocytes, is caused by Epstein-Barr virus in $> 90\%$ of cases, CMV in 5–7% of cases, and *Toxoplasma gondii* in $< 1\%$ of cases. $< 10\%$ atypical lymphocytes are found in other viral diseases (e.g., rubella, roseola, mumps, acute viral hepatitis).

Leukopenia and granulocytopenia are evident during first week. Later, WBC is increased (usually 10,000–20,000/cu mm) because of increased lymphocytes ($\geq 50\%$; ≥ 4500/cu mm is considered essential for diagnosis). Peak changes occur in 7–10 days; many persist for 1–2 months. Increased number of bands and $> 5\%$ eosinophilia are frequent.

Heterophil agglutination (Paul-Bunnell test) is usually more than $1:112$; this is not decreased by more than 1 tube dilution following absorption with guinea pig kidney antigen but usually completely absorbed by beef RBC antigen (the reverse is true in normal persons and in serum sickness). Peak titer occurs in 2–3 weeks; duration is for 4–8 weeks. The agglutination is not related to lymphocytosis or clinical severity. Heterophil antibodies are found in 70% of patients during first week and 80–85% by third week; thus a negative test should be repeated before infectious mononucleosis can be ruled out serologically. Heterophil response is rarely found in children < 3 years old and in only 50% of children 3–8 years old.

> Newer tests using horse instead of sheep RBC have sensitivity $> 96\%$ (e.g., Ortho "Monospot" test); antibodies may be detectable in 75% of cases for up to 18 months, which may be misleading when a subsequent illness occurs; when using sheep or beef RBCs, antibodies are not detected > 3 months after onset of illness.

Evidence of mild hepatitis (e.g., increased serum transaminase, increased urine urobilinogen) is very frequent at some stage but may be transient. Clinical jaundice occurs in $< 10\%$ of patients. Bilirubin enzyme dissociation (normal serum bilirubin or < 2 mg/dl with moderate increase of alkaline phosphatase, SGOT, SGPT) occurs in 75% of cases. If no liver function abnormalities can be found, another diagnosis should be sought.

Serologic test for syphilis, rheumatoid arthritis test, and antinuclear antibodies may show transient false positive results.

Occasional RBCs and albumin are seen in urine.

Hemolytic anemia is rare.

Mild thrombocytopenia is seen in about 50% of early cases, and platelet dysfunction is frequent.

Tests for EBV-specific antibodies are available from state health department laboratories.

See Cytomegalic Inclusion Disease, pp. 603–604.

ACUTE INFECTIOUS LYMPHOCYTOSIS

Markedly increased WBC ($\geq 40,000$/cu mm) is due to lymphocytosis (normal appearance, small-sized lymphocytes).

Heterophil agglutination is negative.

LEUKEMIC RETICULOENDOTHELIOSIS

This is a rare condition of splenomegaly and absence of lymphadenopathy with characteristic pathologic changes in marrow and spleen that often respond to splenectomy but not to chemotherapy.

Diagnosis is established by finding the characteristic cells in the peripheral blood or bone marrow. These cells show a characteristic histochemical reaction of tartrate-resistant acid phosphatase (isoenzyme 5) activity. This isoenzyme 5 may also be increased in the serum.

Hypersplenism causing thrombocytopenia, anemia, and leukopenia of varying degrees is present.

Increased ESR may be present.

Abnormal platelet function may be found.

Leukocyte alkaline phosphatase activity is markedly increased in some patients.

	Leukemic Reticuloendotheliosis	Sézary Syndrome
Involvement of		
Bone marrow	Constant	Exceptional
Skin and lymph node	Uncommon	Constant
Characteristic cell	Hairy cell	Sézary cell

SÉZARY SYNDROME

Syndrome of skin lesion due to infiltration of Sézary cells associated with presence of these cells in peripheral blood

Increased peripheral blood lymphocyte count, >10% of which are atypical lymphocytes (Sézary cells)

Total WBC often increased

ESR, hemoglobin, and platelet counts usually normal

Bone marrow, lymph nodes, and liver biopsy usually normal

CHRONIC GRANULOMATOUS DISEASE

This is a rare, heterogeneous, genetically determined disorder characterized by chronic recurrent infections beginning in the first year of life and causing death by 7 years of age in one-third of patients (polymorphonuclear leukocytes and monocytes ingest normally but fail to kill certain bacteria and fungi).

WBCs show morphologically normal appearance and granules on routine Wright-Giemsa–stained smears.

Failure of these cells to reduce nitroblue tetrazolium on slide test provides a simple rapid diagnosis in patients and in heterozygotes for the X-linked form (carriers).

Prenatal diagnosis has been established using fetal blood obtained before 20 weeks' gestation.

Laboratory findings due to infection (leukocytosis, anemia, increased ESR, elevated gamma globulin levels) are noted.

Serum complement and immunoglobulin levels are normal.

Infections with organisms that usually have low virulence (e.g., *Escherichia coli,* Enterobacteriaceae, *Salmonella, Candida albicans, Serratia marcescens*).

CHÉDIAK-HIGASHI SYNDROME

This is a rare autosomal recessive genetic disease that causes hypopigmentation of skin, hair, and uvea.

Neutrophils contain coarse, deeply staining large granulations in cytoplasm and are present less frequently in other WBCs.

Pancytopenia appears during the (accelerated) "lymphomalike" phase.

Laboratory findings due to frequent severe pyogenic infections and hemorrhage (which cause early death) are noted.

AGRANULOCYTOSIS

In acute fulminant form, WBC is decreased to $\leq$ 2000/cu mm—sometimes as low as 50/cu mm. Granulocytes are 0–2%. Granulocytes may show pyknosis or vacuolization.

In chronic or recurrent form, WBC is down to 2000/cu mm with less marked granulocytopenia.

There is relative lymphocytosis and sometimes monocytosis.

Bone marrow shows absence of cells in granulocytic series but normal erythroid and megakaryocytic series.

ESR is increased.

Hemoglobin and RBC count and morphology, platelet count, and coagulation tests are normal.

Laboratory findings due to infection are noted.

Laboratory findings due to underlying causes (see Aplastic Anemia, p. 332) are noted.

PERIODIC (CYCLIC) NEUTROPENIA

In this rare condition there is a regular periodic occurrence of neutropenia.

> WBC is 2000–4000/cu mm, and granulocytes are as low as 0%.
>
> Monocytosis may occur.
>
> Eosinophilia may occur during recovery.

Bone marrow appearance is variable.

MAY-HEGGLIN ANOMALY

This is an inherited dominant abnormality of WBCs and platelets.

Large, poorly granulated platelets are associated with anomalous area in cytoplasm of all granulocytes (Döhle bodies). Usually no other hematologic abnormalities are present.

The lesion is an asymptomatic familial one. Diagnosis is confirmed by finding Döhle bodies in a parent or sibling.

PELGER-HUËT ANOMALY

This is an autosomal dominant, usually heterozygous, anomaly of WBCs.

Nuclei of granulocytes lack normal segmentation but are shaped like eyeglasses, rods, dumbbells, or peanuts. Coarse chromatin is evident in nuclei of granulocytes, lymphocytes, and monocytes. These cells are present in peripheral blood and bone marrow.

No other hematologic or clinical abnormality is present.

Occasionally cells resembling those in this anomaly are seen following administration of myelotoxic agents in acute and chronic myelogenous leukemia.

ALDER-REILLY ANOMALY
Heavy azurophilic granulation of granulocytes and some lymphocytes and monocytes associated with mucopolysaccharidoses (see
pp. 439, 442) are seen.

HEREDITARY HYPERSEGMENTATION OF NEUTROPHILS
(simple dominant abnormality found in 1% of whites)
Hypersegmentation of neutrophils resembles that seen in pernicious anemia but is a permanent abnormality. Most neutrophils
have four or more lobes.
There is a similar condition that affects only the eosinophilic
granulocytes (hereditary constitutional hypersegmentation of the
eosinophil).
There is also an inherited giant multilobed abnormality of neutrophilic leukocytes.
Hypersegmentation is also found in almost every patient with
chronic renal disease with BUN > 30 mg/dl for more than 3
months.

CONGENITAL ABSENCE OF SPLEEN
Presence of Heinz bodies in 5–20% of RBCs is the most characteris-
tic finding.
Erythroblastosis (2000–40,000/cu mm) may be present, with in-
creased frequency of Howell-Jolly bodies and target cells.
Decreased osmotic fragility may be found.
Same findings in other causes of functional hyposplenism (e.g.,
amyloidosis)

POSTSPLENECTOMY STATE
Howell-Jolly bodies and target cells are seen in peripheral blood
smears.
Heinz bodies can be seen with special stains.
WBC is increased for several weeks in 75% of patients and
indefinitely in 25%.
Lymphocytosis occurs in 50% of patients; some of these may show
increased monocytes, eosinophils, or basophils.
Increased platelets occur in postoperative period.
Decreased serum IgM
Increased risk of overwhelming infection (50% are due to *Streptococcus pneumoniae;* others include *Neisseria meningitidis, E.
coli, Hemophilus influenzae*), with high mortality; DIC is frequent. Risk of infection is greater in infants less than 1 year old,
within 2 years of splenectomy, or if underlying disorder is thalassemia or reticuloendothelial disease.

HYPERSPLENISM
The disease is either secondary to enlarged spleen (see next section)
or "primary" (with no detectable underlying disease).
There are various combinations of anemia, leukopenia, thrombocytopenia associated with bone marrow showing normal or increased cellularity of affected elements (includes primary splenic
pancytopenia and primary splenic neutropenia).
Chromium[51]-tagged RBCs from normal person or from patient are
rapidly destroyed after transfusion, and radioactivity accumulates in spleen.

SOME CAUSES OF SPLENOMEGALY
(see appropriate separate sections)

Congestion (Banti's disease)
>   Cirrhosis of the liver
>   Congestive heart failure
>   Thrombosis or partial occlusion of the portal or splenic veins

Hematologic diseases
>   Infectious mononucleosis
>   Polycythemia vera
>   Leukemias and lymphomas
>   Multiple myeloma, macroglobulinemia
>   Myelofibrosis with myeloid metaplasia (*Teardrop RBCs are pathognomonic.*)
>   Hemolytic anemias (e.g., thalassemias, hereditary spherocytosis, acquired hemolytic anemia, hemolytic disease of newborn)
>   Thrombocytopenic purpuras
>   Pernicious anemia and related macrocytic anemias
>   Primary hypersplenism (see preceding section)

Infections
>   Bacterial (e.g., endocarditis, septicemia, *Salmonella;* granulomas, e.g., tuberculosis, tularemia, brucellosis)
>   Viral (e.g., hepatitis)
>   Rickettsial (e.g., Rocky Mountain spotted fever, typhus)
>   Protozoal (e.g., malaria, kala-azar)
>   Metozoal (e.g., schistosomiasis)
>   Mycotic (e.g., histoplasmosis, blastomycosis, coccidioidomycosis)

Collagen diseases (e.g., SLE, polyarteritis nodosa, Felty's syndrome)

Histiocytoses
>   Gaucher's disease
>   Niemann-Pick disease
>   Histiocytosis X (Hand-Schüller-Christian disease, Letterer-Siwe disease)

Miscellaneous (e.g., sarcoidosis, amyloidosis, gargoylism, hemochromatosis)

Tumors of spleen
>   Cysts (e.g., echinococcus, neoplastic)
>   Primary tumors (e.g., hemangioma, lymphangioma, lymphangiosarcoma)

Needle aspiration of spleen
>   May be useful in diseases without other manifestations, especially tuberculosis, sarcoidosis, Hodgkin's disease, carcinoma, lipid storage diseases (Niemann-Pick and Gaucher's diseases)
>   Contraindicated in hemorrhagic conditions, in patients with septic or tender spleen, or in unconscious patients
>   Caution in presence of leukopenia or mild thrombopenia

Spontaneous rupture of spleen may occur in (see appropriate separate sections)
>   Malaria
>   Chronic myelogenous leukemia
>   Infectious mononucleosis
>   Splenitis

HODGKIN'S DISEASE AND OTHER MALIGNANT LYMPHOMAS

On biopsy of lymph node, the histologic findings establish diagnosis.

Blood findings may vary from completely normal to marked abnormalities.

Moderate normocytic anemia occurs, occasionally of the hemolytic type; may become severe.

WBC is variable and may be normal, decreased, or slightly or markedly increased (25,000/cu mm). Leukopenia, marked leukocytosis, anemia are bad prognostic signs. Eosinophilia occurs in ≅ 20% of patients. Relative and absolute lymphopenia may occur. *If lymphocytosis is present, look for another disease.* Neutrophilia may be found. Monocytosis may be found. These changes may all be absent or may even be present simultaneously or in various combinations. Rarely, Reed-Sternberg cells are found in marrow or peripheral blood smears.

Serum protein electrophoresis: Albumin is frequently decreased. Increased alpha$_1$ and alpha$_2$ globulins suggest disease activity. Decreased gamma globulin is less frequent in Hodgkin's disease than in lymphosarcoma. Gamma globulins may be increased, with macroglobulins present and evidence of autoimmune process (e.g., hemolytic anemia, cold agglutinins, positive LE test).

ESR and CRP are increased during active stages; may be normal during remission.

Laboratory findings due to involvement of other organ systems (e.g., liver, kidney) are noted.

Beware of complicating infections, especially disseminated tuberculosis and fungal and viral (especially herpes zoster and varicella) infections.

MYCOSIS FUNGOIDES

Biopsy of lesion (usually skin) shows microscopic findings that parallel clinical findings.

Laboratory findings are generally not helpful.

Bone marrow may show increase in reticuloendothelial cells, monoblasts, lymphocytes, plasma cells.

Peripheral blood may occasionally show increased eosinophils, monocytes, and lymphocytes.

CLASSIFICATION OF PLASMA CELL DYSCRASIAS

	% Frequency
Plasma cell myeloma	
Multiple myeloma—symptomatic	65
Multiple myeloma—asymptomatic and indolent	2
Localized plasmacytoma	5
Benign idiopathic monoclonal gammopathy	20
Waldenström's macroglobulinemia	8
Heavy-chain diseases	< 1
Primary amyloidosis	< 1

LOCALIZED PLASMACYTOMA

Myeloma proteins are low or normal concentration in serum.

Nonmyeloma immunoglobulin concentration in serum is generally normal.

Following local radiotherapy, level of any myeloma protein is reduced and level of nonmyeloma immunoglobulins may be increased above normal.

IDIOPATHIC ("BENIGN," "ASYMPTOMATIC") MONOCLONAL GAMMOPATHY
(found in 0.5% of normal persons > age 30 and 3% > age 70)
The following changes are present for a period of >5 years.

> Monoclonal serum protein concentration < 3 gm/dl; IgG type in 90% of patients; normal immunoglobulins may be depressed. In contrast, multiple myeloma always shows depression of background immunoglobulins and higher monoclonal serum protein (>3 gm/dl).
>
> Normal serum albumin
>
> <5% plasma cells in bone marrow
>
> Absence of Bence Jones protein, anemia, myeloma bone lesions
>
> Monoclonal light-chain proteinuria may occur (up to 1 gm/24 hours).
>
> May be associated with aging, cholecystitis, neoplasms, many chronic diseases

Periodic reexamination is essential because approximately 10% of these patients will develop myeloma, macroglobulinemia, lymphoma, or amyloidosis within 5 years and 20% at 10 years; no predictive factors permit recognition of this group.

PLASMA CELL LEUKEMIA
WBC usually > 15,000, with > 20% plasma cells varying from typical plasmacytes to immature and atypical forms
Complicates 2% of cases of multiple myeloma
Other findings (see under Multiple Myeloma, below)

MULTIPLE MYELOMA
Very elevated serum total protein is due to increase in globulins (with decreased A/G ratio) in one-half to two-thirds of the patients.
Serum protein immunoelectrophoresis reveals abnormal immunoglobulins in 80% of patients. An immunoelectrophoretic serum or urine monoclonal paraprotein can be identified in > 98% of patients with multiple myeloma.

% of Patients	Show
60%	Serum monoclonal spike
20%	Both serum and urine monoclonal protein
20%	Monoclonal light chains in urine only
<2%	Hypogammaglobulinemia only without serum or urine paraprotein
60%	IgG myeloma protein
20%	IgA myeloma protein
Very rare	IgE myeloma protein
<1%	IgD myeloma protein*

*IgD myeloma is difficult to recognize because serum levels are relatively low; specific antiserum is required to demonstrate IgD; on electrophoresis, IgD is often included in beta globulin peak, and clinical features are the same as in other types of myeloma. *Bence Jones proteinuria is almost always present, and total protein is often normal.*

Bence Jones proteinuria occurs in 35–50% of patients. (Dipstick tests for urine protein will miss Bence Jones protein; see pp. 158, 159.)

Electrophoresis of both serum and urine is abnormal in almost all patients. If only serum electrophoresis is performed, kappa and some lambda light-chain myelomas will be missed.

Bone marrow aspiration usually shows 20–50% plasma cells or myeloma cells, usually in sheets; abnormal plasma cells may be found (flaming cells, morular cells, Mott cells, thesaurocytes); multiple sites may be required.

Hematologic findings

Anemia (normocytic, normochromic; rarely macrocytic) in 60% of patients

Usually normal WBC and platelet count; 40–55% lymphocytes frequently present on differential count, with variable number of immature lymphocytic and plasmacytic forms. Decreased WBC and platelet counts are seen in about 20% of patients, usually with extensive marrow replacement. Eosinophilia may be found.

Rouleaux formation (due to serum protein changes) in 85% of patients, occasionally causing difficulty in cross matching blood

Increased ESR in 90% of patients and other abnormalities due to serum protein changes

Cold agglutinins or cryoglobulins

Hyperviscosity syndrome occurs in 4% of IgG and 10% of IgA myeloma and may be the presenting feature.

Clinical amyloidosis occurs in 15% of cases of multiple myeloma, but monoclonal spikes are present in urine in most, if not all, cases of primary amyloidosis.

Laboratory findings of repeated bacterial infections, especially those due to *Diplococcus pneumoniae, Staphylococcus aureus,* and *E. coli.*

See bone diseases of calcium and phosphorus, Table 29-4, p. 462.

Serum calcium is markedly increased in 25–50% of cases.

Serum phosphorus is usually normal.

Serum alkaline phosphatase is usually normal or slightly increased. Increase may reflect amyloidosis of liver rather than bone disease.

See Kidney in Multiple Myeloma, p. 551.

BUN and creatinine are increased.

Uric acid is increased in 60% of patients, but uric acid stones and gout are rare.

Renal function is decreased in < 50% of patients.

Urinalysis abnormalities appear—albumin, casts, etc.

Renal failure is usually present when there is a marked increase of Bence Jones protein in blood.

Presymptomatic phase (may last many years) may show only

Unexplained persistent proteinuria

Increased ESR

Myeloma protein in serum or urine

Repeated bacterial infections, especially pneumonias (6 times greater incidence)

Amyloidosis (see pp. 639–640)

Table 27-12. Comparison of Diseases with Monoclonal Immunoglobulins

	Multiple Myeloma	Macroglobulinemia	Benign Monoclonal Gammopathy	Heavy Chain Diseases		
				Gamma	Alpha	Mu
Clinical	Bone lesions Anemia Infections	Enlarged LNN, L, S	None	Enlarged LNN, L, S	Intestinal malabsorption	Enlarged LNN, L, S
Bone marrow	Sheets of plasma cells	Lymphocytosis or lymphocytoid plasma cells	Up to 10% plasma cells	Plasma cells or lymphocytoid plasma cells	—	Lymphocytosis or lymphocytoid plasma cells with vacuoles
Monoclonal Ig in serum (electrophoresis)	80%	Present	Present	Present	Present	Present

Bence Jones protein in urine (electrophoresis)	70–80%	80–95%	Rare	Common	Rare	Common
Serum (immunoelectrophoresis)	1 type of M chain[a] 1 type of L chain[b]	Mu chain 1 type of L chain[b]	1 type of M chain[a] 1 type of L chain[b]	Gamma chain No L	Alpha chain No L	Mu chain Free kappa or lambda in two-thirds
Urine (immunoelectrophoresis)	Kappa or lambda	Kappa or lambda	Rare kappa or lambda	Gamma chain	—	Kappa or lambda in two-thirds

LNN = lymph nodes; L = liver; S = spleen.

[a] M chain is gamma, alpha, mu, delta, or epsilon.

[b] L chain is kappa or lambda.

Monoclonal proteins (paraproteins, M proteins) are immunoglobulins synthesized by atypical cells of reticuloendothelial system. Each is a homogeneous product of a single clone of proliferating cells and is expressed as a monoclonal gammopathy. Monoclonal proteins consist of two heavy polypeptide chains of the same class (e.g., gamma, alpha, mu) and subclass and two light polypeptide chains of the same type (either kappa or lambda); may be present in serum, urine, and CSF. Heavy-chain disease is production of only heavy chains without accompanying light chains; light-chain disease is the reverse. They are detected by conventional protein electrophoresis and identified by immunoelectrophoresis.

Table 27-13. Immunochemical Frequency (%) of
Monoclonal Gammopathies

IgG (with/without BJ)	60
IgA (with/without BJ)	15
IgM (with/without BJ)	10–15
Light chain (BJ only)	15
Rare	
IgD (with/without BJ)	1
Heavy chain	1
Gamma heavy-chain disease	
Alpha heavy-chain disease	
Mu heavy-chain disease	
IgE (with/without BJ)	0.1
Biclonal (IgG + IgM)	
Triclonal	

BJ = Bence Jones proteins.

High tumor mass is present when *any* of the following are present.
    Hemoglobin < 8.5 gm/dl
    Corrected calcium > 11.5 mg/dl
    Serum IgG peak > 7 gm/dl or IgA peak > 5 gm/dl
Low tumor mass is present when *all* of the following are present.
    Hemoglobin > 10.5 gm/dl
    Corrected calcium < 11.5 mg/dl
    Serum IgG peak < 5 gm/dl or IgA peak < 3 gm/dl

Corrected calcium (mg/dl) = serum calcium (mg/dl) − serum albumin (gm/dl) + 4.0

Lowered anion gap in IgG myeloma only (due to cationic IgG paraproteins causing retention of excess chloride ion)
Increased incidence of other neoplasms (not known if related to chemotherapy)
    Acute myelomonocytic leukemia, often preceded by sideroblastic refractory anemia, is increasingly seen.
    20% of patients develop adenocarcinoma of GI tract, biliary tree, or breast.

Essential Diagnostic Criteria
1. Bone marrow shows sheets or > 20% plasma cells *and*
2. Abnormality of immunoglobulin formation (monoclonal spike > 4 gm/dl *or* Bence Jones proteinuria > 0.5 gm/24 hours)
    If monoclonal spike is < 4 gm/dl, then substitute criteria:
        Reciprocal depression of normal immunoglobulins or panhypogammaglobulinemia *and* osteolytic bone lesions or plasmacytosis not due to other causes (see p. 113, Plasma Cells).

MACROGLOBULINEMIA
Electrophoresis of serum shows an intense sharp peak in globulin fraction, usually in the gamma zone, and takes PAS stain. The pattern is indistinguishable from that in multiple myeloma.

Acrylic gel electrophoresis shows no penetration by abnormal globulin (therefore it is a macroglobulin).

Ultracentrifugation confirms the macroglobulinemia when > 5–10% of serum components have a sedimentation constant of > 16 Svedberg units (normally such components are < 2%).

Total serum protein and globulin are markedly increased. Immunoelectrophoresis identifies IgM as a component of increased globulin.

ESR is very high.

Rouleaux formation is marked.

There is severe anemia, usually normochromic normocytic, occasionally hemolytic.

WBC is decreased, with relative lymphocytosis; monocytes or eosinophils may be increased.

Bone marrow sections are always hypercellular and show extensive infiltration with atypical "lymphocytes" and also plasma cells.

Lymph node biopsy shows invasion of capsule and loss of architecture as seen in lymphosarcoma in ≅ 50% of patients.

Spleen and liver involvement occurs in ≅ 50% of patients.

Persistent oronasal hemorrhage occurs in ≅ 75% of patients.

Coagulation abnormalities: There may be decreased platelets, abnormal bleeding time, coagulation time, prothrombin time, prothrombin consumption, etc.

50% of patients with Waldenström's macroglobulinemia have hyperviscosity syndrome due to large IgM molecule causing coagulation abnormalities (see previous paragraph).

Macroglobulinemia may be primary Waldenström's or may be associated with neoplasms, collagen diseases, cirrhosis, chronic infections.

HEAVY-CHAIN DISEASE
(a lymphomalike disease with excessive production of heavy-chain proteins)

Serum protein electrophoresis
 Marked decrease in albumin
 Gamma globulin almost absent
 Narrow band of abnormal protein in region of beta or gamma globulin that is similar in serum and urine
 Immunoelectrophoresis—marked decrease of IgG, IgA, IgM

Serum tests
 Reversed A/G ratio
 Positive cephalin flocculation test
 Increased uric acid (> 8.5 mg/dl)
 Increased BUN (30–50 mg/dl)

Hematologic findings
 Anemia almost always present
 Leukopenia and thrombocytopenia common
 Eosinophilia sometimes marked; relative lymphocytosis
 Vacuolated mononuclear cells sometimes seen
 Bone marrow aspiration—many atypical plasma cells and lymphocytes (some patients)

Urine tests
 Trace to 1+ protein
 Negative for Bence Jones protein
 Identical to abnormal serum protein on electrophoresis

Table 27-14. Tests for Immune Deficiency

Arm of the Immune System Deficient	Screening Tests	Definitive Tests[a]	Type of Infection[b]	Suggestive Organism	Example of Immunodeficiency Disease
Antibody	Quantitative IgM, IgG, IgA Rubella titer Isohemagglutinins	Diphtheria-tetanus titer Pneumococcal titer B-lymphocytes Plasma cells	Sinusitis, diarrhea, failure to thrive	S. pneumoniae, nontypeable H. influenzae, Giardia lamblia from gut	Bruton's disease, selective IgA deficiency, hypogammaglobulinemia with normal or increased IgM
Complement	Total hemolytic C3, C4, C5 Factor B	Chemotactic factors Opsonins Immunoelectrophoretic analysis	Sinusitis	S. pneumoniae, Neisseria species	Deficiency of C3, C3b inactivator, Factor B, C6, C7, C8
Phagocytes	WBC and differential count Nitroblue tetrazolium test (NBT) IgE	Chemotaxis Adhesion Aggregation Chemiluminescence Phagocytosis and killing	Osteomyelitis, eczema, stomatitis, furunculosis, liver abscess, draining lymphadenitis	S. aureus, S. epidermidis, C. albicans, S. marcescens	Primary or secondary neutropenia, chronic granulomatous disease, Chédiak-Higashi syndrome
Cell-mediated immunity	Skin tests (e.g., C. albicans)	T-cell rosette Mitogen responses Suppressor or helper cells	Failure to thrive, autoimmune disease, eczema, diarrhea, candidiasis (perineal/oral)	Lungs—CMV, Pneumocystis carinii, varicella-zoster virus, Cryptococcus, Nocardia, recurrent Candida	Wiskott-Aldrich syndrome, ataxia-telangiectasia, thymic hypoplasia, severe combined immunodeficiency disease

[a] At special immunologic centers.
[b] Severe or recurrent pneumonia, acute otitis media in all groups.

SOME CAUSES OF RECURRENT INFECTIONS

Abnormal drainage
  Cystic fibrosis of pancreas
  Tracheoesophageal fistula
  Ureteral stenosis or reflux
Abnormal communication
  Skull fractures
  Dermal sinuses
  Burns, eczema
Foreign bodies
  Artificial heart valves
  Intravascular catheters
  Urinary bladder catheters
Abnormal perfusion
  Diabetes mellitus
  Sickle cell disease
  Atherosclerosis
Abnormalities of immune system (see following pages)
  Immunodeficient diseases are being recognized with increasing frequency as part of well-recognized conditions (e.g., see Table 27-14, p. 376 and Table 27-15, pp. 382–383; lymphomas, SLE, AIDS, nephrosis) *as well as genetically controlled syndromes. The development and increased availability of new tests of deficient immune mechanisms have led to many reports of new conditions and variants of previously described syndromes. Reorganization of the present classification based on improved understanding of these diseases is to be expected, and clinicians should check the most recent literature when working up current cases.*

WISKOTT-ALDRICH SYNDROME

This is a rare immunologic sex-linked recessive condition featuring eczema, repeated infections, and thrombocytopenia.

Platelet count is decreased, with bleeding tendency.
There is marked susceptibility to infections (e.g., bacteria, viruses, fungi, *Pneumocystis carinii*)
Serum IgM is decreased.
Serum IgA is normal or may be markedly increased.
Serum IgG is normal or increased.
Blood lymphocytes are usually decreased in number, especially the small lymphocytes. Depressed number of T cells and mitogen assays.
Incidence of malignancy of the lymphoid system is increased.

CONGENITAL SEX-LINKED HYPOGAMMAGLOBULINEMIA (BRUTON'S DISEASE)

Probably represents a heterogeneous group of defects.
Male patients suffer severe pyogenic infections (commonly due to *S. pneumoniae, H. influenzae, N. meningitidis*) after age 4–6 months.
Serum levels of immunoglobulins are very low (<100 mg/dl).
B cells in peripheral blood detected by surface immunoglobulin techniques are absent or found in very low numbers; however, cells bearing complement receptor (EAC rosettes determination) may be normal.

Plasma cells in lymph nodes and GI tract are absent or found in very low numbers.

T cell numbers and function are intact.

Antibody responses to immunization are usually absent. Live virus vaccination may cause severe disease (e.g., paralytic polio).

HYPOGAMMAGLOBULINEMIA WITH NORMAL OR INCREASED IgM
(sex-linked)

Normal or increased number of IgM-producing B cells and plasma cells

Normal serum IgM

B cells with IgG or IgA are virtually absent.

Serum IgG and IgA are very low.

Normal titers of isohemagglutinins and opsonic antibodies to many polysaccharide-coated bacteria

No IgG antibody response following immunization or infection

Neutropenia is common.

Autoimmune hemolytic anemia and thrombocytopenia are commonly associated findings.

SELECTIVE IgM DEFICIENCY

Decreased serum IgM

Decreased to absent isohemagglutinins

Low levels of opsonins to gram-negative and polysaccharide-coated bacteria

In children and adults who often have serious infections, e.g., sepsis, meningitis

SELECTIVE IgA DEFICIENCY
(a more common immunodeficiency syndrome)

Serum IgA is very low.

Secretory IgA is usually absent.

Peripheral blood lymphocytes bearing IgA, IgM, and IgG are normal.

Plasma cells producing IgA are absent in GI and respiratory epithelium.

Clinical—asymptomatic or recurrent pyogenic respiratory infections; increased incidence of atopic disease, rheumatoid arthritis, lymphonodular hyperplasia of small intestine.

COMMON VARIABLE HYPOGAMMAGLOBULINEMIA
(a more common immunodeficiency syndrome in children and adults)

Serum IgG is decreased.

Other immunoglobulin abnormalities are variable.

Thymus-dependent lymphocyte function may be impaired.

Number of peripheral blood B cells is usually normal, but terminal differentiation into antibody-secreting cells is impaired.

Alternative complement pathway defects

  Special studies show contribution of alternative pathway to opsonization.

  Decreased levels of specific factors (e.g., Factor B) may be found.

  Impaired generation of chemotactic factors or decreased hemolytic activity may occur.

  Severe infections due to *S. pneumoniae, H. influenzae* causing sepsis, pneumonia, meningitis are common.

Due to
>Sickle cell disease with splenic infarction
>Postsplenectomy
>Nephrotic syndrome

COMPLEMENT DEFICIENCIES

Absence of or marked decrease in any of the components of complement will cause absence of or marked decrease in the total hemolytic complement assay, but mild to moderate decrease of an individual component of complement may not alter this total.

Deficiency of early classic pathway components (C1q, r, s, C2, C4)
>Serum shows absence of hemolytic complement activity.
>The affected component is absent or decreased on immunochemical testing.
>Opsonic activity and generation of chemotactic activity are defective.
>Infections are not a problem (due to alternative pathway being intact).
>Symptoms due to collagen vascular disorders (e.g., nephritis, arthritis)

Deficiency of C3 and C5
>Serum shows absence of hemolytic complement activity.
>C3 or C5 is absent or decreased in serum.
>Defective opsonic capacity and chemotactic activity
>Severe recurrent infections (e.g., pneumonia, sepsis, otitis media, chronic diarrhea)
>Often respond to fresh plasma

Deficiency of late classic pathway components (C6, C7, C8)
>Serum shows absence of hemolytic complement activity.
>Normal opsonization and generation of chemotactic factor
>Total absence of individual component
>Recurrent systemic infection due to *N. gonorrhoeae* or *N. meningitidis*

HEREDITARY ANGIOEDEMA

CBC and ESR are usually normal when the manifestation is peripheral or facial angioedema, but they may be abnormal when the manifestation is diarrhea and abdominal pain.

Serum complement-1-esterase inhibitor is either decreased (5–30% of normal) or is functionally inactive. (Test is performed only at reference laboratories.)

BISALBUMINEMIA

Two albumin bands are present on serum protein electrophoresis in clinically healthy homozygotes or carriers.

ALPHA₁ ANTITRYPSIN DEFICIENCY

This is a congenital inherited deficiency associated with familial pulmonary emphysema and liver disease. The heterozygous state occurs in 10–15% of general population who have serum levels of alpha$_1$ antitrypsin $\cong$ 60% of normal; homozygous state occurs in 1:2000 persons who have serum levels $\cong$ 10% of normal.

Pulmonary emphysema occurs in family of 25% of patients; occurs in heterozygotes and homozygotes. Secondary bronchitis and bronchiectasis may occur.

Liver disease occurs in 10–20% of children with this deficiency. Clinical picture may be neonatal hepatitis, prolonged obstructive jaundice during infancy, juvenile cirrhosis, or abnormal liver functions tests (e.g., SGPT) in 50% of apparently healthy asymptomatic patients. Liver biopsy (in both heterozygotes and homozygotes) shows characteristic intracytoplasmic inclusions; these may be found in patients with emphysema without liver disease and in asymptomatic heterozygous relatives, but these inclusions must be searched for and stained specifically, since the rest of the pathology in the liver is not specific.

Decreased serum alpha$_1$ antitrypsin

TUMORS OF THYMUS

(>40% have parathymic syndromes noted below, which are multiple in one-third)

Associated With

Myasthenia gravis in about 35% of cases. May appear up to 6 years after excision of thymoma in 5% of cases. Thymoma develops in 15% of patients with myasthenia gravis. See p. 302.

Acquired hypogammaglobulinemia. 7–13% of adults with this condition have an associated thymoma; does not respond to thymectomy.

Pure red cell aplasia (PRCA) found in approximately 5% of thymoma patients. 50% of cases of PRCA have thymoma, 25% of whom benefit from thymectomy; onset followed thymectomy in 10% of cases. May be accompanied or followed, but not preceded, by granulocytopenia or thrombocytopenia or both in one-third of cases; thymectomy is not useful therapy. PRCA occurs in one-third of patients with hypogammaglobulinemia and thymoma.

Autoimmune hemolytic anemia with positive Coombs' test and increased reticulocyte count

Cushing's syndrome

Multiple endocrine neoplasia (usually Type I)

Systemic lupus erythematosus

Miscellaneous disorders (e.g., giant cell myocarditis, nephrotic syndrome)

Cutaneous disorders (e.g., mucocutaneous candidiasis, pemphigus)

ACQUIRED IMMUNE DEFICIENCY SYNDROME (AIDS)

Due to a retrovirus, human T-cell lymphotropic virus (HTLV-III), also named lymphadenopathy-associated virus (LAV).

Criteria are diagnosed secondary disease that indicates underlying cellular immunodeficiency not due to known causes such as immunosuppressive therapy. These include:

Kaposi's sarcoma in a patient < 60 years old

Opportunistic infections (see p. 381)

Lymphopenia largely due to decreased helper-inducer subset (OKT 4, Leu 3) and increased suppressor subset of T lymphocytes (OKT 8). Normal T4/T8 ratio is 2.0; AIDS patients have ratio of 0.5–1.0 (sensitivity about 85% but low specificity). Lymphopenia is found in 50% of patients with Kaposi's sarcoma and almost all patients with opportunistic infections.

Leukopenia, anemia, idiopathic thrombocytopenia are common.

Decreased T-cell function evidenced

In vivo by
>   Decreased delayed-type hypersensitivity (skin test reactivity)
>   Opportunistic infections (see below)
>   Neoplasms (see below)

In vitro by
>   Decreased ability to help B lymphocytes
>   Decreased cytotoxicity
>   Decreased mitogen responses
>   Decreased mixed lymphocyte reaction

Polyclonal B-cell activation evidenced by
>   Increased serum IgG (see below) and circulating immune complexes
>   Defective response to signals for B-cell activation (e.g., polyclonal mitogens in vitro or de novo response to new antigen)

Other serologic findings: increased levels of
>   Anti-HTLV-III (see p. 154)
>   Acid-labile alpha interferon (previously known in patients with autoimmune disease; found in 63% of homosexual AIDS patients and 29% without AIDS) (more studies are needed to determine value as screening test)
>   Alpha$_1$ thymosin (found in <1% of normal persons, 70–80% of AIDS patients, and 60–70% of patients with chronic reactive lymphadenopathy syndrome)
>   Beta$_2$ microglobulins (also increased in patients with hepatitis, kidney diseases, B-cell malignancies such as multiple myeloma)

Laboratory findings due to opportunistic infections which are most common cause of death (see appropriate separate sections)
>   *Pneumocystis carinii* pneumonia (>50% of patients)
>   Disseminated cytomegalovirus (CMV)
>   Disseminated *Mycobacterium avium-intracellularis*
>   *Candida* esophagitis
>   Mucocutaneous herpes simplex
>   Cryptococcal meningitis
>   Cerebral toxoplasmosis
>   Enteric cryptosporidiosis
>   Milder infections (e.g., herpes zoster, oral candidiasis, tinea, onchomycosis)
>   Opportunistic infections affect respiratory tract in two-thirds of cases and meninges in 10% of cases
>   Progressive multifocal leukoencephalopathy

Laboratory findings due to concomitant neoplasms
>   Kaposi's sarcoma (>30% of patients)
>   Burkitt's lymphoma
>   Cloacal carcinoma of rectum
>   Oropharyngeal carcinoma
>   Non-Hodgkin's lymphoma
>   Hodgkin's disease
>   Angioimmunoblastic lymphadenopathy
>   Lymphoma limited to brain

Laboratory findings due to coexisting diseases
>   Hepatitis B core antigen is positive in > 90% of AIDS patients and 80% of patients with lymphadenopathy syndrome. (Rate of hepatitis B is 10–30 times that of general population in U.S.)

Table 27-15. Classification of Primary Immunologic Defects

Syndrome	Number of Circulating Lymphocytes	Number of Plasma Cells	Immunoglobulin Changes	Thymus	Lymph Node Germinal Center	Lymph Node Paracortical Zone	Other Laboratory Findings
Infantile sex-linked agammaglobulinemia (Bruton's disease)	N	O	Markedly D in all	N	O	N	X; increased frequency of malignant lymphoma
Selective inability to produce IgA	N	IgA-producing plasma cells, especially in lamina propria	IgA is O; others are usually N	N	N	N	May have malabsorption syndrome, steatorrhea, bronchitis
Transient hypogammaglobulinemia of infancy	N	D	IgG is D		O or rare		X
Non-sex-linked primary immunoglobulin deficiencies (e.g., dysgammaglobulinemias—acquired, congenital)	N	V (usually D)	Present, but type and amount are V	N	Usually O _Reticulum hyperplasia_	Often D	X, Z; increased frequency of malignant lymphoma and autoimmune diseases
Agammaglobulinemia with thymoma (Good's syndrome)	Progressively D, often to very low levels	D or O	Markedly D in all	Enlarged (stromal epithelial spindle-cell type)	D or O	May be D	X, Z; thymoma (see p. 380); pure red cell aplasia may occur; eosinophils O or markedly D
Wiskott-Aldrich syndrome (X-linked, recessive immune deficiency with thrombopenia and eczema)	Usually progressively D	N	Usually present, but type and amount are V (frequently IgM is D and IgA is I); IgG usually N	N	May be D	Progressively D in lymphocytes	X, Z; eczema and thrombocytopenia; increased frequency of malignant lymphoma; serum lacks isohemagglutinins; platelets ½ normal size

Disease							Clinical
Ataxia-telangiectasia (Louis-Bar syndrome), autosomal recessive	V (usually slightly D)	V (usually present)	Usually present, but type and amount are V (frequently IgA and IgE are D or O, and D IgG)	Embryonic type (no Hassall's corpuscles or cortical medullary organization)	May be D	Lymphocytes D	Progressive cerebellar ataxia; telangiectasia in tissues; ovarian dysgenesis; increased frequency of malignant lymphoma; frequent pulmonary infections when IgA is D
Primary lymphopenic immunologic deficiency (Gitlin's syndrome)	V–D	V	Always present, but type and amount are V	Hypoplastic (Hassall's corpuscles and lymphoid cells D)	Marked D in tissue lymphocytes; foci of lymphocytes may be present in spleen and lymph nodes		Z
Autosomal recessive alymphocytic agammaglobulinemia (Swiss type agammaglobulinemia; Glanzmann and Riniker's lymphocytophthisis)	Markedly D	O	Markedly D in all	Hypoplastic (Hassall's corpuscles and lymphoid cells O)	Lymphocytes O or markedly D		X, Z; increased frequency of malignant lymphoma
Autosomal recessive lymphopenia with normal immunoglobulins (Nezelof's syndrome)	D	Present	N	Hypoplastic (Hassall's corpuscles and lymphoid cells O)	May be present	Lymphocytes markedly D	Z
DiGeorge's syndrome (thymic aplasia)	V (usually N)	Present	N	Absent	Present	Rare paracortical lymphocytes present	Z; absent parathyroids (tetany of the newborn); frequent cardiovascular malformations

N = normal; O = absent; D = decreased; V = variable; X = recurrent infections with pyogenic organisms; Z = frequent virus, fungus, or *Pneumocystis* infection.
Source: Adapted from M. Seligmann, H. H. Fudenberg, and R. A. Good, A proposed classification of primary immunologic deficiencies. *Am. J. Med.* 45:818, 1968.

Table 27-16. Distribution of Cases of AIDS by Sex and Risk Groups

	Men (%)	Women (%)	Total (%)
Homosexual/bisexual	78	0	73
IV drug user	15	56	17
Haitian	3	8	4
Hemophiliac	1	0	1
Transfusion associated	1	8	4
Heterosexual contact	0	11	1
None of these	3	17	4

Source: Data from Centers for Disease Control. A. S. Fauci, et al. The acquired immunodeficiency syndrome: An update. *Ann. Intern. Med.* 102:800, 1985.

High levels of antibodies against CMV (95% of patients), Epstein-Barr virus (EBV), and human T-cell leukemia virus (HTLV-III) (see p. 154) may be found.

In the absence of other opportunistic diseases, any of the following are considered indicative of AIDS if patient has a positive serologic or virologic test for HTLV-III:

Disseminated histoplasmosis (not confined to lungs or lymph nodes) diagnosed by culture, histology, or antigen detection.

Isosporiasis causing diarrhea longer than 1 month diagnosed by histology or stool examination.

Bronchial or pulmonary candidiasis diagnosed by microscopy or characteristic gross plaques on bronchial mucosa but not by culture alone.

High grade pathologic type of non-Hodgkin's lymphoma (diffuse, undifferentiated) and of B-cell or unknown immunologic phenotype, diagnosed by biopsy.

Histologically confirmed Kaposi's sarcoma in patient > 60 years old.

Chronic lymphoid interstitial pneumonitis in child < 13 years old confirmed histologically.

Increased serum gamma globulins, especially IgG and also IgA; slight IgM increase may occur; associated with opportunistic infection.

Hypoalbuminemia

No single test establishes or rules out the diagnosis.

CHRONIC LYMPHADENOPATHY SYNDROME
Found in homosexual men with lymphadenopathy for > 3 months involving ≥ 2 extrainguinal sites without other illness or drug use known to cause lymphadenopathy. If lymph node is biopsied, shows reactive hyperplasia.

HYPOANABOLIC HYPOALBUMINEMIA
This is an inherited disorder present from birth, without kidney or liver disease. Growth and development are normal. The patient is unaffected except for periodic peripheral edema.

Serum albumin is < 0.3 gm/dl.
Total globulins are 4.5–5.5 gm/dl.

Serum cholesterol is increased.

Albumin synthesis is decreased, with decreased catabolism of IV injected albumin.

CLASSIFICATION OF HEMORRHAGIC DISORDERS

Vascular abnormalities

Congenital (e.g., hereditary hemorrhagic telangiectasia)

Acquired (see Nonthrombocytopenic Purpura, p. 392)

Infection (e.g., bacterial endocarditis, rickettsial infection)

Immunologic (e.g., allergic purpura, drug sensitivity)

Metabolic (e.g., scurvy, uremia)

Miscellaneous (e.g., neoplasms, amyloidosis)

Connective tissue abnormalities

Congenital (e.g., Ehlers-Danlos syndrome)

Acquired (e.g., Cushing's syndrome)

Platelet abnormalities (see sections on thrombocytopenic purpura, thrombocythemia, thrombocytopathies)

Plasma coagulation defects

Causing defective thromboplastin formation

Hemophilia (Factor VIII deficiency)

PTC (Factor IX) deficiency (Christmas disease)

PTA (Factor XI) deficiency

von Willebrand's disease

Causing defective rate or amount of thrombin formation

Vitamin K deficiency (due to liver disease, prolonged bile duct obstruction, malabsorption syndrome, hemorrhagic disease of the newborn, anticoagulant therapy)

Congenital deficiency of Factor II (prothrombin), Factor V (proaccelerin, labile factor), Factor VII (proconvertin, stable factor), Factor X (Stuart factor)

Decreased fibrinogen due to intravascular clotting and/or fibrinolysis

Obstetric abnormalities (e.g., amniotic fluid embolism, premature separation of placenta, retention of dead fetus)

Congenital deficiency of Factor XIII (fibrin-stabilizing factor), congenital afibrinogenemia, hypofibrinogenemia, etc.

Neoplasms (leukemia, carcinoma of prostate, etc.)

Transfusion reactions

Gram-negative septicemia, meningococcemia

Circulating anticoagulants

Heparin therapy

Dysproteinemias, SLE, postpartum state, some cases of hemophilia, etc.

THROMBOCYTOPENIC PURPURA

Due To

Idiopathic thrombocytopenic purpura (ITP; Werlhof's disease; purpura hemorrhagica)

Hematologic disorders

Leukemias

Anemias (aplastic, myelophthisic, pernicious anemia, acquired hemolytic)

Hypersplenism (e.g., Gaucher's disease, Felty's syndrome, sarcoidosis, congestive splenomegaly)

Table 27-17. Screening Tests for Presumptive Diagnosis of Common Bleeding Disorders[a]

Platelet Count	Bleeding Time	Prothrombin Time[b]	Activated Partial Thromboplastin Time[b]	Location of Defect	Most Frequent Causes Acquired	Most Frequent Causes Hereditary
N	N	I	N	Extrinsic pathway[c]	Liver disease, coumarin therapy, vitamin K deficiency, DIC (very rare)	Deficiency of Factor VII (very rare)
N	N	N	I	Intrinsic pathway[d]	Heparin therapy, inhibitors	Hemophilia A or B deficiency of XI, XII, prekallikrein, high-molecular-weight kininogen, Passavoy factor
N[e]	N	I	I	Common or multiple pathways	Heparin therapy, liver disease, vitamin K deficiency, DIC, fibrinogenolysis (very common)	Deficiency of V, X, prothrombin; dysfibrinogenemias (very rare)

D	I	N	N	Thrombocytopenia	ITP, secondary (e.g., drugs)	Aldrich's syndrome, etc.
N or I	I	N	N	Disorder of platelet function	Thrombocythemia, drugs, uremia, dysproteinemias	Thrombasthenia, deficient release reaction
N	I	I	N	Von Willebrand's disease		
N	N	N	N	Vascular abnormality	Allergic purpura, drugs, scurvy, etc.	Deficiency of XIII, telangiectasia

N = normal; I = increased; D = decreased.

a Screening tests may be normal in mild von Willebrand's disease that has borderline or intermittent normal bleeding time, in mild hemophilia, and in Factor XIII deficiency.

b Concentration of factors must be decreased to $\leqq 30\%$ of normal for these tests to be abnormal.

c Extrinsic pathway function depends on Factors VII, X, V, II (prothrombin), I (fibrinogen); is assessed by prothrombin time.

d Intrinsic pathway depends on Factors XII, XI, IX, VIII, X, V, II, I; is assessed by partial thromboplastin time.

3 May be I in acquired disorders that produce abnormalities of platelets and multiple coagulation factors.

Table 27-18. Summary of Coagulation Studies in Hemorrhagic Conditions

Condition	Screening Tests					Accessory Tests		Tests to Identify Deficiency	
	Platelet Count	Bleeding Time	Prothrombin Time	Partial Thromboplastin Time (PTT)	Capillary Fragility (Rumpel-Leede tourniquet test)	Coagulation Time	Clot Retraction	Prothrombin Consumption Time	Thromboplastin Generation Test (TGT)
Thrombocytopenic purpura	D	I	N	N	+	N	Poor	I	I
Nonthrombocytopenic purpura	N	N	N	N	V	N	N	N	N
Glanzmann's thrombasthenia	N[a]	N or I	N		+ or N	N	Poor	I _Corrected by platelet substitute_	I
von Willebrand's disease	N	I or N	N	N or I	N + in severe	V	N	I	V[b]
AHG (Factor VIII) deficiency (hemophilia)	N	N	N	I	N	I N in mild	N	I	I[b]

PTC (Factor IX) deficiency (hemophilia B; Christmas disease)	N	N	N	I[c]	N	I N in mild	N	I	I[c]
Factor X (Stuart) deficiency	N	N	I[c]	I[c]	N	N or slightly I	N	I	I
PTA (Factor XI) deficiency	N	N I in severe	N	I[d]	N	I	N	I	I[d]
Factor XII (Hageman) deficiency	N	N	N	I[d]	N	I	N	I	I[d]
Factor XIII deficiency	N	N	N	N	N	N	N	N	N
Fibrinogen deficiency	N	N I in severe	I	I	N	I	N	N	N
Hypoprothrombinemia	N	N or I	I	I	N	I	N	N	N
Excess dicumarol therapy	N	N I in severe	I	I	N + in severe	I N in mild	N	N	N
Heparin therapy	N	N to I	May be I	I	N	I	N		

Table 27-18. (continued)

Condition	Screening Tests				Accessory Tests				Tests to Identify Deficiency
	Platelet Count	Bleeding Time	Pro-thrombin Time	Partial Thrombo-plastin Time (PTT)	Capillary Fragility (Rumpel-Leede tourni-quet test)	Coagula-tion Time	Clot Retrac-tion	Prothrombin Con-sumption Time	Thrombo-plastin Generation Test (TGT)
Vascular purpura (e.g., Schönlein-Henoch, hereditary hemorrhagic telangiectasia)	N	N	N	N	N	N	N	N	N
Increased antithrom-boplastin	N		I			I		I	May be I and not corrected by absorbed plasma or aged serum
Increased anti-thrombin	N	N	N	N	N	N May be I in severe	N	N[e]	N
Increased anti-fibrinolysin	N	N or I	N	N	N	N or I	Lysis of clot	N[e]	N

D = decreased; I = increased; N = normal; V = variable.
[a] Platelets appear abnormal.
[b] Corrected by absorbed plasma.
[c] Corrected by serum.
[d] Corrected by serum or plasma.
[e] Not useful; may be difficult to do.

Table 27-19. Some Congenital Hemorrhagic Diseases Due to Disorders of Platelet-Vessel Wall

Platelet Defects

Bernard-Soulier syndrome	Moderate thrombocytopenia
	Bleeding time markedly increased
	Large platelets
	Decreased ristocetin-induced agglutination not corrected by vWF
Glanzmann's thrombasthenia	Normal platelet count and morphology
	Increased bleeding time
	Clot retraction absent or much decreased
	No platelet aggregation with any agonists
Pseudo–von Willebrand's disease	Variable mild thrombocytopenia
	Increased bleeding time
	Increased ristocetin-induced agglutination
	Variable plasma immunoreactive vWF
Gray-platelet syndrome	Moderate thrombocytopenia
	Large platelets
	Bleeding time slightly increased
	Platelets agranular on blood smear
	Abnormal platelet aggregation with collagen or thrombin
Dense-granule deficiency syndrome	Normal platelet count
	Normal platelet morphology on blood smear
	Bleeding time variably increased
	Abnormal aggregation with ADP and collagen
Deficiency of platelet enzyme (cyclooxygenase or thromboxane synthetase)	Normal platelet count and morphology
	Abnormal aggregation with ADP, collagen, and arachidonic acid

Plasma Defects

von Willebrand's disease	Normal platelet count and morphology
	Increased bleeding time
	Abnormal ristocetin-induced agglutination
	Abnormal plasma vWF
Afibrinogenemia	Normal platelet morphology
	Mild thrombocytopenia occasionally
	Bleeding time variably increased
	Plasma coagulation abnormalities

Vessel Wall Defects

Genetic disorders of connective tissue	Platelets may be large
	Collagen-induced aggregation may be abnormal

vWF = von Willebrand factor; ADP = adenosine diphosphate.

Thrombotic thrombocytopenic purpura
Massive blood transfusions
May-Hegglin anomaly
Other
Infections (e.g., subacute bacterial endocarditis, septicemia, typhus)
Other diseases (e.g., disseminated lupus erythematosus)
Marrow suppressive agents (e.g., ionizing radiation, benzol, nitrogen mustards and other antitumor drugs)
Drug sensitivity reactions (e.g., chloramphenicol and other antibacterial drugs, tranquilizers, antipyretic drugs, heavy metals)

Laboratory Findings
Decreased platelet count (<100,000/cu mm); no bleeding until < 60,000/cu mm
Positive tourniquet test
Increased bleeding time
Poor clot retraction
Normal coagulation time
Normal partial thromboplastin time
Normal prothrombin time
Bone marrow—normal or increased number of megakaryocytes but without marginal platelets
Blood smear—decreased number of platelets, abnormal appearance of platelets (small or giant or deeply stained)
Normal WBC
Laboratory findings due to hemorrhage
    Increased WBC with shift to left
    Anemia proportional to hemorrhage, with compensatory increase in reticulocytes, polychromatophilia, etc.

NONTHROMBOCYTOPENIC PURPURA
Abnormal platelets
    Thrombocytopathies
    Thrombasthenia
    Thrombocythemia
    Other
Abnormal serum globulins
    Multiple myeloma
    Macroglobulinemia
    Cryoglobulinemia
    Hyperglobulinemia
    Other
Infections (e.g., meningococcemia, subacute bacterial endocarditis, typhoid, Rocky Mountain spotted fever)
Other diseases (e.g., amyloidosis, Cushing's syndrome, polycythemia vera, hemochromatosis, diabetes mellitus, uremia)
Drugs and chemicals (e.g., mercury, phenacetin, salicylic acid, chloral hydrate)
Allergic reaction (e.g., Schönlein-Henoch purpura, serum sickness)
Diseases of the skin (e.g., Osler-Weber-Rendu disease, Ehlers-Danlos syndrome)
von Willebrand's disease
Avitaminosis (e.g., scurvy)
Miscellaneous (e.g., mechanical, orthostatic)
Blood coagulation factors (e.g., hemophilia)

THROMBOTIC THROMBOCYTOPENIC PURPURA
Thrombocytopenic purpura, severe
Microangiopathic hemolytic anemia with
    Increased serum indirect bilirubin, LDH, and serum hemoglobin and decreased serum haptoglobin
    Increased reticulocytes, nucleated RBCs, basophilic stippling and polychromatophilia
    Anemia is normochromic, normocytic.
    Numerous fragmented and misshapen RBCs (burr cells, schistocytes) seen on peripheral smear
    Negative Coombs' test
    Bone marrow shows hyperplasia and prominence of megakaryocytes.
Increased WBCs and neutrophils
Coagulation studies are usually normal.
Abnormal urine findings (RBCs, protein, etc.) with mildly increased BUN and creatinine occur frequently.
SGOT and SGPT may be slightly increased.

PRIMARY HEMORRHAGIC THROMBOCYTHEMIA
Platelets > 800,000/cu mm
No evidence of leukemia or polycythemia in peripheral blood or marrow
Bone marrow—hyperplasia of all elements, with predominance of megakaryocytes and platelet masses, eosinophilia, basophilia
Iron deficiency anemia due to bleeding
Thrombohemorrhagic disease (bleeding—skin, gastrointestinal tract, nose, gums)

GLANZMANN'S THROMBASTHENIA
Probably represents a heterogeneous group of conditions incompletely studied and delineated
Normal platelet count with abnormal platelet morphology (e.g., variation in platelet size, increased platelet size, abnormal clumping and spreading)
Poor clot retraction and increased bleeding time may be present.
Normal coagulation time
TGT and prothrombin consumption tests abnormal but corrected by adding platelet substitute
Capillary fragility sometimes abnormal

VASCULAR ABNORMALITIES CAUSING HEMORRHAGE
Hereditary telangiectasia (Osler-Weber-Rendu disease)
Anaphylactoid purpura (Schönlein-Henoch)
Vascular purpura (associated with uremia, diabetes mellitus, chronic infection, hypertension, postirradiation, etc.) (other conditions, including "vascular pseudohemophilia")
Pigmented purpuric eruptions (e.g., angioma serpiginosum)

ALLERGIC PURPURA
This is called Henoch's purpura when abdominal symptoms are predominant and Schönlein's purpura when joint symptoms are predominant.
Platelet count, bleeding time, coagulation time, and clot retraction are normal.

Tourniquet test may be negative or positive.

WBC and neutrophils may be increased; eosinophils may be increased.

Stool may show blood.

Urine usually contains RBCs and slight to marked protein.

Renal biopsy shows positive immunohistologic findings and typical glomerular histologic changes.

INCIDENCE OF INHERITED CONGENITAL COAGULATION FACTORS

XI	Rare
IX	1:100,000
VIII	1:25,000
VII	1:500,000
X	1:500,000
V	1:1,000,000
II (prothrombin)	Rare
I (fibrinogen)	Rare
XIII	Rare

Autosomal recessive except Factors IX and VIII, which are X-linked recessive, and II.

VON WILLEBRAND'S DISEASE

It is an autosomal dominant hereditary deficiency of a high-molecular-weight plasma protein (von Willebrand factor) that mediates adherence of platelets to injured endothelium.

Difficulty in diagnosis arises from temporal variation in clinical and laboratory findings in an individual patient as well as from patient to patient; since many patients do not have the classic laboratory findings, five clinical variants have been described.

Bleeding time is prolonged using a calibrated template.

Partial thromboplastin time is prolonged.

Platelet adhesiveness to glass beads is decreased. Ristocetin-induced aggregation of platelets is deficient.

Prothrombin time, platelet count, and clot retraction are normal.

Tourniquet test may be positive.

Factor VIII coagulant activity may range from normal to severely reduced (indicated by direct assay, PTT, or TGT tests).

Factor VIII–related antigen measured by special electroimmunoassay is decreased.

Transfusion of normal plasma (or of hemophiliac plasma, cryoprecipitate, serum) causes a rise in Factor VIII activity greater than the amount of Factor VIII infused, which does not peak until 8–10 hours and slowly declines for days; in contrast, hemophilia shows rapid peak and fall after infusion of normal plasma or cryoprecipitate. This response to transfusion is a good diagnostic test in patients in whom diagnosis is equivocal.

Factor VIII levels may increase to normal during pregnancy or use of oral contraceptives with subsidence of hemorrhagic episodes, although bleeding time is often unaffected. Therefore diagnostic evaluation should not be done in the presence of these two circumstances.

Screening of family members may be useful in difficult diagnostic cases even if they are asymptomatic and have no history of unusual bleeding.

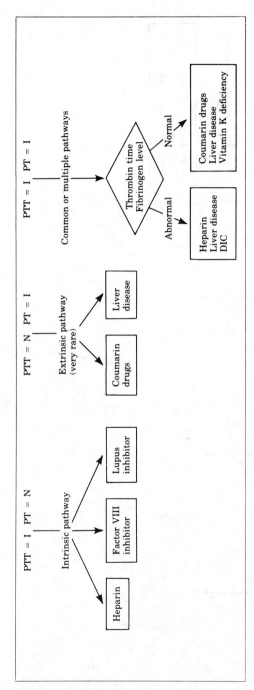

Fig. 27-1. Algorithm for acquired coagulation disorders.

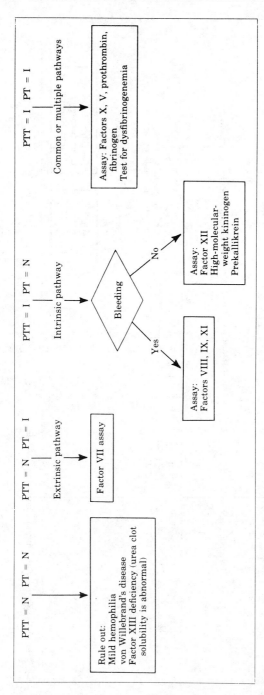

Fig. 27-2. Algorithm for hereditary coagulation disorders.

Table 27-20. Types of von Willebrand's Disease

	Autosomal Dominant Type			Autosomal Recessive
	I	IIa	IIb	
Bleeding time	I	I	I	I
Factor VIII procoagulant activity	D	D or N	D or N	D
Factor VIII–related antigen	D	D or N	D or N	D
Factor VIII von Willebrand's protein	D	D	D or N	D
Ristocetin-induced platelet aggregation	D or N	D	I	D

I = increased; D = decreased; N = normal.

FACTOR V DEFICIENCY (PARAHEMOPHILIA)
Inherited autosomal recessive deficiency syndrome or acquired in association with severe liver disease or DIC.
Prothrombin time and activated partial thromboplastin time are increased but corrected by addition of absorbed plasma.

FACTOR VII DEFICIENCY
Inherited form is autosomal recessive trait and is rare.
Acquired type may be due to liver disease, vitamin K deficiency, or dicumarol therapy.
Prothrombin time is increased but corrected by aged serum.
Activated partial thromboplastin time is normal.

HEMOPHILIA (FACTOR VIII DEFICIENCY; AHG DEFICIENCY)
Classic hemophilia (assay of Factor VIII < 1%) shows increased bleeding time, coagulation time, prothrombin consumption time, and partial thromboplastin time (see Table 27-18).
Moderate hemophilia (assay of Factor VIII 1–5%) shows normal coagulation time and normal prothrombin consumption time but increased partial thromboplastin time.
In mild hemophilia (assay of Factor VIII < 16%) and "sub-hemophilia" (assay of Factor VIII 20–30%), these laboratory tests may be normal.
Abnormal TGT is corrected by absorbed plasma.
Laboratory findings due to hemorrhage and anemia are noted.
Acquired deficiency may occur in DIC and when an inhibitor is present (e.g., some cases of SLE, multiple myeloma, rheumatoid arthritis).

CONGENITAL FACTOR V DEFICIENCY (PARAHEMOPHILIA)
This is an infrequent autosomal recessive defect in which bleeding occurs only in the homozygote.

Table 27-21. Congenital Functional Platelet Disorders

| | Platelet Retention in Glass Bead | Platelet Aggregation | | | |
| | | ADP or Epinephrine | | Risto-cetin | Collagen |
		1st Phase	2nd Phase		
Bernard-Soulier syndrome	D	N	N	D	N
Glanzmann's thrombasthenia	D	D	D	N	D
Release defect	N or D	N	D	N	D
Storage pool disease	N or D	N	D	N	D
von Willebrand's disease	D	N	N	D	N

ADP = adenosine diphosphate; D = depressed; N = normal.
Source: Data from D. J. W. Bowie, Recognition of easily missed bleeding diseases. *Mayo Clin. Proc.* 57:263–264, 1982.

Variable increase in prothrombin time, prothrombin consumption, and coagulation time is not corrected by administration of vitamin K.

CONGENITAL FACTOR VII DEFICIENCY
With this infrequent autosomal trait, bleeding occurs when the gene is homozygous; heterozygotes have little or no manifestations.
Increased prothrombin time (*normal when viper venom is used as thromboplastin; this does not correct prothrombin time in Factor X deficiency*) is not corrected by administration of vitamin K.
Bleeding time, coagulation time, clot retraction, prothrombin consumption, and TGT are normal.

FACTOR IX (PLASMA THROMBOPLASTIN COMPONENTS [PTC]) DEFICIENCY (CHRISTMAS DISEASE; HEMOPHILIA B)
Inherited recessive sex-linked deficiency.
In mild deficiency, only the TGT may be abnormal.
In more severe cases, increased coagulation time, bleeding time, prothrombin consumption time, and partial thromboplastin time are found.
Defect is corrected by frozen plasma just as well as by bank blood.

See Table 27-18.

FACTOR X (STUART-PROWER) DEFICIENCY
This rare autosomal recessive defect resembles Factor VII deficiency; heterozygotes show mild or no clinical manifestations.
Increased prothrombin time (not corrected by use of viper venom as thromboplastin) is not corrected by administration of vitamin K.

Heterozygotes may have only slight increase in prothrombin time.
Acquired form may be associated with amyloidosis, coumarin anticoagulant therapy, vitamin K deficiency, liver trauma.

See Table 27-18.

FACTOR XI (PLASMA THROMBOPLASTIN ANTECEDENT [PTA]) DEFICIENCY
Inherited autosomal recessive deficiency is usually mild; acquired forms are recognized.
In mild form, coagulation may be normal, prothrombin consumption time is slightly increased, and TGT is abnormal.
In severe cases, increased coagulation time, increased prothrombin consumption time, and abnormal TGT are found.

See Table 27-18.

Postoperative bleeding may not begin until several days after surgery.

FACTOR XII (HAGEMAN FACTOR) DEFICIENCY
Coagulation time and prothrombin consumption time are increased; TGT is abnormal.
Specific factor assay is needed to distinguish from Factor XI deficiency.

See Table 27-18.

No hemorrhagic symptoms occur.

CONGENITAL DEFICIENCY OF FACTOR XIII (FIBRIN-STABILIZING FACTOR)
This is an inherited autosomal recessive deficiency with severe coagulation defect.
All standard clotting tests appear normal.
Patient's fibrin clot is soluble in 5M urea.
Whole blood clot is qualitatively friable.
Acquired type may occur in
    Acute myelogenous leukemia
    Liver disease
    Association with hypofibrinogenemia in obstetric complications
    Presence of circulating inhibitors

FIBRINOGEN DEFICIENCY
Congenital
    Afibrinogenemia, hypofibrinogenemia, dysfibrinogenemia
Acquired (see Disseminated Intravascular Coagulation, pp. 400, 402)
    Obstetric (amniotic fluid embolism, meconium embolism, abruptio placentae, septic abortion, missed abortion with prolonged retention, eclampsia)
    Surgical procedures (e.g., prostate, T and A, open heart, lung)
    Neoplasms (e.g., carcinoma of prostate, carcinoma of lung)
    Hematologic conditions (e.g., leukemia, lymphomas, multiple

myeloma, acquired hemolytic anemias, hemolytic transfusion reaction, thrombotic thrombocytopenic purpura)

Other (e.g., cirrhosis, fat embolism, shock, burns, septicemia, drugs, snakebite)

Often associated with depletion of other coagulation factors (e.g., Factors V and VIII, platelets) and presence of circulating anticoagulants

Severe bleeding with failure of blood to clot, abnormal prothrombin time and thrombin time, lysis of clot, decreased platelets, etc.

Fibrinolysis (lysis of sterile whole blood clot in 24 hours)
- Acute hemorrhage
- Severe burns
- Postoperative, obstetric states
- Drug poisoning (e.g., phenobarbital)
- Cirrhosis of liver
- Shock

Inhibition of fibrin formation
- Dysproteinemia and paraproteinemia (e.g., multiple myeloma, macroglobulinemia, cryoglobulinemia)

CONGENITAL AFIBRINOGENEMIA

This is a rare inherited autosomal recessive congenital condition.

Plasma fibrinogen is absent.

Bleeding time is often increased (one-third of patients).

Prothrombin time, activated partial thromboplastin time, and thrombin time are abnormal.

Platelet-to-glass adhesiveness is abnormal unless fibrinogen is added.

CONGENITAL HYPOFIBRINOGENEMIA

Inherited autosomal dominant

Plasma fibrinogen is moderately decreased (usually < 80 mg/dl).

Bleeding and coagulation times are normal.

Blood clots are soft and small.

CONGENITAL DYSFIBRINOGENEMIA

A rare congenital, inherited autosomal dominant condition; it may have no bleeding diathesis.

Fibrin formation is abnormally slow with prolonged plasma thrombin time.

Other coagulation factors are normal.

Due To

Liver disease

Cancer

Fibrinolyis

DIC

DISSEMINATED INTRAVASCULAR COAGULATION (DIC)*
(see Table 27-23, p. 402)

Not only is the clinical picture very variable, but the laboratory findings in a particular patient differ from the textbook compos-

---

*Source: Data from M. Sirridge, Laboratory evaluation of the bleeding patient. *Clin. Lab. Med.* 4:285–301, 1984.

Table 27-22. Effect of Anticoagulant Drugs on Coagulation Tests

Test	Heparin	Warfarin	Aspirin	Dipyridamole/sulfinpyrazone	Urokinase/streptokinase
Platelet count	N[a]	N	N	N	N
Inhibition of platelet aggregation	N or I	N	I	N	I
Bleeding time	N or I	N[b]	I	N	I
Clotting time	I	N[b]	N	N	I
Thrombin time	I	N	N	N	I
Prothrombin time	I	I	N[b]	N	I
PTT	I	N[b]	N	N	I
Fibrinogen	N	N	N	N	D

N = no change; I = increased; D = decreased.
[a] Decreased in 25% of cases.
[b] Increased with high drug dosage.

Table 27-23. Disseminated Intravascular Coagulation (Consumption Coagulopathy)

Determination	% of Cases Abnormal	Abnormal Level for DIC	Mean Values for DIC	Response to Heparin Therapy	Tests
Decreased platelet count (per cu mm)	93	<150,000	52,000	None or may take weeks*	Platelet count, prothrombin time, fibrinogen level are performed first as screening tests; if all three are positive, diagnosis is considered established. If only two of these are positive, diagnosis should be confirmed by at least one of the tests for fibrinolysis.
Increased prothrombin time (seconds)	90	>15	18.0	Becomes normal or falls > 5 sec in few hours to 1 day	
Decreased fibrinogen level (mg/dl)	71	<160	137	Rises significantly (> 40 mg) in 1–3 days	
Latex test for fibrinogen degradation products (titer)	92	>1:16	1:52	Begins to fall in 1 day; if very high, may take > 1 week to become normal	Tests for fibrinolysis
Prolonged thrombin time (seconds)	59	>25	27		
Euglobulin clot lysis time (minutes)	42	<120		Returns to normal	

*Platelet count is not a satisfactory indicator of response to heparin therapy.
Source: Adapted from R. W. Colman, S. J. Robboy, and J. D. Minna, Disseminated intravascular coagulation (DIC): An approach. *Am. J. Med.* 52:679, 1972.

ite, depending on the underlying disease, duration (acute or chronic), and compensatory or overreactive coagulation mechanisms.

Many of the laboratory abnormalities may be present in patients with predisposing conditions (e.g., carcinoma of prostate, inoperable lung carcinoma) in whom DIC is latent; these abnormalities may predict development of DIC precipitated by surgery.

In addition to the findings listed in Table 27-23 (p. 402), the following abnormalities often occur.

Schistocytes in the peripheral blood smear and other evidence of intravascular hemolysis may be present (e.g., increased serum LDH, decreased serum haptoglobin).

Ethanol gelation and protamine gelation tests (that reflect fibrinogen degradation products but are less specific)

Cryofibrinogen may be present.

Observation of the blood clot may show the clot that forms to be small, friable, and wispy because of the hypofibrinogenemia.

Plasma Factors V, VIII, and XIII are usually significantly decreased but are not used for primary diagnosis because of time and technical complexity.

Survival time of radioiodine-labeled fibrinogen and rate of incorporation of ^{14}C-labeled glycine ethyl ester into soluble "circulating fibrin" are sensitive indicators of DIC.

Most sensitive and specific tests
Protamine sulfate or ethanol gelation
Test for fibrin degradation products in serum
Tests for fibrinopeptide A
Serial fibrinogen levels

Less sensitive and specific tests
Prothrombin time (done serially if prolonged)
Activated PTT
Thrombin time
Serial platelet counts

Least sensitive and specific tests
Euglobulin clot lysis
Factor assays
Peripheral blood smear examination

Criteria for specific diagnosis are not well defined.

Repeated prothrombin times (if initially prolonged) and fibrinogen levels are particularly useful. Normal prothrombin time rules out significant consumption coagulopathy.

Clotting time determinations are used to monitor heparin therapy.

Underlying conditions
Tissue injury—pregnancy and obstetric complications (e.g., abruptio placentae, intrauterine fetal death, amniotic fluid embolism), extensive surgery, neoplasms (especially prostate), leukemias, chemotherapy of neoplasia, large traumatic injuries and burns

Endothelial injury—infections, prolonged hypotension

Injury of platelets or RBCs—immunologic hemolytic anemias

Reticuloendothelial system injury—liver disease (cirrhosis, hepatitis), postsplenectomy

Vascular malformations—giant hemangiomas, aortic aneurysm

Suspect clinically in patients with underlying conditions who show bleeding (frequently acute and dramatic), purpura or petechiae, acrocyanosis, arterial or venous thrombosis.

CIRCULATING ANTICOAGULANTS

Various types of anticoagulants may interfere with coagulation at different stages, especially Factor VIII, heparinlike activity, antithromboplastins.

Circulating Anticoagulants Associated with Clinical Disorders

Factor	Disorder
VIII and IX	Following replacement therapy for hereditary deficiency
XI	SLE—very rare
IX	SLE—rare
VIII	SLE, rheumatoid arthritis, drug reaction, asthma, pemphigus, inflammatory bowel disease, postpartum period, advanced age
X	Amyloidosis (tissue binding rather than circulating)
V	Associated with streptomycin administration, idiopathic
X, V	SLE—common
II	Myeloma, SLE
XIII	Associated with isoniazid administration, idiopathic

See Classification of Hemorrhagic Disorders, p. 385, and Table 27-18, pp. 388–390.

CRYOFIBRINOGENEMIA

Plasma precipitates when oxalated blood is refrigerated at 4°C overnight.

May cause erroneous WBC when performed on electronic cell counter.

May be associated with increased alpha$_1$ antitrypsin, haptoglobin, alpha$_2$ macroglobulin (by immunodiffusion technique), and with increased plasma fibrinogen. Not associated with cryoglobulins.

Has been reported in association with many conditions, especially
  Neoplasms
  Thromboembolic conditions

CRYOGLOBULINEMIA

May be associated with
  Immunoproliferative diseases (e.g., multiple myeloma, Waldenström's macroglobulinemia, chronic lymphatic leukemia or lymphoma)
  Collagen diseases (e.g., systemic lupus erythematosus, polyarteritis nodosa, rheumatoid arthritis)
  Autoimmune diseases (e.g., hemolytic anemia)
  Idiopathic
Recurrent purpura occurs.
Cryoprecipitate may be seen in serum.
Rheumatoid factor is present in cryoglobulins.
Serum protein electrophoresis is unremarkable or shows diffuse hyperglobulinemia.
May cause erroneous WBC when performed on electronic cell counter.

Rouleaux formation may occur.

ESR may be increased at 37°C but is normal at room temperature.

Laboratory findings of renal disease may occur (e.g., nephrosis, immune glomerular disease). Renal failure develops in $\cong$ 50%, and marked proteinuria occurs in $\cong$ 25%.

Laboratory findings of liver disease; serologic evidence of hepatitis B virus in 60%

Skin biopsy shows cutaneous vasculitis, often with immune reactants in vessel walls.

Components of complement system (especially C2) are decreased.

Laboratory findings of other associated conditions

Metabolic and Hereditary Diseases

ACID-BASE DISORDERS
In analyzing acid-base disorders, several precautions should be kept in mind.

Determination of pH and blood gases should be performed on *arterial* blood. Venous blood is useless for judging oxygenation but may offer a crude estimate of acid-base status.

The blood specimen should be packed in ice immediately; delay of even a few minutes will cause erroneous results, especially if WBC is high.

Determination of electrolytes, pH, and blood gases ideally should be performed on blood specimens obtained *simultaneously*, since the acid-base situation is very labile.

Repeated determinations may often be indicated because of the development of complications, the effect of therapy, and other factors.

Acid-base disorders are often mixed rather than in the pure form usually described in textbooks. These mixed disorders may represent simultaneously occurring diseases, complications superimposed on the primary condition, or the effect of treatment.

Changes in chronic forms may be notably different from those in the acute forms.

For judging hypoxemia, it is also necessary to know the patient's hemoglobin or hematocrit and whether the patient was breathing room air or oxygen when the specimen was drawn.

Arterial blood gases cannot be interpreted without clinical information about the patient.

Most laboratories measure pH and PCO_2 directly and calculate HCO_3^- using the Henderson-Hasselbalch equation:

$$\text{Arterial pH} = 6.1 + \log \frac{(HCO_3^-)}{0.03 \times PCO_2}$$

where 6.1 is the dissociation constant for CO_2 in aqueous solution and 0.03 is a constant for the solubility of CO_2 in plasma at 37°C.

A normal pH does not ensure the absence of an acid-base disturbance if the PCO_2 is not known.

An abnormal HCO_3^- means a metabolic rather than a respiratory problem; decreased HCO_3^- indicates metabolic acidosis, and increased HCO_3^- indicates metabolic alkalosis. Respiratory acidosis is associated with a $PCO_2 > 45$ mmHg, and respiratory alkalosis is associated with a $PCO_2 < 35$ mmHg. Thus mixed metabolic and respiratory acidosis is characterized by low pH, low HCO_3^-, and high PCO_2. Mixed metabolic and respiratory alkalosis is characterized by high pH, high HCO_3^-, and low PCO_2. (See Table 28-1, Metabolic and Respiratory Acid-Base Changes in Blood.)

In severe metabolic acidosis, respiratory compensation is limited by inability to hyperventilate PCO_2 to < 20 mmHg. In metabolic alkalosis, respiratory compensation is limited by CO_2 retention, which rarely causes PCO_2 > 50–60 mmHg (because CO_2 stimulates respiration very strongly); thus pH is not returned to normal.

Pearls

Pulmonary embolus: Mild to moderate respiratory alkalosis is present unless sudden death occurs. The degree of hypoxia often correlates with the size and extent of the pulmonary embolus. PO_2 > 90 mmHg when breathing room air virtually excludes a lung problem.

Acute pulmonary edema: Hypoxemia is usual. CO_2 is not increased unless the situation is grave.

Asthma: Hypoxia occurs even during a mild episode and increases as the attack becomes worse. As hyperventilation occurs, the PCO_2 falls (usually < 35 mmHg); a normal PCO_2 (>40 mmHg) implies impending respiratory failure; increased PCO_2 in a true asthmatic (not bronchitis or emphysema) indicates impending disaster and the need to consider intubation and ventilation assistance.

Chronic obstructive pulmonary disease (bronchitis and emphysema) may show two patterns—"pink puffers" with mild hypoxia and normal pH and PCO_2 and "blue bloaters" with hypoxia and increased PCO_2; normal pH suggests compensation, and decreased pH suggests decompensation.

Neurologic and neuromuscular disorders (e.g., drug overdose, Guillain-Barré syndrome, myasthenia gravis, trauma, succinylcholine): Acute alveolar hypoventilation causes uncompensated respiratory acidosis with high PCO_2, low pH, and normal HCO_3^-. Acidosis appears before significant hypoxemia, and rising CO_2 indicates rapid deterioration and need for mechanical assistance.

Sepsis: Unexplained respiratory alkalosis may be the earliest sign of sepsis. It may progress to cause metabolic acidosis, and the mixed picture may produce a normal pH; low HCO_3^- is useful to recognize this. With deterioration and worsening of metabolic acidosis, the pH falls.

Salicylate poisoning characteristically shows poor correlation between serum salicylate level and presence or degree of acidemia (because as pH drops from 7.4 to 7.2, the proportion of nonionized to ionized salicylate doubles and the nonionized form leaves the serum and is sequestered in the brain and other organs, where it interferes with function at a cellular level without changing blood levels of glucose, etc.). Salicylate poisoning in adults typically causes respiratory alkalosis, but in children this progresses rapidly to mixed respiratory alkalosis–metabolic acidosis and then to metabolic acidosis (in adults, metabolic acidosis is said to be rare and a near-terminal event).

Isopropyl (rubbing) alcohol poisoning produces enough circulating acetone to produce a positive nitroprusside test (and therefore may be mistaken for diabetic ketoacidosis; thus insulin should not be given until the blood glucose is known). In the absence of a

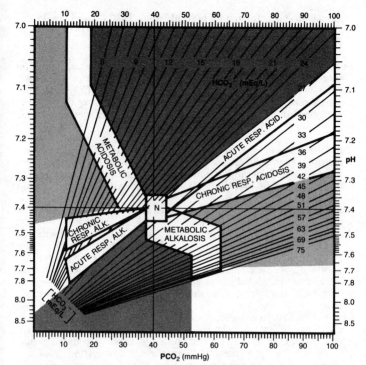

Fig. 28-1. Acid-base map. The values demarcated for each disorder represent a 95% probability range for each *pure* disorder (N = normal). Coordinates lying outside these zones suggest mixed acid-base disorders. (Adapted from M. Goldberg, S. B. Green, M. L. Moss, et al. Computer-based instruction and diagnosis of acid-base disorders. *J.A.M.A.* 223:269–275, 1973. Copyright 1973 American Medical Association.)

history, positive serum ketone test associated with normal anion gap, normal serum HCO_3^-, and normal blood glucose suggests rubbing alcohol intoxication.

Acid-base maps (see Fig. 28-1) are a graphic solution of the Henderson-Hasselbalch equation that predicts the HCO_3^- value for each set of pH/PCO_2 coordinates. They also allow a check of the consistency of arterial blood gas and SMA-6 determinations, since the SMA-6 determines the total CO_2 content, of which 95% is HCO_3^-. These maps contain bands that show the 95% probability range of values for each disorder. If the pH/PCO_2 coordinate is outside the 95% confidence band, then the patient has at least two acid-base disturbances. These maps are of particular use when one of the acid-base disturbances is not suspected clinically. If the coordinates lie within a band, it is not a guarantee of a simple acid-base disturbance.

Data on acid-base disorders from R. C. Klein and S. P. Malloy, Making better use of arterial blood gases. *Diagnosis*, June 1983, p. 48; and N. Flomenbaum, Acid-base disturbances. *Emergency Med.*, Oct. 15, 1980, p. 25.

Table 28-1. Metabolic and Respiratory Acid-Base Changes in Blood

	pH	PCO_2	HCO_3^-
Acidosis			
Acute metabolic	D	N	D
Compensated metabolic	N	D	D
Acute respiratory	D	I	N
Compensated respiratory	N	I	I
Alkalosis			
Acute metabolic	I	N	I
Chronic metabolic	I	I	I
Acute respiratory	I	D	N
Compensated respiratory	N	D	D

D = decreased; N = normal; I = increased.

METABOLIC ACIDOSIS

Laboratory Findings

Serum pH is decreased (< 7.3).

Total plasma CO_2 content is decreased; <15 mEq/L almost certainly rules out respiratory alkalosis.

Serum potassium is frequently increased; it is decreased in renal tubular acidosis, diarrhea, or carbonic anhydrase inhibition.

Azotemia suggests metabolic acidosis due to renal failure.

Urine is strongly acid (pH = 4.5–5.2) if renal function is normal.

In evaluating acid-base disorders, calculate the anion gap (see below).

ANION GAP (AG)

(calculated as NA − [Cl + HCO_3^-]; normal = 8–16 mEq/L)

Increased In

Increased "unmeasured" anions

    Organic (e.g., lactic acidosis, ketoacidosis)

    Inorganic (e.g., administration of phosphate, sulfate)

    Protein (e.g., hyperalbuminemia, transient)

    Exogenous (e.g., salicylate, formate, nitrate, penicillin, carbenicillin)

    Not completely identified (e.g., hyperosmolar hyperglycemic nonketotic coma, uremia, poisoning by ethylene glycol, methanol, salicylates)

Laboratory error

    Falsely increased serum sodium

    Falsely decreased serum chloride or bicarbonate

Decreased unmeasured cations (e.g., hypokalemia, hypocalcemia, hypomagnesemia)

When AG > 12–14 mEq/L, diabetic ketoacidosis is the most common cause, uremic acidosis is the second most common cause, and drug ingestion (e.g., salicylates, methyl alcohol, ethylene glycol, ethyl alcohol) is the third most common cause; lactic acidosis should always be considered when these three causes are ruled out.

Table 28-2. Illustrative Serum Electrolyte Values in Various Conditions

Condition	pH	Bicarbonate	Potassium	Sodium	Chloride
Normal	7.35–7.45	24–26	3.5–5.0	136–145	100–106
Metabolic acidosis					
Diabetic acidosis	7.2	10	5.6	122	80
Fasting	7.2	16	5.2	142	100
Severe diarrhea	7.2	12	3.2	128	96
Hyperchloremic acidosis	7.2	12	5.2	142	116
Addison's disease	7.2	22	6.5	111	72
Nephritis	7.2	8	4	129	90
Nephrosis	7.2	20	5.5	138	113
Metabolic alkalosis					
Vomiting	7.6	38	3.2	150	94
Pyloric obstruction	7.6	58	3.2	132	42
Duodenal obstruction	7.6	42	3.2	138	49
Respiratory acidosis	7.1	30	5.5	142	80
Respiratory alkalosis	7.6	14	5.5	136	112

Decreased In

Decreased unmeasured anion (e.g., hypoalbuminemia is probably commonest cause of decreased anion gap)

Laboratory error

"Hyperchloremia" in bromide intoxication (if chloride determination by colorimetric method)

Hyponatremia due to viscous serum

False decrease in serum sodium; false increase in serum chloride or bicarbonate

Increased unmeasured cations

Hyperkalemia, hypercalcemia, hypermagnesemia

Increased proteins in multiple myeloma, paraproteinemias, polyclonal gammopathies (these abnormal proteins are positively charged and lower the AG)

Increased lithium, TRIS buffer (tromethamine)

Anion gap > 30 mEq/L almost always indicates organic acidosis even in presence of uremia. Anion gap = 20–29 mEq/L occurs in absence of identified organic acidosis in 25% of patients.

Anion gap is rarely > 23 mEq/L in chronic renal failure.

Simultaneous changes in ions may cancel each other out, leaving anion gap unchanged (e.g., increased Cl and decreased HCO_3^-).

Anion gap may provide a clue to the presence of a mixed rather than simple acid-base disturbance.

CAUSES OF METABOLIC ACIDOSIS

With Increased Anion Gap (> 15 mEq/L)

Lactic acidosis—commonest cause of metabolic acidosis with increased anion gap (AG frequently > 25 mEq/L) (see following section)

Renal failure (AG < 25 mEq/L)

Ketoacidosis

Diabetes mellitus (AG frequently > 25 mEq/L)

Associated with alcohol abuse (AG frequently 20–25 mEq/L)

Starvation (AG usually 5–10 mEq/L)

Others

Salicylate poisoning (AG frequently 5–10 mEq/L; higher in children)

Methanol poisoning (AG frequently > 20 mEq/L)

Ethylene glycol poisoning (AG frequently > 20 mEq/L)

Paraldehyde (AG frequently > 20 mEq/L)

With Normal Anion Gap

(hyperchloremic acidosis)

Decreased serum potassium

Renal tubular acidosis

Acquired (e.g., drugs, hypercalcemia)

Inherited (e.g., cystinosis, Wilson's disease)

Carbonic anhydrase inhibitors (e.g., acetazolamide, mafenide)

Increased loss of alkaline body fluids (e.g., diarrhea, loss of pancreatic or biliary fluids)

Ureteral diversion (e.g., ileal bladder or ureter, ureterosigmoidostomy)

Normal or increased serum potassium
    Hydronephrosis
    Early renal failure
    Administration of HCl (e.g., ammonium chloride)
    Hypoadrenalism (diffuse, zona glomerulosa, or hyporeninemia)
    Renal aldosterone resistance
    Sulfur toxicity

In lactic acidosis the increase in AG is usually greater than the decrease in HCO_3^-, in contrast to diabetic ketoacidosis in which the increase in AG is identical to the decrease in HCO_3^-.

LACTIC ACIDOSIS
Should be considered in any metabolic acidosis with increased anion gap (>15 mEq/L). Diagnosis is confirmed by exclusion of other causes of metabolic acidosis and serum lactate $\geqq 5$ mEq/L (upper limit of normal $= 1.6$ for plasma and 1.4 for whole blood). Considerable variation in literature in limits of serum lactate and pH to define lactic acidosis.
Exclusion of other causes by
    Normal serum creatinine and BUN *(Increased acetoacetic acid [but not beta-hydroxybutyric acid] will cause false increase of creatinine by colorimetric assay.)*
    Osmolar gap < 10 mOsm/L
    Negative nitroprusside reaction *(Nitroprusside test for ketoacidosis measures acetoacetic acid but not beta-hydroxybutyric acid; thus blood ketone test may be negative in diabetic ketoacidosis.)*
    Urine negative for calcium oxalate crystals
    No known ingestion of toxic substances
Laboratory findings due to underlying diseases (e.g., diabetes mellitus, renal insufficiency, etc.)
Laboratory tests for monitoring therapy
    Arterial pH, pCO_2, HCO_3^-, serum electrolytes every 1–2 hours until patient is stable
    Urine electrolytes every 6 hours
Associated or compensatory metabolic or respiratory disturbances (e.g., hyperventilation or respiratory alkalosis may result in normal pH)

CLASSIFICATION OF LACTIC ACIDOSIS
Type A due to clinically apparent tissue hypoxia
    Acute hemorrhage
    Shock or hypotension
    Severe acute congestive heart failure
    Severe anemia
    Asphyxia
    Hypoxemia
    Carbon monoxide poisoning
Type B (without clinically apparent tissue hypoxia)
    Diabetes mellitus
    Uremia
    Liver disease
    Infections
    Various malignancies (e.g., leukemia, lymphoma)—may respond to antitumor chemotherapy

Convulsions
Alkaloses

Drugs and toxins
    Diguanides (especially pheniformin for treatment of diabetes; this was most common cause before removed from market in 1977)
    Ethanol, methanol, ethylene glycol
    Salicylates (especially in adults may be combined with respiratory alkalosis)
    Others (e.g., fructose, sorbitol, xylitol, streptozocin)
Hereditary enzyme defects
    Type I glycogenesis (glucose 6-phosphate dehydrogenase deficiency)
    Fructose-1,6-diphosphatase deficiency
    Pyruvate carboxylase deficiency
    Pyruvate dehydrogenase deficiency
    Methylmalonic aciduria
D-Lactic acidosis
With a typical clinical picture (acute onset following nausea and vomiting, altered state of consciousness, hyperventilation, high mortality), the following laboratory findings occur.
    Decreased serum bicarbonate
    Low serum pH, usually 6.98–7.25
    Increased serum potassium, often 6–7 mEq/L
    Serum chloride normal or low with increased anion gap
    WBC is increased (occasionally to leukemoid levels).
    Increased serum uric acid is frequent (up to 25 mg/dl in lactic acidosis)
    Increased serum phosphorus. Phosphorus-creatinine ratio > 3 indicates lactic acidosis either alone or as a component of other metabolic acidosis.
    Increased SGOT, LDH, and phosphorus in serum

METABOLIC ALKALOSIS

Due To
Loss of acid
    Vomiting, gastric suction, gastrocolic fistula
    Diarrhea in mucoviscidosis (rarely)
    Aciduria secondary to potassium depletion
Excess of base due to administration of
    Absorbable antacids (e.g., sodium bicarbonate)
    Salts of weak acids (e.g., sodium lactate, sodium or potassium citrate)
Some vegetable diets
Potassium depletion (causing sodium and H^+ to enter the cells)
    Gastrointestinal loss (e.g., chronic diarrhea)
    Lack of potassium intake (e.g., anorexia nervosa, IV fluids without potassium supplements for treatment of vomiting or postoperatively)
    Diuresis (e.g., mercurials, thiazides, osmotic diuresis)
    Extracellular volume depletion and chloride depletion
    All forms of mineralocorticoid excess (e.g., primary aldosteronism, Cushing's syndrome, administration of steroids, large amounts of licorice)

Table 28-3. Upper Limits of Arterial Blood pH and Bicarbonate Concentrations (expected for blood PCO$_2$ values)

Arterial Blood		
PCO$_2$ (mmHg)	pH	Bicarbonate (mEq/L)
20	7.66	22.8
30	7.53	25.6
40	7.47	27.3
60	7.29	27.9
80	7.18	28.9

Values shown are the upper limits of the 95% confidence bands.
Source: Data from F. L. Coe, Metabolic alkalosis. *J.A.M.A.* 238:2288, 1977.

Glycogen deposition
Chronic alkalosis
Potassium-losing nephropathy

Laboratory Findings
Serum pH is increased.
Total plasma CO$_2$ is increased (bicarbonate > 30 mEq/L).
PCO$_2$ is normal or slightly increased.
Serum pH and bicarbonate above those predicted by the PCO$_2$ (by nomogram or Table 28-3)
Serum potassium is usually decreased, which condition is the chief danger in metabolic alkalosis.
Serum chloride is relatively lower than sodium.
BUN may be increased.
Urine pH is > 7.0 (≦ 7.9) if potassium depletion is not severe and concomitant sodium deficiency (e.g., vomiting) is not present. With severe hypokalemia (< 2.0 mEq/L), urine may be acid in presence of systemic alkalosis.
When the urine chloride is low (< 10 mEq/L) and the patient responds to chloride treatment, the cause is more likely loss of gastric juice, diuretic therapy, or rapid relief of chronic hypercapnia. Chloride replacement is completed when urine chloride remains > 40 mEq/L.
When the urine chloride is high (> 20 mEq/L) and the patient does not respond to NaCl treatment, the cause is more likely hyperadrenalism or severe potassium deficiency.

RESPIRATORY ACIDOSIS
Laboratory findings differ in acute and chronic conditions.

Acute
Due to decreased alveolar ventilation
Pneumonia
Pneumothorax

Pulmonary edema
Foreign body aspiration
Laryngospasm, bronchospasm
Mechanical ventilation
General anesthesia
Oversedation

Acidosis is severe (pH 7.05–7.10) but HCO_3^- concentration is only 29–30 mEq/L.

Severe mixed acidosis is common in cardiac arrest when respiratory and circulatory failure cause marked respiratory acidosis and severe lactic acidosis.

Chronic

Due to chronic obstructive or restrictive disease

Nerve disease (e.g., poliomyelitis)
Muscle disease (e.g., myopathy)
Central neurologic disorder (e.g., brain tumor)
Restriction of thorax (e.g., musculoskeletal, scleroderma)
Pulmonary disease (e.g., prolonged pneumonia, primary alveolar hypoventilation)

Acidosis is not usually severe.

Beware of commonly occurring mixed acid-base disturbances (e.g., chronic respiratory acidosis with superimposed acute hypercapnia resulting from acute infection, such as bronchitis or pneumonia).

Superimposed metabolic alkalosis (e.g., due to diuretics or vomiting) may exacerbate the hypercapnia.

RESPIRATORY ALKALOSIS

Due To

Hyperventilation

CNS disorders (e.g., infection, tumor, trauma, CVA)
Salicylate intoxication
Fever
Gram-negative bacteremia
Liver disease
Pulmonary disease (e.g., pneumonia, pulmonary emboli, asthma)
Mechanical overventilation
Congestive heart failure
Hypoxia (e.g., decreased barometric pressure, ventilation-perfusion imbalance)

Laboratory Findings

Acute hypocapnia—usually only a modest decrease in plasma HCO_3^- concentrations and marked alkalosis
Chronic hypocapnia—usually only a slight alkaline pH

MIXED ACID-BASE DISTURBANCES
(must always be interpreted with clinical data and other laboratory findings)

Respiratory Acidosis With Metabolic Acidosis

Examples: Acute pulmonary edema, cardiopulmonary arrest (lactic acidosis due to tissue anoxia and CO_2 retention due to alveolar hypoventilation)

Acidemia may be extreme with pH < 7.0 ($H^+ > 100$ mEq/L) $HCO_3^- < 26$ mEq/L. Failure of HCO_3^- to increase $\geqq 3$ mEq/L for each 10 mmHg rise in $PaCO_2$ suggests metabolic acidosis with respiratory acidosis.

Mild metabolic acidosis superimposed on chronic hypercapnia caus-
ing partial suppression of HCO_3^- may be indistinguishable from
adaptation to hypercapnia alone.

Metabolic Acidosis With Respiratory Alkalosis
Examples: Rapid correction of severe metabolic acidosis, salicylate intoxication, gram-negative septicemia, initial respiratory alkalosis with subsequent development of metabolic acidosis

pH may be normal or decreased.
Hypocapnia remains inappropriate to decreased HCO_3^- for several hours or more.

Respiratory Acidosis With Metabolic Alkalosis
Examples: Chronic pulmonary disease with CO_2 retention developing metabolic alkalosis due to administration of diuretics, severe vomiting, or sudden improvement in ventilation ("posthypercapnic" metabolic alkalosis)

Decreased or absent urine chloride indicates that chloride-responsive metabolic alkalosis is a part of the picture.
In clinical setting of respiratory acidosis but with normal blood pH and/or HCO_3^- higher than predicted, complicating metabolic alkalosis may be present.

Respiratory Alkalosis With Metabolic Alkalosis
Examples: Hepatic insufficiency with hyperventilation plus administration of diuretics or severe vomiting; metabolic alkalosis with stimulation of ventilation (e.g., sepsis, pulmonary embolism, mechanical ventilation) that causes respiratory alkalosis
Marked alkalemia with decreased PCO_2 and increased HCO_3^- is diagnostic.

Acute and Chronic Respiratory Acidosis
Examples: Chronic hypercapnia with acute deterioration of pulmonary function causing further rise of PCO_2

HCO_3^- in intermediate range between acute and chronic respiratory acidosis *(similar findings in chronic respiratory acidosis with superimposed metabolic acidosis or acute respiratory acidosis with superimposed metabolic alkalosis)*

Coexistence of Metabolic Acidoses of Hyperchloremic Type and Increased Anion Gap Type
May be suspected by plasma HCO_3^- that is lower than is explained by the increase in anions (e.g., anion gap $= 16$ mEq/L and $HCO_3^- = 5$ mEq/L)
Examples are uremia and proximal RTA, lactic acidosis with diarrhea, excessive administration of NaCl to patient with organic acidosis.

Table 28-4. Laboratory Findings in Some Syndromes Associated With Persistent Hypokalemia

	Serum Renin	Serum Aldosterone	Hypertension
Primary hyperaldosteronism	D	I	+
Secondary hyperaldosteronism	I	I	+
Malignant hypertension	I	I	+
Renovascular hypertension	I	I	+
Pseudoaldosteronism	D	N or D	+
Bartter's syndrome	I	I	N
Cushing's syndrome, ACTH-secreting tumor	D	V	+
17-Hydroxylase deficiency	D	D	+
Licorice ingestion	D	D	+
Liddle's syndrome	D	D	+
Excess corticosterone, deoxycorticosterone	D	D	+
Periodic paralysis	N		N
Fanconi's syndrome		N	N
Renal tubular acidosis	I	N	N
Salt-losing nephritis		I	+
Renal tumor	N	N	N
Renin-secreting tumor	I	I	+
Familial hypokalemia with renal interstitial fibrosis	I	N	N

D = decreased; I = increased; N = normal; V = variable; + = hypertension present.
See elsewhere in text for other findings in these conditions.
Source: Adapted from W. Z. Potter et al, *Am. J. Med.* 57:971, 1974; and P. J. Cannon, Recognizing and treating cardiac emergencies due to potassium imbalance. *J. Cardiovasc. Med.*, April 1983, p. 467.

PROTEIN-CALORIE MALNUTRITION*

Adult Kwashiorkor

Occurs in patients whose protein intake is inadequate in presence of low or normal caloric intake and whose catabolism is increased (e.g., trauma, severe burns); may develop quickly

Decreased serum albumin (2.1–3.0 mg/dl in moderate; < 2.1 mg/dl in severe)

Decreased total iron binding capacity (TIBC) or serum transferrin (100–150 mg/dl in moderate; < 100 mg/dl in severe)

Decreased thyroxine-binding prealbumin

*Source: M. Haider and S. Q. Haider, Assessment of protein-calorie malnutrition. *Clin. Chem.* 30:1286–1299, 1984.

All serum complement components except C4 and sometimes C5 are decreased.

Decreased total lymphocyte count (800–1200 in moderate; < 800 in severe; normal = 2000–3500/cu mm) evidencing diminished immunologic resistance *(should always be interpreted with total WBC count)*

Diminished delayed hypersensitivity reaction (measured by skin testing)

Normal anthropometric measurements (e.g., creatinine-height, index, triceps skinfold, arm circumference measurements)

Clinically, may show pitting edema, ascites, enlarged liver, diarrhea

These laboratory tests all have low sensitivity and specificity or are not easily available.

Marasmus

Chronic deficiency in total energy intake as in wasting illnesses (e.g., cancer)

Normal serum protein levels

Impaired immune function

Clinically, show severe wasting of skeletal muscle and fat; edema is distinctively absent. May progress to marasmic kwashiorkor.

Marasmic Kwashiorkor

Shows features of both marasmus and kwashiorkor

Severe form of malnutrition that occurs when stress is superimposed on starved, chronically ill patients

Laboratory findings due to underlying diseases (e.g., cancer) or complications (e.g., infection)

NUTRITIONAL DWARFISM

Serum proteins, amino acids, and BUN are usually normal.

Anemia is not prominent.

Laboratory changes due to underlying conditions (e.g., intestinal malabsorption, chronic vomiting, congenital heart disease, chronic infections, chronic renal insufficiency) are present.

SCURVY (VITAMIN C DEFICIENCY)

Plasma level of ascorbic acid is decreased—usually 0 in frank scurvy. Normal is 0.5–1.5 mg/dl, but lower level does not prove diagnosis.

Ascorbic acid in buffy coat is decreased—usually absent in clinical scurvy. Normal is 30 mg/dl.

Tyrosyl compounds are present in urine (detected by Millon's reagent) in patients with scurvy but are absent in normal persons after protein meal or administration of tyrosine.

Serum alkaline phosphatase is decreased; serum calcium and phosphorus are normal.

Rumpel-Leede test is positive.

Microscopic hematuria is present in one-third of patients.

Stool may be positive for occult blood.

Laboratory findings due to associated deficiencies (e.g., anemia due to folic acid deficiency) are present.

BERIBERI (THIAMINE DEFICIENCY)

Increased blood pyruvic acid level

Decreased thiamine level in blood and urine; becomes normal within 24 hours after therapy begins (thus baseline levels should be established first)

Laboratory findings due to complications (e.g., heart failure)

Laboratory findings due to underlying conditions (e.g., chronic diarrhea, inadequate intake)

VITAMIN A DEFICIENCY

Decreased plasma level of vitamin A. <25 IU/ml is significantly low. *Elevated carotenoids may cause false low values for vitamin A.*

RIBOFLAVIN DEFICIENCY

Decreased riboflavin level in plasma, RBCs, WBCs

PELLAGRA (NIACIN DEFICIENCY)

Decreased excretion of niacin metabolites (nicotinamide) in 6- or 24-hour urine sample

Plasma tryptophan level markedly decreased

PYRIDOXINE (VITAMIN B_6) DEFICIENCY

Decreased pyridoxic acid in urine

Decreased serum levels of vitamin B_6

FOLIC ACID DEFICIENCY

Table 27-4, p. 337.

COPPER DEFICIENCY

Nutritional Copper Deficiency

Found in patients on parenteral nutrition and in children recovering from severe protein-calorie malnutrition fed iron-fortified milk formula with cane sugar and cottonseed oil

Anemia not responsive to iron and vitamins

Leukopenia with WBC < 5000/cu mm and neutropenia (<1500/cu mm)

Copper administration corrects neutropenia in 3 weeks and anemia responds with reticulocytosis.

Decreased copper and ceruloplasmin in plasma and decreased hepatic copper confirm diagnosis.

"Kinky Hair" Syndrome

Syndrome of neonatal hypothermia, feeding difficulties, and sometimes prolonged jaundice; at 2–3 months, seizures and progressive change of hair from normal to steel-wool light color; striking facial appearance, increasing mental deterioration, infections, failure to thrive, death in early infancy; changes in elastica interna of arteries

Decreased copper in serum and liver; normal in RBCs

Increased copper in amniotic fluid, cultured fibroblasts, and amniotic cells

ZINC DEFICIENCY

Occurs In

Acrodermatitis enteropathica (rare autosomal recessive disease of
  infancy)
Inadequate nutrition (e.g., parenteral alimentation)
Excessive requirements
Decreased absorption or availability
Increased losses
Iatrogenic
Plasma zinc levels do not always reflect nutritional status.
Measurement of zinc in hair may be helpful.
Decreased or very excessive urinary zinc excretion may be helpful.

CLASSIFICATION OF SOME INHERITED METABOLIC CONDITIONS

Disorders of carbohydrate metabolism
    Diabetes mellitus
    Pentosuria
    Fructosuria
    Familial lactose intolerance
    Galactosemia
    Glycogen storage diseases
    Mucopolysaccharidoses
    Other
Disorders of amino acid metabolism
    Phenylketonuria
    Tyrosinosis
    Maple syrup urine disease
    Alkaptonuria
    Other
Disorders of purine and pyrimidine metabolism
    Gout
    Orotic aciduria
    Beta-aminoisobutyric aciduria
    Other
Disorders of lipid metabolism
    Essential familial hypercholesterolemia
    Inherited deficiency of lipoprotein lipase
Disorders of porphyrin metabolism
Disorders of metabolism involving metals
    Wilson's disease
    Hemochromatosis
    Periodic paralysis
    Adynamia episodica hereditaria
    Other
Disorders of renal tubular function
    Fanconi's syndrome of cystinosis
    Vitamin D–resistant rickets of primary hypophosphatemia
    Cystinuria
    Renal glycosuria
    Other
Disorders of serum enzymes
    Hypophosphatasia
    Other

Disorders of plasma proteins
    Analbuminemia
    Agammaglobulinemia
    Atransferrinemia
    Other
Disorders of blood
    Coagulation diseases (e.g., hemophilias)
    RBC glucose-6-PD deficiency
    Hemoglobinopathies and thalassemias
    Hereditary spherocytosis
    Hereditary nonspherocytic hemolytic anemia
    Other

DETECTING HETEROZYGOUS CARRIERS OF SOME DISORDERS*

Disorder	Abnormality
Duchenne type of muscular dystrophy	Increased serum CK
Gout	Increased serum uric acid
Wilson's disease	Abnormality detected by ^{48}Cu studies
Glucose-6-PD deficiency	Decreased glucose-6-PD in RBCs
Orotic aciduria	Decreased orotidylic decarboxylase in RBCs
Hemoglobinopathies (e.g., thalassemia)	Abnormality detected by hemoglobin electrophoresis
Tay-Sachs disease	Decreased serum fructose 1-phosphate aldolase
Glycogen storage disease (Type III)	Decreased amylo-1, 6-glucosidase in leukocytes
Glycogen storage disease (von Gierke's, Type I)	Decreased glucose-6-phosphate in intestinal mucosa
Phenylketonuria	Prolonged increase in serum phenylalanine after phenylalanine load
Argininosuccinic aciduria	Decreased argininosuccinase in RBCs and increased argininosuccinic acid in urine
Cystathioninuria	Increased cystathionine in urine
Cystinurea	Increased cystine and lysine in urine
Homocystinuria	Decreased cysthathionine synthetase in liver
Histidinemia	Decreased histidase in skin
Hyperoxaluria	Abnormality detected by special radioisotope study
Galactosemia	Decreased galactose-1-p-uridyl transferase in RBCs

*Source: Data from D.Y.Y. Hsia, The diagnosis of carriers of disease-producing genes. *Ann. N.Y. Acad. Sci.* 134:946, 1966.

HYPERLIPIDEMIAS

Primary Hyperlipidemias
(see Table 28-5, pp. 424–427)

Familial hypercholesterolemia (familial Type II hyperlipoproteinemia)

> Homozygous—serum cholesterol is very high (e.g., 600–1000 mg/dl) with corresponding increase in low-density lipoproteins (LDL). Both parents are heterozygous. Clinical manifestations of increased cholesterol (xanthomata, corneal arcus, ischemic heart disease that causes death usually before age 30 years). Neonatal diagnosis requires finding increased LDL cholesterol in cord blood; serum cholesterol is unreliable. Because of marked variation in serum cholesterol levels during first year of life, diagnosis should be deferred until 1 year old. Prenatal diagnosis of homozygous fetus can be made by estimation of binding sites on fibroblasts cultured from amniotic fluids; useful when both parents are heterozygous.

> Heterozygous—increased serum cholesterol (300–500 mg/dl) and LDL with similar change in a parent or first-degree relative; serum triglycerides and very-low-density lipoproteins (VLDL) are normal in 90% and slightly increased in 10% of these cases.

Familial combined hyperlipidemia (IIA, IIB, IV, V)

> There may be any combination of increased LDL and VLDL and chylomicrons; HDL is often low; different family members may have increased serum cholesterol or triglycerides or both.

> Premature atherosclerosis occurs later in life than with familial hypercholesterolemia.

> Xanthomatosis is rare.

Familial dysbetalipoproteinemia (Type III hyperlipoproteinemia)

> Excess of abnormal lipoprotein (beta-VLDL) is present; cholesterol and triglycerides are both increased.

> Xanthomas are present.

> Atherosclerosis is more common in peripheral than coronary arteries.

Polygenic hypercholesterolemia (Type IIA)

> Cholesterol elevation may be mild to marked. LDL is increased.

> Premature atherosclerosis is frequent.

> Xanthomatosis is rare.

Familial hypertriglyceridemia (Type IV)

> Elevated plasma triglycerides and VLDL with normal LDL.

> Distinction from familial combined hyperlipidemia is made only by extensive family screening.

Secondary Hyperlipidemias

Poorly controlled diabetes mellitus

> Most common findings—increase in VLDL with increased serum triglycerides and less marked increase in cholesterol

> Less common findings—as above with increase in chylomicrons also

> Least common—normal pattern despite poor control

Hypothyroidism

> Most common pattern is Type II with increased LDL and serum cholesterol.

Less common pattern is Type III.
Serum cholesterol is not always increased.
Rapidly becomes normal with treatment

Nephrotic syndrome
Increased serum cholesterol is usual.
Increased LDL is common.
Increased VLDL and therefore increased serum triglyceride may also occur.

Hepatic glycogenoses
Increased serum lipoprotein is common in any of the forms, but the pattern cannot be used to differentiate the type of GSD.
Predominant increase in VLDL in glucose-6-phosphatase deficiency
Predominant increase in LDL in debrancher and phosphorylase deficiencies

Obstructive liver disease
Increased serum cholesterol is common until liver failure develops. The type of lipoproteinemia is variable.
In intrahepatic biliary atresia, there is often increase in lipoprotein X with marked increase in serum cholesterol and even more marked increase in serum phospholipids.

Hyperlipoproteinemia of "affluence" (dietary)

PHENYLKETONURIA

Inherited absence of phenylalanine hydroxylase activity in liver causes increased blood and urine phenylalanine along with metabolites; associated with mental retardation.

For screening of newborns, urine amounts of phenylpyruvic acid may be insufficient for detection by colorimetric methods when blood level is < 15 mg/dl. May not appear in urine until 2–3 weeks of age.

Preliminary blood-screening tests (inhibition assay, fluorometry, paper chromatography) detect levels > 4 mg/dl.

To confirm diagnosis of phenylketonuria, administer 100 mg of ascorbic acid, and collect blood and urine 24 hours later.

Phenylketonuria
Serum phenylalanine is > 15 mg/dl.
Serum tyrosine is < 5 mg/dl *(is never increased in phenylketonuria)*.
Urine phenylalanine is > 100 μg/ml.
Orthohydroxyphenylacetic acid is present in urine.
Phenylpyruvic acid in urine is significant (gives positive ferric chloride test) but may not be present in some patients.

Abnormalities of tyrosine metabolism (e.g., incomplete development of tyrosine oxidizing system, especially in premature or low-birth-weight infants)
Serum phenylalanine is > 4 mg/dl (5–20 mg/dl).
Serum tyrosine is between 10 and 75 mg/dl.
Tyrosine metabolites in urine are ≤ 1 mg/ml (parahydroxyphenyl-lactic and parahydroxyphenylacetic acids can be distinguished from orthohydroxyphenylacetic acid by paper chromatography).
Orthohydroxyphenylacetic acid is absent from urine.

Without administration of ascorbic acid, 25% of premature infants may have increased serum phenylalanine and tyrosine for several

Table 28-5. Comparison of Types of Hyperlipoproteinemia

Point of Comparison	Type I (rarest)	Type IIa (relatively common)	Type IIb (relatively common)	Type III (relatively uncommon)	Type IV (most common)	Type V (uncommon)
Origin	Exogenous hyperlipidemia due to deficient lipoprotein lipase		Overindulgence lipidemia		Endogenous hyperlipidemia	Mixed endogenous and exogenous hyperlipidemia (combined Types I and IV)
Definition	Familial fat-induced hyperglycidemia	Hyperbetalipoproteinemia (hypercholesterolemia)	Combined hyperlipidemia (mixed hyperlipidemia)	Carbohydrate-induced hyperglyceridemia with hypercholesterolemia	Carbohydrate-induced hyperglyceridemia without hypercholesterolemia	Combined fat and carbohydrate-induced hyperglyceridemia
Age	Usually under age 10			Not known under age 25	Only occasionally seen in children	
Gross appearance of plasma	On standing: supernatant creamy, infranatant clear	Clear (no cream layer on top)	No cream layer on top; clear to turbid infranatant	Clear, cloudy, or milky	Slightly turbid to cloudy Unchanged on standing	Markedly turbid On standing: supernatant creamy, infranatant milky
Serum cholesterol	Normal or slightly increased	Markedly increased (300–600 mg/dl)	Markedly increased (300–600 mg/dl)	Markedly increased (300–1000 mg/dl)	Normal or slightly increased	Increased (250–500 mg/dl)

Serum triglycerides	Markedly increased (usually > 2000 mg/dl)	Normal	Increased ≦ 400 mg/dl	Markedly increased (200–1000 mg/dl)	Markedly increased (500–1500 mg/dl)	Markedly increased (500–1500 mg/dl)
Appearance of lipoprotein components visualized by electrophoresis[a]						
Chylomicron	Marked I	0	0	0	0	I
Beta-lipoprotein[b]	N or D	I	I	I — Floating beta	N or I	N or I
Prebetalipoprotein[c]	N or D	N	I	I	I	I
Alpha-lipoprotein[d]						
Other laboratory abnormalities	Glucose tolerance usually normal			Hyperglycemia; glucose tolerance often abnormal; serum uric acid increased	Glucose tolerance often abnormal; serum uric acid often increased	Glucose tolerance usually abnormal; serum uric acid usually increased
Triglyceride-cholesterol ratio	8	1	Variable	<2	1–5	> 5

Table 28-5. (continued)

Point of Comparison	Type I (rarest)	Type IIa (relatively common)	Type IIb (relatively common)	Type III (relatively uncommon)	Type IV (most common)	Type V (uncommon)
Lipid changes resembling primary hyperlipidemias Diet		Very high cholesterol diet	Same as Type IIa		Caffeine or alcohol before testing	
Drugs		Triglyceride-lowering drugs in Types III and IV	Same as Type IIa	Triglyceride-lowering drugs in Type IV	Cholesterol-lowering drugs Chlorothiazide Birth control pills or estrogens	
Primary disease		Myxedema Nephrosis Obstructive liver disease Stress Porphyria Anorexia nervosa Idiopathic hypercalcemia	Same as Type IIa	Myxedema Dysgammaglobulinemia Liver disease	Nephrotic syndrome Hypothyroidism Pregnancy Glycogen storage disease	Myeloma Macroglobulinemia Nephrosis

0 = absent; N = normal; I = increased; D = decreased.

[a] Chylomicrons are mainly dietary triglycerides.

[b] Beta-lipoproteins (LDL) are mainly cholesterol.

[c] Prebetalipoproteins (VLDL) are composed of endogenous triglycerides synthesized in liver plus cholesterol.

[d] Alpha-lipoproteins (high-density lipoproteins [HDL]) are cholesterol scavengers derived from liver and gut.

[e] Intermediate-density lipoproteins (IDL) are remnants of VLDL catabolism.

Mild elevation of serum triglycerides (up to 250 mg/dl) probably does not represent increased risk for any disease. Range of 250–500 mg/dl may be a marker for patients with genetic forms of hyperlipoproteinemias who need specific therapy because of increased cardiovascular risk. >500 mg/dl should be labelled "hypertriglyceridemia" with danger of pancreatitis; >1000 mg/dl carries substantial risk of pancreatitis.

Obtain blood only after at least 12–14 hours' fasting and when patient has been on usual diet for at least 2 weeks.

Rule out diabetes and pancreatitis in all groups.

Increased susceptibility to coronary artery disease occurs in Types II, III, IV; accelerated peripheral vascular disease in Type III.

Xanthomas appear in Types I, II, III.

Abdominal pain occurs in Types I, V.

If dietary or drug treatment has begun, it may not be possible to classify the lipoproteinemia or the classification may be erroneous.

Type IIb is overindulgence hyperlipemia; shows increased cholesterol and triglycerides, with increased beta and prebeta; can only be distinguished from Type III by detecting abnormal beta-migrating lipoprotein in serum fraction with density > 1.006.

Source: Data from Office of Medical Application of Research, NIH. Treatment of hypertriglyceridemia. *J.A.M.A.* 251:1196–1200, 1984.

Table 28-6. Summary of Primary Overflow Aminoacidurias (increased blood concentration with overflow into urine)

Disease	Increased Blood Amino Acids	Urine Abnormalities*	Other Laboratory Findings
Phenylketonuria	Phenylalanine	o-Hydroxyphenylacetic acid; phenylpyruvic, acetic, and lactic acids	Blood tyrosine does not rise after phenylalanine load
Maple syrup urine disease Severe infantile form	Valine, leucine, isoleucine, alloisoleucine	Branched chain keto acids in great excess; urine has odor of maple syrup	
Intermittent form	Same	Ketoaciduria and urine odor present only during attacks	
Hypervalinemia	Valine		
Homocystinuria	Methionine; homocystine slightly increased	Homocystine in great excess in urine	Blood cystine low; vascular accidents, Marfan-like syndrome, osteoporosis
Tryptophanemia	Tryptophan	Decreased excretion of kynurenin after tryptophan load	
Hyperlysinemia	Lysine	Ornithine, gamma-aminobutyric acid, and ethanolamine in excess	
Congenital lysine intolerance	Lysine, arginine		Ammonia intoxication
Tyrosinosis	Tyrosine; methionine may be markedly increased	p-Hydroxyphenylpyruvic, acetic, and lactic acids; methionine may be prominent	Generalized aminoaciduria, renal glycosuria, renal rickets, cirrhosis; Fanconi's syndrome

Cystathioninuria	Cystathionine slightly increased	Cystathionine (may be > 1 gm/day)	Congenital acidosis, thrombocytopenia, pituitary gland abnormalities
Hyperglycinemia Severe infantile	Glycine (other amino acids may be elevated)	Acetone	May have ammonia intoxication, ketosis, neutropenia, and osteoporosis
With hypo-oxaluria	Glycine	Decreased oxalate excretion	
Argininosuccinic aciduria	Argininosuccinic acid ($\leqq 4$ mg/dl)	Argininosuccinic acid (2.5–9.0 gm/day)	Ammonia intoxication
Citrullinemia	Citrulline		Liver disease, ammonia intoxication; may have low BUN
Ornithinemia	Ornithine	Ornithine may be normal	Ammonia intoxication
Histidinemia	Histidine (alanine may also be increased)	Alanine may be increased; imidazolepyruvic, acetic, and lactic acids	Urocanic acid absent in sweat and urine after oral histidine load
Carnosinuria		Carnosine (20–100 mg/day)	
Hyper-beta-alaninemia	Beta-alanine, gamma-aminobutyric acid (GABA)	Beta-aminoisobutyric acid, GABA and taurine in excess	Beta-alanine and GABA increased in CSF
Hyperprolinemia Type I	Proline	Hydroxyproline, glycine elevated	May have hereditary nephritis
Type II	Proline	Δ^1-Pyrroline-5-carboxylate, hydroxyproline, glycine elevated	No nephritis

Table 28-6. (continued)

Disease	Increased Blood Amino Acids	Urine Abnormalities*	Other Laboratory Findings
Hydroxyprolinemia	Hydroxyproline	No excretion of Δ^1-pyrroline-3-hydroxy-5-carboxylate or gamma-hydroxyglutamic acid after hydroxyproline load	
Hypophosphatasia	Phosphoethanolamine slightly elevated ($\cong 0.4$ mg/dl)	Phosphoethanolamine ($\geqq 150$ mg/day)	Bone disease

*In addition to overflow aminoaciduria:

Mental retardation is often present in these patients.

For proper interpretation of aminoaciduria, avoid all drugs and medications for 3–4 days (unless immediate diagnosis is required), since they may cause renal tubular damage with aminoaciduria or may produce confusing spots on chromatograms. Use fresh urine specimens without urinary tract infection or else amino acid pattern may be abnormal. Since aminoaciduria may occur with various acute illnesses, repeat amino acid chromatogram after recovery from acute illness to avoid misdiagnosis.

Some aminoacidurias may not be clinically significant (e.g., newborn aminoaciduria, glycinuria, beta-aminoisobutyric aciduria).

Source: Data from M. D. Efron and M. G. Ampola, The aminoacidurias. *Pediatr. Clin. North Am.* 14:881, 1967.

weeks (but reversed in 24 hours after ascorbic acid administration) and increased urine tyrosine and tyrosine derivatives.

Similar blood and urine findings not reversed by administration of ascorbic acid may occur in untreated galactosemia, tyrosinemia, congenital cirrhosis, and giant-cell hepatitis; jaundice occurs frequently.

Serum serotonin (5-hydroxytryptophan) is decreased.

Urine 5-HIAA excretion is decreased.

MAPLE SYRUP URINE DISEASE (KETOACIDURIA)
(metabolic block in degradation of ketoacids of branched chain amino acids)

Urine has maple syrup odor

Chromatography of urine shows greatly increased urinary excretion of ketoacids of leucine, isoleucine, and valine.

The disease may be severe or intermittent.

HOMOCYSTINURIA

This is an inborn error of methionine metabolism with deficient cystathionine synthetase in liver and brain with inability to change homocystine to cystathionine.

Urine excretion of homocystine is increased (positive nitroprusside screening test).

Level of homocystine and methionine is increased in serum and also increased in CSF.

Laboratory findings due to associated clinical conditions (e.g., mental retardation, Marfan's syndrome, osteoporosis, thromboembolic accidents, mild variable hepatocellular dysfunction) are noted.

TYROSINOSIS

There is increased urinary excretion of p-hydroxyphenylpyruvic acid (due to deficiency of p-hydroxyphenylpyruvic oxidase) (chromatography of urine). *Also increased in myasthenia gravis, liver disease, ascorbic acid deficiency, malignancies.*

Acetic and lactic acids and methionine may be increased in urine.

Increased blood tyrosine; methionine may be markedly increased.

Laboratory findings due to Fanconi's syndrome and hepatic cirrhosis are noted.

CYSTATHIONINURIA
(rare disorder of intermediate metabolism of methionine)

Increased cystathionine in urine

HYPERGLYCINEMIA

Long-chain ketosis (without hypoglycemia) and ketonuria accentuated by leucine ingestion

Neutropenia

Thrombocytopenia

Hypogammaglobulinemia

Increased glycine in blood and urine

Osteoporosis

ARGININOSUCCINIC ACIDURIA

Argininosuccinic acid is increased in urine; may also be increased in blood and CSF.

Serum alkaline phosphatase may be increased.

Table 28-7. Summary of Renal Transport Aminoacidurias (blood amino acids normal or low)

Disease	Amino Acids Increased in Urine
Oasthouse urine disease (methionine malabsorption syndrome)	Methionine (may not be much increased on normal diet but is on high-methionine diet); smaller amounts of valine, leucine, isoleucine, tyrosine, and phenylalanine
Hartnup disease	Neutral (monoamine, monocarboxylic) amino acids; basic amino acids, methionine, proline, hydroxyproline, and glycine normal or only slightly increased
Glycinuria (may be harmless; may be heterozygous for benign prolinuria; may be associated with many conditions)	Glycine
Severe prolinuria (Joseph's syndrome)	Proline, hydroxyproline, and glycine in great excess ($\leqq 3$ gm/day proline)
Benign prolinuria	Proline, hydroxyproline, and glycine ($\leqq 600$ mg/day proline)
Cystine-lysinuria Type I (renal calculi) Type II Type III	Cystine and dibasic amino acids
Isolated cystinuria (familial hypoparathyroidism—incidental?)	Cystine

Source: Data from M. D. Efron and M. G. Ampola, The aminoacidurias. *Pediatr. Clin. North Am.* 14:881, 1967.

Fasting blood ammonia is normal but may be markedly increased after eating.

Heterozygous carriers show increased argininosuccinic acid in urine and decreased argininosuccinase in RBCs.

CITRULLINEMIA
(rare condition of metabolic block in citrulline utilization and associated mental retardation)

Increased citrulline in blood and also CSF and urine

Laboratory findings due to liver disease

HISTIDINEMIA
(rare inherited disorder)

Blood histidine is increased.

Histidine, imidazole acetic, imidazole lactic, and imidazole pyruvic acids are increased in urine; alanine may be increased.

Urine may show positive Phenistix test because of imidazole pyruvic acid.
With oral histidine load, no FIGLU appears in urine.

HYPERPROLINEMIA
Increased proline in blood
Increased glycine and hydroxyproline in urine

HYDROXYPROLINEMIA
Increased hydroxyproline in blood

OASTHOUSE URINE DISEASE
(distinctive odor of urine)
Increase of various amino acids in blood and also in urine (e.g., phenylalanine, tyrosine, methionine, valine, leucine, isoleucine)

HARTNUP DISEASE
(hereditary abnormality of tryptophan metabolism)
Urine chromatography shows greatly increased amounts of indolacetic acid, alpha-N (indole-3-acetyl) glutamine, and tryptophan.

JOSEPH'S SYNDROME (SEVERE PROLINURIA)
Urine shows marked increase in proline, hydroxyproline, and glycine.
Heterozygotes may show mild prolinuria.

BENIGN PROLINURIA
Increased proline, hydroxyproline, and glycine appear in urine.
Heterozygotes may show glycinuria but not prolinuria.
Prolinuria may occur in association with various diseases; may be harmless.

CYSTINURIA
(failure of renal tubular reabsorption and of intestinal uptake of cystine and dibasic amino acids)
Increased cystine in urine (20–30 times normal)
Increased urinary arginine, lysine, and ornithine
Cystine renal stones

BETA-AMINOISOBUTYRIC ACIDURIA
(familial recessive disorder of thymine metabolism)
Increased beta-aminoisobutyric acid in urine (50–200 mg/24 hours)

May also occur in leukemia due to increased breakdown of nucleic acids.

FAMILIAL IMINOGLYCINURIA
(inherited autosomal defect of renal transport; may be associated with mental retardation)
Increased urine glycine
Increased urine imino acids (proline, hydroxyproline)

METHYLMALONIC ACIDURIA
(very rare inborn error of metabolism with neonatal metabolic acidosis and mental and somatic retardation)
Metabolic acidosis
Increased methylmalonic acid in urine and blood

Long-chain ketonuria
Intermittent hyperglycinemia
All findings accentuated by high-protein diet or supplemental ingestion of valine or isoleucine
Neutropenia
Possibly, thrombocytopenia

Methylmalonic aciduria also occurs in vitamin B_{12} deficiency.

FAMILIAL LECITHIN–CHOLESTEROL ACYLTRANSFERASE DEFICIENCY
(rare genetic disorder of adults)
Anemia with large RBCs that are frequently target cells
Proteinuria
Serum cholesterol level normal but cholesterol esters virtually absent

PRIMARY OXALOSIS
(rare familial disease)
Increased serum and urinary oxalic acid
Increased urinary glycolic and glyoxylic acid
Calcium oxalate renal calculi and nephrocalcinosis with extrarenal deposition of calcium oxalate
Uremia causes death.
Manifestations of hyperoxaluria are the same, but extrarenal calcium oxalate deposits are absent.

L-GLYCERIC ACIDURIA
(genetic variant of primary hyperoxaluria; autosomal trait that causes disease only when homozygous)
Renal calculi composed of calcium oxalate
Increased urinary oxalic acid (3–5 times normal)
L-Glyceric acid in urine (not found in normal urine)

CYSTINOSIS
Children
    Renal Fanconi's syndrome
        Phosphaturia
        Decreased serum phosphorus
        Decreased serum calcium (usually normal)
        Decreased serum potassium due to high urine potassium
        Hyperchloremic acidosis *(Renal calcinosis develops in renal tubular acidosis but not in cystinosis.)*
        Generalized aminoaciduria (similar to that seen in lead and other heavy-metal poisoning, Wilson's disease, and vitamin D deficiency)
        Glycosuria with normal blood sugar; frequently ketonemia and ketonuria
        Vitamin D–resistant rickets *(In vitamin D–resistant rickets of primary hypophosphatemia, there is no aminoaciduria; severe rickets develops before azotemia appears.)*
        (Renal hypophosphatemia, aminoaciduria, and glycosuria begin at age 6 months.)

Polyuria with low specific gravity; proteinuria sometimes present

Progressive loss of glomerular function with increasing azotemia and death from uremia, usually before age 10

Cystine crystals in bone marrow and in tissues (especially reticuloendothelial system)

Serum uric acid sometimes decreased

Adults (benign disease)

Urinary tract calculi

Cystinuria (cystine crystals in urine; > 200 mg of cystine in 24-hour urine)

SECONDARY AMINOACIDURIA

Severe liver disease

Renal tubular damage due to

Lysol

Heavy metals

Maleic acid

Burns

Galactosemia

Wilson's disease

Scurvy

Rickets

Fanconi's syndrome (e.g., outdated tetracycline, multiple myeloma, inherited)

Neoplasm

Cystathionine excretion in neuroblastoma of adrenal gland; ethanolamine excretion in primary hepatoma

GALACTOSEMIA

(inherited defect of galactose-1-phosphate uridyl transferase in liver and in RBCs that converts galactose to glucose; therefore accumulation of galactose-1-phosphate)

Jaundice (onset at age 4–10 days)

Liver biopsy—dilated canaliculus filled with bile pigment with surrounding rosette of liver cells

Galactosuria—detected by nonspecific reducing tests; identified by chromatography

General ammoaciduria—identified by chromatography

Proteinuria

Galactosemia (equal to total reducing sugar minus glucose-oxidase sugar)

Serum glucose—*apparently* elevated in fasting state but falls as galactose increases; development of hypoglycemia possible

Galactose tolerance test—positive but is unnecessary for diagnosis and may be hazardous because of induced hypoglycemia and hypokalemia

Lack of RBC galactose-1-phosphate uridyl transferase

CONGENITAL FRUCTOSE INTOLERANCE

This is a severe familial genetic disease of infancy due to defect involving fructose-1-phosphoaldolase and fructose-1,6-diphospho-aldolase; it resembles galactosemia.

Fructose in urine of 100–300 mg/dl gives a positive test for reducing substances (Benedict's reagent, Clinitest) but not with glucose-oxidase methods (Clinistix, Tes-Tape). Identify fructose by paper chromatography.

Aminoaciduria and proteinuria may be present.

Fructose tolerance test shows prolonged elevation of blood fructose and marked decrease in serum glucose. Serum phosphorus shows rapid prolonged decrease.

Hypoglycemia with convulsions and coma follows ingestion of fructose.

Increased serum bilirubin and cirrhosis may occur.

BENIGN FRUCTOSURIA

This is a benign asymptomatic disorder due to fructokinase deficiency.

Large amount of fructose in urine gives a positive test for reducing substances (Benedict's reagent, Clinitest) but not with glucose-oxidase methods (Clinistix, Tes-Tape).

Identify fructose by paper chromatography.

Fructose tolerance test shows that blood fructose increases to 4 times more than in normal persons, blood glucose increases only slightly, and serum phosphorus does not change.

ALKAPTONURIA

Recessive inherited absence of liver homogentisic acid oxidase causes excretion of homogentisic acid in urine.

Urine becomes brown-black on standing and reduces Benedict's solution and Fehling's solution, but glucose-oxidase methods are negative.

Ferric chloride test is positive.

An oral dose of homogentisic acid is largely recovered in the urine of affected patients but not in normal persons.

SUCROSURIA

Urine specific gravity is very high ($\leqq 1.07$).

Urine tests for reducing substances are negative.

Sucrosuria may follow IV administration of sucrose or the purposeful addition of cane sugar to urine.

PENTOSURIA

Pentosuria is due to a block in oxidation of glucuronic acid; the patient can metabolize only the sixth carbon, excreting the 5-carbon fraction as pentose.

Urinary excretion of L-xylulose is increased (1–4 gm/day), and the increase is accentuated by administration of glucuronic acid and glucuronogenic drugs (e.g., aminopyrine, antipyrine, menthol).

Differential Diagnosis

Alimentary pentosuria—arabinose or xylose excreted after ingestion of large amount of certain fruits (e.g., plums, cherries, grapes)

Healthy normal persons—small amounts of D-ribose in urine

Healthy normal persons—trace amounts of ribulose in urine

Muscular dystrophy—small amounts of D-ribose in urine (some patients)

MANNOHEPTULOSURIA
Mannoheptulose in urine after the eating of avocados occurs in some persons; not clinically important.

INTESTINAL DEFICIENCY OF SUGAR-SPLITTING ENZYMES (MILK ALLERGY; MILK INTOLERANCE; CONGENITAL FAMILIAL LACTOSE INTOLERANCE; LACTASE DEFICIENCY; DISACCHARIDASE DEFICIENCY)
Familial disease that often begins in infancy with diarrhea, vomiting, failure to thrive, malabsorption, etc.; patient becomes asymptomatic when lactose is removed from diet.

Oral lactose tolerance test shows a rise in blood sugar < 20 mg/dl in blood drawn at 15, 30, 60, 90 minutes (usual dose = 50 gm).

In diabetics, blood sugar may increase > 20 mg/dl despite impaired lactose absorption. Test may also be influenced by impaired gastric emptying or small bowel transit.

If test is positive, repeat using glucose and galactose (usually 25 gm each) instead of lactose; subnormal rise indicates a mucosal absorptive defect; normal increase (>25 gm/dl) indicates lactase deficiency only.

Biopsy of small intestine mucosa shows low level of lactose in homogenized tissue. Is used to assess other diagnostic tests but is seldom required except to exclude secondary lactase deficiency with histologic studies.

Hydrogen breath test (measured by gas chromatography) is noninvasive, rapid, simple, sensitive, quantitative. Patient expires into a breath-collecting apparatus; complete absorption causes no increase of H_2 formed in colon to be excreted in breath. Malabsorption causes H_2 production by fermentation in colon that is proportional to amount of test dose not absorbed. False-negative test in $\cong$ 20% of patients due to absence of H_2-producing bacteria in colon or prior antibiotic therapy.

After ingestion of milk or 50–100 gm of lactose, stools have a pH of 4.5–6.0 (normal pH is > 7.0) and are sour and frothy. Fecal studies are of limited value in adults.

Lactose in urine amounts to 100–2000 mg/dl. It produces a positive test for reducing sugars (Benedict's reagent, Clinitest) but a negative test with glucose-oxidase methods (Tes-Tape, Clinistix).

CLASSIFICATION OF PORPHYRIAS
Congenital Erythropoietic Porphyria
Very rare, autosomal recessive, probably due to decreased activity of uroporphyrinogen III cosynthetase in RBCs. Usual onset in infancy, extreme cutaneous photosensitivity with mutilation, red urine and teeth with ultraviolet fluorescence of urine, teeth, and bones.

Normocytic, normochromic, anicteric hemolytic anemia that tends to be mild; may be associated with hypersplenism.

Urine—marked increase of uroporphyrin is characteristic; coproporphyrin shows lesser increase. Excretion of porphobilinogen and delta-aminolevulinic acid is normal.

Stool—marked increase of porphyrins, especially coproporphyrins

RBCs and plasma—marked increase of uroporphyrins

Porphyria Cutanea Tarda

Most common porphyrin disorder. Autosomal dominant deficiency of hepatic and RBC uroporphyrinogen decarboxylase. Associated with alcoholic liver disease and hepatic siderosis. Skin changes and photosensitivity are present. Acquired form may be due to hepatoma, cirrhosis, chemicals (an epidemic in Turkey was caused by contamination of wheat by hexachlorobenzene).

Laboratory findings of underlying liver disease

Liver biopsy shows morphologic changes of underlying disease and fluorescence under ultraviolet light.

Serum iron and transferrin saturation are often increased.

Urine—marked increase of uroporphyrin with only slight increase of coproporphyrin and ratio of uroporphyrin-coproporphyrin > 7.5.

Stool—slight increase of coproporphyrin

Erythropoietic Protoporphyria

Relatively common type of porphyria due to autosomal dominant deficiency of heme synthetase activity in bone marrow, reticulocytes, liver, and other cells

Mild anemia with slight hypochromia is common.

Laboratory findings due to liver disease and gallstones may be found.

Urine—porphyrins within normal limits

RBCs—marked increase of free protoporphyrin in symptomatic patients (may also be increased in iron deficiency anemia and lead poisoning in Zn chelate form but nonchelated in protoporphyria). May be normal or slightly increased in asymptomatic carriers. Examination of dilute blood by fluorescent microscopy may show rapidly fading fluorescence in variable part of RBCs.

Stool—protoporphyrin is usually increased in symptomatic patients and in some carriers even when carrier RBC porphyrins are normal.

Acute Intermittent Porphyria

Most frequent and severe form of porphyria in U.S. Is autosomal dominant deficiency of uroporphyrinogen I synthetase in RBCs, liver, and other cells. Adult onset with episodes of abdominal pain, neurologic, and mental symptoms that may be precipitated by certain drugs (especially barbiturates, alcohol, and sulfonamides), infection, starvation, and certain steroids; no photosensitivity.

Urine may be of normal color when fresh and become brown, red, or black on standing.

Urine—marked increase of porphobilinogen and, to a lesser extent, of delta-aminolevulinic acid; these decrease during remission but are rarely normal. Coproporphyrin and uroporphyrin may be increased.

Stool—protoporphyrin and coproporphyrin are usually normal.

During acute attack, there may be slight leukocytosis, decreased serum sodium, chloride, and magnesium, and increased BUN.

Liver function tests are normal except for BSP retention.

Other frequent laboratory abnormalities are increased serum cholesterol, hyperbetalipoproteinemia (Type IIa), increased serum iron, abnormal glucose tolerance, increased T-4, and TBG without hyperthyroidism.

Variegate Porphyria

Autosomal dominant condition probably due to deficiency of protoporphyrinogen oxidase causes episodes of abdominal pain and neuropsychiatric symptoms that cannot be distinguished from acute intermittent porphyria but are almost always precipitated by a drug. Skin changes of excessive mechanical fragility of sun-exposed areas.

Stool—characteristic change is marked increase of protoporphyrin and coproporphyrin, which is found during attack, remission, or only with skin manifestations.

Urine—marked increase of delta-aminolevulinic acid and porphobilinogen during an acute attack, which are usually normal after acute episode or with only skin manifestations (in contrast to acute intermittent porphyria).

Hereditary Coproporphyria

Autosomal dominant deficiency of coproporphyrinogen oxidase in WBC, liver, and other cells. Two-thirds of patients are latent. Acute attacks resemble acute intermittent and variegate porphyrias and may be precipitated by drugs (e.g., barbiturates, sedatives, anticonvulsants); skin photosensitivity may occur.

Stool—coproporphyrin is always increased; very markedly during an acute attack. Protoporphyrin is normal or only slightly increased.

Urine—coproporphyrin is markedly increased and is usually normal during remission.

RBC, but not plasma, protoporphyrins are also increased in iron deficiency anemia and lead intoxication. Screening tests using fluorescence microscopy of RBCs or Wood's lamp viewing of treated whole blood may also be positive in iron deficiency anemia, lead intoxication, and other dyserythropoietic states.

GENETIC MUCOPOLYSACCHARIDOSES

Mucopolysaccharide Type	Mucopolysaccharide Excreted in Urine
I (Hurler's syndrome)	Chondroitin sulfate B and heparitin sulfate
II (Hunter's syndrome)	Chondroitin sulfate B and heparitin sulfate
III (Sanfilippo's syndrome)	Heparitin sulfate
IV (Morquio-Ullrich syndrome)	Keratosulfate
V (Scheie's syndrome)	Chondroitin sulfate B
VI (Maroteaux-Lamy syndrome)	Chondroitin sulfate B
VII (I-cell disease)	Chondroitin sulfate B and heparitin sulfate
VIII (Lipomucopolysaccharidoses)	Keratosulfate and heparitin sulfate

All mucopolysaccharide diseases show metachromatically staining inclusions of mucopolysaccharides in circulating polynuclear leukocytes (Reilly granulations) or lymphocytes, cells of inflammatory exudate, and bone marrow cells (most consistently in clasmatocytes). Mucopolysaccharide is also deposited in various parenchymal cells.

Table 28-8. Comparison of Porphyrias

	Enzyme Deficiency	Mode of Inheritance	Usual Age (yr) of Onset	RBC			Feces			Urine			
				Uroporphyrin	Coproporphyrin	Protoporphyrin	Uroporphyrin	Coproporphyrin	Protoporphyrin	δ-aminolevulinic acid	Porphobilinogen	Uroporphyrin	Coproporphyrin
Hepatic													
Acute intermittent porphyria	Uroporphyrinogen I synthetase	AD	Puberty to 30	N	N	N	N	N	N	+[a]	++[a]	++[a]	+[a]
Variegate porphyria	Protoporphyrinogen oxidase	AD	<30	N	N	N	N	(+)	+	++[a]	++[a]	++[a,c]	++[a]
Hereditary coproporphyria	Coproporphyrinogen oxidase	AD	<10	N	N	N	N	(++)[b]	N	+[a]	±[a]	+[a,d]	++[a]
Porphyria cutanea tarda	Uroporphyrinogen decarboxylase	AD[e]	>40	N	N	N	±	±[b]	N	N	N	++[c]	±

			Congenital										
Erythropoietic Congenital porphyria	AR	Uroporphyrinogen III cosynthetase		N	(+)	+	+	N	N	++	N	N	++	+
Protoporphyria	AD	Heme synthetase	<6	N	(+)	N	N	+	++	+	N	N	N	N
Coproporphyria	AD	Coproporphyrinogen oxidase	<10	+	±	+	N	N	N	+	N	N	N	N

Circle = the significant test in differential diagnosis, AR = autosomal recessive, AD = autosomal dominant, N = normal, + = increased, ± = slightly increased, ++ = marked increase.

a During acute attack; may be absent during remission.

b Fecal protoporphyrin > coproporphyrin in variegate porphyria, but fecal protoporphyrin < coproporphyrin in cutanea tarda.

c Urine uroporphyrin:coproporphyrin < 1 in variegate porphyria and > 7.5 in cutanea tarda.

d In hereditary coproporphyria, urine coproporphyrin is greater than uroporphyrin.

e Some cases are chemically induced without genetic predisposition.

Excess production of porphyrins is associated with cutaneous photosensitivity.
Excess production of only porphyrin precursors is associated with neurologic symptoms.
Excess production of both is associated with both types of clinical symptoms.

In a recent report of 106 patients with variegate porphyria, 25 also showed a porphyrin excretory pattern of porphyria cutanea tarda. (Day, R. S., et al. Coexistent variegate porphyria and porphyria cutanea tarda. *N. Engl. J. Med.* 307:36–41, 1982.)

GENETIC DISEASES OF MUCOPOLYSACCHARIDE METABOLISM

Morquio-Ullrich syndrome

Excess excretion of keratosulfate in urine associated with aortic valvular disease, osteochondrodystrophy, and cloudy cornea

Scheie's syndrome

Excess excretion of chondroitin sulfate B in urine associated with aortic valve disease (usually regurgitation) and cloudy cornea

Hurler's syndrome (gargoylism)

Excess excretion of chondroitin sulfate B and mucopolysaccharide in urine Alder-Reilly anomaly—azurophil granules in cytoplasm of myeloid cells (occasionally lymphocytes and monocytes)

Fibrosis of heart valves with functional changes

VON GIERKE'S DISEASE (TYPE I GLYCOGEN STORAGE DISEASE; GLUCOSE-6-PHOSPHATASE DEFICIENCY)

May appear in first days or weeks of life.

After overnight fast, hypoglycemia, increased blood lactate, and pyruvate with metabolic acidosis, ketonemia, and ketonuria. (Recurrent acidosis is commonest cause for hospital readmission.)

Blood glucose is markedly decreased.

Blood triglycerides, cholesterol, and serum free fatty acids are markedly increased.

Mild anemia is present.

There is increased serum uric acid (due to depressed renal tubular function by increased blood lactic acid) causing clinical gout.

Table 28-9. Classification of Glycogenoses (Glycogen Storage Diseases [GSD])

Frequency of Types (GSD%)	Type	Clinical Name	Enzyme Defect
20	I	Classic von Gierke's disease	Deficiency of liver glucose 6-phosphatase
20	II	Pompe's disease	Defect in lysosomal alpha-1,4-glucosidase
30	III	Forbes' disease (debrancher deficiency, limit dextrinosis)	Deficiency of amylo-1,6-glucosidase (debranching enzyme)
< 1	IV	Andersen's disease (brancher deficiency, amylopectinosis)	Absence of amylo-(1,4 → 1,6)-transglucosidase (branching enzyme)
5	V	McArdle's disease of muscle	Absence of muscle phosphorylase
25	VI		Deficiency of liver phosphorylase
	VII		Deficiency of muscle phosphofructokinase

Serum phosphorus and alkaline phosphatase are decreased.

Urine glucose is increased.

Urinary nonspecific amino acids are increased, without increase in blood amino acids.

Other renal function tests are relatively normal.

Liver function tests (other than related to carbohydrate metabolism) are relatively normal.

Glucose tolerance may be normal or diabetic type; diabetic type is more frequent in older children and adults.

Functional tests

Administer 1 mg of glucagon intravenously after 8-hour fast. A 50–60% increase in blood glucose appears in 10–20 minutes in the normal person. No increase occurs in infants or young children with von Gierke's disease; delayed response may occur in older children and adults.

Administer the galactose or fructose intravenously. No rise in blood glucose occurs in von Gierke's disease, but normal rise occurs in limit dextrinosis (Type III GSD).

Biopsy of liver

Histology is not diagnostic; shows vacuolization of hepatic cells and abundant glycogen granules. Confirm with Best's stain.

Biochemical studies

Glycogen content > 4% by weight.

Glucose-6-phosphatase is absent or markedly decreased.

Glycogen is biochemically normal.

Other enzymes (other GSD) are present in normal amounts.

Biopsy of jejunum

Intestinal glucose-6-phosphatase is decreased or absent.

Biopsy of muscle shows no abnormality of enzyme activity or glycogen content.

Type IB

Shows all the changes of von Gierke's disease except that liver biopsy does not show deficiency of glucose-6-phosphatase.

POMPE'S DISEASE (TYPE II GLYCOGEN STORAGE DISEASE; GENERALIZED GLYCOGENOSIS; ALPHA-GLUCOSIDASE DEFICIENCY GLYCOGENOSIS)

Features of the disease are imbecility, varying neurologic defects, muscle hypotonia, cardiac enlargement, and frequent liver enlargement.

Fasting blood sugar, GTT, glucagon responses, and rises in blood glucose after fructose infusion are normal. No acetonuria is present.

General hematologic findings are normal.

Staining of circulating leukocytes for glycogen shows massive deposition.

Confirm diagnosis by muscle biopsy, specific enzymatic assays, glycogen structure analysis (these are special studies).

TYPE III GLYCOGEN DEPOSITION DISEASE (FORBES' DISEASE; DEBRANCHER DEFICIENCY; LIMIT DEXTRINOSIS)

This is a familial disease with enlarged liver, retarded growth, chemical changes, and benign course.

Serum cholesterol is increased.

Acetone appears in urine.

Fasting hypoglycemia occurs.

There is a diabetic type of glucose tolerance curve with associated glucosuria.

Infusions of galactose and fructose cause a normal hyperglycemic response.

Fasting blood sugar does not show expected rise after administration of subcutaneous glucagon or epinephrine but does increase 2 hours after high-carbohydrate meal.

Confirm diagnosis by biochemical findings of increased liver glycogen, abnormal glycogen structure, absence of detectable amylol, 6-glucosidase activity with normal phosphorylase and glucose-6-phosphatase. RBC glycogen is often increased.

Serum uric acid is normal or slightly increased.

TYPE IV GLYCOGEN DEPOSITION DISEASE (ANDERSEN'S DISEASE; BRANCHER DEFICIENCY; AMYLOPECTINOSIS)

This extremely rare fatal condition is due to absence of amylo-(1,4 → 1.6)-transglucosidase.

Liver function tests may be altered (e.g., slight increase in bilirubin, reversed A/G ratio, increased SGOT, decreased serum cholesterol).

There may be a flat blood glucose response to epinephrine and glucagon.

There may be increased WBC and decreased hemoglobin.

Biopsy of liver may show a cirrhotic reaction to the presence of polysaccharide of abnormal structure, which stains with Best's carmine and periodic acid–Schiff stain but has a very low glycogen content.

TYPE V GLYCOGEN DEPOSITION DISEASE (MCARDLE SYNDROME; MCARDLE-SCHMID-PEARSON DISEASE; MYOPHOSPHORYLASE DEFICIENCY)

This is a familial autosomal recessive disease showing very limited ischemic muscle exercise tolerance in the presence of normal appearance of muscle.

Epinephrine or glucagon causes a normal hyperglycemic response.

Biopsy of muscle is microscopically normal in young; vacuolation and necrosis are seen in later years. Increased glycogen is present. Absence of phosphorylase is demonstrated by various techniques.

Following exercise that quickly causes muscle cramping and weakness, the regional blood lactate and pyruvate does not increase (in a normal person it increases 2–5 times). Similar abnormal response occurs in Type III involving muscle and in Types VII, VIII, X.

Myoglobulinuria may occur after strenuous exercise.

TYPE VI GLYCOGEN STORAGE DISEASE (HEPATIC PHOSPHORYLASE DEFICIENCY)

Enlarged liver present from birth is associated with hypoglycemia.

Hypoglycemia is mild to moderate.

Serum cholesterol and lactic acid are mildly increased.

Serum uric acid is moderately increased.

Liver function tests are normal, except for mobilization of glycogen.

Fructose tolerance is normal.

Response to glucagon and epinephrine is variable but tends to be poor.

Leukocyte phosphorylase activity is decreased, but muscle phosphorylase is normal. Liver phosphorylase is decreased.

TYPE VII GLYCOGEN STORAGE DISEASE (MUSCLE PHOSPHOFRUCTOKINASE DEFICIENCY)

Fasting hypoglycemia is marked.

Other members of family may have reduced tolerance to glucose.

RBCs show 50% decrease in phosphofructokinase activity.

Biopsy of muscle shows marked decrease (1–3% of normal) in phosphofructokinase activity.

TYPE O GLYCOGEN STORAGE DISEASE

This is a very rare condition.

Blood glucose is markedly decreased, causing hypoglycemic seizures and mental retardation.

Glucagon administration causes no increase in blood glucose (see von Gierke's disease, p. 442), but ingestion of food causes a rise in 2–3 hours.

Biopsy of liver shows marked decrease in glycogen synthetase.

FAMILIAL PAROXYSMAL PERITONITIS (FAMILIAL MEDITERRANEAN FEVER; "PERIODIC DISEASE")

WBC is increased (10,000–20,000/cu mm), and there may be increased eosinophils during an attack but a return to normal between attacks.

ESR is increased during an attack but normal between attacks.

Mild normocytic normochromic anemia is occasionally seen.

Serum glycoprotein is increased in patients and their relatives.

Increased alpha$_2$ globulin and fibrinogen are common.

Amyloidosis develops in 10–40% of patients; it is not related to frequency or severity of clinical attacks.

Etiocholanolone is increased in urine and blood during attacks in a few patients.

FAMILIAL DYSAUTONOMIA (RILEY-DAY SYNDROME)

This condition is due to an autosomal recessive trait occurring in Ashkenazi Jews, who show difficulty in swallowing, corneal ulcerations, insensitivity to pain, motor incoordination, excessive sweating, diminished gag reflex, lack of tongue papillae, progressive kyphoscoliosis, pulmonary infections, etc.

Urine vanillylmandelic acid (VMA) (3-methoxy-4-hydroxymandelic acid) may be low, and homovanillic acid (HVA) increased.

In asymptomatic carriers, urine VMA may be lower than in healthy adults.

BATTEN'S DISEASE (BATTEN-SPIELMEYER-VOGT DISEASE)

(autosomal recessive type of juvenile amaurotic idiocy)

Azurophilic hypergranulation of leukocytes occurs in patients and in heterozygous and homozygous members of their families. In Giemsa- and Wright-stained smears, it resembles toxic granulation but differs by the absence of supravital staining in Batten's disease and by normal leukocyte alkaline phosphatase activity

Table 28-10. Classification of Gangliosidoses

Clinical Name	Enzyme Defect	Major Lipid Accumulation	Signs and Symptoms
Gaucher's disease	Beta-glucosidase	Glucocerebroside	Spleen and liver enlargement Erosion of long bones and pelvis Mental retardation only in infantile form
Niemann-Pick disease	Sphingomyelinase	Sphingomyelin	Liver and spleen enlargement Mental retardation About 30% with red spot in retina
Krabbe's disease (globoid leukodystrophy)	Beta-galactosidase	Galactocerebroside	Mental retardation Almost total absence of myelin Globoid bodies in white matter of brain Increased CSF protein (150–300 mg/dl)
Metachromatic leukodystrophy	Arylsulfatase A	Sulfatide	Mental retardation Psychological disturbances in adult form Nerves stain yellow-brown with cresyl violet dye CSF normal or increased CSF protein ($\leqq$ 200 mg/dl) (see p. 294)

Disease	Enzyme deficiency	Accumulating substance	Symptoms
Ceramide lactoside lipidosis	Beta-galactosidase	Ceramide lactoside	Slowly progressing brain damage Liver and spleen enlargement
Fabry's disease	Alpha-galactosidase	Ceramide trihexoside	Reddish-purple skin rash Kidney failure Pain in lower extremities
Tay-Sachs disease	Hexosaminidase A	Ganglioside GM_2	Mental retardation Red spot in retina Blindness Muscular weakness
Tay-Sachs variant (Sandhoff's disease)	Hexosaminidase A and B	Globoside (and ganglioside GM_2)	Same as Tay-Sachs disease but progresses more rapidly
Generalized gangliosidosis	Beta-galactosidase	Ganglioside GM_1	Mental retardation Liver enlargement Skeletal deformities About 50% with red spot in retina
Fucosidosis	Alpha-fucosidase	H-isoantigen	Cerebral degeneration Muscle spasticity Thick skin

(markedly increased in toxic granulation). This granulation occurs in $\geq$ 15% of neutrophils.

GAUCHER'S DISEASE

Gaucher's cells appear in bone marrow aspiration, needle biopsy, or aspiration of spleen, liver, or lymph nodes.

Serum acid phosphatase is increased (if substrate for test is different from that for prostatic acid phosphatase; i.e., use phenyl phosphate or *p*-nitrophenylphosphate instead of glycerophosphate). It may return to normal following splenectomy.

Serum cholesterol and total fats are normal.

Laboratory findings due to involvement of specific organs
> Spleen—hypersplenism occurs with anemia (normocytic normochromic), leukopenia (with relative lymphocytosis; monocytes may be increased), and/or thrombocytopenia.
> Bone—serum alkaline phosphatase may be increased.
> Liver—serum SGOT may be increased.
> Spinal fluid—GOT may be increased.

NIEMANN-PICK DISEASE

Foamy histiocytes may be found in bone marrow aspiration and may appear in peripheral blood terminally.

Peripheral blood lymphocytes and monocytes may be vacuolated (2–20% of cells). WBC is variable.

Rectal biopsy may show changes in ganglion cells of myenteric plexus.

Laboratory findings due to involvement of specific organs
> Anemia is due to hypersplenism or microcytic anemia associated with anisocytosis, poikilocytosis, and elliptocytosis.
> SGOT may be increased in serum and spinal fluid.
> Enzyme changes in CSF are same as in Tay-Sachs disease, except that LDH is normal (see next section).

Acid phosphatase is increased (same as in Gaucher's disease—see preceding section).

Serum aldolase is increased.

LDH is normal in serum and CSF.

HISTIOCYTOSIS X

Letterer-Siwe Disease

Bone marrow aspiration or biopsy of lymph node may show characteristic histiocytes and histologic changes.

Progressive normocytic normochromic anemia is present.

Hemorrhagic manifestations (thrombocytopenia) occur.

Hand-Schüller-Christian Disease

Diabetes insipidus may occur.

Histologic examination of skin, bone, etc., is diagnostic.

Anemia, leukopenia, thrombocytopenia may or may not be present.

Eosinophilic Granuloma

Biopsy of bone is diagnostic.

Blood is normal; eosinophilia is unusual.

Development of leukopenia and thrombocytopenia suggests poorest prognosis.

DOWN'S SYNDROME (TRISOMY 21; MONGOLISM)

Karyotyping shows 47 chromosomes with trisomy 21 in most patients (see p. 195).

Increased leukocyte alkaline phosphatase staining reaction

Leukocytes show decreased incidence of drumsticks (see p. 194) and mean lobe counts.

Serum acid phosphatase may be decreased.

Incidence of leukemia is increased.

D_1 TRISOMY (TRISOMY 13)

In peripheral blood smears, most of the neutrophilic leukocytes show an increased number of anomalous nuclear projections compared to those of normal persons. The nuclear lobulation may appear abnormal (nucleus may look twisted without clear separation of individual lobes, coarse lumpy chromatin, etc.).

Fetal hemoglobin may persist longer than normal (i.e., be increased).

Endocrine Diseases

HYPERTHYROIDISM

Serum triiodothyronine (T-3) concentration on radioimmunoassay (RIA) and resin uptake are increased in 65–85% of patients.

Serum total thyroxine (T-4) and free thyroxine are increased. With a typical clinical picture of hyperthyroidism, serum T-4 > 16 μg/dl confirms the diagnosis.

Free thyroxine index (FTI) (serum T-4 concentration by RIA times T-3 resin uptake) is the best initial screening test, since it is not affected by alterations in thyroxine-binding protein sites. Is increased in about 90% of hyperthyroid patients.

Serum thyroxine-binding globulin (TBG) is normal.

Radioactive iodine uptake (RAIU) is increased. It is relatively more affected at 1, 2, or 6 hours than at 24 hours. It may be normal with recent iodine ingestion. RAIU is no longer useful for diagnosis of hyperthyroidism but should be performed prior to administration of therapeutic dose of ^{131}I.

Salivary excretion and urinary excretion of RAI are increased.

Iodine tolerance test shows increased utilization of iodine.

Serum cholesterol is decreased, and total lipids are usually decreased.

Glucose tolerance is decreased with early high peak and early fall. Hyperglycemia and glycosuria are present.

Liver function tests show impairment.

Creatine excretion in urine and creatine tolerance are increased. Normal serum creatine almost excludes hyperthyroidism.

Urinary and fecal excretion of calcium are increased.

Serum total and ionized calcium is increased in > 10% of patients. Serum phosphorus is normal. Parathormone level is not increased.

Unusual laboratory manifestations of hyperthyroidism include increased alkaline phosphatase, hypoproteinemia, malabsorption, anemia.

Thyroid suppression test: T-3 administration decreases RAIU in normal persons but not in hyperthyroid persons. Is largely replaced by TRH stimulation test (see pp. 83–85).

Serum TSH is decreased in all forms of thyrotoxicosis except the very rare cases of pituitary neoplasms that secrete TSH; therefore, routine measurement of TSH is not indicated in overt thyrotoxicosis. TRH administration does not cause a significant rise in serum TSH in hyperthyroid patients as it does in normal persons; a normal rise (> 2 μU/ml) virtually excludes hyperthyroidism (see p. 83). This test may be indicated in the following situations:

Hyperthyroid patients in whom associated nonthyroid conditions result in only slight elevation of serum T-4 and T-3.

Euthyroid Graves' disease presenting with only exophthalmos (unilateral or bilateral). *TRH stimulation test may sometimes be normal in these patients, and T-3 suppression test may be required.*

Elderly patients with or without symptoms of hyperthyroidism may have serum T-4 and T-3 in upper normal range.

Euthyroid sick syndrome (see p. 453)—generally serum TSG is normal with a relatively normal TSH response to TRH.

T-3 toxicosis—causes 5% of cases of hyperthyroidism

Should be suspected in patients with clinical thyrotoxicosis in whom usual laboratory tests are normal (serum T-4, FTI, 24-hour RAI, TBG, and thyroxine-binding albumin [TBPA]), but serum T-3 is increased.

RAIU is autonomous (not suppressed by T-3 administration).

Abnormal TRH test

Factitious hyperthyroidism—self-induced hyperthyroidism by ingestion of thyroxine (T-4) or Cytomel (T-3).

Increased serum T-4 or T-3, depending on which drug is ingested

RAIU is low when all other thyroid function tests indicate hyperthyroidism.

Augmented RAIU after TSH administration, whereas patients with subacute and painless thyroiditis usually do not have any response to TSH administration.

Serum thyroglobulin is depressed to low-normal level or undetectable (therefore may be useful to distinguish from early or recovery phases of subacute thyroiditis, in which it is increased).

Normal serum T-4 levels may be found in hyperthyroid patients with

T-3 thyrotoxicosis

Factitious hyperthyroidism due to T-3 (Cytomel)

Decreased binding capacity due to hypoproteinemia or ingestion of certain drugs (e.g., phenytoin, salicylates)

Increased serum T-4 levels may be found in euthyroid patients with increased serum TBG (see pp. 80–81).

Thyroid Storm

Thyroid function test values may be somewhat higher than in uncomplicated thyrotoxicosis but are useless for differentiation.

Transient hyperglycemia is common.

Abnormal liver function tests are common.

Mild to moderate hypercalcemia is common.

Abnormal serum electrolytes are common.

Hyperthyroidism With Decreased RAIU (<3%)

Factitious thyrotoxicosis*

Iodine-induced hyperthyroidism (jodbasedow)†,‡

Graves' disease with iodine excess

Subacute thyroiditis

Lymphocytic thyroiditis with spontaneous resolving hyperthyroidism (silent thyroiditis)†

---

*TSH injection causes a normal increase ≥ 50% of RAIU.

†TSH injection does not cause a normal increase ≥ 50% of RAIU.

‡Urinary iodine > 2000 µg/24 hours.

Metastatic functioning thyroid carcinoma*
Struma ovarii*

Hyperthyroidism With Increased RAIU (> 12%)
Graves' disease (diffuse toxic goiter)
Plummer's disease (toxic multinodular goiter)
Toxic adenoma (uninodular goiter)
TSH-producing pituitary tumor (TSH > 4 μU/ml)
Hyperthyroidism and chronic lymphocytic thyroiditis (see pp. 458–459)
Trophoblastic tumor
Thyrotropin-producing neoplasms (e.g., choriocarcinoma, hydatidiform mole, embryonal carcinoma of testis)

HYPOTHYROIDISM
Serum T-4 and free thyroxine concentration are decreased. T-4 > 7 μg/dl almost certainly excludes hypothyroidism.
Serum T-3 concentration (RIA) is decreased (may be normal in ≅ 20% of hypothyroid patients), and serum T-3 resin uptake is decreased (may be normal in ≦ 50% of hypothyroid patients). *Thus serum T-4 is a better test for diagnosis of hypothyroidism than T-3.*
Free thyroxine index is increased.
Serum T-3/T-4 ratio is increased.
Serum TBG is normal.
RAIU is usually decreased and is not helpful in diagnosis.
Salivary excretion and urinary excretion of RAI are decreased.
Iodine tolerance test shows decreased utilization of iodine.
Serum cholesterol is increased (may be useful to follow effect of therapy, especially in children).
Glucose tolerance is increased (oral GTT is flat; IV GTT is normal); fasting blood sugar is decreased.
Serum calcium is sometimes increased.
Serum alkaline phosphatase is decreased.
Serum LDH, SGOT, CK are increased in 40–90% of cases.
Serum carotene is increased.
Normocytic normochromic anemia is present.
Serum iron and total iron-binding capacity (TIBC) may be decreased.
Serum sodium is decreased in approximately 50% of cases.
CSF protein may be increased.
Luteinizing hormone (LH) may be decreased, and urine 17-ketosteroids (17-KS) and 17-hydroxyketosteroids (17-OHKS) may be increased.
Proteinuria is seen in about 8% of cases.
Laboratory findings indicative of pernicious anemia and primary adrenocortical insufficiency occur with increased frequency in primary hypothyroidism.
Serum myoglobin is significantly increased in 90% of untreated, long-term hypothyroid patients; inversely proportional to serum T-3 and T-4. Gradual decrease after T-4 therapy begins with return to normal before TSH becomes normal.
Serum TSH is increased in proportion to degree of hypofunction; is at least 2 times and often 10 times normal value. A single determination is usually sufficient to establish the diagnosis.

*TSH injection causes a normal increase ≧ 50% of RAIU.

Since increased serum TSH is earliest evidence of hypothyroidism, it should be measured to document subclinical hypothyroidism and begin early therapy in patients with Graves' disease treated with RAI or surgery or with chronic thyroiditis.

TSH is especially useful in cases where T-4 and FTI are not diagnostic; the TSH is generally considered essential to confirm the diagnosis of hypothyroidism.

Serum TSH should always be measured prior to treatment in all patients with hypothyroidism to distinguish primary from secondary or tertiary types, since the latter two are often associated with secondary adrenal insufficiency, which could be lethal if unrecognized.

Administration of TRH causes a greater increase in serum TSH in primary than in pituitary hypothyroidism (see pp. 83–85 and Table 29-3, p. 458).

TSH stimulation (20 units/day for 3 days) increases RAIU to $\cong$ normal (20%) in pituitary but not in primary hypothyroidism. Diagnosis of primary hypothyroidism is unlikely if RAIU increases substantially after administration of TSH.

Myxedema coma—hypoglycemia, hyponatremia and findings due to adrenocortical insufficiency may be found.

CSF protein is elevated (100–340 mg/dl) in 25% of cases of myxedema.

Levothyroxine is now considered the treatment of choice, since adequate replacement results in normal serum T-4 and T-3 concentrations. When hypothyroidism is due to thyroid failure, the dose of levothyroxine is gradually increased, and the adequacy of therapy is determined when serum T-4 increases to normal and TSH decreases to normal range. TSH response to TRH also returns to normal if originally abnormal, but this test is generally not necessary. When hypothyroidism is secondary or tertiary, serum T-4 is used to judge adequacy of therapy, as the TSH is not useful.

When levothyroxine is used for TSH suppression in patients with thyroid cancer, nodular disease, or chronic thyroiditis, the decreased TSH cannot be distinguished from normal levels; therefore levothyroxine dose is increased until serum T-4 is normal and TSH is undetectable, or an abbreviated TRH test is performed with a single TSH measurement 15 minutes after injection of TRH—if TSH is undetectable, then TSH secretion is considered adequately suppressed.

Thyroid hormone status should be reassessed at least yearly in treatment of hypothyroidism.

EUTHYROID SICK SYNDROME (LOW T-3 SYNDROME, LOW T-4 SYNDROME)*
(wide variety of nonthyroidal acute and chronic conditions such as infection, liver disease, cancer, starvation, renal failure, heart failure, severe burns, trauma, surgery may be associated with abnormal thyroid function tests in euthyroid patients)

Low T-3 syndrome is the most common.

Decreased serum T-3 with increased reversed T-3 (rT-3)

*Source: J. E. Morley, M. F. Slag, K. K. Elson, and R. B. Shafer, The interpretation of thyroid function tests in hospitalized patients. *J.A.M.A.* 249:2377–2379, 1983; and M. Blum, Thyroid function and disease in the elderly. *Hosp. Pract.,* Oct. 1981, p. 105.

With progressive illness, tendency is for fall in total T-4 and T-4 binding globulin with increase of free T-4. Thus T-3 uptake increases, and FTI (T-7) tends to remain normal.

Serum TSH is typically normal, as is TSH response to TRH.

Increased T-4 syndrome is most common in acute psychiatric admissions (20%), especially in the presence of certain drugs (e.g., amphetamines, phencyclidine); increased values tend to decrease during first 2 weeks after admission as patient improves. Is rarer in acutely ill patients (e.g., acute hepatitis).

Increased serum T-4, FTI (T-7), and T-3

TRH test is often not useful due to flat TSH response commonly seen in melancholia patients.

See Table 29-1, Differential Diagnosis of Euthyroid Sick Syndrome

2% of hospitalized elderly patients have unsuspected hyperthyroidism, and another 2% have unsuspected hypothyroidism; 0.5% of psychiatric hospital admissions have unsuspected hypothyroidism. In addition, thyroid function tests can be affected by the common use of diuretics and low-salt diet (causing iodine deficiency and spurious increase of RAIU) and by many factors that change protein binding of thyroid hormone (see p. 82, Serum Thyroxine-

Table 29-1. Differential Diagnosis of Euthyroid Sick Syndrome

	Euthyroid Sick Syndrome	Primary Hypothyroidism	Primary Hypothyroidism with Concomitant Illness
Serum T-4	N or D	D	D
Serum T-3 uptake	I	D	
Serum T-3	D	N or D	D
T-7 (FTI)	I, N, or D	D	D
Reverse T-3	I	D	D, N, or I
Serum TSH	N	I	I, occasionally N
TSH response to TRH	N or D	I	I

N = normal; D = decreased; I = increased.

Definitely increased T-3 uptake associated with decreased serum T-4 strongly indicates euthyroid sick syndrome, whereas in hypothyroidism T-3 uptake tends to be decreased.

In hypothyroidism with concomitant illness, T-3 uptake tends to increase into normal range but not above normal.

Serum TSH is increased in primary hypothyroidism as the earliest and most specific test; in contrast, basal and TRH-stimulated TSH are typically normal in euthyroid sick syndrome.

Reverse T-3 may be a useful discriminator in many euthyroid sick patients without renal failure, but it is not as useful as serum TSH.

Pituitary hypothyroidism may be difficult to distinguish, since serum TSH is low and not responsive to TRH, which is a common pattern in euthyroid sick patients.

Table 29-2. Thyroid Function Tests in Various Conditions

Disease	Total Serum Thyroxine (T-4)	Serum T-3 (concentration)	Serum T-3 Uptake	Free Thyroxine ("normalized") (FTI, T-7)	Serum Thyroxine-Binding Globulin (TBG)	Radioactive Iodine Uptake (RAIU)	Serum TSH	TRH Test
Hypothyroidism	D	D	D	D	N or I	D	I[a]	A[b]
Euthyroid sick (low T-3) syndrome	N or D	D	I	I, N, or D	N	N	N	N or D
Hyperthyroidism	I	I	I	I	N	I	D	A
T-3 thyrotoxicosis	N	I	N or slightly I	N	N	N or I	D	A
Administration of Thyroxine (factitious hyperthyroidism)[c]	I	V	I	I	N	D	D	A
Inorganic iodine	N	N	N	N	N	D	N	A
Radiopaque contrast media[d]	N	N	N	N	N	D	N	

Table 29-2. (continued)

Disease	Total Serum Thyroxine (T-4)	Serum T-3 (concentration)	Serum T-3 Uptake	Free Thyroxine ("normalized") (FTI, T-7)	Serum Thyroxine-Binding Globulin (TBG)	Radioactive Iodine Uptake (RAIU)	Serum TSH	TRH Test
Estrogen and antiovulatory drugs	I	I	D	N	I	I	N	N
Testosterone	D	D	I	N	D	D	N	N
ACTH and corticosteroids	D	N or D	I	N	D	D	N or D	N
Dilantin or large doses of salicylates	D	D	I	N	D		N	N
Pregnancy	I	I	D	N	I	X	N	N
With hyperthyroidism	I	I	N	I	I	X	N	A

With hypothyroidism	D	D or N	D	D	I	X	I	A
Hereditary increase of TBG in euthyroid state	I	I	D	N	I	I	N	N
Hereditary decrease of TBG in euthyroid state	D	D	I	N	D	D	N	N
Granulomatous thyroiditis	V or I	V or D	V or I	V or I	N	D	V or I	
Adenomatous thyroid goiter	N	N	N	N	N	N	N	
Thyroid neoplasm (nonfunctional)	N	N	N	N	N	N	N	
Nephrosis[e]	D	D	I	N	D	May be I	N	

N = normal; D = decreased; I = increased; A = abnormal; X = contraindicated in pregnancy; V = variable.

[a] Increased serum TSH is diagnostic of primary hypothyroidism; TSH is decreased in secondary and tertiary hypothyroidism.

[b] TRH stimulation test is normal in euthyroid state, increased response in primary hypothyroidism, blunted or no response in pituitary hypothyroidism, delayed response in hypothalamic etiology.

[c] RAIU is decreased when all other thyroid function tests indicate hyperfunction.

[d] Invalidates RAIU results.

[e] Thyroid function tests are altered due to loss of TBG in urine.

Table 29-3. Laboratory Tests in Differential Diagnosis of Primary and Secondary Hypothyroidism

Test	Panhypopituitarism	Primary Myxedema
Serum TSH	Decreased	Increased
Serum TSH response to TRH administration	Absent	Normal or exaggerated
Response to administration of thyrotropic hormone	Responds with increase in RAIU	No response
Urine 17-ketosteroids	Absent	Low
Response to insulin	Prompt decrease in blood sugar; fails to return to normal	Usually delayed fall in blood sugar and sometimes delayed return to normal

Binding Globulin). These are not included in euthyroid sick syndrome.

No single test is clearly diagnostic, especially in elderly and acutely or severely ill patients.

THYROID FUNCTION DURING PREGNANCY
RAIU is contraindicated.

In hyperthyroidism, both serum T-3 uptake and T-4 are increased, but in the pregnant euthyroid patient or euthyroid patient taking birth control pills or estrogens, the T-4 is increased and the T-3 uptake is decreased. Hyperthyroidism may be indicated by the failure of the T-3 uptake to decrease during pregnancy.

T-3 uptake gradually decreases (as early as 3–6 weeks after conception) until the end of the first trimester and then remains relatively constant. It returns to normal 12–13 weeks postpartum. Failure to decrease by the eighth to tenth week of pregnancy may indicate threatened abortion (one should know the patient's normal nonpregnant level).

ACUTE STREPTOCOCCAL THYROIDITIS
WBC and polynuclear leukocytes are increased.

ESR is increased.

The 24-hour RAIU is usually decreased but sometimes is normal.

HASHIMOTO'S THYROIDITIS (CHRONIC LYMPHOCYTIC THYROIDITIS)
Thyroid function may be normal; occasionally a patient passes through a hyperthyroid stage. 15–20% of patients develop hypothyroidism, but Hashimoto's disease is a very unlikely cause of hypothyroidism in the absence of thyroglobulin and microsome antibodies.

Antithyroglobulin (tanned RBCs) and antimicrosomal antibodies are found in 60–70% of these cases. Antithyroglobulin titers are usually quite high. (See Thyroid Antibody Tests, pp. 85–86.)

Serum TSH is increased in one-third of persons who are clinically euthyroid and in those with clinical hypothyroidism, many of whom have normal T-4, T-3, and T-7.

Iodide-perchlorate discharge test exceeding 10% of gland radio-iodine (abnormal) in 60–80% of cases

RAIU may be higher than expected in hypothyroidism.

Radioiodine scan may show involvement of only a single lobe (more common in younger patients).

Response to TSH distinguishes primary and secondary hypothyroidism. If thyroid uptake for each lobe is measured separately after TSH, a difference between the lobes may demonstrate lobar thyroiditis when total uptake is apparently normal.

Laboratory findings of hypothyroidism, when present (see pp. 452–453 and Table 29-3, p. 458), are noted.

Biopsy of thyroid may be performed.

SILENT THYROIDITIS (LYMPHOCYTIC THYROIDITIS WITH SPONTANEOUSLY RESOLVING HYPERTHYROIDISM)

This is a form of hyperthyroidism described recently that now composes up to 25% of all cases of hyperthyroidism; hyperthyroidism resolves spontaneously in several weeks to months and is often followed by a transient hypothyroidism during recovery period; common in postpartum period; multiple episodes may occur. Pathologic changes are less severe than in Hashimoto's thyroiditis, but the latter cannot be ruled out in biopsy specimens.

Hyperthyroid phase

Increased serum T-4, T-3, T-3 resin uptake, FTI (T-7). Become normal in 10 days with prednisone therapy.

RAIU is very low (<3%); not increased after TSH administration.

Serum TSH is low with complete suppression of TSH response to TRH.

Urine iodide level is 2–5 times higher than normal (due to leakage of iodinated material from thyroid).

Antithyroglobulin antibodies (tanned RBCs) are increased in about 25% of patients (positive in all patients if use more sensitive RIA method); antimicrosomal antibodies are increased in about 60% of patients. Titers usually between 1:100 and 1:250,000 and rarely in the very high ranges of Hashimoto's thyroiditis.

ESR increased in 50% of patients to range of 20–40 mm/hour.

CBC and serum proteins are normal.

Recovery phase

Serum T-4 and T-3 fall into normal range, but RAIU and TSH response to TRH remain suppressed.

Hypothyroid phase (occurs in 20–30% of patients)

Antithyroid antibody titers are highest during this phase (especially in postpartum patients). Gradually decrease with time; 50% become negative within 6 months.

Serum T-4 and T-3 gradually return to normal.

RAIU, serum TSH, TRH test begin to normalize toward the end of this phase, and urinary iodide falls to normal levels (50–200 μg/day).

DE QUERVAIN'S THYROIDITIS (SUBACUTE THYROIDITIS)
(probably of viral origin)
RAIU is decreased; may be zero in early stages. It is not increased by TSH administration during active phase. It may be > 50% for several weeks after recovery.

ESR is increased.

WBC is normal or decreased.

Biopsy of thyroid confirms diagnosis.

Antithyroglobulin antibodies (tanned RBCs) may be present for up to several months at levels of about 1:320), but the titer is never as high as in Hashimoto's thyroiditis. The level falls with recovery.

Serum T-3 and T-4 may be increased if thyroiditis is extensive.

Thyroid scan may show decreased uptake in involved areas.

RIEDEL'S CHRONIC THYROIDITIS
Biopsy of thyroid confirms diagnosis.

Some patients may have laboratory findings of hypothyroidism.

SIMPLE NONTOXIC DIFFUSE GOITER
No specific laboratory findings.

SINGLE OR MULTIPLE NODULAR GOITERS
Isotope scanning of thyroid may show decreased ("cold") or increased ("hot") uptake.

Functioning solitary adenoma may produce hyperthyroidism.

In multinodular goiter, TSH level is rarely increased; usually is normal or low-normal range.

Fine-needle aspiration biopsy will produce a definitive diagnosis in 85% of cases of thyroid nodules.

CARCINOMA OF THYROID
Serum T-3, T-4, TSH are almost always normal in untreated patients. Rarely, evidence of hyperthyroidism may be found with large masses of follicular carcinoma.

Basal serum calcitonin may be increased in patients with medullary carcinoma of the thyroid even when there is no palpable mass in the thyroid. Calcium infusion and/or pentagastrin injection are used as provocative tests in patients with normal basal levels in whom there is a high index of suspicion of medullary carcinoma of thyroid; normally should not rise above 0.2 ng/ml (see Serum Calcitonin, p. 94). Serum calcitonin levels are also useful to detect incomplete removal, recurrence, or presence of metastases in medullary thyroid carcinoma.

Serum thyroglobulin levels are increased in most patients with differentiated thyroid carcinoma but not in undifferentiated or medullary carcinoma. May not be increased with small occult differentiated carcinoma. May be useful to detect presence and possibly the extent of residual, recurrent, or metastatic differentiated carcinoma. *Increased levels may be found in patients with nontoxic nodular goiter; presence of autoantibodies interferes with the test.* (See Serum Thyroglobulin, p. 95.)

Serum carcinoembryonic antigen (CEA) may be increased in medullary carcinoma and may correlate with tumor size or extent of disease.

Laboratory findings due to associated lesions (e.g., pheochromocytoma and parathyroid tumors) (*10–20% of cases of medullary carcinoma of thyroid occur as an inherited familial disease as part of multiple endocrine neoplasia [MEN]* [see pp. 513–514]) and to production of additional substances (e.g., ACTH, serotonin, histaminase) by medullary carcinoma.

RAIU is almost always normal.

Radioactive scan of thyroid (see p. 86)

Needle biopsy of thyroid nodule

PRIMARY HYPERPARATHYROIDISM

Due to parathyroid adenoma in 80% of cases, hyperplasia in 15%, and parathyroid carcinoma in < 5% of cases; no test can differentiate these.

Serum calcium is increased. Repeated determinations may be required to demonstrate increased levels. Rapid decrease after excision of adenoma may cause tetany during next few weeks, especially when serum alkaline phosphatase is increased. Drug-induced hypercalcemia should be reevaluated after discontinuation for 1–2 months; cessation of thiazides may unmask primary hyperparathyroidism.

Serum total protein and albumin must always be measured simultaneously, as marked decrease may cause a decrease in calcium.

Normal calcium level may occur with coexistence of conditions that decrease serum calcium level (e.g., high-phosphate intake, malabsorption, acute pancreatitis, nephrosis, infarction of parathyroid adenoma); also beware of laboratory error as a cause of "normal" serum calcium.

High-phosphate intake can abolish increased serum and urine calcium and decreased serum phosphorus; low-phosphate diet unmasks these changes.

Serum phosphorus is decreased (< 3 mg/dl). It may be normal in the presence of high-phosphorus intake or renal damage with secondary phosphate retention. It may be normal in one-half of patients, even without uremia. Low serum phosphorus supports the diagnosis of primary hyperparathyroidism, an increased level supports the diagnosis of nonparathyroid hypercalcemia, but a normal level is not useful.

Serum alkaline phosphatase is normal in 50% of patients with primary hyperparathyroidism and only slightly increased in the rest; infrequently is markedly increased in the presence of bone disease. There is a slow decrease to normal after excision of adenoma. Increase > 2 times upper limit of normal favors hypercalcemia of malignancy rather than hyperparathyroidism.

Urine calcium is increased (> 400 mg on a normal diet; 180 mg on a low-calcium diet). Urine calcium increase is found in only 70% of patients with hyperparathyroidism. Urine calcium excretion is often > 500 mg/24 hours in malignancy, sarcoidosis, hyperthyroidism. Is < 50–100 mg/24 hours in benign familial hypocalciuric hypercalcemia.

Urine phosphorus is increased unless there is renal insufficiency or phosphate depletion (especially due to commonly used antacids containing aluminum). Phosphate loading unmasks the increased urine phosphorus of hyperparathyroidism.

Polyuria is present, with low specific gravity.

Serum chloride is increased (> 102 mEq/L; < 99 mEq/L in other

Table 29-4. Laboratory Findings in Various Diseases of Calcium and Phosphorus Metabolism[a]

Disease	Serum Calcium[b]	Serum Phosphorus	Serum Alkaline Phosphatase	Urine Calcium[c]	Urine Phosphorus
Hyperparathyroidism[d]	I (>11 mg/dl in 90%)	D (<3 mg/dl in 90%)	I (N if no bone disease)	I	I
Hypoparathyroidism	D	I	N	D	D[e]
Pseudohypoparathyroidism	D	I	N; occasionally D	D	D[e]
Pseudopseudohypoparathyroidism	N	N	N	N	N
Secondary hyperparathyroidism (renal rickets)	V	I	I or N	D or I	D
Vitamin D excess	I	I or D	N or I	I	I
Rickets and osteomalacia	D or N	D or N	I	D	D
Osteoporosis	N	N	N	N or I	N
Polyostotic fibrous dysplasia	N	N	N or I	N	N

Paget's disease	N	N or I	I	N or I	I
Metastatic neoplasm to bone	N or I	V	N or I	V	I
Multiple myeloma	N or I	V	N or I	N or I	N or I
Sarcoidosis	N or I	N or I	N or I	I	N
Fanconi's syndrome or renal loss of fixed base	D or N	D	N or I	I	I
Histiocytosis X (Letterer-Siwe, Hand-Schüller-Christian, eosinophilic granuloma)	N	N	N or I	N or I	N
Hypercalcemia and excess intake of alkali (Burnett's syndrome)	I	I or N	N	N	N
Solitary bone cyst	N	N	N	N	N

N = normal; D = decreased; I = increased; V = variable.

[a] See Serum Parathyroid Hormone, p. 90.

[b] Serum calcium. Repeated determinations may be required to demonstrate abnormalities. Serum total protein level should always be known. See also response to corticoids on p. 102.

[c] Urine calcium. Patient should be on a low-calcium diet (e.g., Bauer-Aub).

[d] See Table 29-5, p. 467.

[e] See Ellsworth-Howard Test, p. 102.

types of hypercalcemia). Hyperparathyroidism patients tend toward hyperchloremic (nonanion gap) acidosis, whereas other hypercalcemic patients tend toward alkalosis. Chloride-phosphorus ratio > 33 supports the diagnosis of hyperparathyroidism and < 30 contradicts this diagnosis.

Cortisone suppression test (e.g., administer hydrocortisone 40 mg 3 times daily for 10 days, then withdraw slowly for 5 days; measure serum calcium at 5, 8, and 10 days). Positive suppression test is fall of corrected serum calcium > 1.0 mg/dl.

>   Test is positive in 77% of nonparathyroid causes of hypercalcemia (e.g., sarcoidosis, vitamin D intoxication, metastatic carcinoma, multiple myeloma) and in 50% of cases of hyperparathyroidism with osteitis fibrosa.

>   Test is negative in hyperparathyroidism without osteitis fibrosa (77% of cases) and in familial benign hypercalcemia.

Serum alpha$_2$ and beta$_1$ globulins are slightly increased but return to normal after parathyroidectomy. *Serum protein electrophoresis should always be performed in hyperparathyroidism to rule out multiple myeloma and sarcoidosis.*

Uric acid is increased in $> 15\%$ of patients. Uric acid level is not affected by cure of hyperparathyroidism, but a postoperative gout attack may occur.

Increased hydroxyproline in serum and urine may occur with bone disease but is not as useful as serum alkaline phosphatase for detection of bone disease.

Increased ESR is infrequent in hyperparathyroidism (may be due to infection or moderate renal insufficiency). Marked increase occurs in multiple myeloma.

Indirect studies of parathyroid function (e.g., phosphate deprivation, calcium infusion, tubular reabsorption of phosphate) are often borderline, and interpretation is difficult with any significant degree of renal insufficiency (see pp. 102–103).

Serum parathyroid hormone (PTH) level is elevated. Must always be measured concurrently with serum calcium, since PTH level in the upper normal range may be inappropriately high in relation to a distinctly increased calcium level, which is consistent with hyperparathyroidism. PTH level > 2 times upper limit of normal is almost always due to primary hyperparathyroidism. Failure to detect PTH in the presence of simultaneous hypercalcemia militates against the diagnosis of primary hyperparathyroidism and surgical exploration of the parathyroid glands. In general, nonparathyroid disease causing hypercalcemia (e.g., sarcoidosis, vitamin D intoxication, hyperthyroidism, milk-alkali syndrome, most malignancies) will have a low or suppressed PTH value. (See Fig. 29-1.)

>   *PTH C-terminal fragment is not the biologically active one but is more sensitive index of hyperparathyroidism than the active N-terminal fragment; normal ranges vary depending on which fragment is being measured. Lithium-induced hypercalcemia resembles that of familial hypocalciuric hypercalcemia in that both show increased PTH levels and low urine calcium concentrations.*

Serum 1,25-hydroxyvitamin D may be elevated in primary hyperparathyroidism and in sarcoidosis. Serum 25-hydroxyvitamin D may be useful to establish vitamin D intoxication, especially in factitious cases.

Urinary cyclic AMP (adenosine monophosphate) may be high in primary hyperparathyroidism but low in vitamin D intoxication and sarcoidosis. May also be increased in many cases of malignancy but not usually increased in multiple myeloma or other hematologic malignancies. Is not increased in hypercalcemia induced by PTH. An elevated level that falls to normal range within 6 hours after surgery is said to provide functional confirmation of successful parathyroidectomy.

Hyperparathyroidism must always be ruled out in the presence of

Renal colic and stones or calcification (2–3% have hyperparathyroidism) (see Table 30-5, p. 543)

Peptic ulcer (occurs in 15% of patients with hyperparathyroidism)

Calcific keratitis

Bone changes (present in 20% of patients with hyperparathyroidism)

Jaw tumors

Clinical syndrome of hypercalcemia (nocturia, hyposthenuria, polyuria, abdominal pain, adynamic ileus, constipation, nausea, vomiting) *(present in 20% of patients with hyperparathyroidism; only clue to diagnosis in 10% of patients with hyperparathyroidism)*

Multiple endocrine neoplasia (e.g., islet cell tumor of pancreas, pituitary tumor, pheochromocytoma (see pp. 513–514)

Relatives of patients with hyperparathyroidism or "asymptomatic" hypercalcemia

Mental aberrations

A changing clinical spectrum of hyperparathyroidism has resulted from earlier detection of hypercalcemia by multiphasic screening.

50% of cases are asymptomatic (most show only mild elevation of calcium).

20% of cases have renal stones.

6% of cases show osteitis fibrosa cystica.

15% of cases have peptic ulcer.

"Asymptomatic" hypercalcemia is detected by routine multiphasic screening in 1–2% of tests.

21–38% of hospitalized patients had no documented clinical cause found for hypercalcemia.

Malignancy caused one-third to two-thirds of hospitalized cases in different series.

Hyperparathyroidism caused 15–50% of cases in different series.

SECONDARY HYPERPARATHYROIDISM

This is a diffuse hyperplasia of parathyroid glands usually secondary to chronic advanced renal disease.

Laboratory findings due to underlying causative disease are noted.

Classic findings in renal osteodystrophy are

Serum calcium is low or normal.

Serum phosphorus is increased.

Serum alkaline phosphatase is increased.

These levels can also be used to monitor response to treatment with calcitriol or alphacalcidiol.

Serum parathormone level is increased.

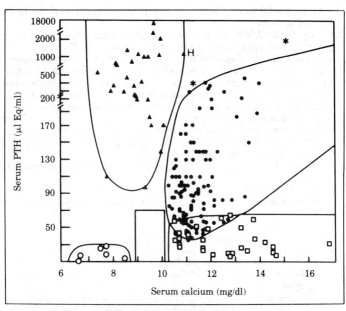

Fig. 29-1. Distribution of patients according to serum calcium and serum PTH. The values of patients with primary hyperparathyroidism are indicated by ●, with malignancies by □, with renal failure by ▲, with parathyroid carcinoma by *, with hypoparathyroidism by ○, and hypernephroma by H. The empty rectangle represents the normal range. (From *Mayo Medical Laboratories Test Catalog, 1984*. Rochester, MN: Mayo Medical Laboratories, 1984.)

Table 29-5. Comparison of Types of Excess Parathormone Production

Laboratory Tests	Ectopic Parathyroid Hormone Production	Primary Hyperparathyroidism
Cause	Epidermoid or large cell carcinoma of bronchus, hypernephroma of kidney, cancer of ovary, colon	Primary hyperplasia, adenoma, carcinoma of parathyroids
Serum calcium	Very high: >14 mg/dl in 75% of patients Suppressed by cortisone in 25–50% of patients	Moderately high: >14 mg/dl in 25% of patients Rarely suppressed by cortisone
Serum chloride	Low: <99 mEq/L	High: >102 mEq/L
Serum chloride-phosphorus ratio	<30	>33
Serum bicarbonate	Often increased	Normal or low

Table 29-5. (continued)

Laboratory Tests	Ectopic Parathyroid Hormone Production	Primary Hyperparathyroidism
Serum alkaline phosphatase	Increased in 50% of patients, even when bone x-rays are negative	Seldom increased unless bone disease is present
Serum phosphorus	Normal or low	Normal or low
Urine calcium	Often >400 mg/24 hours	Usually <400 mg/24 hours
Serum parathormone	Increased but less than in primary hyperparathyroidism for the calcium level	Increased
Nephrolithiasis and x-ray changes in bone	Absent	Common
Anemia and other findings due to malignancy	Present*	Absent

*Many patients with malignancy are at least mildly anemic, normal hemoglobin level may favor the diagnosis of primary hyperparathyroidism rather than cancer.

Patients with malignancy, receiving thiazides, or with other causes of hypercalcemia may have concurrent hyperparathyroidism.

Hypercalcemia occurs in about 20–35% of patients with breast cancer, about 70% of cases of multiple myeloma, about 10–15% of cases of lung cancer, rare in lymphoma and leukemia.

Malignancy-associated hypercalcemia in at least some patients shows increased nephrogenous cAMP (also seen in 90% of cases of primary hyperparathyroidism) but differs by showing strikingly decreased levels of 1,25-vitamin D and markedly increased fractional excretion of urinary calcium.

Multiple tests are necessary in differential diagnosis of hypercalcemia.

Occult cancer should be ruled out as the cause of hypercalcemia in the presence of

Serum alkaline phosphatase > 2 times upper limit of normal

Increased serum phosphorus

Serum chloride-phosphorus ratio < 30:1

Anemia

Serum calcium > 14.5 mg/dl without florid hyperparathyroidism

Hypercalcemia concurrent with absent serum PTH level

Positive cortisone suppression test in absence of osteitis fibrosa

Urine calcium > 500 mg/24 hours

FAMILIAL HYPOCALCIURIC HYPERCALCEMIA (FAMILIAL BENIGN HYPERCALCEMIA)

(rare familial autosomal dominant disorder of chronic lifelong hypercalcemia with onset before age 10 years with low incidence of renal stones, kidney damage, peptic ulcer; no response to parathyroidectomy)

Has many of same biochemical findings as primary hyperparathyroidism, including elevated parathormone level in 20% of cases, but lower than those in typical primary hyperparathyroidism.

Mean rate of calcium excretion in urine is only one-third that in primary hyperparathyroidism.

Urine calcium excretion is decreased despite hypercalcemia.

50–100 mg/24 hours in familial hypocalciuric hypercalcemia

50–150 mg/24 hours in normal persons

Increased (often > 250 mg/24 hours) in two-thirds of patients with hyperparathyroidism

Increased (often > 500 mg/24 hours) in patients with malignancies

Serum magnesium is mildly increased in 50% of patients.

Renal function is maintained with normal creatinine clearance.

Serum 25-hydroxyvitamin D is normal and 1,25-dihydroxyvitamin D is proportional to parathormone level.

Urinary cAMP is increased in about one-third of patients.

MILK-ALKALI (BURNETT'S) SYNDROME

Increased serum calcium without hypercalciuria

Decreased serum phosphorus

Normal serum alkaline phosphatase

Mild alkalosis

Renal insufficiency with azotemia (increased BUN)

Metastatic calcinosis

HYPOPARATHYROIDISM

Serum calcium is decreased (as low as 5 mg/dl). *More than one-third of these patients may present as "epileptics."* Hypoparathyroidism should be ruled out in presence of mental and emotional changes, cataracts, faulty dentition in children, associated changes in skin and nails (e.g., moniliasis is frequent).

Serum phosphorus is increased (usually 5–6 mg/dl; as high as 12 mg/dl).

Serum alkaline phosphatase is normal or slightly decreased.

Urine calcium is decreased (Sulkowitch's test is negative).

Urine phosphorus is decreased. Phosphate clearance is decreased (see p. 102).

Serum parathyroid hormone level is decreased (see p. 90).

Injection of potent parathyroid extract (200 units IV) causes urine phosphorus to increase ≧ 10 times within 3–5 hours. In a normal person the increase in urine phosphorus is 5–6 times. In pseudohypoparathyroidism, the urine phosphorus is not increased > 2 times (see Ellsworth-Howard test, p. 102).

Alkalosis is present.

Congenital form may be associated with thymic aplasia (DiGeorge's syndrome) (see p. 383).

Serum uric acid is increased.

There is a flat oral GTT (due to poor absorption).

CSF is normal, even with mental or emotional symptoms or with calcification of basal ganglia.

PSEUDOHYPOPARATHYROIDISM

Serum calcium, phosphorus, and alkaline phosphatase are the same as in hypoparathyroidism but cannot be corrected by (or they respond poorly to) administration of parathyroid hormone (see reference to Ellsworth-Howard test in the preceding section).

Serum parathyroid hormone level is elevated.

Cyclic AMP excretion in urine increases up to 100 times 2 hours after IV administration of parathormone in primary hypoparathyroidism but much less marked increase in pseudohypoparathyroidism.

PSEUDOPSEUDOHYPOPARATHYROIDISM

Serum and urine calcium, phosphorus, and alkaline phosphatase are normal.

Response to parathyroid hormone is normal.

Clinical anomalies are the same as in pseudohypoparathyroidism.

PRIMARY HYPOPHOSPHATEMIA

This is a familial but occasionally sporadic condition of intrinsic renal tubular defect in phosphate resorption.

Serum phosphorus is always decreased in the untreated patient.

Serum calcium is usually normal.

Serum alkaline phosphatase is often increased.

Bone biopsy shows a characteristic pattern of demineralization around osteocyte lacunae.

HYPOPHOSPHATASIA

This rare genetic disease of bone mineralization with x-ray changes and clinical syndromes is found in infants, children, and adults.

Serum alkaline phosphatase is decreased to $\cong 25\%$ of normal (may vary from $0 \leqq 40\%$ of normal); is not correlated with severity of disease. Due to bone and sometimes liver isoenzymes.

Serum and urine levels of phosphoethanolamine are increased (may be normal in asymptomatic heterozygotes).

Serum calcium is increased in severe cases.

Serum phosphorus is normal.

Treatment with corticosteroids usually causes an increase in serum alkaline phosphatase (but it never attains normal level) with a marked fall in serum calcium; phosphoethanolamine excretion in urine continues high.

PSEUDOHYPOPHOSPHATASIA

(clinical syndrome resembling hypophosphatasia)

Serum alkaline phosphatase is normal.

SYNDROME OF FAMILIAL HYPOCALCEMIA, LATENT TETANY, AND CALCIFICATION OF BASAL GANGLIA

This rare clinical syndrome has features resembling those of pseudohypoparathyroidism, pseudopseudohypoparathyroidism, and basal cell nevus syndrome.

Hypocalcemia is not responsive to parathormone administration.

Parathormone administration produces a phosphate diuresis.

DECREASED TISSUE CALCIUM WITH TETANY

The tetany, associated with normal serum calcium, magnesium, potassium, and CO_2, responds to vitamin D therapy.

Special radioactive calcium studies show decreased tissue calcium pool that returns toward normal with therapy.

VITAMIN D INTOXICATION

Serum calcium may be increased.

Serum phosphorus is usually also increased but sometimes is decreased, with increased urinary phosphorus.

Serum alkaline phosphatase is decreased.
Serum parathormone level is low or undetectable.
Urine calcium excretion is increased.
Renal calcinosis may lead to renal insufficiency and uremia.

MAGNESIUM DEFICIENCY TETANY SYNDROME
Serum magnesium is decreased (usually < 1 mEq/L).
Serum calcium is normal (slightly decreased in some patients)
Blood pH is normal.
Tetany responds to administration of magnesium but not of calcium.

CLASSIFICATION OF DIABETES MELLITUS AND OTHER HYPERGLYCEMIC DISORDERS
(National Diabetes Data Group, 1979)
I and II are idiopathic diabetes mellitus.

  I Insulin-dependent type (IDDM) (formerly called juvenile diabetes or ketosis-prone or brittle diabetes mellitus)—represents 10–20% of diabetic patients
 II Non-insulin-dependent type (NIDDM)—represents 80–90% of diabetic patients
      Not obese NIDDM
        Insulin-treated for hyperglycemia
        Not insulin treated
      Obese NIDDM—represents ≅ 75% of NIDDM
        Insulin-treated for hyperglycemia (formerly called maturity-onset or ketosis-resistant diabetes mellitus)
        Not insulin treated
 III Gestational diabetes (GDM)—see p. 471.
 IV Impaired glucose tolerance (IGT)—replaces terms "latent" or "chemical" diabetes
  V Previous abnormality of glucose tolerance (PrevAGT)—this term recognizes the imperfect reproducibility of the oral GTT.
 VI Potential abnormality of glucose tolerance (PotAGT)—high risk subjects without demonstrable abnormality; replaces terms "prediabetes," "potential diabetes"
VII Glucose intolerance associated with certain conditions and syndromes (e.g., Cushing's syndrome, acromegaly, chronic pancreatitis, hemochromatosis, pheochromocytoma, miscellaneous drugs and chemicals)

See sections on diabetic nephrosclerosis, papillary necrosis, infection of genitourinary tract, lipoproteins, etc.

COMPARISON OF INSULIN-DEPENDENT AND NON-INSULIN-DEPENDENT DIABETES MELLITUS

Insulin-Dependent (IDDM) (formerly called juvenile, brittle, or ketosis-prone diabetes)	**Non-Insulin-Dependent (NIDDM)** (formerly called adult-onset, stable, maturity-onset, diabetes of youth)
Deficiency of insulin production due to beta-cell destruction by antibody or cell-mediated mech-	Possible contributing factors: genetic, environmental, decreased number of beta cells, peripheral insulin resistance

Insulin-Dependent (IDDM)
(formerly called juvenile, brittle, or ketosis-prone diabetes)

Non-Insulin-Dependent (NIDDM)
(formerly called adult-onset, stable, maturity-onset, diabetes of youth)

    anisms or some other unknown cause
Prone to ketosis
Very low serum C-peptide levels

Resistant to ketosis
Normal or increased serum C-peptide levels

GESTATIONAL DIABETES MELLITUS

Hyperglycemia that develops for the first time during pregnancy; most will return to normal glucose tolerance after delivery. Diagnosis is necessary for short-term identification of increased risk of fetal morbidity.

All pregnant women > age 25 years should be screened between 24 and 33 weeks' gestation with serum glucose taken 1 hour after ingestion of 50 gm of glucose. Values < 135 mg/dl are considered normal; > 182 mg/dl are considered definitely abnormal; 135–182 mg/dl are suspicious and indicate a standard 3-hour GTT.

Diagnosis is made if at least two of the following glucose levels are found on oral GTT with 100-gm glucose loading dose:

Fasting	>105 mg/dl
1 hour	>190 mg/dl
2 hours	>165 mg/dl
3 hours	>145 mg/dl

DIABETIC KETOACIDOSIS

Blood glucose is increased (usually > 300 mg/dl)

Plasma acetone is increased (4+ reaction when plasma is diluted 1:1 with water)

    Highly elevated glucose (500–800 mg/dl or more) suggests non-ketotic hyperosmolar hyperglycemia (because glucose levels become very high only when extracellular fluid volume is markedly decreased).

Volume and electrolyte depletion (due to glucose-induced osmotic diuresis)

    Absence of volume depletion should arouse suspicion of other possibilities (e.g., hypoglycemic coma, other causes of coma).

    Very low sodium (120 mEq/L) is usually due to hypertriglyceridemia and hyperosmolality although occasionally may be dilutional due to vomiting and water intake.

Azotemia is present (BUN is usually 25–30 mg/dl); creatinine may be proportionally increased > BUN due to methodologic interference.

Metabolic acidosis (pH < 7.25 and/or bicarbonate < 10 mEq/L). Whole spectrum of patterns from pure hyperchloremic acidosis to wide-anion-gap acidosis. May cause initial serum potassium to be increased.

WBC is increased (often > 20,000/cu mm) even without infection.

Serum amylase may be increased (may originate from salivary glands rather than pancreas) in up to 20% of patients.

Serum osmolality is slightly increased.
Decreased serum phosphate in 10% of cases
Changes due to complications in treatment
    Hypoglycemia
    Hypokalemia
    Alkalosis
    Nonketotic hyperglycemic coma (see p. 47)
        Underlying precipitating medical problem (e.g., myocardial infarction, infection)

See Metabolic Acidosis, pp. 409–412; Lactic Acidosis, pp. 412–413; Hyperosmolar State, pp. 47–48.

Look for precipitating factors, especially infection.

SOME HETEROGENEOUS GENETIC DISEASES ASSOCIATED WITH HYPERGLYCEMIA
Alstrom's syndrome
Ataxia-telangiectasia
Diabetes mellitus
Friedreich's ataxia
Hemochromatosis
Herrmann's syndrome
Hyperlipoproteinemias (three different types)
Isolated growth hormone deficiency
Laurence-Moon-Bardet-Biedl syndrome
Lipoatrophic diabetes
Myotonic dystrophy
Optic atrophy
Prader-Willi syndrome
Refsum's syndrome
Schmidt's syndrome
Werner's syndrome

PRADER-WILLI SYNDROME
This condition is characterized by mental retardation, muscular hypotonia, obesity, short stature, and hypogonadism associated with diabetes mellitus.
Diabetes mellitus frequently develops in childhood and adolescence but is insulin-resistant, responds to oral hypoglycemic drugs, and is not accompanied by acidosis.

CLASSIFICATION OF ISLET CELL TUMORS OF PANCREAS
Insulin-secreting beta-cell tumor (may be benign or malignant, primary or metastatic) produces hyperinsulinism with hypoglycemia (see next section for laboratory findings and differential diagnosis).
Non-insulin-secreting non-beta-cell tumor (benign or malignant, primary or metastatic) may produce several types of syndromes.
    Zollinger-Ellison syndrome (see p. 475)
    Profuse diarrhea with hypokalemia and dehydration
        Profuse diarrhea with hypokalemia (and sometimes periodic paralysis) may occur as a separate syndrome without peptic ulceration. (*Some of the patients have histamine-fast achlorhydria.*) Diabetic glucose tolerance curves may occur in some patients because of chronic

Table 29-6. Differential Diagnosis of Diabetic Coma

Condition	Serum Glucose (mg/dl)	Serum Ketones (undiluted)	Arterial pH	Serum Osmolality (mOsm/kg)	Serum Lactate (mmol/L)	Plasma Insulin
Diabetic ketoacidosis	300–1000	+ + + +	D	300–350	2–3	0–L
Lactic acidosis	100–200	0	D	N–300	≧7	L
Alcoholic ketoacidosis	40–200	+ + + +	D	290–310	2–6	L
Hyperosmolar coma	500–2000	0/+	N	320–400	1–2	Some
Hypoglycemia	10–40	0	N	285 ± 6	Low	I

D = decreased; L = low; N = normal; I = increased; 0 = none; + = small amount; up to + + + + = large amount.
Normal serum lactate = 0.6–1.1 mmol/L.

Lactic acidosis occurs in one-third of patients with diabetic ketoacidosis.

Hyperosmolar coma and alcoholic ketoacidosis may occur in diabetic ketoacidosis.

potassium depletion. May be associated with multiple endocrine adenomas.

Nonspecific diarrhea

Steatorrhea (due to inactivation of pancreatic enzymes by acid pH)

PRIMARY ENDOCRINE-SECRETING TUMORS OF PANCREAS

Cell Type	Hormone Secreted	Tumor
B cell	Insulin	Insulinoma (see below)
D cell	Gastrin	Gastrinoma (see p. 475)
A cell	Glucagon	Glucagonoma (see p. 475)
H cell	Vasoactive intestinal peptide (VIP)	Vipoma (see p. 475)
D cell	Somatostatin	Somatostatinoma (see p. 475)
HPP cell	Human pancreatic polypeptide (HPP)	HPP-secreting tumor (very rare tumor)

Other rare endocrine secreting tumors have been identified as causing ectopic ACTH syndrome, atypical carcinoid syndrome, SIADH, ectopic hypercalcemia syndrome.

INSULINOMA
(tumor of pancreatic islet beta-cell origin; most often benign solitary tumors; occasionally may be part of MEN I, see pp. 513–514)

In patients with fasting hypoglycemia, insulinoma should be considered the cause until another diagnosis can be proved.

Fasting 24–36 hours will provoke hypoglycemia in 80–90% of these patients; 72 hours of fasting will provoke hypoglycemia in > 95% of these patients especially if punctuated with exercise. Low serum glucose and high serum insulin establishes the diagnosis, i.e., insulin level is inappropriately elevated for the degree of hypoglycemia (in normal persons, insulin level becomes < 5 μU/ml or undetectable). Serum C-peptide is similarly inappropriately elevated, in contrast to factitious hypoglycemia. In women, serum glucose during fasting can fall to 20–30 mg/dl and return to normal without treatment; in men, a fall in serum glucose to < 50 mg/dl is considered abnormal.

Serum insulin-glucose ratio > 0.3 when serum glucose > 50 mg/dl indicates inappropriate hyperinsulinism, and this usually indicates insulinoma if factitious hypoglycemia is ruled out.

Serum insulin values are not useful in reactive hypoglycemia but should always be performed in cases of fasting hypoglycemia.

Occasional patients with insulinoma have very low serum insulin levels; their serum shows very high proinsulin level that interferes with the insulin immunoassay giving falsely low values.

Stimulation tests are usually not necessary and may be dangerous if serum glucose < 50 mg/dl.

Tolbutamide tolerance test—see p. 98 and Table 13-8, p. 99.

Glucagon stimulation test: Administer 1 mg of glucagon IV during 1–2 minutes; measure serum insulin 3 times at 5-minute intervals and then twice at 15-minute intervals. Patients with insulinoma show an exaggerated response of serum immuno-reactive insulin. Serum insulin > 100 μU/ml after glucagon stimulation in a patient with fasting hypoglycemia and inappropriate insulin secretion strongly suggests insulinoma.

Infusion of exogenous insulin to reduce serum glucose level will also suppress the secretion of insulin and of C-peptide in normal persons but not in patients with insulinoma. C-peptide level usually remains elevated if insulinoma is present but falls to undetectable level if beta-cell function is normal.

GLUCAGONOMA

Diabetes mellitus

Anemia

Increased serum level of glucagon (difficult laboratory measurement and must also differentiate glucagon-like immunoreactivity, gut glucagon, and pancreatic glucagon). Serum proglucagon is also increased occasionally.

Clinical clue is association of dermatitis (necrolytic migratory erythema) with insulin-requiring diabetes.

Increased serum insulin level is characteristic.

VIPOMA

Voluminous watery diarrhea (6–10 L/day) with dehydration

Hypokalemia that may be associated with hypokalemic nephropathy

Metabolic acidosis

Hypercalcemia in 50% of cases

Abnormal oral GTT

Increased plasma vasoactive intestinal peptide (VIP)

Achlorhydria or hypochlorhydria

This clinical syndrome has also been seen with islet cell hyperplasia, bronchogenic carcinoma, pheochromocytoma, ganglioneuroblastoma.

SOMATOSTATINOMA
(rare condition)

Diabetes mellitus that improves after resection of the tumor

Hypochlorhydria

Steatorrhea

Occasionally anemia is present.

ZOLLINGER-ELLISON SYNDROME (GASTRINOMA)
(see also Serum Gastrin, pp. 93–94)

Increased basal serum gastrin. >500 pg/ml is highly suggestive for gastrinoma in absence of achlorhydria or renal failure. <100 pg/ml is unlikely to be gastrinoma. 100–500 pg/ml occurs in ≅ 40% of gastrinoma patients and ≅ 10% of ulcer patients without gastrinoma. For this indeterminate range, provocative tests should be performed.

IV injection of secretin (1–2 units/kg body weight) will provoke an increase of serum gastrin ≧ 110 pg/ml within 10 minutes. Some ulcer patients may increase serum gastrin ≦ 100 pg/ml. Serum gastrin decreases in most nongastrinoma patients. Negative response occurs in ≅ 5% of gastrinoma patients.

Other provocative tests such as IV injection of calcium gluconate (4 mg of Ca^{2+}/kg) or a standard test meal are not as sensitive or specific as secretin test. Response after calcium infusion is positive if serum gastrin $\geq$ 395 pg/ml.

There is a large volume of highly acid gastric juice in the absence of pyloric obstruction; it is refractory to vagotomy and subtotal gastrectomy* (see Gastric Analysis, pp. 174–175).

Basal acid output > 15 mEq/hour and ratio of basal acid output–maximal output > 0.6 strongly favors gastrinoma, but false positive and false negative results are common. Gastric analysis does not improve the diagnostic ability of the basal serum gastrin and is probably not indicated for diagnosis of gastrinoma in a patient with active ulcer disease.

Hypokalemia is frequently associated with chronic severe diarrhea that may be a clue to this diagnosis.

Steatorrhea occurs rarely.

Serum albumin may be decreased.

Laboratory findings due to peptic ulcer of stomach, duodenum, or proximal jejunum (e.g., perforation, fluid loss, hemorrhage) are noted. *25% of these patients have ulcers in unusual locations or have multiple ulcerations. A tendency toward rapid or severe recurrence of ulcer after adequate therapy is a clue to Zollinger-Ellison syndrome.*

> Gastrinomas are non-beta-cell tumors arising in pancreas.
>
> *Tumors are multiple in 28% of all patients.*
>
> *Adenomas are multiple in 29% of patients and may be ectopic (e.g., in duodenal wall).*
>
> *Tumors are malignant in 62% of patients; 44% of patients have metastases.*
>
> *Diffuse hyperplasia occurs in 10% of patients.*

This syndrome is associated with hyperparathyroidism in 20% of patients and frequently with adenomas of other endocrine glands, adrenal and pituitary (e.g., insulinoma) (see Multiple Endocrine Neoplasia, pp. 513–514).

CLASSIFICATION OF HYPOGLYCEMIA

Reactive
> Alimentary
> Diabetes mellitus (mild maturity-onset)
> Idiopathic
> Rare conditions (e.g., hereditary fructose intolerance, galactosemia, familial fructose and galactose intolerance)

Fasting (spontaneous)—almost always indicates organic disease
> Liver—parenchymal disease or enzyme defect
> Pancreatic
>> Insulinoma (pancreatic islet cell tumor)
>> MEN-I
>> Pancreatic hyperplasia
> Deficiency of hormones that oppose insulin (e.g., decreased function of thyroid, anterior pituitary, or adrenal cortex)
> Large extrapancreatic tumors (80% are intra- or retroperitoneal fibromas or sarcomas)

---

*12-hour nocturnal secretion shows acid of > 100 mEq/L and volume of > 1500 ml; baseline secretion is > 60% of the secretion caused by histamine or betazole stimulation.

Factitious (see next section)
    Insulin
    Sulfonylureas
    Alcohol
    Salicylates
    Propanolol (rare)

Diagnosis of reactive hypoglycemia requires
    Hypoglycemia symptoms associated with low blood glucose and
        alleviation by ingestion of glucose
    Diagnosis should not be made only on glucose tolerance test,
        since 25% of healthy young men may have postprandial glu-
        cose < 50 mg/dl and 2–3% of subjects may have < 40 mg/dl.
Diagnosis of insulinoma by
    Increased plasma insulin and C-peptide during hypoglycemic
        episode stimulated by fasting (up to 72 hours may be neces-
        sary) or tolbutamide tolerance test. Increased insulin-glucose
        ratio.

    *Serum insulin rarely reaches these high levels in patients with
    reactive hypoglycemia.*

    Failure to suppress C-peptide by hypoglycemia induced by ex-
        ogenous insulin administration
    Proinsulin > 30% of serum insulin after overnight fast suggests
        insulinoma. (May also be increased in renal disease.)

Following overnight fast, normal ranges are
    Serum insulin: 1–25 μU/ml
    Serum proinsulin: <25% of total measurable insulin
    Serum C-peptide: 1–2 ng/ml
    Ratio of insulin to glucose: < 0.3 (up to 0.35 in obese persons).
        During fasting, ratio decreases in healthy persons and in-
        creases in insulinoma patients.

FACTITIOUS HYPOGLYCEMIA

Due To Insulin Abuse

Insulin antibodies appear whenever insulin administration has oc-
    curred for more than a few weeks but are almost never present in
    persons not taking insulin (rarely occurs on an autoimmune
    basis).
During hypoglycemic episode, high insulin and low C-peptide levels
    in serum confirm diagnosis of exogenous insulin administration
    (diagnostic triad). (Increased *endogenous* insulin secretion is al-
    ways associated with increased C-peptide secretion.)
Insulin-glucose ratio > 0.3 in serum (normal is < 0.3). Increased
    ratio is also seen in autonomous production due to insulinoma.
Extreme elevations of serum insulin (e.g., >1000 μU/ml) suggest
    factitious hypoglycemia (fasting levels in patients with in-
    sulinoma rarely exceed 200 μU/ml).

Due To Sulfonylureas

May be anticipated to cause increased serum C-peptide levels and
    therefore mimic insulinoma more closely than insulin abuse.
Specific chemical assay can identify the agent.

Table 29-7. Differentiation of Hypoglycemic Symptoms

Criteria for Diagnosis	Anxiety State	Reactive Hypoglycemia*
5-Hour GTT	Blood glucose level not usually < 50 mg/dl	Blood glucose level falls to < 40 mg/dl
Symptoms	Not related to blood glucose level	Coincide with low blood glucose level
Response of plasma cortisol level to low blood glucose level	No plasma cortisol response	Plasma cortisol level doubles within 90 minutes after hypoglycemic symptoms or low blood glucose level occurs

*Reactive hypoglycemia refers to low blood glucose level during 5-hour GTT (not during fasting) and may be due to alimentary conditions (e.g., peptic ulcer) or diabetes mellitus, or it may be idiopathic.

ADRENAL FUNCTION TESTS

Daily infusion of 50 units of ACTH for 5 days, with before and after measurement of 24-hour urines for 17-ketosteroids (KS), 17-hydroxyketosteroids (OHKS) *(Protect possible Addison's disease patient with 1 mg of dexamethasone.)*

Complete primary adrenal insufficiency (Addison's disease)—no increase in urine steroids or increase of < 2 mg/day

Incomplete primary adrenal insufficiency—less than normal increases on all 5 days or slight increase on first 3 days that may be followed by decrease on days 4 and 5

Secondary adrenal insufficiency due to pituitary hypofunction—"staircase" response of progressively higher values each day

Secondary adrenal insufficiency due to chronic steroid therapy—may require prolonged ACTH testing to elicit the "staircase" response; may produce increments only in 17-OHKS but not in 17-KS

Normal = 3–5 times increase on first day and further increase next day

Do not do metyrapone test until this test proves that adrenals are sensitive to ACTH.

Measurement of circulating eosinophil count before and after ACTH stimulation

Normal

Decrease of 80% if previous baseline was > 100 cells/cu mm and no parasitic eosinophilia

Adrenal insufficiency

Decrease of < 25%

LABORATORY TESTS FOR EVALUATION OF ADRENAL-PITUITARY FUNCTION IN PATIENTS WITH HYPERADRENALISM

Adrenocortical Reserve (stimulation of adrenal cortex by administration of ACTH)

Functioning adrenal cortex is indicated by increased blood and urine 17-OHKS above patient's previous baseline level.

> Normal adrenocortical reserve—an increase of 3–5 times is shown the first day and a further increase the next day.
>
> Adrenocortical hyperplasia—test is often not helpful in diagnosis of Cushing's syndrome.
>
> Hypopituitarism—a slight increase is shown the first day and a greater increase the next day.

Nonfunctioning adrenal cortex is indicated by no increase of blood and urine 17-OHKS.

> Adenoma of adrenal cortex—lack of response almost always means autonomous tumor.
>
> Carcinoma of adrenal cortex—lack of response almost always means autonomous tumor; there is an associated characteristic marked increase over baseline of urinary neutral 17-KS.
>
> Addison's disease

Pituitary-Adrenal Suppression (suppression of pituitary ACTH secretion by administration of dexamethasone)

Functioning pituitary-adrenal system is indicated by decrease in blood and urine 17-OHKS.

> Normal pituitary-adrenal system—Urinary 17-OHKS falls to < 2.5 mg/24 hours, and plasma cortisol decreases (< 5 μg/dl) after both lower and higher dose schedules of dexamethasone.
>
> Cushing's disease (pituitary dysfunction causing adrenal hyperplasia)—urinary 17-OHKS falls to < 2.5 mg/24 hours, and plasma cortisol decreases to < 5 μg/dl only after higher but not after lower dose of dexamethasone (80% of cases).
>
> Adrenal adenoma or carcinoma or ectopic ACTH syndrome—urinary 17-OHKS and plasma cortisol are not decreased after high or low doses of dexamethasone.

Pituitary Reserve (adrenal suppression of pituitary secretion of ACTH inhibited by administration of metyrapone)

Functioning adrenal-pituitary system is indicated by increased urine 17-OHKS to twice the previous baseline level with

> Normal adrenal glands
>
> Pituitary Cushing's disease—increase may be 5–6 times baseline level.

Nonfunctioning adrenal-pituitary system (Long-standing production of excessive cortisol by adrenal tumor decreases pituitary reserve and responsiveness. Therefore ACTH is not secreted and there is no increase in urinary 17-OHKS and 17-KS.)

> Adenoma or carcinoma of adrenal cortex
>
> Ectopic ACTH syndrome
>
> Addison's disease, hypopituitarism

CAUSES OF CUSHING'S SYNDROME*

Pituitary	68%
Pituitary tumor	40%
No pituitary tumor	28%
Adrenal	17%
Adenoma	9%
Carcinoma	8%
Nodular hyperplasia	?
Ectopic neoplasms (e.g., lung)	15%

Adrenal cause is predominant in children, in whom adrenal carcinoma is found in 65% of patients less than age 15 years.

In adults, pituitary causes 75% of cases in women of childbearing age, but ectopic neoplasm causes most of the cases in men.

CUSHING'S SYNDROME

The first and best test to establish the diagnosis is presence of excessive cortisol production, indicated by (1) increased plasma cortisol with (2) loss of normal diurnal variation, (3) increased urinary free cortisol, (4) increased urinary metabolites of cortisol (17-KS, 17-OHKS) *(17-OHKS includes both Porter-Silber and ketogenic steroids)*.

> Increased plasma cortisol is most convenient and inexpensive screening measurement; however, 60% of cases of Cushing's syndrome may have normal values, and false positive results are frequent in obese patients.

> Increased urinary free cortisol (>100 µg/24 hours) is particularly valuable when plasma results are ambiguous, as it is not increased in obesity or estrogen therapy.

> Cushing's syndrome is strongly suggested in the presence of
>> Elevated plasma cortisol level (>30 µg/dl) at 8 A.M.–10 A.M.
>> Elevated plasma cortisol level (>15 µg/dl, i.e., $<50\%$ fall) after 4 P.M.
>> Elevated plasma cortisol level (>10 µg/ml) at 8 A.M. following dexamethasone 1 mg orally at 12 midnight
>> Virtually all patients with Cushing's syndrome show this absence of diurnal variation, but one-half of obese patients and two-thirds of normal-weight patients without Cushing's syndrome also show this absence of diurnal variation (due to depression, stress, alcoholism, etc.), and this has been used for diagnosis of endogenous depression (see p. 300).
>> Urinary 17-KS may be normal in 35% of patients with Cushing's syndrome but increased (>25 mg/24 hours) in 20% of obese persons without Cushing's.
>> Urinary 17-OHKS is increased (>10 mg/24 hours) in virtually all patients with Cushing's syndrome but increased in 20% of obese persons without Cushing's and in some patients with hyperthyroidism. Night collection sample $>$ day sample (reverse is true in normal persons). ACTH

*Source: Data from E. M. Gold, The Cushing syndromes: Changing views of diagnosis and treatment. *Ann. Intern. Med.* 90:829–844, 1979.

stimulation test produces lowest 17-OHKS in Cushing's syndrome due to adrenal carcinoma and the highest 17-OHKS due to adrenal adenoma.

If any of these are abnormal, then dexamethasone suppression test should be performed.

Increased urinary 17-ketogenic steroids (> 20 mg/24 hours).

Some patients have no clinical Cushing's syndrome despite high levels of plasma cortisol and urinary 17-OHKS.

Basal plasma ACTH level is low or undetectable in Cushing's syndrome due to adrenal disease (e.g., tumor) or exogenous steroid. High or high-normal range in pituitary Cushing's syndrome but rarely > 200 pg/ml, whereas two-thirds of patients with ectopic ACTH production have levels > 200 pg/ml. The other one-third of patients with ectopic ACTH production usually have moderately elevated values (100–200 pg/ml). In these cases, different ACTH levels between blood obtained simultaneously from the jugular and peripheral veins suggest pituitary hypersecretion of ACTH; dexamethasone suppression test is also indicated. Diurnal variation should be absent in ectopic ACTH syndrome.

Dexamethasone suppression test—see p. 300.
ACTH stimulation test—see p. 478.
Metyrapone test—see p. 479.

Urinary steroid findings in different etiologies of Cushing's syndrome:
  Increased urinary 17-OHKS by metyrapone administration is positive in
    100% of adrenal hyperplasias without tumor
    50% of adrenal adenomas
    25% of adrenal carcinomas
  Increased urinary 17-OHKS > 4 times normal in
    63% of patients with Cushing's syndrome
    3% of patients without Cushing's syndrome
    65% of patients with Cushing's syndrome due to ectopic ACTH syndrome
    3% of patients with Cushing's syndrome due to adrenal hyperplasia without tumor
  Increased urinary 17-KS > 4 times normal in
    50% of adrenal carcinomas (higher values increase likelihood of diagnosis of adrenal carcinoma; >100 mg/24 hours is virtually diagnostic)
    15% of cases of ectopic ACTH syndrome
    3% of adrenal hyperplasias without tumors
  Urinary 17-KS is normal or low in
    70% of adrenal adenomas
    50% of adrenal hyperplasias
    10% of adrenal carcinomas
  Urinary 17-KS is usually > 20 mg/24 hours in adrenal carcinomas and < 20 mg/24 hours in adrenal adenomas that cause Cushing's syndrome.
When total urinary 17-KS is elevated, the source may be determined by fractionation. Gonadal dysfunction is indicated by increased androsterone and etiocholanolone without elevation of

dehydroepiandrosterone and 11-oxy-17-KS; this is especially useful when serum testosterone is borderline increased.

Fractionation may differentiate between adrenal hyperplasia and carcinoma. Increased total 17-KS is due to elevation of all of the 17-KS in adrenal hyperplasia. In adrenal carcinoma, most of the increase is usually due to dehydroepiandrosterone.

Plasma renin activity is increased; suppressed activity suggests ectopic ACTH syndrome or adrenal adenoma or carcinoma (causing increased secretion of DOC or aldosterone).

Glucose tolerance is diminished.

> Glycosuria appears in 50% of patients.
> Fasting blood glucose may be elevated.
> GGT is frequently diabetic in type.
> Insulin tolerance is increased.
> Occasional polydipsia and polyuria are seen.

Usually moderate increase in serum sodium and decrease in serum potassium are found.

Hypokalemic alkalosis occurs in $\cong$ 10% of patients.

Hypokalemic alkalosis may indicate extra-adrenal neoplasia (e.g., bronchogenic carcinoma) causing increased production of ACTH with simultaneous increased secretion of mineralocorticoids and glucocorticoids; occurs in 30–50% of such patients.

Urine potassium is increased; sodium is decreased.

Salivary sodium-potassium ratio is decreased.

Hematologic changes are as follows:

> WBC is normal or increased.
> Relative lymphopenia is frequent (differential is usually < 15% of cells).
> Eosinopenia is frequent (usually < 100/cu mm).
> Hematocrit is usually normal; if increased, it indicates an androgenic component.

Osteoporosis causes changes.

> Serum and urine calcium may be increased.

BUN may be increased.

Urine creatine is increased.

Serum gamma globulins may be decreased and alpha$_2$ globulin may be moderately increased.

FACTITIOUS CUSHING'S SYNDROME

Increased plasma and urinary cortisol

Plasma ACTH is low or undetectable.

These findings may also occur in adrenal Cushing's syndrome. Differentiate by history of ingestion or, in some cases, determination of synthetic steroid analogues by specific plasma assays.

ADRENAL FEMINIZATION

This condition occurs in adult males with adrenal tumor (usually unilateral carcinoma, occasionally adenoma) that secretes estrogens.

Urinary estrogens are markedly increased.

17-KS is normal or moderately increased and cannot be suppressed by low doses of dexamethasone when due to adrenal tumor.

17-OHKS is normal.

Biopsy of testicle shows atrophy of tubules.

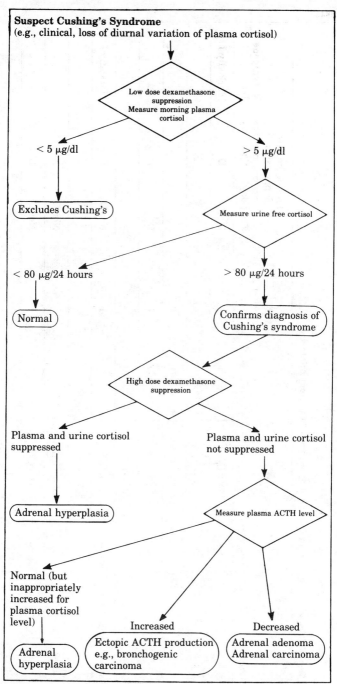

Suspect Cushing's Syndrome
(e.g., clinical, loss of diurnal variation of plasma cortisol)

Low dose dexamethasone suppression
Measure morning plasma cortisol

< 5 μg/dl → Excludes Cushing's

> 5 μg/dl → Measure urine free cortisol

< 80 μg/24 hours → Normal

> 80 μg/24 hours → Confirms diagnosis of Cushing's syndrome

High dose dexamethasone suppression

Plasma and urine cortisol suppressed → Adrenal hyperplasia

Plasma and urine cortisol not suppressed → Measure plasma ACTH level

Normal (but inappropriately increased for plasma cortisol level) → Adrenal hyperplasia

Increased → Ectopic ACTH production e.g., bronchogenic carcinoma

Decreased → Adrenal adenoma Adrenal carcinoma

Fig. 29-2. Sequence of laboratory tests in diagnosis of Cushing's syndrome.

Table 29-8. Differential Diagnosis of Cushing's Syndrome of Different Etiologies

Condition	Component		Baseline	After ACTH Stimulation	Dexamethasone Suppression 2 mg/day	Dexamethasone Suppression 8 mg/day	Metyrapone Test
Normal	Urine	17-OHKS	Higher	I	D	D	Markedly I
		17-KS	in				
		Free cortisol	A.M.				
	Plasma	Cortisol	than	I	D	D	
		ACTH	in P.M.				
Pituitary hyperfunction (Cushing's disease)	Urine	17-OHKS	I	I	Not D	D	Markedly I
		17-KS	I				
		Free cortisol	I		Not D	Not D	
	Plasma	Cortisol	I[a]	I	Not D	D	
		ACTH	I[a]				

Condition	Specimen	Measurement					
Ectopic ACTH syndrome (e.g., cancer of bronchus)	Urine	17-OHKS	I	NC or may be I	Not D	Not D	Not I
		17-KS	I			Not D	
		Free cortisol	I		Not D	Not D	
	Plasma	Cortisol	I[a]	NC or may be I	Not D	Not D	
		ACTH	I[a]				
Adrenal adenoma	Urine	17-OHKS	I	V[b]	Not D	Not D	Not I
		17-KS	Usually D (< 20 mg/24 hr)				
		Free cortisol	I	V[b]	Not D	Not D	
	Plasma	Cortisol	I[a]	V[b]	Not D	Not D	
		ACTH	D[a]				
Adrenal carcinoma	Urine	17-OHKS	I	Not I	Not D	Not D	Not I
		17-KS	Usually I (> 20 mg/24 hr)				
		Free cortisol	I	Not I	Not D	Not D	

Table 29-8. (continued)

Condition	Component		Baseline	After ACTH Stimulation	Dexamethasone Suppression 2 mg/day	Dexamethasone Suppression 8 mg/day	Metyrapone Test
	Plasma	Cortisol	I^a	Not I	Not D	Not D	Not I
		ACTH	D^a				
	Urine	17-OHKS	D	V	Not D	Not D	Not I
		17-KS					
		Free cortisol					
Steroid therapy	Plasma	Cortisol	I^a	Not I	Not D	Not D	

I = increased; D = decreased; V = variable; NC = no change.
^{a}No diurnal variation.
^{b}Not I in autonomous tumors, I in incompletely autonomous tumors.

Table 29-9. Comparison of Different Forms of Congenital Adrenal Hyperplasia

| | Enzyme Deficiency | | | | | |
| | Hydroxylase Deficiency | | | | | |
Laboratory Test	21-	11-	17-	18-	Desmolase	3-Beta-OH-Dehydrogenase
Pregnenolone	I	I	I	N or I	D	I
Progesterone	I	I	I	N or I	D	D
17-OH-progesterone	I*	I*	D*	N	D*	D*
17-OH-pregnenolone	I	I	D	N	D	I*
DHEA	I	I	D	N	D	I
DHEAS	I*	I*	D*	N*	D*	I*
Deoxycorticosterone	D*	I*	I*	I	D*	D
Corticosterone	D	D	N or I	I*	D	D
11-Deoxycortisol	D*	I*	D*	N	D*	D
Cortisol	D or N	D or N	D	N*	D	D
Aldosterone	D or N	D	D	D*	D	D
Androstenedione	I	I	D	N	D	D
ACTH	I	I	I	N	I	I
17-KS	I	I	D	N	D	I

I = increased; D = decreased; N = normal; DHEA = dehydroepiandrosterone; DHEAS = dehydroepiandrosterone sulfate.
*Most useful differential tests.
More than 90% of cases are due to 21-hydroxylase deficiency.
Source: Data from H. N. Mandell and M. Johnson, Laboratory Medicine in Clinical Practice. Boston: John Wright—PSG, 1983.

ALDOSTERONISM (PRIMARY)

Excessive mineralocorticoid hormone secretion by adrenal cortex causes renal tubules to retain sodium and excrete potassium. The classic biochemical abnormalities are urinary aldosterone, plasma renin, and serum potassium changes.

	Sensitivity (%)	Specificity (%)
Potassium, <4.0 mEq/L	100	64
Stimulated renin, <2.5 ng/ml/3 hr	100	88
Suppressed aldosterone, >10 ng/dL	98	92
Sequential, 1, 2, and 3	98	99

Hypokalemia (usually <3.0 mEq/L) is alleviated by administration of spironolactone* and by sodium restriction but not by potassium replacement therapy. May be normal in cases of shorter duration before classic clinical picture develops ($\cong$20% of cases initially). Hypokalemia not related to use of diuretics or laxatives in a hypertensive patient is the first indication of this condition. Hypokalemia is usually less in hyperplasia than adenoma, but considerable overlap occurs.

Saline infusion causes significant fall in serum potassium and in corrected potassium clearance. This hypokalemia induced by sodium loading is a reliable screening test.

Plasma renin is markedly decreased (normal or increased in secondary aldosteronism). It cannot be stimulated by use of salt restriction and upright posture to deplete plasma volume. Plasma renin levels are not decreased in at least 10% of patients with primary aldosteronism.

Urinary aldosterone is increased on normal-salt diet (not detectable on all days); cannot be reduced by high-sodium intake and DOCA administration. 24-hour urinary aldosterone is best initial screening procedure (normal salt intake, no drugs).

Saline infusion (2 L normal saline in 4 hours) suppresses plasma aldosterone to < 5 ng/dl in hypertensive patients without primary aldosteronism but not in patients with primary aldosteronism. (Plasma aldosterone level is first increased by having patient in upright position for 2 hours.) Since plasma aldosterone levels vary from moment to moment, a single specimen may not properly reflect adrenal secretion.

Renin-aldosterone ratio $\geqq$ 30 in random blood sample in patient not on medication is said to indicate primary aldosteronism.

Measurement of aldosterone in blood from periphery and both adrenal veins confirms the diagnosis by elevated level from side of lesion; opposite side has level close to that in peripheral blood. This also distinguishes unilateral adenoma from bilateral adenomas and hyperplasia and indicates location of lesion for surgeon.

It has been suggested that cortisol be measured simultaneously and aldosterone-cortisol ratio be calculated in blood from each adrenal vein and upper and lower vena cava (simultaneous measurements verify source of blood and correct for dilution). In unilateral

---

*Administration of spironolactone for 3 days increases serum potassium > 1.2 mEq/L. It also increases urine sodium and decreases urine potassium. Negative potassium balance reoccurs in 5 days. It increases urinary aldosterone (this is variable in hypertensive and normal people).

adenoma, aldosterone-cortisol ratio in blood from the adrenal vein is > 2 times higher on the affected side, and the ratio on the uninvolved side is less than in the lower inferior vena cava. In hyperplasia, the ratios on both sides are similar and are greater than in the lower inferior vena cava. Diagnosis of adenoma rather than hyperplasia is also suggested if plasma aldosterone decreases when patient is in upright posture and by a diurnal rhythm with lower evening plasma aldosterone levels.

Urine is neutral or alkaline (pH > 7.0) and not normally responsive to ammonium chloride load. Its large volume and low specific gravity are not responsive to vasopressin or water restriction (decreased tubular function, especially reabsorption of water). There is hyperkaluria even with low potassium intake. Sodium output is reduced.

There is absence of hyponatremia or slight hypernatremia, hypochloremia, and alkalosis (CO_2 content > 25 mEq/L; blood pH tends to increase).

Glucose tolerance is decreased in ≦ 50% of patients.

Plasma cortisol and ACTH are normal.

Urine 17-KS and 17-OHKS are normal.

Serum magnesium falls.

Total blood volume increases because of increased plasma volume.

Sodium level in sweat is low.

Salivary Na/K ratio < 0.65 is consistent with diagnosis, but a higher ratio does not exclude it.

Caused By

Single benign cortical adenoma (70% of patients)

Multiple benign cortical adenomas (15% of patients)

Bilateral cortical hyperplasia (9% of patients)

Normal size adrenal gland with normal architecture or focal nodular hyperplasia (6% of patients)

Rarely, adrenal carcinoma or heterotopic adrenal tissue

ALDOSTERONISM (SECONDARY)

Due To

Decreased effective blood volume
    Congestive heart failure
    Cirrhosis with ascites (aldosteronism 2000–3000 mg/day)
    Nephrosis
    Sodium depletion

Hyperactivity of renin-angiotensin system
    Renin-producing renal tumor (see p. 554)
    Bartter's syndrome (see below)
    Toxemia of pregnancy
    Malignant hypertension
    Renovascular hypertension
    Oral contraceptive drugs

NORMOTENSIVE SECONDARY HYPERALDOSTERONISM (BARTTER'S SYNDROME)

Hypokalemia with renal potassium wasting

Chloride-resistant metabolic alkalosis

Increased plasma renin is a characteristic feature.

Frequently there is decreased serum magnesium and increased uric acid.

Table 29-10. Laboratory Differentiation of Primary and Secondary Aldosteronism

Testing Procedure	Primary Aldosteronism	Secondary Aldosteronism
Etiology	Usually due to tumor (adenoma more frequent than carcinoma); may be due to bilateral hyperplasia	1. Edematous conditions (e.g., cirrhosis, nephrosis, congestive heart failure) 2. Hypertension (e.g., essential, malignant, renovascular renal artery stenosis) 3. Renal tubular dysfunction (e.g., renal tubular acidosis, Fanconi's syndrome) 4. Hemorrhage
Blood electrolytes	Hypokalemia, usually with acidosis and hypernatremia	Depends on underlying condition
Plasma renin	Markedly D	N or I
Urinary 17-OHKS and 17-KS	Usually N; may be I in adrenal carcinoma	N
Urinary aldosterone	Markedly I	Markedly I
Aldosterone administration	Escapes from sodium retention after initial rise in serum sodium	Causes increased edema
Salt-loading	Does not suppress aldosterone secretion (as in normal person) and increases potassium excretion	
Low-sodium diet	Usually reduces potassium excretion	
Deoxycorticosterone administration	In adenoma, aldosterone level is *not* suppressed; in bilateral adrenal hyperplasia, aldosterone level *is* suppressed	

D = decreased; N = normal; I = increased.

Increased circulating angiotensin II and urine aldosterone in the absence of edema, hypertension, or hypovolemia
Renal concentrating defect resistant to ADH

PSEUDOHYPERALDOSTERONISM (LIDDLE'S SYNDROME)
Familial disorder with clinical manifestations closely resembling those due to aldosterone-producing adrenal adenoma
Hypokalemia due to renal potassium wasting
Metabolic alkalosis
Hypertension

All are corrected by long-term administration of diuretics that cause natriuresis and renal potassium retention (e.g., triamterene or amiloride) and by restriction of sodium.

Aldosterone secretion and excretion are greatly reduced.

PSEUDOALDOSTERONISM DUE TO INGESTION OF LICORICE (AMMONIUM GLYCYRRHIZATE)
(excessive ingestion causes hypertension due to sodium retention)

Decreased serum potassium

Decreased aldosterone excretion in urine

Decreased plasma renin activity

HYPOFUNCTION OF RENIN-ANGIOTENSIN-ALDOSTERONE SYSTEM
(differs from Addison's disease and congenital adrenal hyperplasia, which have deficiency of glucocorticoids as well as of mineralocorticoids)

Infrequent condition due to

> Rare congenital or acquired defect in aldosterone biosynthesis (renin normal or increased)
> Prolonged administration of heparin (very rare)
> Removal of unilateral aldosterone-secreting tumor (usually transient)
> Autonomic nervous system dysfunction; aldosterone deficiency causes impaired renal sodium conservation but without hyperkalemia
> Idiopathic hyporeninism

Hyperkalemia, urinary sodium loss, extracellular volume depletion corrected by administration of mineralocorticoids

Normal adrenal glucocorticoid response to ACTH stimulation test

Low 24-hour urinary excretion of aldosterone (normal = 3–32 μg/24 hours), with normal dietary intake of sodium and potassium; subnormal aldosterone response to sodium restriction

Mild hyperchloremic metabolic acidosis

Renal function frequently impaired (creatinine clearance rate may be 25–70 ml/minute)

Laboratory findings of associated diseases (e.g., diabetes mellitus, gout, pyelonephritis)

Table 29-11. Comparison of Pathologic Hypofunction of Renin-Angiotensin-Aldosterone System and Low-Renin Hypertension

Pathologic Hypofunction of Renin-Angiotensin-Aldosterone System	Low-Renin Hypertension
Hyperkalemia	Normal or low serum potassium
Urinary sodium loss	Sodium retention
Extracellular volume depletion	Increase in extracellular volume
Hypotension; may be normal	Persistent hypertension
Low renin-angiotensin-aldosterone activity	Low plasma renin activity with normal plasma and urinary levels of aldosterone

Table 29-12. Laboratory Tests in Differential Diagnosis of Benign Pheochromocytoma and Neural Crest Tumors (Neuroblastoma, Ganglioneuroma)

Urinary Levels of	Pheochro-mocytoma	Neural Crest Tumor (neuroblastoma, ganglioneuroma)
Catecholamines	I	I
VMA	I	I
Metanephrines	I	I
Dopamine	N*	I
HVA	N*	I

I = increased; N = normal.
*I in malignant pheochromocytoma.

Pseudohypoaldosteronism is a heterogeneous group of disorders with signs and symptoms of aldosterone deficiency, but aldosterone levels are increased, and it is not ameliorated by exogenous mineralocorticoid.

PHEOCHROMOCYTOMA

Blood and urine levels of catecholamines (norepinephrine and, to a lesser extent, epinephrine; normetanephrine and metanephrine) are increased, usually even when patient is asymptomatic and normotensive; rarely are increases found only following a paroxysm. However, the diagnosis is never ruled out by a normal level, and repeated testing may be necessary. Blood should be drawn in the unstressed supine patient.

Plasma catecholamines drop markedly after 5 minutes if RBCs are not separated from plasma.

Urine VMA (vanillylmandelic acid, a catecholamine metabolite) excretion is considerably increased. Because this determination is simpler than for catecholamines, it has been more commonly used. Beware of false increase due to foods (e.g., vanilla, fruits, especially bananas, coffee, tea) and drugs (e.g., vasopressor agents) ingested within 72 hours before the test (see p. 168). Beware of nonspecific techniques for VMA assay that fail to detect 30% of cases of pheochromocytoma.

Hyperglycemia and glycosuria are found in 50% of patients during an attack.

Glucose tolerance test frequently shows a diabetic type of curve.

Thyroid function tests are normal.

Urine changes are secondary to sustained hypertension.

Plasma renin activity is increased.

≦ 15% of pheochromocytomas are malignant; 15% are extra-adrenal; 10% are multiple. Familial inheritance in 10–20% of patients. Extensive surgical exploration may be required. Rarely, this syndrome is due to hyperplasia of the adrenal medulla.

"Incidental" pheochromocytomas have been discovered.

Occurs in $\cong$ 0.1–0.2% of hypertensive population of U.S.

5% of patients with pheochromocytoma have normal blood pressure most or all of the time.

NEUROBLASTOMA, GANGLIONEUROMA, GANGLIOBLASTOMA
Urinary levels of catecholamines (norepinephrine, normetanephrine, dopamine, VMA, and HVA [homovanillic acid]) are increased.
Excretion of epinephrine is not increased.

Not all methods include dopamine in measurement of total catecholamines.

Not all patients have increased urinary levels of catecholamines VMA and HVA.
   If only 1 of these substances is measured, only $\cong$ 75% of cases are diagnosed.
   If VMA and HVA or VMA and total catecholamines are measured, 95–100% of cases are diagnosed.
These tests are also useful for differentiating Ewing's tumor and metastatic neuroblastoma of bone and to show response to therapy (surgery, irradiation, or chemotherapy), which should bring return to normal in 1–4 months. Continued elevation indicates need for further treatment.

ADDISON'S DISEASE
(chronic adrenal insufficiency)
Serum potassium is increased.
Serum sodium and chloride are decreased.
Sodium-potassium ratio is < 30:1.
Blood volume is decreased; hematocrit level is increased (because of water loss).
BUN may be moderately increased.

Table 29-13. Laboratory Differentiation of Primary and Secondary Adrenal Insufficiency

Determination	Primary Adrenal Insufficiency	Adrenal Insufficiency Secondary to Hypopituitarism
After ACTH stimulation (see p. 478)		
Urinary 17-OHKS and 17-KS levels	No responsive increase	Marked "staircase" response
Eosinophil count (decreases 80–90% daily in normal person)	Decreased < 20%	Decrease depends on degree of insufficiency
Blood ACTH level	Increased	Decreased

Fasting hypoglycemia is present, with a flat oral glucose tolerance curve and insulin hypersensitivity. IV GTT shows a normal peak followed by severe prolonged hypoglycemia.

Neutropenia and relative lymphocytosis are common.

Eosinophilia is present (300/cu mm). *(A total eosinophil count of < 50 is evidence against severe adrenocortical hypofunction.)*

Normocytic anemia is slight or moderate but difficult to estimate because of decreased blood volume.

Increased blood ACTH (200–1600 pg/ml) with wide variation between morning and evening levels in primary adrenal hypofunction but decreased or absent ACTH in pituitary (secondary) hypoadrenalism. Increased ACTH level is quickly suppressed by replacement therapy.

Decreased blood cortisol (<5 µg/dl in 8–10 A.M. specimen) is useful screening test. High or high-normal result excludes both primary and secondary adrenocortical insufficiency. Low or borderline result is indication for ACTH stimulation test.

Injection of ACTH (e.g., 0.25 mg of Cosyntropin IM or IV) should cause an increase in blood cortisol > 2 times baseline level at any of 30-, 60-, or 90-minute intervals in normal persons. >50% increase excludes primary but not secondary (pituitary) adrenocortical failure. Almost total lack of response indicates primary insufficiency even if 8 A.M. blood cortisol level is low-normal.

Prolonged ACTH infusion should be performed to evaluate longstanding adrenal insufficiency. 24-hour urine 17-OHKS is measured daily for 4 days; on each of last 3 days, patient is given 8-hour ACTH infusion (e.g., 0.25 mg of Cosyntropin). Normal response is 4–5 times increase by third day. Complete unresponsiveness indicates primary insufficiency. Subnormal response suggests secondary insufficiency.

Metyrapone inhibition test is performed if ACTH test causes some increase in blood cortisol. (10 mg/kg body weight is administered to adults and 15 mg/kg to children, orally every 4 hours for 6 doses or single oral dose of 2–3 gm of metyrapone at 11 P.M. followed by blood measurement at 8 A.M.) Normal response ≧ 2 times increase in urinary 17-OHKS next day and increase in plasma 11-deoxycortisol ≧ 7 µg/dl at 8 A.M. (Concomitant fall in plasma cortisol indicates that metyrapone dose has effectively blocked 11-beta-hydroxylation.) Subnormal response occurs in secondary (pituitary) adrenocorticol insufficiency. Normal response excludes ACTH deficiency. Abnormal response *by itself* indicates adrenocortical insufficiency but does not distinguish between primary and secondary types.

Cortisol treatment will interfere with all of the above tests and must be discontinued for prior 24–48 hours. Dexamethasone will interfere with metyrapone test and plasma ACTH levels.

Laboratory tests for associated conditions

  Primary adrenocortical insufficiency may be caused by congenital adrenal hyperplasia (see p. 487) or associated with hypoaldosteronism.

  Secondary (pituitary) insufficiency may be associated with laboratory findings of hypothyroidism (see p. 458), hypogonadism (see p. 501), etc.

Urine 17-OHKS is absent or markedly decreased.

Urine 17-KS is markedly decreased.

Urine 17-KGS is markedly decreased.

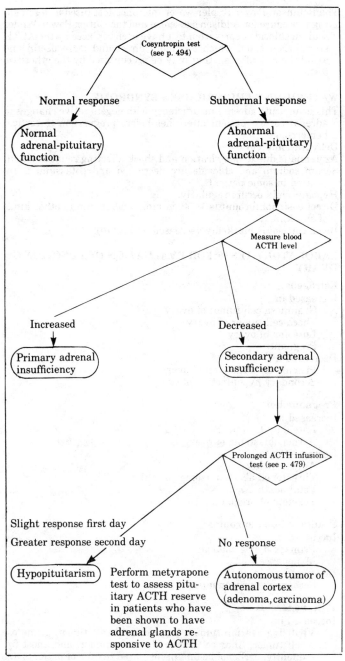

Fig. 29-3. Sequence of laboratory tests in diagnosis of adrenal insufficiency.

The Robinson-Power-Kepler water tolerance test (used as a screening procedure for Addison's disease) and the Cutler-Power-Wilder sodium chloride deprivation test have been replaced by the ACTH stimulation tests, which are more direct and more useful and avoid the risk of crisis that may be precipitated by the other two tests.

WATERHOUSE-FRIDERICHSEN SYNDROME

This is an acute adrenal insufficiency with degenerative changes in adrenal cortex; patient often dies before progression to cortical hemorrhage.

Dehydration occurs.

Azotemia is due to dehydration and shock affecting renal function.

Serum sodium and chloride are decreased and potassium is increased in some patients.

Hypoglycemia occurs regularly.

Direct eosinophil count is > 50/cu mm (<50/cu mm in other kinds of shock).

Blood cortisol is markedly decreased (<5 µg/dl).

LABORATORY TESTS FOR EVALUATION OF FUNCTION OF OVARY

Estrogens
Increased in
    Granulosa cell tumor of ovary
    Theca-cell tumor of ovary
    Luteoma of ovary
    Pregnancy
Decreased in
    Primary hypofunction of ovary
    Secondary hypofunction of ovary

Pregnanediol
Increased in
    Luteal cysts of ovary
    Arrhenoblastoma of ovary
Decreased in
    Amenorrhea
    Threatened abortion (some patients)
    Fetal death
    Toxemia of pregnancy

Pituitary Gonadotropins
Increased in
    Primary hypogonadism
    Menopause
Decreased in
    Secondary hypogonadism

17-Ketosteroids
Increased in
    Virilizing ovarian tumors (e.g., adrenal rest tumor, granulosa cell tumor, hilar cell tumor, Brenner tumor, and, most frequently, arrhenoblastoma); increased in 50% of patients and normal in 50% of patients

Decreased in
> Primary ovarian agenesis

OVARIAN TUMORS

Feminizing Ovarian Tumors (e.g., granulosa cell tumor, thecoma, luteoma)
Pap smear of vagina and endometrial biopsy show high estrogen effect and no progestational activity; no signs of ovulation during reproductive phase.
Urinary FSH is decreased (inhibited by increased estrogen).
Urine 17-KS and 17-OHKS are normal.
Pregnanediol is absent.

Masculinizing Ovarian Tumors
(e.g., arrhenoblastoma, hilar cell tumors, adrenal rest tumors)
Pap smear of vagina shows decreased estrogen effect.
Endometrial biopsy shows moderate atrophy of endometrium.
Urine FSH (gonadotropins) is low.
Urine 17-KS is normal or may be slightly increased in arrhenoblastoma. They may be markedly increased in adrenal tumors of ovary ("masculinovoblastoma"). The higher the urine 17-KS level, the greater the likelihood of adrenocortical carcinoma; >100 mg/24 hours is virtually diagnostic. It may be moderately increased in Leydig cell tumors.

> *In arrhenoblastoma there may be an increase of androsterone, testosterone, etc., excreted in urine even though the 17-KS is not much increased. Urine 17-KS normal or slightly increased associated with plasma testosterone in male range is almost certainly due to ovarian tumor.*

> *In adrenal cell tumors of ovary, laboratory findings may be the same as in hyperfunction of adrenal cortex with Cushing's syndrome, etc.*

In some cases there are no endocrine effects from these tumors.
Some cases of arrhenoblastoma with masculinization also show evidence of increased estrogen formation.

Struma Ovarii
About 5–10% of cases are hormone-producing. Classic findings of hyperthyroidism may occur. These tumors take up radioactive iodine. *(Simple follicle cysts may also take up radioactive iodine.)*

Primary Chorionepithelioma of Ovary
Urinary chorionic gonadotropins are markedly increased.
Estrogen and progesterone secretion may be much increased.

Nonfunctioning Ovarian Tumors
Only effect may be hypogonadism due to replacement of functioning ovarian parenchyma.

PRECOCIOUS PUBERTY IN GIRLS

Due To
Diseases of central nervous system (usually floor of the third ventricle) with involvement of the posterior hypothalamus (e.g., tuber-

culous meningitis, epidemic encephalitis, other inflammations, tumors, tuberous sclerosis [more frequent in boys])

Polyostotic fibrosis dysplasia (Albright's syndrome)

Ovarian tumors (e.g., teratomatous choriocarcinomas, granulosa cell tumors, theca-cell tumors, luteomas)

Adrenal adenoma or carcinoma, which may secrete estrogen and be associated with feminization without virilization in rare cases

Iatrogenic cause of accidental ingestion or inunction of estrogens

Laboratory Findings

Pap smear of vagina indicates estrogen effect.

Pituitary gonadotropin is usually low, with ovarian and adrenal lesions.

Increased 17-KS and estrogen excretion (above normal adult level) occur, with feminizing adrenal tumors.

Chorionic gonadotropin titers are increased in choriocarcinoma. *(Not all choriocarcinomas produce gonadotropin.)*

STEIN-LEVENTHAL SYNDROME (POLYCYSTIC OVARIAN DISEASE)

Serum luteinizing hormone (LH) is increased (> 35 mIU/ml) in approximately ≅ 60% of patients in association with normal or low follicle-stimulating hormone (FSH) level. Abnormally high LH/FSH ratio (> 2) is more consistently abnormal than is either measurement alone.

Plasma testosterone is increased ≦ 200 μg/dl (> 200 μg/dl usually indicates an androgen-producing tumor).

Plasma androstenedione is increased.

Approximately 85% of these patients have one or more abnormalities of serum LH/FSH ratio, testosterone, or androstenedione. Hyperandrogenism does not differentiate condition from congenital adrenal hyperplasia.

Urinary 17-KS is somewhat increased (higher values occur in congenital virilizing adrenal hyperplasia and hyperadrenalism due to Cushing's syndrome). Dexamethasone administration for 5 days causes partial suppression in cases of ovarian origin, but complete suppression suggests adrenal origin. Administration of gonadotropin increases urinary 17-KS.

Biopsy of ovary is consistent with increased androgen effect but is not specific; ovarian visualization and biopsy are not routine part of diagnosis.

Plasma cortisol, urinary 17-OHKS, and 17-KGS are normal.

Because of erratic daily fluctuations of LH and androgens, daily plasma specimens for 3–5 days may be necessary.

Increased serum LH (> 35 mIU/ml), LH/FSH > 2, and mild increase of ovarian androgen level are sufficient for diagnosis in presence of the symptoms and clinical signs. Laboratory tests may be helpful in defining pathogenesis, following course of treatment, or ruling out adrenal or ovarian tumors.

Increased serum LH with normal or decreased FSH may occur in simple obesity, hyperthyroidism, liver disease.

SOME CAUSES OF GENERAL HIRSUTISM
Polycystic ovary syndrome (Stein-Leventhal syndrome) (common)
Idiopathic (common)
Drugs (e.g., phenytoin, corticosteroids, androgens, diazoxide, minoxidil)
Endocrine conditions
    Virilizing ovarian tumors
    Virilizing adrenal tumors
    Virilizing congenital adrenal hyperplasia
    Cushing's syndrome
    Acromegaly
    Hypothyroidism

"CONSTITUTIONAL" HIRSUTISM IN WOMEN
With normal menses and fertility, urine 17-KS is normal.
With amenorrhea, hypomenorrhea, or oligomenorrhea, urine 17-KS may be slightly increased.

LABORATORY TESTS IN DIFFERENTIAL DIAGNOSIS OF PATIENTS WITH HIRSUTISM AND DIMINISHED MENSES

Urinary 17-Hydroxyketosteroids
Normal
    Constitutional hirsutism
    Stein-Leventhal syndrome
    Mild adrenogenital syndrome
    Masculinizing tumor of ovary
Increased
    Cushing's syndrome

Urinary 17-Ketosteroids
Normal
    Constitutional hirsutism
    Stein-Leventhal syndrome
    Masculinizing tumor of ovary
    Cushing's syndrome
Slight increase
    Constitutional hirsutism
    Stein-Leventhal syndrome
    Mild adrenogenital syndrome
    Cushing's syndrome
Marked increase
    Masculinizing tumor of adrenal gland
    Adrenogenital syndrome

Urinary 17-Ketosteroids Decreased by Daily Prednisone
Poor response
    Constitutional hirsutism
    Stein-Leventhal syndrome
    Masculinizing tumor of ovary
Good response
    Adrenogenital syndrome

Urinary 17-Ketosteroids Further Decreased by Daily Stilbestrol and Prednisone
No response
    Constitutional hirsutism

Masculinizing tumor of ovary
Adrenogenital syndrome
Response
Stein-Leventhal syndrome (testosterone level also decreases)

SOME COMMON CAUSES OF PRIMARY AMENORRHEA/DELAYED MENARCHE

Gonadal disorders (60% of all causes)
  Gonadal dysgenesis (75% of gonadal disorders)
  Testicular feminization syndrome
  Polycystic ovaries
  Resistant ovary syndrome
Genital tract disorders (35–40% of all causes)
  Imperforate hymen
  Uterine agenesis
  Vaginal agenesis
  Transverse vaginal septum
Pituitary disorders (rare)
  Hypopituitarism
  Adenomas (prolactin secreting)
Hypothalamic disorders (rare)
  Anatomic lesions (e.g., craniopharyngioma)
  Functional disturbance of hypothalamic-pituitary axis (e.g., anorexia nervosa, emotional stress)
Systemic disorders
  Hypothyroidism
  Congenital adrenal hyperplasia
  Debilitating chronic diseases (e.g., malnutrition, congenital heart disease, renal failure, collagen diseases)

SECONDARY AMENORRHEA

If increased LH and normal FSH
  Polycystic ovarian disease (Stein-Leventhal syndrome)
  Early pregnancy
  Ectopic gonadotropin production by neoplasm (e.g., lung, gastrointestinal tract)
If increased LH and increased FSH
  Ovarian failure
If decreased LH and decreased FSH
  Pituitary or hypothalamic impairment
  Clomiphene citrate should be administered for 5–10 days; if gonadotropin level rises or menses return, cause is probably hypothalamic
  Administer hypothalamic luteinizing hormone–releasing factor (LRF); normal or exaggerated response in hypothalamic amenorrhea (cause in 80% of patients); smaller or no response in pituitary tumor or dysfunction

TURNER'S SYNDROME (OVARIAN DYSGENESIS)

Barr bodies are negative (male) in 80% of patients.
Chromosomal pattern—45 chromosomes (monosomy X with XO; or if XX, one X is abnormal; or XO mosaic)
Because of the frequency with which 45 X cells are admixed with 46 XX cells, it is impossible to exclude the diagnosis (i.e., 45 X karyotype) by either buccal smear or chromosome analysis alone.

Biopsy of ovary shows connective tissue stroma with rare follicular
structure.
Vaginal smear and endometrial biopsy are atrophic.
17-KS and 17-OHKS are normal.
ACTH is normal.
FSH is increased.
T-3, etc., are usually normal.

*About 60% of patients with primary amenorrhea have Turner's syn-
drome or sometimes testicular feminization.*

TURNER'S SYNDROME IN THE MALE
Biopsy of testicle reveals dysgenetic tubules with few or no germ
cells.
Chromosomal pattern—46 chromosomes (XY pattern with very defective Y that is equivalent to XO)

MENOPAUSE (FEMALE CLIMACTERIC)
Urinary gonadotropin is increased.
Urinary estrogens are decreased.
Urinary 17-KS is decreased.
Plasma gonadotropin is increased.

SECONDARY OVARIAN INSUFFICIENCY
Urinary gonadotropin is decreased or absent.

GALACTORRHEA-AMENORRHEA
10–25% of women with galactorrhea and normal menses have increased serum prolactin levels.
10–15% of women with amenorrhea but without galactorrhea have
increased serum prolactin levels.
75% of women with both galactorrhea and amenorrhea/oligo-
menorrhea have increased serum prolactin levels.
Women may also present with hirsutism, infertility.

**Table 29-14. Laboratory Differentiation of Primary and Secondary (to
Pituitary Defect) Hypogonadism**

Determination	Primary Hypogonadism	Hypogonadism Secondary to Pituitary Defect
Level of FSH and gonadotropin in urine	High	Low
After administration of gonadotropins		
17-KS excretion	Does not increase	Increases
Clinical evidence of hypogonadism	Does not subside	Subsides with Increased sperm count Increased estrogenic effect in woman's Pap smear

Men present with loss of libido, impotence, oligospermia, low serum
testosterone levels, and sometimes galactorrhea.

Serum prolactin levels (see p. 91)

> Normal < 25 ng/ml in women; lower in men and children
>
> 100–200 ng/ml is strong evidence of pituitary tumor in non-
> pregnant women.
>
> >300 ng/ml is virtually diagnostic of pituitary tumor in non-
> pregnant women.
>
> TRH stimulation of patients without pituitary tumors usually
> doubles serum prolactin level, but most patients with pitu-
> itary tumors do not respond to TRH stimulation. Enhanced
> responsiveness in hypothyroidism and blunted prolactin rise
> in chronic renal failure. Unresponsiveness to TRH or meto-
> clopramide indicates pituitary prolactin insufficiency as in
> panhypopituitarism.
>
> Serum samples should be collected under basal conditions with
> minimal stress and by pooling 3 blood samples collected at 20-
> minute intervals for one assay; all drugs should be discon-
> tinued for at least 2 weeks before testing.

In absence of drug ingestion, most cases of hyperprolactinemia are
due to pituitary adenoma (almost always benign)

> Multiple basal prolactin levels have replaced stimulation and
> suppression tests for diagnosis of prolactinoma (along with
> exclusion of other causes of increased serum prolactin).

LABORATORY TESTS FOR EVALUATION OF FUNCTION OF TESTICLE

Chorionic Gonadotropins in Urine

Increased in

> Choriocarcinoma
>
> Seminoma

Serum Alpha-Fetoprotein (AFP)

Serum AFP levels > 40 ng/ml are found in 75% of patients with
teratocarcinoma.

90% of patients with testicular tumors are positive for AFP or urinary chorionic gonadotropin, or both; these are valuable for gaug-
ing efficacy of chemotherapy. 30% of patients receiving intensive
chemotherapy apparently have a complete clinical remission;
AFP levels may remain elevated although lower than pretreatment levels.

Serum AFP is not increased in pure seminoma without teratomatous component.

Pituitary Gonadotropins in Urine

Increased in

> Primary hypogonadism

Decreased in

> Secondary hypogonadism

17-Ketosteroids in Urine
(indicative of adrenal rather than testicular status)

Increased in

> Interstitial cell tumor

Decreased in
    Primary hypogonadism
    Secondary hypogonadism

Plasma Testosterone
Decreased in
    Primary hypogonadism
    Secondary hypogonadism

Semen Analysis
Sterile males usually show
    Volume of < 3 ml
    < 20 million sperm/ml
    < 25% motility

Biopsy of Testicle
Evidence of atrophy in sterility study
Diagnosis of tumor

Normal spermatogenesis associated with normal endocrine findings in patient with aspermia and infertility suggests a mechanical obstruction to sperm transport that may be correctable.

Chromosome Analysis
Turner's syndrome (gonadal dysgenesis)—usually negative for Barr bodies
Klinefelter's syndrome—positive for Barr bodies
Pseudohermaphroditism—chromosomal sex corresponding to gonadal sex

TESTICULAR CANCER
Serum markers for alpha-fetoprotein and human chorionic gonadotropin (HCG) (beta chain) may be elevated in conditions other than testicular cancer (see p. 91 and 137).
Increased serum HCG (>1–2 ng/ml or >5–10 mIU/ml) is found in 40–60% of patients with nonseminomatous tumors and in some patients with apparently pure seminoma. In the latter case, immunochemical staining of paraffin-embedded tumor should be performed, since isolated syncytiotrophoblastic cells may show the hormone but are not by themselves evidence of choriocarcinoma.
Increased serum alpha-fetoprotein (>20 ng/ml) is found in 70% of patients with teratocarcinoma or embryonal carcinoma.
Both markers should always be measured simultaneously. 40% of patients with nonseminomatous tumors have elevation of only one marker.
20–30% of patients have false negative results preoperatively despite tumor (usually microscopic) in the retroperitoneal lymph nodes. Therefore, lymphadenectomy should not be omitted simply because of normal marker levels.
False positive elevation of marker levels is rare.
The most important use is for follow-up after surgery or chemotherapy.
Failure of increased preoperative levels to fall after surgery suggests metastatic disease and the need for chemotherapy. Rise of

levels that had previously declined to normal suggests recurrent tumor even with no other evidence of disease.

Negative markers are not useful for differential diagnosis of scrotal mass, but elevated levels indicate testicular cancer.

GERMINAL APLASIA
Buccal smears are normal (negative for Barr bodies).
Chromosomal pattern is normal.
Urinary gonadotropin is normal.
Urinary pituitary gonadotropin is increased.
17-KS is decreased.
There is azoospermia.
Biopsy of testicle shows that Sertoli's and Leydig's cells are intact and germinal cells are absent.

KLINEFELTER'S SYNDROME
Buccal smears are positive for Barr bodies.
Biopsy of testicle shows atrophy, with hyalinized tubules lined only by Sertoli's cells, clumped Leydig's cells, and failure of spermatogenesis.
There is azoospermia.
Abnormal chromosomal pattern. XY males have an extra X; usually XXY; may have additional X (e.g., XXYY, XXXY, XXXXY).
Testosterone levels are usually decreased.
Urinary gonadotropin level is elevated.

MALE CLIMACTERIC
There is decreased testosterone level in blood (< 300 ng/ml) and urine (< 100 μg/24 hours).
Urinary gonadotropin level is elevated. (Gonadotropin is decreased when low testosterone level is due to pituitary tumor, gout, or diabetes.)

ACROMEGALY AND GIGANTISM
(usually due to eosinophilic adenoma of pituitary)
Serum growth hormone is increased. (Avoid stress before and during venipuncture because stress stimulates secretion of growth hormone.)
> Fasting levels above 5 ng/ml in men are suggestive but not diagnostic of acromegaly.
> Most patients of both sexes show a fall of < 50% during glucose tolerance test, whereas normal subjects show almost complete suppression of growth hormone (or to < 5 ng/ml) by induced hyperglycemia.

IV ACTH administration may cause excessive increase in urine 17-KS but normal 17-OHKS excretion.
Adrenal virilism and increased urine 17-KS are common in women.
Urine 17-KS, 17-KGS, and pituitary gonadotropins are usually normal or may be slightly changed but not diagnostically useful.
Rare associated endocrinopathies are hyperthyroidism, hyperparathyroidism, pheochromocytoma, insulinoma.
Glucose tolerance is impaired in most patients. Mild diabetes mellitus that is insulin-resistant is found in < 15% of patients.
Serum phosphorus is increased for age of patient in 40% of cases.
Serum alkaline phosphatase may be increased.
Urine calcium is increased.

Urine hydroxyproline is increased.
Biopsy of costochondral junction evidences active bone growth.
CBC and ESR are normal.
In inactive cases, all secondary laboratory findings may be normal.
In late stage, panhypopituitarism may develop.

PITUITARY GROWTH HORMONE DEFICIENCY

There may be isolated deficiency with dwarfism or associated with
  TSH deficiency, with ACTH deficiency, or with TSH and ACTH
  deficiencies.
Serum growth hormone levels are decreased (<1.0 ng/ml) with no
  response 4 hours after oral glucose load, and serum growth hormone level increases to >10 ng/ml after IV insulin (0.1 unit/kg)
  is administered.
Functional tests
> Draw serum at 0, 30, 60, 90, and 120 minutes.
> Insulin (regular crystalline, IV, 0.05 to 0.3 unit/kg body weight)
>   should normally produce at least 2 times increase in serum
>   growth hormone level and 3 times increase in serum prolactin
>   level at 60-minute peak. This is the most reliable challenge
>   for growth hormone secretion.
> Levodopa (500 mg orally) should normally produce at least 2
>   times increase in serum growth hormone level at 60-minute
>   peak.
> Arginine (0.5 gm/kg body weight as 5% solution IV over 30
>   minutes) should normally produce at least 3 times increase in
>   serum growth hormone and at least 2 times increase in serum
>   prolactin level at 30- to 60-minute peak.
> Failure to produce the minimal responses indicated above indi-
>   cates a lesion of pituitary or hypothalamus but does not dif-
>   ferentiate between them.
> About one-fourth of patients with normal growth hormone se-
>   cretory capacity are unable to secrete growth hormone in re-
>   sponse to provocative tests indicated above, at any given
>   time. Therefore, at least two of these tests should be used to
>   confirm diagnosis of growth hormone deficiency.
> A normal response is at least 10 ng/ml peak value; 5–10 ng/ml
>   is indeterminate, $\leqq 5$ ng/ml is subnormal.

Decreased fasting blood sugar (<50 mg/dl) is frequent; responds to
  growth hormone therapy.
Serum phosphorus and alkaline phosphatase are decreased in pre-
  pubertal child but normal in adult-onset cases.
TSH deficiency (see Serum TSH, pp. 82–83; Hypothyroidism, pp.
  452–3; and Table 29-3, p. 458)
ACTH deficiency (see tests of adrenal function and adrenal-
  pituitary function, p. 478)
Gonadotropins are decreased or absent from urine in postpubertal
  patients (but increased levels occur in primary hypogonadism).

May Be Due To

Pituitary
> Congenital hypoplasia or absence, atrophy, fibrosis, cystic
>   changes with calcification, etc.

Hypothalamus
> Progressive degenerative changes, which may cause multiple
>   deficiency or isolated growth hormone deficiency types

Familial and genetic types
Isolated growth hormone deficiency or multiple deficiency types

HYPOPITUITARISM

Due To

Hypothalamic dysfunction
Idiopathic
Panhypopituitarism
Isolated growth hormone deficiency
Partial growth hormone deficiency (some forms of "constitutional short stature" with delayed onset of adolescence)
Suprasellar lesions
Psychosocial dwarfism
Pituitary disease
Pituitary necrosis secondary to postpartum hemorrhage (Sheehan's syndrome)
Craniopharyngioma, chromophobe adenoma, eosinophilic adenoma
Meningioma
Metastatic tumor (especially breast, lung)
Granulomatous lesions (e.g., sarcoidosis, Hand-Schüller-Christian syndrome)
See sections on secondary insufficiency of gonads, thyroid, adrenals. All of these may be involved or only one (usually gonadal first).
See Diabetes Insipidus (Central), p. 508.
Other conditions (e.g., trauma, infection)
Familial pituitary deficiency
End-organ resistance to growth hormone (normal or increased serum growth hormone with low somatomedin level)
Laron dwarfs (somatomedin levels are often undetectable and fail to rise when growth hormone is administered).
Protein-calorie malnutrition (e.g., kwashiorkor)

Serum somatomedin-C levels are 5–15% of normal in most hypopituitary dwarfs and 4–12 times normal in all active acromegaly patients.

ANOREXIA NERVOSA

No diagnostic or typical laboratory profile. Findings may be compensatory regulatory changes secondary to nutritional deprivation rather than primary hypothalamic dysfunction.
Prerenal azotemia with increased BUN and serum creatinine
Laboratory findings of hypothyroidism may be found in some patients (decreased T-3 and T-4 but normal TSH).
Basal growth hormone levels may be elevated as in other forms of protein-calorie malnutrition; response to stimulation tests is usually normal.
Plasma prolactin level is normal.
Plasma luteinizing and follicle-stimulating hormone concentrations are sometimes decreased.
Adrenal function abnormalities (e.g., normal or increased plasma corticoids, absence of diurnal variation of glucocorticoids, hyperresponsive ACTH test, low 17-KS and 17-KGS in urine; no adrenal insufficiency)

Atrophic vaginal smear
Elevated serum carotene (>250 mg/dl) and cholesterol
Leukopenia
Anemia is unusual.
Normal ESR
With marked loss of body weight, serum protein, potassium, and phosphorus may be decreased.
Vitamin deficiencies are rare.

DISEASES OF HYPOTHALAMUS

Due To
Neoplasms (primary or metastatic cancer, craniopharyngioma) (most frequent cause)
Inflammation (e.g., tuberculosis, encephalitis)
Trauma (e.g., basal skull fractures, gunshot wounds)
Intracranial xanthomatosis
Other

Manifestations
Sexual abnormalities are the most frequent manifestations of hypothalamic disease.
> Precocious puberty
> Hypogonadism (frequently as part of Fröhlich's syndrome)
Diabetes insipidus is a frequent but not an early manifestation of hypothalamic disease.

FRÖHLICH'S SYNDROME (ADIPOSOGENITAL DYSTROPHY)
Usually this is a transient functional disorder of the hypothalamus.
No deficiency of ACTH, TSH, or growth hormone is seen.
If there is a thyroid or adrenal hypofunction, an organic lesion, especially craniopharyngioma, should be suspected.

PRECOCIOUS PUBERTY IN BOYS
Precocious puberty occurs occasionally in boys with hepatoblastoma.
Urine contains chorionic gonadotropin-like substance.
There is secondary Leydig's cell hyperplasia.

See Pineal Tumors (below) and Diseases of Hypothalamus (above).

PINEAL TUMORS
Boys—precocious puberty in 30% of patients
Girls—delayed pubescence

Diabetes insipidus occurs occasionally.

CAUSES OF HYPONATREMIAS
Isotonic
> Hyperlipidemia (plasma looks milky)
> Hyperproteinemia (e.g., myeloma, macroglobulinemia)
Hypertonic
> Hyperglycemia (each increase of blood sugar of 100 mg/dl decreases serum sodium by 1.6 mEq/L)
> Excess mannitol treatment
Hypotonic
> Hypervolemic (e.g., congestive heart failure, cirrhosis, ne-

phrotic syndrome)—usually clinical edema. Urine is concentrated, urine sodium < 20 mEq/L. Serum uric acid and BUN tend to be increased.

Hypovolemic (excessive loss of fluids, e.g., GI tract, burns, fistulas, ascites, renal salt-wasting, excess diuretics)—urine is concentrated and urine sodium < 10 mEq/L except for patients on diuretics or with salt-wasting. Serum uric acid and BUN tend to be increased.

Normovolemic (e.g., SIADH, low reset osmostat syndrome, potassium depletion, renal failure, water poisoning)—usually no edema is present. Large amounts of sodium appear in urine.

Hyponatremic patients with BUN < 10 mg/dl and uric acid < 3.0 mg/dl should be considered to have SIADH or reset osmostat until proved otherwise.

"ESSENTIAL" HYPERNATREMIA

This condition is due to a hypothalamic lesion (e.g., infiltration of histiocytes, neoplasm) that causes impaired osmotic regulation but intact volume regulation of antidiuretic hormone secretion.

Serum sodium shows sustained but fluctuating elevations, corrected by administration of antidiuretic hormone but not corrected by fluid administration.

Serum osmolality is increased.

Serum creatinine, BUN, and creatinine clearance are normal.

There is spontaneous excretion of random specimens of urine that may be very concentrated or very dilute and opposite to plasma osmolality.

DIABETES INSIPIDUS (CENTRAL)

Due To

Idiopathic (now causes < 50% of cases)

Supra- and intrasellar tumors

> Histiocytosis X (eosinophilic granuloma) is most common.
> Neoplasms (e.g., craniopharyngioma, metastatic carcinoma of breast, cyst)
> Granulomatous lesions (e.g., sarcoidosis, tuberculosis)

Trauma, with or without basal skull fracture; neurosurgical procedures

Vascular lesions (e.g., aneurysms, thrombosis)

Meningitis, encephalitis, hypoxemic encephalopathy

Heredity (causes ≅ 1% of cases)

Large urine volume (4–15 L/24 hours) is characteristic.

Low urine specific gravity (usually < 1.005) and osmolality (50–200 mOsm/kg) is found.

Increased plasma osmolality (> 295 mOsm/kg)

Plasma vasopressin level is decreased.

Dehydration test fails to increase urine specific gravity or osmolality, and plasma osmolality remains elevated. After administration of vasopressin, urine osmolality will double.

Partial central diabetes insipidus shows intermediate values between complete central and normal.

See Table 29-16, p. 511.

Table 29-15. Comparison of Hyponatremia Due To Various Causes

Cause	Urine Sodium	Urine Osmolarity	BUN
Hypervolemic (e.g., congestive heart failure, cirrhosis, nephrotic syndrome)			
Early	D (usually < 10–15 mEq/L)	I (usually > 350–400 mOsm/L)	N
Late	D with isotonic urine is ominous finding	(> 200 mmol/kg)	I disproportionate to creatinine
Hypovolemic			
Extrarenal Gastrointestinal Skin (burns, sweat) Third space	D (< 10 mEq/L)	I (> 400 mOsm/L)	N
Renal Diuretic (most common) Chronic renal disease (especially interstitial) Mineralocorticoid deficiency	I (> 20 mEq/L)	Isotonic to plasma If severe volume contraction, 300–450 mOsm/kg	Usually I
Normovolemic			
SIADH (almost always) (see p. 512)	I (> 20 mmol/L)	I (> 200 mmol/kg) D in plasma	Often D (< 8–10 mg/dl)
Reset Osmostat (see p. 510)	V	V	V (N or D)

I = increased; D = decreased; V = variable.

NEPHROGENIC DIABETES INSIPIDUS

Due To

Chronic renal failure (e.g., glomerulonephritis, pyelonephritis, gout, analgesic nephropathy, polycystic kidneys, nephrosclerosis)

Diuretic phase of acute tubular necrosis

Following renal transplant or relief of urinary tract obstruction

Primary hyperaldosteronism

Sickle cell anemia

Multiple myeloma, amyloidosis, Sjögren's syndrome

Drugs (e.g., lithium, demeclocycline)

Prolonged potassium depletion and hypokalemia (Condition is reversed by restoring potassium level to normal.)

Prolonged hypercalciuria, usually with hypercalcemia (Condition is reversed by restoring the calcium level to normal.)

Hereditary renal tubular unresponsiveness to vasopressin due to X-linked genetic defect; severe form occurs in males; family history of this condition is frequent.

Laboratory findings are the same as in hypophyseal (central) diabetes insipidus except that nephrogenic type shows
Normal or increased plasma vasopressin level
Dehydration test does not cause urine osmolality to rise above plasma osmolality.
Dehydration test causes the plasma vasopressin level to increase.
Urine osmolality does not rise with subsequent injection of vasopressin.

See Table 29-16, p. 511.

DIABETES INSIPIDUS DUE TO HIGH-SET OSMORECEPTOR

This is a rare entity in which the set point for stimulating release of ADH is $\geq$ 300 mOsm/kg instead of the normal 285 mOsm/kg level. As plasma osmolality rises, patient becomes thirsty and drinks fluids, thereby diluting the plasma before it reaches the higher set level to stimulate release of ADH, initiating cycle of polyuria and polydipsia. If thirst center is also impaired, patient develops essential hypernatremia (see p. 508).

Plasma osmolality after dehydration is significantly higher than in normal state.

Urine osmolality does not change after administration of vasopressin.

PSYCHOGENIC POLYDIPSIA

Excessive intake of water causes loss of medullary sodium and urea to renal venous blood and abnormally reduced tonicity of renal medulla.

Test dose of vasopressin often shows failure to concentrate urine, simulating nephrogenic diabetes insipidus. However, the test will be normal when performed after restoration of normal hypertonicity of renal medulla by a period of high-sodium and low-water intake.

Table 29-16. Comparison of Different Types of Diabetes Insipidus

	After Dehydration[a]				After Pitressin,[b] Urine Osmolality (% change)	Plasma Vasopressin (pg/ml)
	Urine Specific Gravity	Urine Osmolality (mOsm/kg)	Plasma Osmolality (mOsm/kg)			
Normal	≥ 1.015	700–1400	288–291		No change (< 5%)	1.3–4.1
Central diabetes insipidus (complete)	< 1.010	50–200	310–320		Doubles (> 100%)[c]	< 1.1
Central diabetes insipidus (partial)	1.010–1.015	250–500	295–305		Increases (9–67%)[c]	
Nephrogenic diabetes insipidus	< 1.010	100–200	310–320		No change[d]	12–13 (> 2.7 in high Ca/low K type)
"High-set" osmoreceptor diabetes insipidus	≥ 1.015	700–1400	300–305		No change	
Primary (psychogenic) polydipsia	≥ 1.015	700–1200			No change after medullary washout; normal increase after high sodium diet	3.0–7.5

[a] Dehydration test: No fluid intake for 4–18 hours, measure urine osmolality and/or specific gravity hourly, weigh patient (or urine) frequently to avoid loss of > 3% of body weight (if > 3% of body weight, measure plasma and urine osmolality, and terminate test to avoid hypotension). After 3 successive hourly urine osmolality determinations indicate no further change (i.e., have reached a plateau), administer 5 units of vasopressin (Pitressin) subcutaneously, and 60 minutes later, measure urine osmolality.

[b] 1 hour after subcutaneous injection of 5 units of aqueous Pitressin.

[c] Useful to distinguish partial from complete central diabetes insipidus.

[d] Therefore differs from diabetes insipidus.

Plasma vasopressin levels must always be interpreted relative to plasma osmolality.

SYNDROME OF INAPPROPRIATE SECRETION OF ANTIDIURETIC HORMONE (SIADH)

Decreased serum sodium and osmolality

Increased urine sodium (> 20 mmol/L) with inappropriately high urine osmolality (> 200 mmol/kg)

Increased ratio of urine-serum osmolality

Normal serum potassium, CO_2, BUN, and creatinine

Decreased serum chloride

No evidence of cardiac, liver, kidney, adrenal, pituitary disease, or hypovolemia and not on drug therapy (especially diuretics)

Increased plasma vasopressin that is inappropriately elevated for the degree of plasma osmolality

Clinical and biochemical response to fluid restriction but not to administration of isotonic or hypertonic saline

Due To

CNS disease of all types (e.g., neoplastic, degenerative, infective, trauma, vascular, psychogenic)

Advanced endocrinopathies (e.g., myxedema, ACTH deficiency, adrenal insufficiency)

Neoplasms (most commonly oat cell carcinoma of lung; adenocarcinoma of lung, carcinoma of pancreas, carcinoma of duodenum, lymphoma)

Pulmonary infection (e.g., tuberculosis, pneumonia, chronic infections, aspergillosis)

Miscellaneous (e.g., acute intermittent porphyria, postoperative state)

Idiopathic

Various drugs

    Oral hypoglycemic agents (chlorpropamide, tolbutamide, phenformin, metformin)

    Antineoplastic agents (vincristine, cyclophosphamide)

    Diuretics (chlorothiazide)

    Sedatives, analgesics (morphine, barbiturates, acetaminophen)

    Psychotropic drugs (amitriptyline, phenothiazines)

    Miscellaneous (clofibrate, isoproterenol, nicotine)

NONENDOCRINE NEOPLASMS CAUSING ENDOCRINE SYNDROMES

Tumors secrete polypeptides that have hormonal activity.

Cushing's syndrome* due to

    Bronchogenic carcinoma and carcinoid

    Thymoma

    Hepatoma

    Carcinoma of ovary

    Also carcinoma of thyroid, pancreas, etc.

Hypoglycemia—patients show variable sensitivity to tolbutamide.

    Not associated with decreased serum phosphorus as in insulin-induced hypoglycemia.

---

*Cushing's syndrome due to these neoplasms cannot be distinguished from Cushing's syndrome due to excessive pituitary secretion of ACTH by use of dexamethasone suppression test or metyrapone test.

Bronchogenic carcinoma
Carcinoma of adrenal cortex (6% of patients)
Hepatoma (23% of patients)
Fibrosarcoma (most frequently)
Thyrotoxicosis—signs and symptoms are rare, but PBI, RAIU, etc., are increased.
Tumors of GI tract, hematopoietic, pulmonary, etc.
Trophoblastic tumors in women
Choriocarcinoma of testis
Precocious puberty in boys
Hepatoma
Hypercalcemia simulating hyperparathyroidism*
Renal carcinoma
Squamous cell carcinoma of upper respiratory tract
Carcinoma of breast (occurs in 15% of patients with bone metastases)
Malignant lymphoma, etc.

See also Carcinoid Syndrome (below), Precocious Puberty in Girls (p. 497), Precocious Puberty in Boys (p. 507), Secondary Polycythemia (p. 359), Inappropriate Secretion of Antidiuretic Hormone (p. 512).

CARCINOID SYNDROME
The syndrome occurs in patients with malignant carcinoids (argentaffinomas).
Urinary level of 5-hydroxyindoleacetic acid (5-HIAA) (a metabolite of serotonin) is increased, usually when tumor is far advanced (i.e., large liver metastases), but may not be increased despite massive metastases. Useful in confirming diagnosis in only 5–7% of patients with a carcinoid tumor.
Blood serotonin may be increased (> 0.4 μg/ml).
VMA and catecholamines in urine are at normal levels.
Laboratory findings due to other aspects of carcinoid syndrome are noted (e.g., pulmonary valvular stenosis, tricuspid valvular insufficiency, heart failure, liver metastases, electrolyte disturbances).

MULTIPLE ENDOCRINE NEOPLASIA (MEN SYNDROME)

	Wermer's Syndrome (MEN I)	Sipple's Syndrome (MEN II)
Characteristic neoplasms	Pituitary adenoma	Medullary thyroid carcinoma
	Islet cell adenoma or carcinoma	Pheochromocytoma
	Parathyroid adenoma or hyperplasia	Parathyroid adenoma or hyperplasia

---

*Serum calcium level is $\leqq 21$ mg/dl; less marked increase with renal tumors. Serum phosphorus is decreased in $> 50\%$ of patients. Alkaline phosphatase is frequently increased but not difficult to evaluate because of liver metastases. Serum proteins are not consistently abnormal. Urine calcium and phosphorus and renal tubular reabsorption of phosphate are not useful in differential diagnosis.

Associated neoplasms	Adrenal cortical adenoma	Mucosal neuroma
	Renal cortical adenoma	
	Thyroid carcinoma or hyperplasia	
	Carcinoid	
	Lipoma	
	Gastric polyp	
	Mediastinal endocrine neoplasm	
	Gastrinoma (see p. 475)	

Genitourinary Diseases

RENAL GLYCOSURIA
(glycosuria when serum glucose is < 180 mg/dl)
Due to proximal tubular damage
    Fanconi's syndrome
    Heavy-metal poisoning
    Nephrotic phase of glomerulonephritis
Due to increased glomerular filtration rate (GFR) without tubular
    damage
    Pregnancy
Oral and IV glucose tolerance tests normal
Ketosis absent

RENAL DISEASES THAT MAY BE FOUND WITHOUT PROTEINURIA
Congenital abnormalities
Renal artery stenosis
Obstruction of GU tract
Pyelonephritis
Stone
Tumor
Polycystic kidneys
Hypokalemic nephropathy
Hypercalcemic nephropathy
Prerenal azotemia

PROTEINURIA PREDOMINANTLY GLOBULIN RATHER THAN ALBUMIN
Multiple myeloma
Macroglobulinemia
Primary amyloidosis
Adult Fanconi's syndrome (some patients)

CAUSES OF PROTEINURIA
Benign: orthostatic, functional (e.g., fever, exercise), idiopathic
    transient proteinuria
Overload: myeloma (immunoglobulin light chains [Bence Jones]),
    monocytic leukemia (lysozyme)
Tubular: see p. 520.
Glomerular: see p. 520.

FUNCTIONAL PROTEINURIA
Occurs in 10% of hospital medical patients; associated with high
    fever, congestive heart failure, hypertension, stress, exposure to
    cold, strenuous exercise
Usually < 2 gm/day; transient; disappears with recovery from pre-
    cipitating cause
Progressive renal disease is not present.

Table 30-1. Urinary Findings in Various Diseases

Disease	Volume	Specific Gravity	Protein[a]	RBCs[b]	WBCs and Epithelial Cells[b]	Casts[c,d]	Comment
Normal	600–2500	1.003–1.030 0 (0.05 gm)	0 (0.05 gm)	0–occ. (0–0.130)	0–0.65	0–occ. (2000/24 hrs)	
Acute febrile states	D	I	Trace to +			Few	
Orthostatic proteinuria	N	N	I (up 1 gm)	N (0–0.130)	0–3	V; H & G	Normal when recumbent; abnormalities after upright posture
Glomerulonephritis Acute	D	I	2–4+ (0.5–5.0)	1–4+ (1–1000)	1–400	2–4+; H & G; *RBC, epithelial, mixed RBC & epithelial*	Gross hematuria or "smoky" urine
Latent			(0.1–2.0)	(1–100)	1–20	*RBC*, H & G	

Nephrosis ("nephrotic stage")	D	I	4+ (4–40)	0–few (0.5–50)	20–1000	*Epithelial, fatty, waxy;* H & G	Fat-laden epithelial cells, anisotropic fat in epithelial cells and casts
Terminal	I or D	D; fixed	1–2+ (2–7)	Trace–1+ (0.5–10)	1–50	1–3+ *Broad, waxy,* H & G, epithelial	
Pyelonephritis Acute	N	N	0–2+ (0.5–2)	Few (0–1)	20–2000	*WBC,* H & G, *bacteria*	Bacteria, many WBCs in clumps
Chronic	N or D	N or D	2–4+ (0–5)	Few (0–1)	0.5–50.0	Same as acute; often few or none	Same as acute; findings may be intermittent
Renal tuberculosis			(0.1–3)	(1–20)	1–50	WBC, H & G	Tubercle bacilli
Disseminated lupus erythematosus	V	N or D	1–4+ (0.5–20.0)	1–4+ (1–100)	1–100	1–4+ RBC, *fatty, waxy;* H & G	

Table 30-1. (continued)

Disease	Volume	Specific Gravity	Protein[a]	RBCs[b]	WBCs and Epithelial Cells[b]	Casts[c,d]	Comment
Toxemia of pregnancy	D	I	3–4+ (0.5–10.0)	0–1+ (0–1)	1–5	3–4+ H & G	
Malignant hypertension	V	D; fixed	1–2+ (1–10)	Trace–1+ (1–100)	1–200	1–2+ H & G, RBC, fatty	Increasing uremia with minimal or marked proteinuria and hematuria
Benign hypertension	N or I	N or D	0–1+	0–trace (1–5)		0–1+ H & G	
Congestive heart failure	D	I	1–2+	0–1+		1+ H & G	

						Frequently associated: pyelonephritis and nephrosclerosis
Intercapillary glomerulosclerosis (Kimmelstiel-Wilson syndrome)		1–4 + (2–20)	(0–1)	1–30	Epithelial, fatty, H & G	Frequently associated: pyelonephritis and nephrosclerosis
Lower nephron nephrosis Acute	D I		1–4+	1–4+	RBC; H & G, epithelial	
Diuretic	I	0.5–10.0	(0–1)	1–100	Broad, waxy, epithelial, H & G	

D = decreased; I = increased; occ. = occasionally; N = normal; V = variable; H & G = hyaline and granular casts.

a Protein = quantitative values in ( ) given as gm/24 hours.

b = quantitative values given as cells $\times 10^6/24$ hours.

c Cast requires examination of fresh or preserved urine and acid pH.

d Italics denote most important or diagnostic finding.

IDIOPATHIC TRANSIENT PROTEINURIA

Commonly found in routine urinalysis of asymptomatic healthy children and young adults initially but not subsequently

Progressive renal disease is not present.

ORTHOSTATIC (POSTURAL) PROTEINURIA

First morning urine before arising shows high specific gravity but no protein.

Protein only appears after person is upright; usually < 1.5 gm/day.

Urine microscopy is normal.

Is usually considered benign and slowly disappears with time but is still present in 50% of persons 10 years later

Progressive renal insufficiency does not occur.

Occurs in 15% of apparently healthy young men and 3% of otherwise healthy persons and some patients with resolving acute pyelonephritis or glomerulonephritis

Renal biopsy, electron microscopy, and immunofluorescent stains show pathologic changes in some patients.

SOME GLOMERULAR CAUSES OF PROTEINURIA

Immune complexes (e.g., nephritis of SLE, poststreptococcal glomerulonephritis, membranous glomerulonephritis)

Antiglomerular basement membrane antibodies (e.g., Goodpasture's syndrome)

Deposition of abnormal material (e.g., amyloidosis, diabetes mellitus)

Pyelonephritis

Vascular disease (e.g., hypertension, congestive heart failure)

Congenital (e.g., Alport's syndrome of progressive interstitial nephritis and progressive nerve deafness)

Unknown etiology (e.g., lipoid nephrosis)

Physiologic (e.g., orthostatic, exercise, fever)

SOME TUBULAR CAUSES OF PROTEINURIA*

Fanconi's syndrome

Renal tubular acidosis

Medullary cystic disease

Pyelonephritis

Cystinosis

Wilson's disease

Oculocerebral renal syndrome

Renal transplantation

Sarcoidosis

Cadmium toxicity

Balkan nephropathy

POSTRENAL PROTEINURIA

Primarily associated with epithelial tumors of bladder or renal pelvis

---

*Proteinuria refers to protein excretion of > 150 mg/day.

Significant proteinuria in adults: > 300 mg/24 hours

in children: > 10 $mg/m^2/24$ hours

Proteinuria > 1000 mg/24 hours makes diagnosis of renal parenchymal disease very likely.

Degree of proteinuria related to size and invasiveness; generally <
1 gm/day (similar to pyelonephritis) and includes IgM

RENAL TUBULAR ACIDOSIS
(glomerular function is either normal or relatively less impaired)

Primary Proximal Renal Tubular Acidosis
Usually occurs in males

Only clinical manifestation is retarded growth; renal and metabolic
complications are absent.

Good prognosis with clinical response to alkali therapy, which is
usually not permanently required

Caused by defect in bicarbonate reabsorption

> Low plasma bicarbonate concentration with hyperchloremic
> acidosis
>
> Alkaline urine that becomes acid if extracellular bicarbonate
> level is decreased below the patient's maximum reabsorptive
> limit
>
> Normal urine pH in the absence of bicarbonate in the urine

Secondary Proximal Renal Tubular Acidosis May Be Due To
Idiopathic or secondary Fanconi's syndrome (cystinosis, Lowe's syndrome, tyrosinemia, glycogen storage disease, Wilson's disease,
hereditary fructose intolerance, heavy-metal intoxication, toxic
effect of drugs such as outdated tetracycline)

Vitamin D–deficient rickets

Medullary cystic disease

Following renal transplantation

Nephrotic syndrome, multiple myeloma, renal amyloidosis

Primary Distal Renal Tubular Acidosis
(Butler-Albright syndrome)

Occurs predominantly in females (70%)

Often presents with complications (e.g., nephrocalcinosis, renal calculi, rickets, and osteomalacia) as well as growth retardation

Caused by inability of tubular cell to secrete enough H^+

> Hyperchloremic acidosis, hypokalemia, low plasma bicarbonate
> concentration
>
> Alkaline urine (pH 6.5–7.0) that persists at any level of plasma
> bicarbonate. Ammonium loading test shows inability to
> acidify urine below pH 6.5 and depressed rates of excretion of
> titratable acid and ammonium.
>
> Absence of other tubular defects
>
> Laboratory findings due to complications (e.g., nephrocal-
> cinosis, nephrolithiasis, interstitial nephritis)

Secondary Distal Tubular Acidosis May Also Be Due To
Increased serum globulins (especially gamma) (e.g., SLE, Sjögren's
syndrome, Hodgkin's disease, sarcoidosis, chronic active hepatitis, cryoglobulinemia)

Potassium depletion nephropathy

Pyelonephritis

Medullary sponge kidney

Ureterosigmoidostomy

Hereditary insensitivity to antidiuretic hormone (vasopressin)

Various renal diseases (e.g., obstructive uropathy, hypercalcemia,

potassium-losing disorders, medullary cystic disease, polyar-
teritis nodosa, amyloidosis, Sjögren's syndrome)
A variety of genetically transmitted disorders (e.g., Ehlers-Danlos
syndrome, Fabry's disease, hereditary elliptocytosis)
Starvation, malnutrition
Hyperthyroidism
Hyperparathyroidism
Vitamin D intoxication

*An incomplete or mixed tubular acidosis may be seen in obstructive
uropathy and in hereditary fructose intolerance.*

**Type 4 Renal Tubular Acidosis (a variety of conditions) Is
Characterized By**
Mild to moderate renal impairment
Hyperchloremic acidosis
*Hyper*kalemia
Acid urine pH
Reduced ammonium secretion
Frequently, tendency to lose sodium in urine
Some patients have decreased mineralocorticoid secretion due to

**Table 30-2. Differentiation of Distal and Proximal Renal Tubular
Acidosis**

	Distal (type 1)	Proximal (type 2)
Hypokalemia	Severe	Mild–moderate
Response to K⁺ therapy	Good	Poor
Bicarbonate Tm	Normal	Decreased
Bicarbonate loss in urine	Small	Large
Serum bicarbonate concentration	May be very low (<16 mEq/L)	Usually > 16–18 mEq/L
Urine pH when serum HCO_3^-:		
>20 mEq/L	> 5.5	> 5.5
< 15 mEq/L	> 5.5	May be < 5.4
Amount of HCO_3^- needed to correct acidosis	<2 mEq/kg/day	> 5 mEq/kg/day
Response to alkali therapy	Good	Poor
Glycosuria	Absent	Often present
Aminoaciduria	Absent	Often present
Hypercalciuria	Often present	Usually absent
Urinary citrate	Low	Normal
Fanconi's syndrome	No	Yes
Nephrocalcinosis	Often present	Rare
Nephrolithiasis	Often present	Absent
Renal insufficiency	Often present	Absent
Bone disease	Often present	Absent

isolated hypoaldosteronism; others have decreased tubular response to aldosterone.

ACUTE RENAL FAILURE

Early Stage

Urine is scant in volume (often < 50 ml/day) for $\leq$ 2 weeks; anuria for > 24 hours is unusual. Urine usually bloody (because RBCs and protein are present, specific gravity may be high). Urine sodium concentration is usually > 50 mEq/L.

WBC is increased even without infection.

BUN rises $\leq$ 20 mg/dl/day in transfusion reaction. It rises $\leq$ 50 mg/dl/day in overwhelming infection of severe crushing injuries. Serum creatinine is increased.

Hypocalcemia may occur.

Disproportionately increased serum phosphorus and creatinine indicate tissue necrosis.

Serum amylase and lipase may be increased without evidence of pancreatitis.

Metabolic acidosis is present.

Second Week

Urine becomes clear several days after onset of acute renal failure, and there is a small daily increase in volume. Daily volume of 400 ml indicates onset of tubular recovery. Daily volume of 1000 ml occurs in several days or $\leq$ 2 weeks. RBCs and large hematin casts are present. Protein is slight or absent.

Azotemia increases. BUN continues to rise for several days after onset of diuresis.

Metabolic acidosis increases.

Serum potassium is increased (because of tissue injury, failure of urinary excretion, acidosis, dehydration, etc.). ECG changes are always found when serum potassium is > 9 mEq/L but are rarely found when it is < 7 mEq/L.

Serum sodium is often decreased, with increased extracellular fluid volume.

Anemia usually appears during second week.

Bleeding tendency is frequent, with decreased platelets, abnormal prothrombin consumption, etc.

Diuretic Stage

Large urinary potassium excretion may cause decreased serum potassium level.

Urine sodium concentration is 50–75 mEq/L.

Serum sodium and chloride may increase because of dehydration from large diuresis if replacement of water is inadequate.

Hypercalcemia may occur in some patients with muscle damage.

Azotemia disappears 1–3 weeks after onset of diuresis.

Later Findings

Anemia may persist for weeks or months.

Pyelonephritis may first occur during this stage.

Renal blood flow and glomerular filtration rate do not usually become completely normal.

Recovery from renal cortical necrosis complicating pregnancy may be followed by renal calcification, contracted kidneys, and death from malignant hypertension in 1–2 years.

If there is complete anuria for > 48 hours, suspect urinary tract obstruction, bilateral renal vascular thrombi or emboli, cortical necrosis, or acute glomerulonephritis.

Suspect cortical necrosis if proteinuria is > 3–4 gm/L, BUN does not fall, and diuresis does not occur.

Suspect urinary tract obstruction if recurrent oliguria and increasing azotemia occur during period of diuresis.

Due To
Ischemic conditions
    Trauma
    Hemorrhage
    Shock
    Transfusion reaction
    Myoglobinuria
    Pancreatitis, gastroenteritis
Nephrotoxicity and hypersensitivity reaction
    Heavy metals (e.g., mercury, lead, arsenic, cadmium, bismuth)
    Organic solvents (e.g., carbon tetrachloride, ethylene glycol)
    Antibiotics (e.g., aminoglycosides, tetracyclines, penicillins, amphotericin)
    X-ray contrast media, especially in diabetic persons
    Pesticides, fungicides
    Others (e.g., phenylbutazone, phenytoin, calcium, uric acid)
Glomerular and vascular disease
    Acute poststreptococcal glomerulonephritis
    Rapidly progressive glomerulonephritis
    SLE
    Polyarteritis nodosa
    Subacute bacterial endocarditis
    Schönlein-Henoch purpura
    Goodpasture's syndrome
    Malignant hypertension
    Hemolytic-uremic syndrome
    Drug-related vasculitis
Large-vessel disease
    Bilateral renal vein thrombosis
    Renal artery occlusion (embolism, thrombosis, stenosis)
60% of cases of acute renal failure occur during or immediately after surgery, most often with cardiac or aneurysm surgery.
10% of cases are associated with obstetric problems.
30% of cases are associated with medical conditions, usually due to nephrotoxins or renal ischemic mechanisms.
Often, combined mechanisms (e.g., crushing injury with myoglobinemia plus shock, shock plus intravascular hemolysis from transfusion reaction or bacteremia or infusion of distilled water during prostatectomy)

Indications for Artificial Dialysis in Acute Renal Failure
Uncontrollable hyperkalemia
Increasing acidosis in which congestive heart failure contraindicates sodium administration
Simplified treatment of oliguria in presence of severe infection, tissue damage, etc.

Urinary Diagnostic Indices in Acute Renal Failure
(see Table 30-3)

These indices may be difficult or impossible to interpret if mannitol or diuretics have been administered.

Urinary sodium levels between 20 and 40 mEq/L may be found in all forms of acute renal failure.

Fractional excretion of sodium (FE_{Na})

$$= \frac{\text{urine sodium}}{\text{plasma sodium}} \div \frac{\text{urine creatinine}}{\text{plasma creatinine}} \times 100$$

is an index of renal ability to conserve sodium and represents percent of filtered sodium to reach the urine. Is considered the most reliable test to distinguish prerenal azotemia from acute tubular necrosis with oliguria.

Renal failure index (RFI) = urine sodium $\div \dfrac{\text{urine creatinine}}{\text{plasma creatinine}}$

measures Na conservation and concentrating ability.

Diagnostic indices in patients with reversible acute obstructive uropathy often resemble indices in acute tubular necrosis or prerenal azotemia; indices in obstructive uropathy depend on duration of obstruction and severity of azotemia. Indices are not useful for diagnosis of presence or absence of obstruction in cases of acute renal failure.

These diagnostic indices are often intermediate, and considerable overlapping of values is frequent, especially at time of initial evaluation. Even the total profile may not be useful in the individual case. Indices (especially RFI and FE_{Na}) are chiefly of value in *oliguric* patients for the early differentiation of prerenal azotemia from acute tubular necrosis; nonoliguric acute renal failure patients frequently have intermediate values between prerenal azotemia and oliguric renal failure. Differences between prerenal azotemia and acute tubular necrosis by these indices are particularly blurred in elderly patients as well as those with hypertensive or diabetic nephrosclerosis or other chronic parenchymal renal diseases.

Specimens for urinary indices should be obtained before onset of treatment if possible; several therapies may make results uninterpretable, especially administration of mannitol or furosemide. It is not necessary to obtain a timed 12- or 24-hour urine specimen, since the patient with acute renal failure cannot vary urine sodium or osmolality significantly from hour to hour; a random specimen is sufficient.

Urine sediment

   Renal tubular cells (or cellular casts) and pigmented granular casts indicate acute tubular necrosis.

   Sediment may be normal in interstitial nephritis, prerenal or postrenal azotemia.

   Eosinophils may be found in acute interstitial nephritis.

   RBC casts indicate glomerulonephritis, vasculitis, or microembolic disease.

   RBCs indicate blood from lower GU tract or from glomerulus.

   Myoglobin casts indicate myoglobinuria.

   WBCs in hyaline casts indicate renal parenchymal infection rather than lower GU tract infection.

Table 30-3. Urinary Diagnostic Indices in Acute Renal Failure

	Prerenal Azotemia	Acute Oliguric (acute tubular necrosis)	Acute Nonoliguric	Acute Obstructive	Acute Glomerulo-nephritis
Urine specific gravity	H (>1.015)	L (<1.010)			
Urine osmolality (mOsm/kg H$_2$O)	H > 500 (518 ± 35)	L < 350 (369 ± 20)	L (343 ± 17)	L (393 ± 39)	L (385 ± 61)
U/P Osmolality	>1.5	< 1.2	< 1.2		
Urine Na (mEq/L)	L < 20 (18 ± 3)	H > 40 (68 ± 5)	H > 40 (50 ± 5)	H > 40 (68 ± 10)	(22 ± 6)
U/P urea N	>8 (18 ± 7)	<3 (3 ± 0.5)	(7 ± 1)	>8 (8 ± 4)	>8 (11 ± 4)

U/P creatinine	> 40 (45 ± 6)	< 20 (17 ± 2)	< 20 (17 ± 2)	< 20 (16 ± 4)	< 20 (43 ± 7)
Renal failure index	< 1 (90% of cases) (0.6 ± 0.1)	> 2 (95% of cases) (10 ± 2)	(4 ± 0.6)	> 2 (8 ± 3)	< 1 (0.4 ± 0.1)
Fractional Na excretion (FE_{Na})	< 1 (85–94% of cases) (0.4 ± 0.1)	> 3 (7 ± 1.4)	> 3 (3 ± 0.5)	> 3 (6 + 2)	< 1 (0.6 ± 0.2)
BUN/creatinine ratio	> 15:1	≅ 10:1	≅ 10:1	> 15:1	≅ 10:1

H = high; L = low.

Source: Data from T. R. Miller et al, Urinary diagnostic indices in acute renal failure: A prospective study. *Ann. Intern. Med.* 89:47, 1978; D. E. Oken, On the differential diagnosis of acute renal failure. *Am. J. Med.* 71:916, 1981; and R. W. Schrier, Acute renal failure: Pathogenesis, diagnosis, and management. *Hosp. Pract.* (March 1981), p. 93.

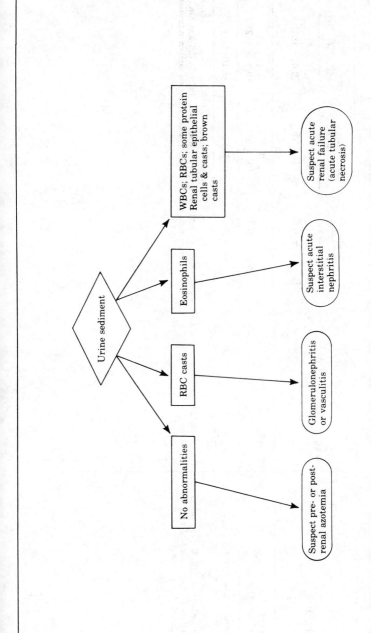

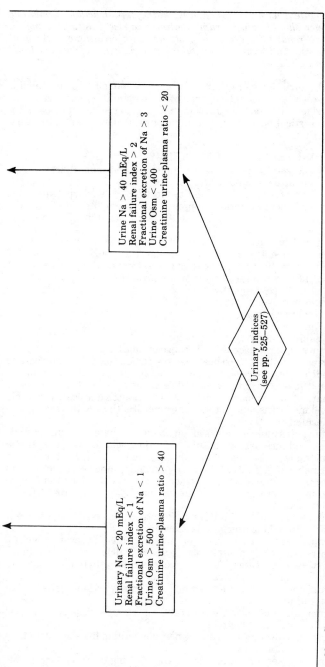

Fig. 30-1. Sequence of laboratory tests in differential diagnosis of acute renal failure. Data from R. W. Schrier, Acute renal failure: Pathogenesis, diagnosis, and management. *Hosp. Pract.*, March 1981, p. 93.)

In a patient with two functioning kidneys, obstruction of only one ureter should cause serum creatinine to rise ≅ 50% to 2 mg/dl; acute renal failure that is postrenal with creatinine > 2 mg/dl suggests that obstruction is bilateral or patient has only one functioning kidney.

Total anuria for more than 2 days is uncommon in acute tubular necrosis and should suggest other possibilities (e.g., ruptured bladder, GU tract obstruction, micro- or large-vessel disease, renal cortical necrosis, glomerulonephritis, allergic interstitial nephritis).

CHRONIC RENAL INSUFFICIENCY

BUN and serum creatinine are increased and renal function tests are impaired (see pp. 103–108).

Loss of renal concentrating ability (nocturia, polyuria, polydipsia) is an early manifestation of progressive renal functional impairment. Specific gravity is usually same as that of glomerular filtrate.

Abnormal urinalysis is usually the first finding. Variable abnormalities include proteinuria, hematuria, pyuria, granular and cellular casts and may be found in asymptomatic patients.

Hypotonic urine unresponsive to vasopressin may occur in
>   Obstructive uropathy
>   Chronic pyelonephritis
>   Nephrocalcinosis
>   Amyloidosis
>   Familial nephrogenic diabetes insipidus

Serum sodium is decreased (because of tubular damage with loss in urine, vomiting, diarrhea, diet restriction, etc.). The decrease is indicated by increased urine sodium levels (> 5–10 mEq sodium/ L). It may occur in any renal disease, especially when polyuria is marked, but is more common with obstructive uropathy, chronic pyelonephritis, and interstitial nephritis than with chronic glomerulonephritis.

Serum potassium is increased (on account of dietary sodium restriction and increased potassium ingestion, acidosis, oliguria, tissue breakdown). Decreased serum potassium with increased loss in urine (> 15–20 mEq/L) occurs in primary aldosteronism. It may occur in malignant hypertension, tubular acidosis, Fanconi's syndrome, nephrocalcinosis, diuresis during recovery from tubular necrosis.

Acidosis (due to renal failure to secrete acid as NH_4^+ and to reabsorb filtered bicarbonate) is present.

Serum calcium is decreased (because of decreased serum albumin, increased serum phosphorus, decreased calcium absorption in intestine, etc.). Tetany is rare. Secondary parathyroid hyperplasia may occur, but hypercalcemia is not found.

Serum phosphorus increases when creatinine clearance falls to ≅ 25 ml/minute.

Serum alkaline phosphatase may be normal or may be increased with renal osteodystrophy.

Serum magnesium increases when glomerular filtration rate falls to < 30 ml/minute.

Increase in serum uric acid is usually < 10 mg/dl. Secondary gout is rare. If clinical gout and family history of gout are present or if serum uric acid level is > 10 mg/dl, rule out primary gout nephropathy.

Increased serum amylase occurs frequently; baseline level should be obtained in dialysis patients to evaluate episodes of abdominal pain, since these patients have an increased incidence of pancreatitis.

Serum CK may be increased; a subset of uremic patients have persistent elevations of CK-MB fraction without evidence of cardiac disease.

Increased serum triglycerides, cholesterol, and VLDL lipoprotein (prebeta) is common as renal failure progresses.

Blood organic acids, phenols, indoles, certain amino acids, etc., are increased.

Normochromic normocytic anemia is usually proportionate to the degree of azotemia.

Bleeding tendency is evident. There may be decreased platelets, increased capillary fragility, abnormal TGT and prothrombin consumption (possible platelet defect), normal bleeding and clotting time.

Gastrointestinal hemorrhage from ulcers anywhere in GI tract may be severe.

Laboratory findings due to uremic pericarditis, pleuritis, and pancreatitis are noted. (BUN is usually > 100 mg/dl).

Laboratory findings due to uremic meningitis are noted ($\cong 50\%$ of these patients have increased CSF protein or leukocytes; protein may be reduced by hemodialysis; pleocytosis is not related to degree of azotemia).

Serum albumin and total protein are decreased. *When there is edema without hypoproteinemia or heart failure, rule out acute glomerulonephritis, toxemia of pregnancy, excess fluid intake in oliguria during acute tubular necrosis or terminal renal failure.*

Due To (see appropriate separate sections)
Primary renal disease
    Vascular lesions
        Nephrosclerosis, benign or malignant
        Renal artery stenosis or thrombosis
        Renal vein thrombosis
        Acute ischemic tubular necrosis, renal cortical necrosis
    Glomerular lesions—glomerulonephritis
    Tubular or interstitial lesions
        Infectious—chronic pyelonephritis, tuberculosis
        Other
            Fanconi's syndrome and renal tubular acidosis
            Heavy-metal poisoning
            Analgesic abuse
            Irradiation nephritis
            Chronic interstitial nephritis
    Congenital
        Polycystic disease
        Congenital hypoplastic kidneys
Systemic diseases involving the kidney
    Collagen diseases
        SLE
        Polyarteritis nodosa
        Scleroderma

Subacute bacterial endocarditis
Goodpasture's syndrome
Allergic purpura, etc.
Metabolic diseases
Diabetes mellitus
Gout
Amyloidosis
Hypercalcemic nephropathy
Hypokalemic nephropathy
Urinary tract obstruction
Neoplasms (e.g., carcinoma of cervix)
Stones
Retroperitoneal fibrosis
Prostatic enlargement
Urethral stricture
Congenital urethral or bladder defects
Other
Multiple myeloma
Sickle cell anemia
Hemoglobinurias (e.g., paroxysmal nocturnal)
Nephrotoxicity causes up to 20% of cases of chronic renal failure
and is a major cause of very rapid deterioration of renal function.

Chief Causes of Chronic Renal Failure Presenting for Dialysis

Glomerulonephritis	44%
Diabetic nephropathy	15%
Nephrosclerosis and renal vascular disease	12%
Congenital or hereditary disease (including polycystic kidney)	10%
Chronic pyelonephritis	6%
Others and unknown	15%

Chronic Renal Failure With Normal Urine May Occur In
Nephrosclerosis (e.g., aging, hypertension).
Renal tubular acidosis
Interstitial nephritis
Hypercalcemia
Potassium deficiency
Uric acid nephropathy
Obstruction (including retroperitoneal fibrosis)

POSTSTREPTOCOCCAL ACUTE GLOMERULONEPHRITIS IN CHILDREN

Evidence of infection with Group A beta-hemolytic *Streptococcus* by
Culture of throat
Serologic findings indicative of recent streptococcal infection
Antistreptolysin O titers (ASOT) of > 250 Todd units (increased in 80% of patients). Rise begins 10–14 days after
infection, peaks in 4–6 weeks, declines in next 4–6
months. Titer unreliable *after Streptococcus pyoderma.*

*Increased in ≅ 20% of cases of MPGN. Early use of penicillin
prevents rise of ASOT in either condition.*

Usually develops 7–21 days after a beta-hemolytic streptococcal
infection.

Antihyaluronidase
Antidesoxyribonuclease-beta
Antistreptokinase
Antidiphosphopyridine-nucleotidase
Antinicotinamide-adeninedenucleotidase, etc.
Combined use of serologic tests will establish recent streptococcal infection in virtually all cases.

Urine

Hematuria—gross or only microscopic. Microscopic hematuria may occur during the initial febrile upper respiratory infection (URI) and then reappear with nephritis in 1–2 weeks. It lasts 2–12 months; usual duration is 2 months.

RBC casts show glomerular origin of hematuria.

WBC casts and WBCs show inflammatory nature of lesion.

Granular and epithelial cell casts are present.

Fatty casts and lipid droplets occur several weeks later; not related to hyperlipemia.

Proteinuria is usually < 2 gm/day (but may be ≦ 6–8 gm/day). May disappear while RBC casts and RBCs still occur.

Oliguria is frequent.

Azotemia is found in ≅ 50% of patients.

Glomerular filtration rate usually shows greater decrease than renal blood flow; therefore filtration factor is decreased.

PSP excretion is normal in cases of mild to moderate severity; increases with progression of disease.

ESR is increased.

Leukocytosis is present, with increased polynuclear neutrophils.

There is mild anemia, especially when edema is present (may be due to hemodilution, bone marrow depression, or increased destruction of RBCs).

Serum proteins are normal or there is nonspecific decrease of albumin and increase of alpha$_2$ and sometimes of beta and gamma globulins.

Serum cholesterol may be increased.

Serum complement falls 24 hours before onset of hematuria and rises to normal within about 8 weeks when hematuria subsides.

Antihuman kidney antibodies are present in serum in 50% of patients.

Decreased urinary aldosterone occurs in the presence of edema.

Renal biopsy shows characteristic findings with electron microscopy and immunofluorescence.

Azotemia with high urine specific gravity and normal PSP excretion usually means acute glomerulonephritis.

Clinical Course

Patients usually recover in 2–4 weeks; 10% die within a few months. A second attack is unusual after repeated urinalysis is normal. Marked proteinuria for > 4 months suggests poor prognosis.

Acute nephritis in > 50% of cases of Schönlein-Henoch anaphylactoid purpura has a poorer initial prognosis and more often becomes chronic.

Acute glomerulonephritis in adults causes death or becomes chronic in 25–50% of patients. There may be a long latent period with only proteinuria and abnormal microscopic urinary findings.

Table 30-4. Classification of Glomerulonephritis

Glomerular Disorder	Situations in Which May Be Found	Hematuria		Proteinuria		Renal Function D	Comment
		Micro Present (% of cases)	RBC Casts Present (% of cases)	1–3 gm Present (% of cases)	>3 gm Present (% of cases)		
IgA nephropathy (Berger's disease)	Focal proliferative GN	100	50	75	25	25% or NS; N in 75%	
IgM mesangial nephropathy		50	Rare	50	50	>75% or NS	
Acute GN secondary to infection (focal GN)	SBE, bacterial pneumonia, viral infections, infection of implanted devices	100	50	75	25	100%	
Crescentic (rapidly progressive) GN Anti-GBM	Goodpasture's syndrome in 2/3 of patients	100	50	50	50	100%	90% have HLA-DR2 antigen.
Immune complex	SLE, mixed cryoglobulinemia, Schönlein-Henoch purpura	100	50	50	50	100%	

Category	Subtype							Comments
Non-immune complex								
GN and vasculitis	Wegener's granulomatosis, polyarteritis	100	50	50	50	100%		
	Wegener's granulomatosis, Schönlein-Henoch purpura, mixed cryoglobulinemia; Goodpasture's syndrome may occur							
Systemic lupus erythematosus (SLE)	Mesangial	15	50	10	50		N	Most frequent type in SLE.
	Focal proliferative	50		25	85		N or D	
	Membranous	50			75		N or D	
	Diffuse proliferative (<25% of SLE patients)	75					Usually D; uremia develops in 50–75%	
	Minimal change disease	Lipid nephrosis, nil disease	20			100	N	85% respond to steroid therapy. Most common cause of NS in children.
	Focal sclerosis	75		25	75		Usually D	Frequent cause of NS.

Table 30-4. (continued)

Glomerular Disorder	Situations in Which May Be Found	Hematuria		Proteinuria		Renal Function D	Comment
		Micro Present (% of cases)	RBC Casts Present (% of cases)	1–3 gm Present (% of cases)	>3 gm Present (% of cases)		
Membranous nephropathy	Usually idiopathic; occasionally due to heavy-metal toxicity (e.g., gold, mercury); persistent hepatitis B infection, other viruses (e.g., measles, varicella, Coxsackie), other infections (e.g., malaria, syphilis, leprosy, schistosomiasis), neoplasias (e.g., colon carcinoma, lymphoma, leukemia, sarcoidosis, SLE, others	50		25	75	N early; D late	Frequent cause of NS. Strong association with HLA-DR3. Spontaneous remission in 25–50%. Persistent proteinuria without progression in 25%. Progressive glomerular sclerosis causing renal failure in 50%. Common in adults; uncommon in children.

Membranoproliferative GN Type I (idiopathic)	SBE, essential cryo-globulinemia, Schön-lein-Henoch purpura, SLE, sickle cell disease, hepatitis and cirrhosis, C2 deficiency, alpha₁ antitrypsin deficiency, infected shunts (*Staphylococcus*, *Corynebacterium*)	75	25	50	50	Usually D; NS at onset in 75%	Renal failure within 5 years common in adults but may be delayed 10–20 years. Persistent marked proteinuria is poor prognostic sign. Renal vein thrombosis may occur.
Type II (idiopathic)	Infection with strepto-cocci, pneumococci, *Candida*, lipodys-trophy						

GN = glomerulonephritis; NS = nephrotic syndrome; SBE = subacute bacterial endocarditis; D = decreased; N = normal.

Goodpasture's syndrome occurs in < 5% of cases of GN.

Source: Data from W. A. Border and R. J. Glassock, Progress in treating glomerulonephritis. *Drug Therapy*, April 1981, p 97; T. R. Miller, et al., Urinary diagnostic indices in acute renal failure: A prospective study. *Ann. Intern. Med.* 89:47, 1978; D. E. Oken, On the differential diagnosis of acute renal failure. *Am. J. Med.* 71:916, Dec. 1981.

537

RAPIDLY PROGRESSIVE NONSTREPTOCOCCAL GLOMERULONEPHRITIS

Preceded by nonstreptococcal respiratory or gastrointestinal viral illness in many patients. Occasionally in SLE, subacute bacterial endocarditis, polyarteritis.

No cultural or serologic (e.g., ASOT) evidence of recent streptococcus infection.

Oliguria with urine volume often < 400 ml/day.

Hematuria is often gross.

RBCs, WBCs, and casts are present in urine.

Proteinuria is usually > 3 gm/day.

Azotemia is usually marked, with BUN > 80 mg/dl and serum creatinine > 10 mg/dl (in poststreptococcal type, BUN is usually 30–100 mg/dl and serum creatinine 1.5–4.0 mg/dl).

Serum complement levels are normal.

Renal biopsy and immunofluorescent antibody findings.

Prognosis is poorer than in poststreptococcal glomerulonephritis.

FOCAL PROLIFERATIVE GLOMERULONEPHRITIS

Attacks of hematuria usually occur at height of upper respiratory infection (bacterial or viral).

Serum IgA is often increased.

Azotemia is usually absent.

Proteinuria is slight or absent.

Prognosis is usually good, especially in children, but progressive nephritis causing renal failure is more common in adults.

MEMBRANOPROLIFERATIVE GLOMERULONEPHRITIS

Marked proteinuria and nephrotic type of syndrome is found in 70% of patients.

Normal serum C4 but prolonged or permanent depression of C3 is found in 60–80% of patients; clinical course is not related to serum complement levels.

Clinical course may be clinically active, or there may be periods of remission; 50% have chronic renal insufficiency in 10 years.

Renal biopsy and immunofluorescent antibody findings.

GFR < 80 ml/min/1.73 m^2 in two-thirds of patients

ACUTE INTERSTITIAL NEPHRITIS

(may occur following Group A beta-hemolytic streptococcal infection or as complication of drug therapy [especially antibiotics, allopurinol, and street drugs] or idiopathic)

Increased WBC, neutrophils, and bands

Increased absolute eosinophil count and blood IgE

Anemia with hemoglobin as low as 6.5 gm/dl; no evidence of hemolysis or iron deficiency; negative indirect Coombs' test; normal bone marrow. Anemia resolves when renal function becomes normal.

ESR is increased.

Serum IgG is usually increased; serum complement is normal.

Varying degrees of renal insufficiency with increased BUN and creatinine, hyponatremia, hyperchloremic metabolic acidosis, decreased serum albumin

Oliguria may occur.

Urinalysis

    Low osmolality and specific gravity

Microscopic hematuria

Proteinuria is usually mild to moderate, < 1.0 gm/m^2/24 hours, unless nephrotic syndrome is present.

Pyuria is minimal or absent; bacteriuria is absent and cultures negative. Eosinophils may be found.

Casts are uncommon.

Glycosuria without hyperglycemia and reduced TRP may occur.

Enlarged, poorly functioning kidneys may be demonstrated by IVP, ultrasound, or renal scan.

Nephrotic syndrome may occur.

Biopsy of kidney establishes the diagnosis and is usually more severe than indicated by urinalysis and renal studies.

Long-term prognosis is good in children but poor in adults.

BERGER'S DISEASE (IgA-IgG NEPHROPATHY)
(a focal proliferative glomerulonephritis, immunologic mediation)

Painless recurrent gross hematuria and minimal proteinuria, often associated with (rather than following by 4–10 days) an acute nonstreptococcal upper respiratory or GI tract infection. Recurrent episodes of gross hematuria commonly occur with acute infections. Microhematuria is usually present between acute exacerbations.

Disease may be progressive in up to 10% of adults.

NEPHROTIC SYNDROME

Characterized By

Marked proteinuria—usually > 4.5 gm/day; usually exclusively albuminuria in children with lipoid nephrosis, but in glomerulonephritis, high- and low-molecular-weight proteins are present.

Decreased serum albumin—usually < 2.5 gm/dl—and total protein

Increased serum cholesterol (free and esters)—usually > 350 mg/dl. (Low or normal serum cholesterol occurs with poor nutrition and suggests poor prognosis.)

Increased serum phospholipids, neutral fats, triglycerides, low-density beta-lipoproteins, and total lipids

Serum alpha$_2$ and beta globulins are markedly increased, gamma globulin is decreased, alpha$_1$ is normal or decreased. If gamma globulin is increased, rule out systemic disease (e.g., SLE).

Urine containing doubly refractive fat bodies as seen by polarizing microscopy; many granular and epithelial cell casts

Hematuria—may be present in 50% of patients but is usually minimal and not part of syndrome

Azotemia—may be present but not part of syndrome

Changes secondary to proteinuria and hypoalbuminemia (e.g., decreased serum calcium, decreased serum ceruloplasmin, increased fibrinogen)

Increased ESR due to increased fibrinogen

Changes due to primary disease (see p. 540)

Increased susceptibility to infection (most frequently peritonitis) during periods of edema

Serum C3 complement is normal in idiopathic lipoid nephrosis but decreased when there is underlying glomerulonephritis.

Associated renal vein thrombosis has been reported in 5–62% of patients, especially when due to membranous nephropathy, membranoproliferative glomerulonephritis, lipoid nephrosis, rapidly progressive glomerulonephritis.

Associated neoplasm in 10% of adults and 15% > age 60 years
In adult with minimal-change nephrotic syndrome without evident cause, first rule out Hodgkin's disease. With membranous lesion, carcinoma may be more likely.

Etiology
Renal
Glomerulonephritis (>50% of patients)
Lipoid nephrosis (10% in adults; 80% in children)
Systemic
Diabetic glomerulosclerosis (15% of patients)
SLE (20% of patients)
Amyloidosis (primary and secondary)
Schönlein-Henoch purpura
Multiple myeloma
Goodpasture's syndrome
Berger's disease
Polyarteritis
Takayasu's syndrome
Sarcoidosis
Sjögren's syndrome
Dermatitis herpetiformis
Venous obstruction
Obstruction of inferior vena cava (thrombosis, tumor)
Constrictive pericarditis
Tricuspid stenosis
Congestive heart failure
Infections
Bacterial (poststreptococcal glomerulonephritis, bacterial endocarditis; syphilis, leprosy, etc.)
Viral (hepatitis B; also cytomegalovirus, infectious mononucleosis, varicella)
Protozoal (malaria, toxoplasmosis)
Parasitic (schistosomiasis, filiariasis)
Allergic (e.g., serum sickness, bee sting)
Neoplastic (e.g., Hodgkin's disease; carcinoma of colon, lung, stomach, and others; lymphomas and leukemia)
Toxic (e.g., heavy metals; penicillamine, mephenytoin, other drugs)
Hereditary/familial (e.g., Alport's syndrome, Fabry's disease, sickle cell disease)
Miscellaneous
Preeclampsia
Chronic allograft rejection
Others

CHRONIC GLOMERULONEPHRITIS

Various Clinical Courses
Early death after marked proteinuria, hematuria, oliguria, progressive increasing uremia, anemia
Intermittent or continuous or incidental proteinuria, hematuria with slight or absent azotemia, and normal renal function tests (may develop into late renal failure or may subside)
Exacerbation of chronic nephritis (with accentuation of proteinuria, hematuria, and decreased renal function) shortly following streptococcal upper respiratory infection
Nephrotic syndrome (see p. 539)

Compared to pyelonephritis, chronic glomerulonephritis shows lipid droplets and epithelial and RBC casts in urine, more marked proteinuria (> 2–3 gm/day), poorer prognosis for equivalent amount of azotemia.

NEPHROSCLEROSIS

"Benign" nephrosclerosis ("essential hypertension")

Urine contains little or no protein or microscopic abnormalities.

10% of patients develop marked renal insufficiency.

"Accelerated" nephrosclerosis ("malignant hypertension")

Syndrome may occur in the course of "benign" nephrosclerosis, glomerulonephritis, unilateral renal artery occlusion, or any cause of hypertension.

Increasing uremia is associated with minimal or marked proteinuria and hematuria.

RENAL CALCULI

(autopsy incidence = 1.12%; cause of death = 0.38%)

Calcium oxalate alone or with phosphate is the constituent of kidney stones in 65% of patients in the United States.

35% of patients have increased urinary calcium, i.e., > 250 mg/24 hours in females and > 300 mg/24 hours in males (50–75% of hyperparathyroidism patients have renal calculi; ≅ 5% of patients with nephrolithiasis have primary hyperparathyroidism).

20–30% of patients have

Bone diseases—destructive (e.g., metastatic tumor) or osteoporosis (e.g., immobilization, Paget's disease, Cushing's syndrome)

Milk-alkali (Burnett's) syndrome

Hypervitaminosis D

Sarcoidosis

Renal tubular acidosis—Type I (hypercalciuria, highly alkaline urine, serum calcium usually normal)

Hyperthyroidism

Other

50–60% of patients have idiopathic hypercalciuria (p. 542).

Oxalate is the constituent of renal calculi in 65% of all patients, but hyperoxaluria is a relatively rare cause of these calculi and is due to primary hyperoxaluria (see p. 542).

Magnesium ammonium phosphate is the constituent of renal calculi in 15% of patients. It occurs almost exclusively in patients with recurrent urinary tract infections by urea-splitting organisms, particularly *Proteus* species (but should rule out *Klebsiella, Pseudomonas, Serratia, Enterobacter),* and in patients with persistently alkaline urine.

Cystine stones form when urine contains > 300 mg/day of cystine in congenital familial cystinuria. Urine shows cystine crystals. Cyanide-nitroprusside test is positive. Causes 1–2% of all stones.

Uric acid is present in calculi in 10% of patients.

Gout—25% of patients with primary gout and 40% of patients with marrow-proliferative disorders have calculi.

Urine is more acid than normal (e.g., patients with chronic diarrhea, ileostomy).

> 50% of patients with urinary calculi have normal serum and urine uric acid levels.

Xanthine is present in children with inborn error of metabolism.
Hereditary glycinuria is a rare familial disorder associated with renal calculi.

Microscopic hematuria is found in 80% of patients.
In renal colic, hematuria and proteinuria are present, and there is an increased WBC due to associated infection.

IDIOPATHIC HYPERCALCIURIA
Increased 24-hour excretion of urinary calcium
>   >300 mg in males or >250 mg in females
>   >4 mg/kg (either sex)
>   >140 mg/gm of urinary creatinine is most useful in short or obese patients.
Normal blood calcium levels.
Serum 1,25-dihydroxyvitamin D_3 levels are usually high.
Absence of underlying cause of hypercalciuria (see p. 165); may be familial
Occurs in ≅ 40% of patients who form calcium renal stones
Occurs in 5–10% of general population
Two types
>   "Renal": Hypercalciuria persists despite absent dietary calcium in intestine following fasting (see below). One-tenth as common as absorptive type.
>   "Absorptive": 2-hour urine collection after fasting shows calcium-creatinine ratio < 0.11, but in renal hypercalciuria is > 0.15. 24-hour urine falls to < 200 mg/24 hours following low-calcium diet (400 mg/day) for 3–4 days.

PRIMARY HYPEROXALURIA
Rare, autosomal recessive inherited disorder of glyoxylate metabolism causing
>   Calcium oxalate renal lithiasis, interstitial nephritis, uremia
>   Urinary oxalate is usually > 100 mg/24 hours unless renal function is diminished.

SECONDARY HYPEROXALURIA
Due To
Increased oxalate in diet
Ingestion of oxalate precursors (e.g., ascorbic acid, ethylene glycol)
Methoxyflurane anesthesia
Primary diseases of ileum with normal colon absorption (e.g., bypass surgery, Crohn's disease) causing increased absorption of dietary oxalate. Urinary oxalate is usually 50–100 mg/24 hours.

OBSTRUCTIVE UROPATHY
(unilateral or bilateral; partial or complete)
Partial obstruction of both kidneys may cause increasing azotemia with normal or increased urinary output (due to decreased renal concentrating ability).
Partial obstruction may cause inexplicable wide variations in BUN and urine volume in patients with azotemia. PSP excretion is less in first 15-minute period than in any later period. There is considerable PSP excretion after the 2-hour test period.
In unilateral obstruction, BUN usually remains normal unless underlying renal disease is present.

Table 30-5. Characteristic Features in Differential Diagnosis of Hypercalciuria*

Measurement	Primary Hyperparathyroidism	Absorptive Hypercalciuria	Renal Hypercalciuria	Normocalciuric Nephrolithiasis
Serum calcium	I	N	N	N
Urine calcium Fasting	I	N	I	N
After calcium load	I	I	I	N or I
Urine cyclic AMP Fasting	I in 30%	N	Usually I	N
After calcium load	I in 82%	N	N	N
Serum parathormone	I	N	I	N

N = normal; I = increased.
*See reference given as source for normal values and test procedures.
*Source: Data from C.Y.C. Pak et al., A simple test for the diagnosis of absorptive, resorptive and renal hypercalciurias. *N. Engl. J. Med.* 292:497, 1975.

Laboratory findings due to superimposed infection or underlying disease are noted.

Laboratory findings due to underlying disease

Obstruction of bladder (e.g., benign prostatic hypertrophy, carcinoma of prostate or bladder, urethral stricture, neurogenic bladder dysfunction [multiple sclerosis, diabetic neuropathy])

Obstruction of both ureters (e.g., infiltrating neoplasm [especially of uterine cervix], bilateral calculi, congenital anomalies, retroperitoneal fibrosis)

If ureter is obstructed > 4 months, functional recovery is unlikely. When obstruction is relieved, most functional recovery takes place in 2–3 weeks; then there is continued improvement for several months.

PYELONEPHRITIS

Bacteriuria (see p. 157–158). Colony count of > 100,000/ml of urine (properly collected) indicates active infection. If the count is 10,000 to 100,000/ml, it should be repeated. Bacteria seen on Gram's stain of uncentrifuged urine indicates bacteriuria.

A culture should be performed for identification of the specific organism and determination of antibiotic sensitivity.

Microscopic examination of urine sediment: WBC casts are very suggestive of pyelonephritis. Glitter cells may be seen.

Pyuria is present in only 50% of patients with chronic urinary tract infection and asymptomatic bacteriuria. Bacteriuria and pyuria are often intermittent; in the chronic atrophic stage of pyelonephritis, they are often absent.

Urine concentrating ability is decreased relatively early in chronic infection compared to other renal diseases.

Albuminuria is usually < 2 gm/24 hours (≦2+ qualitative) and therefore helps to differentiate pyelonephritis from glomerular disease, in which albuminuria is usually > 2 gm/24 hours. Albuminuria may be undetectable in a very dilute urine associated with fixed specific gravity.

There is a decrease in 24-hour creatinine clearance before a rise in BUN and blood creatinine takes place.

Hyperchloremic acidosis (due to impaired renal acid excretion and bicarbonate reabsorption) occurs more often in chronic pyelonephritis than in glomerulonephritis.

Renal blood flow and glomerular filtration show parallel decrease proportional to progress of renal disease. Comparison of function in right and left kidneys shows more disparity in pyelonephritis than in diffuse renal disease (e.g., nephrosclerosis, glomerulonephritis).

Fluctuation in renal insufficiency (e.g., due to recurrent infection, dehydration) with considerable recovery is more marked and frequent in pyelonephritis than in other renal diseases.

Laboratory findings of associated diseases, e.g., diabetes mellitus, urinary tract obstruction (stone, tumor, etc.), neurogenic bladder dysfunction, are present.

Laboratory findings due to sequelae (e.g., papillary necrosis, bacteremia) are present.

When urine cultures are persistently negative in the presence of other evidence of pyelonephritis, specific search should be made for tubercle bacilli (e.g., culture, guinea pig inoculation).

"Cured" patient should be followed with routine periodic urinalysis and colony count for at least 2 years because asymptomatic recurrence of bacteriuria is common.

TUBULOINTERSTITIAL NEPHROPATHY
Three basic patterns of functional disturbance depending on site of injury: proximal tubular acidosis, distal tubular acidosis, medullary (reduced ability to concentrate urine, causing nephrogenic diabetes insipidus in most severe form)

Due To
Bacterial infection (e.g., acute and chronic pyelonephritis)
Drugs (e.g., acute interstitial nephritis [see pp. 538–539], analgesic nephropathy)
Immune disorders (e.g., acute interstitial nephritis [see pp. 538–539], transplant rejection, associated with glomerulonephritis, Sjögren's syndrome)
Metabolic disorders (e.g., urate, hypercalcemic, hypokalemic, oxalate nephropathies)
Heavy metals (e.g., lead, cadmium)
Physical factors (e.g., obstructive uropathy, radiation nephritis)
Neoplasia (e.g., myeloma kidney, infiltration in leukemia and lymphoma)
Hereditary renal diseases (e.g., medullary cystic disease, familial interstitial nephritis, Alport's syndrome)
Miscellaneous conditions (e.g., granulomatous diseases [sarcoidosis, tuberculosis, leprosy], Balkan nephropathy)

LABORATORY FINDINGS THAT FAVOR CHRONIC TUBULOINTERSTITIAL RATHER THAN GLOMERULOVASCULAR RENAL DISEASE
Minimal or absent proteinuria
Moderate polyuria
Hyperchloremic metabolic acidosis
Severe sodium wasting
Disproportionate hyperkalemia
Mild or absent hypertension

PAPILLARY NECROSIS OF KIDNEY
Findings of associated diseases
    Diabetes mellitus
    Urinary tract infection
    Chronic overuse of phenacetin
Sudden diminution in renal function; occasionally oliguria or anuria with acute renal failure
Hematuria

RENAL ABSCESS
(due to metastatic infection not related to previous renal disease)
Urine
    Trace of albumin
    Few RBCs (may have transient gross hematuria at onset)
    No WBCs
    Very many gram-positive cocci in stained sediment
WBC high (may be > 30,000/cu mm)

Complications
Sudden rupture into renal pelvis—urine suddenly cloudy and contains very many WBCs and bacteria
Renal carbuncle formation
Rupture into perirenal space
Secondary pyelonephritis

PERINEPHRIC ABSCESS
Laboratory findings due to underlying or primary diseases
> Hematogenous from distant foci (e.g., furuncles, infected tonsils) usually due to staphylococci and occasionally streptococci
>
> Direct extension from kidney infection (e.g., pyelonephritis, pyonephrosis) due to gram-negative rods and occasionally tubercle bacilli
>
> Infected perirenal hematoma (e.g., due to trauma, tumor, polyarteritis nodosa) due to various organisms

Urine changes due to underlying disease
> Urine may be normal and sterile. *(Do acid-fast smear and culture for tubercle bacilli.)*

Increased polynuclear leukocytes
Increased ESR
Positive blood culture (some patients)

RENAL TUBERCULOSIS
Should be ruled out when there is unexplained albuminuria, pyuria, microhematuria, but cultures for pyogenic bacteria are negative, especially in presence of TB elsewhere
Urine culture for TB
Guinea pig inoculation

See Table 30-1, pp. 516–519.
See Tuberculosis, pp. 580–581, for general findings.

HORSESHOE KIDNEYS
Laboratory findings due to complications
> Renal calculi
> Pyelonephritis
> Hematuria

POLYCYSTIC KIDNEYS
Polyuria is common.
Hematuria may be gross and episodic or an incidental microscopical finding (50% of patients).
Proteinuria may be an incidental finding of routine analysis (75% of patients).
Renal calculi may be associated (10% of patients).
Superimposed pyelonephritis is frequent (33% of patients).
Death occurs within 5 years after BUN rises to 50 mg/dl (33% of patients).
Death usually occurs in early infancy or in middle age when superimposed nephrosclerosis of aging or pyelonephritis has exhausted renal reserve.
Cerebral hemorrhage causes death in 10% of patients; intracranial berry aneurysms are frequently associated.
Autosomal dominant transmission

Diagnosed 1 : 3,000 patients
Accounts for 5% of the hemodialysis population
Increased incidence of gout in patients with polycystic kidneys
Anemia of renal failure is less severe than in other forms of kidney
    disease.

MEDULLARY CYSTIC DISEASE
Anemia is often severe and out of proportion to degree of renal
    failure.
Polyuria
Salt-losing syndrome
Death from renal insufficiency (may take many years)

Urinalysis shows minimal or no proteinuria; presence of RBCs,
    WBCs, casts, or bacteria is rare. Specific gravity may be de-
    creased.
Serum alkaline phosphatase may be increased when bone changes
    occur.

SPONGE KIDNEY
Findings due to complications
    Hematuria
    Infection
    Renal calculi within cysts
Disease asymptomatic, not progressive

HEREDITARY NEPHRITIS
May be classified into two types
    Angiokeratoma corporis diffusum (familial condition of abnor-
        mal glycolipid deposition in glomerular epithelial cells, ner-
        vous system, heart, etc.)
        Proteinuria begins in second decade.
        Urine may contain lipid globules and foam cells.
        Uremia occurs by fourth or fifth decade.
    Familial autosomal dominant disease associated with nerve
        deafness and lens defects (Alport's syndrome) is rare. Renal
        disease is progressive.
        Hematuria, gross or microscopic, is common; more marked
            after occurrence of unrelated infection. Other laboratory
            findings are the same as in other types of nephritis.

ARTERIAL INFARCTION OF KIDNEY
Microscopic or gross hematuria is usual.
BUN is normal unless other renal disease is present.
In some cases, urine shows no albumin or abnormal sediment at
    time of analysis.
WBC, SGOT, SGPT are increased if area of infarction is large; peak
    by second day; return to normal by fifth day.
Serum and urine LDH may be increased markedly.
Increased serum LDH is the most sensitive enzyme abnormality.
CRP and serum LDH peak on third day; return to normal by tenth
    day.
Changes in serum enzyme levels, WBC, CRP, ESR are similar in
    time changes to those in myocardial infarction.
Plasma renin activity may rise on second day, peak about 11th day,
    and remain elevated for more than a month.

Increased serum alkaline phosphatase occurs in about one-third of cases and is the least discriminating enzyme abnormality.

Laboratory findings due to infarction of other organs (e.g., brain, heart)

RENAL VEIN THROMBOSIS

Hematuria

Microscopic pyuria

Proteinuria and decreased creatinine clearance show marked variability from day to day.

Postprandial glycosuria

Nephrotic syndrome (see pp. 539–540)

Hyperchloremic acidosis (renal tubular acidosis)

Hyperosmolarity

Oliguria and uremic death if infarction is extensive

Anemia is common.

Platelet count may be decreased.

Increased fibrin degradation products in blood may be > 3 times normal limits (consumptive coagulopathy/DIC).

Laboratory findings due to thromboembolic disease elsewhere (e.g., pulmonary)

Laboratory findings due to underlying causative conditions (e.g., hypernephroma, metastatic cancer, trauma, amyloidosis, diabetic glomerulosclerosis, hypertension, papillary necrosis, DIC, sickle cell disease, polycythemia, heart failure, etc.)

See Nephrotic Syndrome, pp. 539–540.

RENAL ARTERIOVENOUS FISTULA

Hematuria

Laboratory findings due to congestive heart failure and hypertension

RENAL CHANGES IN BACTERIAL ENDOCARDITIS

There are three types of pathologic changes: diffuse subacute glomerulonephritis, focal embolic glomerulonephritis, microscopic or gross infarcts of kidney.

Laboratory findings due to bacterial endocarditis are noted (see pp. 209–210).

Albuminuria is almost invariably present, even when no renal lesions are found.

Hematuria (usually microscopic, sometimes gross) is usual at some stage of the disease, but repeated examinations may be required.

Renal insufficiency is frequent (15% of cases during active stage; 40% of fatal cases).

BUN is increased—usually 25–75 mg/dl.

Renal concentrating ability is decreased.

AZOTEMIA DUE TO CARDIAC FAILURE*

Parallels the degree of heart failure

Serum creatinine rarely > 4 mg/dl even when BUN > 100 mg/dl in pure prerenal azotemia.

---

*May also occur in other functional forms of acute renal failure (e.g., hepatorenal syndrome, volume contraction).

Urine is hypertonic (increased osmolality) with low sodium concentration (<10 mEq/L).

Protein excretion is frequently increased but rarely > 2 gm/24 hours.

Urine sediment may contain granular or hyaline casts, but cellular or pigmented casts are conspicuously absent.

In contrast:

Acute tubular necrosis (may complicate cardiac failure; due to cardiogenic shock, excessive use of diuretics or vasodilators) shows

Urine osmolality approaches that of plasma.

Urine sodium is usually high (40–80 mEq/L).

Urine sediment contains many renal tubular cells and casts and many narrow (often pigmented) casts.

KIDNEY DISORDERS IN GOUT

Kidney stones occur in 15% of patients with gout; may occur in absence of arthritis.

Early renal damage is indicated by decreased renal concentrating ability, mild proteinuria, and decreased PSP excretion.

Later renal damage is shown by slowly progressive azotemia with slight albuminuria and slight or no abnormalities of urine sediment.

Arteriolar nephrosclerosis and pyelonephritis are usually associated.

Renal disease causes death in ≦ 50% of patients with gout.

It has been suggested that acute uric acid nephropathy may be differentiated from other forms of acute renal failure if ratio of urine urate–urine creatinine > 1.0 in an adult (many children under age 10 years have ratio > 1.0).

KIMMELSTIEL-WILSON SYNDROME (DIABETIC INTERCAPILLARY GLOMERULOSCLEROSIS)

The disease usually occurs after associated diabetes mellitus has been present > 10 years; it is not related to control of diabetes. Occasionally it is associated only with prediabetes.

Proteinuria is usual (may be earliest clinical clue) and may be marked (often more than 5 gm/day). Nephrotic syndrome is often associated.

Urine shows many hyaline and granular casts and double refractile fat bodies. Hematuria is rare.

Serum protein is decreased.

Azotemia develops gradually after several years of proteinuria.

Biopsy of kidney is diagnostic.

Laboratory findings are those due to frequently associated infections of the urinary tract.

See sections on diabetes mellitus, acidosis, papillary necrosis, urinary tract infection, diabetic neuropathy.

RENAL DISEASE IN POLYARTERITIS NODOSA

Renal involvement occurs in 75% of patients.

Azotemia is often absent or only mild and slowly progressive.

Albuminuria is always present.

Hematuria (gross or microscopic) is very common. Fat bodies are frequently present in urine sediment.

There may be findings of acute glomerulonephritis with remission or early death from renal failure.

Always rule out polyarteritis in any case of glomerulonephritis, renal failure, or hypertension that shows unexplained eosinophilia, increased WBC, or laboratory evidence of involvement of other organ systems.

NEPHRITIS OF SYSTEMIC LUPUS ERYTHEMATOSUS (SLE)

Renal involvement occurs in two-thirds of patients with SLE.
Nephritis of SLE may occur as acute, latent, or chronic glomerulonephritis, nephrosis, or asymptomatic albuminuria.
Urine findings are as in chronic active glomerulonephritis.
Azotemia or marked proteinuria usually indicates death in 1–3 years.
Signs of SLE (e.g., positive LE test) may disappear during active nephritis, nephrosis, or uremia.
Examination of needle biopsy should always include immunofluorescent and electron as well as light microscopy. May show membranous glomerulonephritis, diffuse proliferative glomerulonephritis, focal proliferative glomerulonephritis, or mesangial lesions.

Table 30-6. Comparison of Clinical and Morphologic Types of SLE Nephritis

	Mesangial Changes (% of Pts)	Focal Proliferative GN (% of Pts)	Diffuse Proliferative GN (% of Pts)	Membranous GN (% of Pts)
% of total pts	39	27	16	18
Hematuria, pyuria	13	53	78	50
Proteinuria	36	67	89	100
Nephrotic syndrome	0	27	56	90
Azotemia	13	20	22	10
Decreased complement	54	77	100	75
Increased anti-DNA	45	75	80	33
Decreased complement & increased anti-DNA	36	63	80	33
Hypertension	22	40	56	50
Prognosis	Better	Worse	Worse	Better

Source: Appel, GB. The course of management of lupus nephritis. *Intern. Med.* 2:82, Feb 1981

RENAL DISEASE IN SCLERODERMA

Renal involvement occurs in two-thirds of patients; one-third die of renal failure.

Proteinuria may be minimal and is usually < 2 gm/day; this may be the only finding for a long time.

Azotemia usually signals death within a few months.

Terminal oliguria or anuria may occur.

TOXEMIA OF PREGNANCY

Proteinuria varies from a trace to very marked ($\leqq$ 800 mg/dl, equivalent to 15–20 gm/day). > 15 mg/dl may indicate early toxemia.

RBCs and RBC casts are not abundant; hyaline and granular casts are present.

BUN, renal concentrating ability, and PSP excretion are normal unless the disease is severe or there is a prior renal lesion. *(BUN usually decreases during normal pregnancy because of increase in glomerular filtration rate.)*

Serum uric acid is increased (decreased renal clearance of urate) in 70% of patients in absence of treatment with thiazides, which can produce hyperuricemia independent of any disease.

Serum total protein and albumin commonly are markedly decreased.

There may be multiple clotting deficiencies in severe cases.

Biopsy of kidney can establish diagnosis; rules out primary renal disease or hypertensive vascular disease.

GFR and renal plasma flow are 10–30% less than in normal pregnancy but may appear normal, increased, or decreased compared to rates in nonpregnant women. (Normally GFR increases gradually to a maximum of 40% more than nonpregnant level by 32nd week, then decreases slightly until term. Renal plasma flow is not so markedly increased. Therefore the filtration fraction—GFR/RPF ratio—increases slightly.)

Tubular reabsorption of sodium, water, urea, and uric acid is increased (perhaps on account of decreased GFR). Sodium excretion is decreased $\geqq$ 35%.

Beware of associated or underlying conditions—hydatidiform mole, twin pregnancy, prior renal disease.

KIDNEY IN MULTIPLE MYELOMA

Renal function is impaired in > 50% of patients: usually there is loss of renal concentrating ability and azotemia.

Proteinuria is very frequent and is due to albumin and globulins in urine; Bence Jones proteinuria may be intermittent.

There is severe anemia out of proportion to azotemia.

Occasional changes due to altered renal tubular function are present.

    Renal glycosuria, aminoaciduria, decreased serum uric acid, renal potassium wasting

    Renal loss of phosphate with decreased serum phosphorus and increased alkaline phosphatase

    Nephrogenic diabetes insipidus

    Oliguria or anuria with acute renal failure precipitated by dehydration

Changes due to associated amyloidosis are found (see pp. 639–640).

Changes due to associated hypercalcemia are found.

See Multiple Myeloma, pp. 370–374.

PRIMARY OR SECONDARY AMYLOIDOSIS OF KIDNEY

Persistent proteinuria that varies from mild, with or without hematuria, to severe, with nephrotic syndrome.

Vasopressin-resistant polyuria is present if the medulla alone is involved (rare).

See Amyloidosis, pp. 639–640.

SICKLE CELL NEPHROPATHY

Gross and microscopic hematuria is common.

Early decrease of renal concentrating ability is evident even with normal BUN, GFR, and renal plasma flow; it occurs in sickle cell trait as well as the disease, but progressive nephropathy occurs only with the disease. The decrease is temporarily reversed in children by transfusion but not in adults.

RENAL DISEASE IN ALLERGIC (SCHÖNLEIN-HENOCH) PURPURA

Urine is abnormal in 50% of patients, but renal biopsy is abnormal in most (usually a focal proliferative glomerulonephritis).

Clinical picture varies from minimal urinary abnormalities to severe, rapidly progressive nephritis that is indistinguishable from glomerulonephritis. Nephrotic syndrome may occur. Chronic course, with remissions and exacerbations and permanent renal damage, may occur.

Serum complement is normal.

Platelet count is normal.

HEMOLYTIC-UREMIC SYNDROME

Usually occurs in a child less than age 2 years who develops urinary findings of acute glomerulonephritis after several days of gastroenteritis.

Severe hemolytic anemia is present at onset or within a few days; hemoglobin is often < 6 gm/dl. Burr RBCs are always seen in peripheral blood smear.

Platelet count is usually decreased.

WBC is normal.

Coombs' test is negative.

Serum complement is normal.

Laboratory findings indicate progressive renal disease or recovery.

Azotemia, with BUN frequently > 100 mg/dl.

HEPATORENAL SYNDROME

Oliguria

Azotemia

Concentrated urine with high specific gravity, urine-plasma osmolality ratio > 1.0

Decreased urine sodium to < 10 mEq/L (often 1–2 mEq/L)

Urine is acid; small amount of protein, few casts, few RBCs may be found.

Usually appears in patients with decompensated cirrhosis and ascites, especially following fluid loss (e.g., GI hemorrhage, diarrhea, forced diuresis).

Must differentiate from acute tubular necrosis in which urine has low fixed specific gravity and high sodium content and a characteristic sediment may be found.

HYPERCALCEMIC NEPHROPATHY
Diffuse nephrocalcinosis is the result of prolonged increase in serum and urine calcium (due to hyperparathyroidism, sarcoidosis, vitamin D intoxication, multiple myeloma, carcinomatosis, milk-alkali syndrome, etc.).

Urine is normal or contains RBCs, WBCs, WBC casts; proteinuria is usually slight or absent.

Early findings are decreased renal concentrating ability and polyuria.

Later findings are decreased GFR, decreased renal blood flow, azotemia.

Renal insufficiency is insidious and slowly progressive; it may sometimes be reversed by correcting hypercalcemia.

See various primary causative diseases.

IRRADIATION NEPHRITIS
Exposure (one or both kidneys) to > 2300 rads for 6 weeks or less
Latent period is > 6 months.
Slight proteinuria is present.
Hematuria and oliguria are absent.
Refractory anemia is present.
Progressive uremia is found; may be reversible later.
Renal biopsy

LABORATORY CRITERIA FOR KIDNEY TRANSPLANTATION
Donor: Three successive urinalyses and cultures must be negative.
Donor and recipient must show
    ABO and Rh blood group compatibility
    Leukoagglutinin compatibility
    Platelet agglutinin compatibility

ANALGESIC NEPHROPATHY
See Phenacetin—Chronic Excessive Ingestion, p. 648.

LABORATORY FINDINGS OF KIDNEY TRANSPLANT REJECTION
Total urine output is decreased.
Proteinuria is increased.
Cellular or granular casts appear.
Urine osmolality is decreased.
Blood urea nitrogen and creatinine rise.
Hyperchloremic renal tubular acidosis may be an early sign of rejection or indicate smoldering rejection activity.
Renal clearance values decrease.
Sodium iodohippurate ^{131}I renogram is altered.
Biopsy of kidney shows a characteristic microscopic appearance and is the definitive way to diagnose rejection.

LEUKOPLAKIA OF RENAL PELVIS
Cell block of urine shows keratin or keratinized squamous cells.

CARCINOMA OF RENAL PELVIS AND URETER
Hematuria is present.
Renal calculi are associated.
Urinary tract infection is associated.
Cytologic examination of urinary sediment for malignant cells is
  necessary.

HYPERNEPHROMA OF KIDNEY
Even in the absence of the classic loin pain, flank mass, and
  hematuria, hypernephroma should be ruled out in the presence of
  these *unexplained* laboratory findings.
> Abnormal liver function tests (in absence of metastases to liver)
>   found in 40% of these patients, e.g., increased serum alkaline
>   phosphatase, prolonged prothrombin time, altered serum pro-
>   tein values (decreased albumin, increased alpha$_2$ globulin)
> Hypercalcemia
> Polycythemia
> Leukemoid reaction
> Refractory anemia and increased ESR
> Amyloidosis
> Cushing's syndrome
> Salt-losing syndrome
For laboratory assistance in diagnosis
> Exfoliative cytology of urine for tumor cells
> Test for increased urine LDH level
> Radioisotope scan of kidney

Needle biopsy is not recommended.

RENIN-PRODUCING RENAL TUMORS
**(hemangiopericytomas of juxtaglomerular apparatus; Wilms' tumor;
rarely lung cancer)**
Plasma renin activity is increased, with levels significantly higher
  in renal vein from affected side.
Plasma renin activity responds to changes in posture but not to
  changes in sodium intake.
Plasma renin activity maintains circadian rhythm despite marked
  elevation.
Secondary aldosteronism is evident, with hypokalemia, etc. (see pp.
  489–490).
Laboratory changes (and hypertension) are reversed by removal of
  tumor.

BENIGN PROSTATIC HYPERTROPHY
Laboratory findings are those due to urinary tract obstruction and
  secondary infection.

PROSTATITIS
Most frequently due to
> *Escherichia coli*
> *Proteus mirabilis*
> *Pseudomonas*
> *Klebsiella*
> *Streptococcus faecalis*
> *Staphylococcus aureus*

The acute form usually shows laboratory findings of infected urine (WBCs in centrifuged sediment of last portion of voided specimen; positive culture).

In the chronic form, prostatic fluid usually shows > 10–15 WBCs (pus cells). Cultures are frequently positive (see bacteria listed above). Chronic "nonbacterial" type may be due to organisms that are difficult to culture (e.g., *Ureaplasma,* chlamydiae, trichomonads, CMV, or herpes virus) or to interpret (e.g., *Staphylococcus epidermidis,* diphtheroids, or micrococci)

Laboratory findings due to associated or complicating conditions (e.g., epididymitis) may be present.

POSTVASECTOMY STATUS

Sperm count may fall to low levels after 3 or 4 ejaculations and then rise abruptly before falling again.

Ten ejaculations may be required before sperm count reaches 0.

Three consecutive azoospermic specimens are recommended before dispensing with contraception.

Reanastomosis of the vas deferens may occur.

NONSPECIFIC URETHRITIS

Urethritis is diagnosed if smear of urethral discharge shows > 4 PMNs/1000 × field.

In absence of urethral discharge, an early-morning urine specimen is collected. An initial 10-ml specimen is centrifuged and compared to the rest of the sample. If the first specimen shows more PMNs (>15 PMNs/400 × field) than the later sample, urethritis is diagnosed. If equal numbers of PMNs are present in both specimens, the inflammation is higher up in the GU tract. If no PMNs are present, urethritis is unlikely. Sediment of the first specimen should also be examined for *Trichomonas vaginalis.*

Gram stains will show gram-negative intracellular diplococci in > 95% of cases of gonorrhea. When only some extracellular diplococci are seen, subsequent cultures are positive for *Neisseria gonorrhoeae* in < 15% of patients. *Chlamydia* and *Ureaplasma* cannot be identified on Gram stains, and cultures must be done at specialized laboratories. Culture in cells is currently the most sensitive and specific test for chlamydial infection and is usually positive within 48 hours.

When Gram stains and cultures for gonorrhea are negative, the presumptive diagnosis is nongonococcal urethritis, and *Chlamydia trachomatis* causes about 50% of such cases. *This is the most frequent venereal disease and is estimated to be 2 times more frequent than gonorrhea.*

Ureaplasma urealyticum probably causes 20–30% of cases of urethritis in males.

Candida albicans, T. vaginalis, herpes simplex, and cytomegalovirus probably cause 10–15% of cases of nongonococcal urethritis.

In VD clinics, up to 50% of males with gonococcal urethritis have concomitant *C. trachomatis* present. Chlamydiae are responsible for 70% of postgonococcal urethritis. In VD clinics, *C. trachomatis* can be cultured from 20–30% of females.

In males, a positive gram-stained smear establishes the diagnosis of gonorrhea and a culture is not necessary, but in females, a positive smear should be confirmed by culture on appropriate media (i.e., Gram stains are highly sensitive and specific in males but not in females).

In sexually active men with no symptoms or laboratory findings of urethritis, chlamydial infection is found in < 3%.

In sexually active young men, acute epididymitis is almost always due to sexually transmitted disease (STD); 70–80% are due to *C. trachomatis*, and 10% are due to gonorrhea. Laboratory findings of urethritis will usually be found even if patient is asymptomatic. *Escherichia coli* is the most common pathogen in men > 35 years old.

Sexually active women with symptoms of lower urinary tract infection, pyuria (> 15 WBCs/hpf) but sterile urine cultures probably have chlamydial infection. If coliforms or staphylococci are found, bacterial cystitis is likely even if < 100,000/cu mm.

Mycoplasma hominis may cause pyelonephritis, pelvic inflammatory disease, and postpartum febrile complications.

Laboratory findings of complications
    Prostatitis (20% of patients)
    Epididymitis (3% of patients)
    Urethral stricture (<5% of patients)
    Reiter's syndrome (2% of patients)
    Cervicitis, cervical erosion, cytologic atypia on Papanicolaou smear, salpingitis
    Sterility
    Acute proctitis (see p. 240)

SOME CAUSES OF SEXUALLY TRANSMITTED DISEASES

Bacteria
Neisseria gonorrhoeae
Chlamydia trachomatis
Treponema pallidum
Ureaplasma urealyticum
Mycoplasma hominis
Haemophilus ducreyi
Calymmatobacterium granulomatis
Shigella sp.
Campylobacter fetus
Gardnerella vaginalis (?)
Streptococcus Group B (?)

Viruses
Herpes simplex
Hepatitis A and B
Cytomegalovirus
Genital wart
Molluscum contagiosum

Protozoa
Treponema vaginalis
Entamoeba histolytica
Giardia lamblia

Ectoparasites
Crab louse
Scabies mite

VULVOVAGINITIS

Due To

Bacteria, especially gonococcus (see pp. 567–568); also *Gardnerella vaginalis*

  Vaginal pH > 4.5 (using pH indicator paper) in > 80% of cases (found in one-third of normal women)

  Wet mount of vaginal discharge shows "clue cells" (vaginal epithelial cells coated with bacilli).

  Alkalinization of vaginal discharge with 10% KOH produces a fishy odor (due to release of amines).

  Positive culture on HB or chocolate agar (may also be found in asymptomatic women)

  Gram stain and Papanicolaou smear may also suggest this diagnosis.

Fungi, especially *Candida albicans*, diagnosed by culture on Nickerson's or Sabouraud's medium and also by identification on Papanicolaou smears

Trichomonas, diagnosed by hanging drop preparation; often seen in routine urinalysis on microscopic examination

Local cause is most common (e.g., poor hygiene, pinworms, scabies, foreign body).

In nongonorrheal cases, smear shows more epithelial cells and fewer WBCs compared to gonorrhea. Gram stain may show many or few bacteria, which are often mixed (i.e., gram-positive and gram-negative; cocci and bacilli).

CARCINOMA OF PROSTATE

Increased serum acid phosphatase indicates local extension or distant metastases. It is increased in 60–75% of patients with bone metastases, 20% of patients with extension into periprostatic soft tissue but without bone involvement, 5% of patients with carcinoma confined to gland. Occasionally it remains low despite active metastases. Increased serum acid phosphatase shows pronounced fall in activity within 3–4 days after castration or within 2 weeks after estrogen therapy is begun; may return to normal or remain slightly elevated; failure to fall corresponds to the failure of clinical response that occurs in 10% of the patients. Most patients with invasive carcinoma show a significant increase in serum acid phosphatase after massage or palpation; this rarely occurs in patients with normal prostate, benign prostatic hypertrophy, or in situ carcinoma, or in patients with prostate carcinoma who are receiving hormone treatment.

Prostatic acid phosphatase (PAP) is nearly always increased with a palpable prostatic nodule. Specificity > 94% but may be normal in poorly differentiated or androgen-insensitive prostate carcinomas. Is not useful for screening of general or asymptomatic population for prostate cancer. If PAP assay is elevated in presence of a negative biopsy, the biopsy should be repeated. Elevated PAP assay should return to normal 1 week following surgery or radiotherapy for carcinoma palpable on rectal examination; failure to do so suggests the presence of metastatic lesions. Not increased in nonprostate diseases listed on p. 61–62.

Alkaline phosphatase is increased in 90% of patients with bone metastases. Increases with favorable response to estrogen therapy or castration and reaches peak in 3 months, then declines.

Recurrence of bone metastases causes new rise in alkaline phosphatase.

Anemia is present.

Carcinoma cells may appear in bone marrow aspirates.

Fibrinolysins are found in 12% of patients with metastatic prostatic cancer; occur only with extensive metastases and are usually associated with hemorrhagic manifestations; they show fibrinogen deficiency and prolonged prothrombin time.

Urinary tract infection and hematuria occur late.

Needle biopsy of suspicious nodules in prostate is called for.

Cytologic examination of prostatic fluid is not generally useful.

CARCINOMA OF BLADDER

Hematuria is present.

Biopsy of tumor should be taken.

Cytologic examination of urine for tumor cells is useful for Grades II, III, and IV carcinoma but not for Grade I, which has a high false positive rate. It may be of value in screening dye workers in chemical industry.

	Sensitivity*	
	First Urine Specimen	**Third Urine Specimen**
Grade I	None	20%
		(many false positives)
Grade II	30%	80%
Grade III	65%	85%
Grade IV	92%	98%

Urinary LDH level may be useful in screening studies to discover asymptomatic patients with neoplasm of GU tract.

Laboratory findings due to complications will stem from infection or from obstruction of ureter.

Laboratory findings due to preexisting conditions (e.g., schistosomiasis, stone, or infection)

RETROPERITONEAL FIBROSIS

ESR is increased.

Leukocytosis is present.

Occasionally eosinophilia occurs.

Serum protein and A/G ratio are normal; if the person is chronically ill, total protein may be decreased.

Gamma globulins may be increased.

Anemia is present.

Laboratory findings due to ureteral obstruction are made.

The condition may be primary, due to angiomatous lymphoid hamartoma, or secondary to administration of methysergide.

CARCINOMA OF UTERUS

Carcinoma of the Corpus

Cytologic examination (Pap smear) is positive in $\cong$ 70% of patients;

---

*False positives may occur due to atypia in chronic cystitis, calculi, irradiation, chemotherapy (e.g., myleran).

a false negative result occurs in 30% of patients. Therefore a
negative Pap smear does not rule out carcinoma.

Pap smear from aspiration of endometrial cavity is positive in 95%
of patients. Endometrial biopsy may be helpful, but a negative
result does not rule out carcinoma.

Diagnostic curettage is the only way to rule out carcinoma of the
endometrium.

Carcinoma of the Cervix

Pap smear for routine screening in the general population may be
positive for carcinoma of the cervix in $\cong$ 6 of every 1000 women
(prevalence); only 7% of these lesions are invasive. The prevalence rate is greatest in certain groups:

> Women ages 21–35 years, with peak in 31st to 35th year
> Black and Puerto Rican women
> Women who use birth control pills rather than diaphragm for
> contraception
> Women with early onset or long duration of sexual activity

*Vaginal pool Pap smear has an accuracy rate of $\cong$ 80% in detect-
ing carcinoma of the cervix. Smears from a combination of
vaginal pool, exocervical, and endocervical scrapings have an
accuracy rate of 95%.*

*After an initial abnormal smear, the follow-up smear taken in
the next few weeks or months may not always be abnormal;
there is no clear explanation for this finding. Biopsy shows
important lesions of the cervix in some of these patients. Therefore an abnormal initial smear requires further investigation
of the cervix regardless of subsequent cytologic reports.*

Late Cases

Laboratory findings due to obstruction of ureters with pyelonephritis, azotemia, etc., may be present.

General effects of cancer are found.

RUPTURED TUBAL PREGNANCY

Increased WBC usually returns to normal in 24 hours. Persistent
increase may indicate recurrent bleeding. 50% of patients have
normal WBC; 75% of the patients have WBC < 15,000/cu mm.
Persistent WBC > 20,000/cu mm may indicate pelvic inflammatory disease.

Anemia is present but often precedes the tubal pregnancy in im-
poverished populations. Progressive anemia may indicate continuing bleeding into hematoma. Absorption of blood from
hematoma may cause increased serum bilirubin.

Pregnancy tests are positive in $\cong$ 50% of patients; however, the
beta-subunit HCG assay is positive in $\cong$ 95% of patients.

ALTERED LABORATORY TESTS DURING PREGNANCY
(by term unless otherwise specified)

RBC hemoglobin and hematocrit decrease approximately 15%.

RBC volume increases 20%, but plasma volume increases 45%.

WBC increases 66%.

ESR increases markedly during pregnancy, making this a useless
diagnostic test during pregnancy.

Serum iron decreases 40% in patients not on iron therapy.

Serum transferrin increases 40% and percent saturation decreases up to 70%.

Serum total protein decreases 1 gm/dl during first trimester; remains at that level.

Serum albumin decreases 0.5 gm/dl during first trimester; decreases 0.75 gm/dl by term.

Serum alpha$_1$ globulin increases 0.1 gm/dl.

Serum alpha$_2$ globulin increases 0.1 gm/dl.

Serum beta globulin increases 0.3 gm/dl.

Serum ceruloplasmin increases 70%.

Fasting blood glucose decreases 5–10 mg/dl by end of first trimester.

Renal function changes are difficult to assess because they are based on body surface and because of changes in plasma volume during pregnancy.

BUN and creatinine decrease 25%, especially during first half of pregnancy.

BUN of 18 mg/dl and creatinine of 1.2 mg/dl are definitely abnormal in pregnancy, although normal in nonpregnant women.

Serum uric acid decreases 35% in first trimester; returns to normal by term.

Serum cholesterol increases 30–50%.

Serum triglycerides increase 100–200%.

Serum phospholipid increases 40–60%.

Serum CK decreases 15% by 20 weeks; then returns to normal.

Serum alkaline phosphatase is increased 200–300%.

Serum leucine aminopeptidase (LAP) may be moderately increased throughout pregnancy.

Serum lipase decreases 50%.

Serum pseudocholinesterase decreases 30%.

Serum calcium decreases 10%.

Serum magnesium decreases 10%.

Serum osmolality decreases 10 mOsm/kg during first trimester.

Serum vitamin B$_{12}$ level decreases 20%.

Serum folate decreases 50% or more. Overlap of decreased and normal range of values often makes this test useless in diagnosis of megaloblastic anemia of pregnancy.

Serum T-3 uptake is decreased and T-4 is increased. T-7 (T-3 × T-4) is normal. TBG is increased.

No changes are found in serum levels of
    Sodium
    Potassium
    Chloride
    Phosphorus
    Amylase
    LDH
    ICD
    SGOT
    SGPT
    Acid phosphatase
    Alpha-hydroxybutyrate dehydrogenase (α-HBD)

Occasionally cold agglutinins may be positive and osmotic fragility increased.

Urine volume may increase ≦ 25% in last trimester.

Proteinuria is common ($\cong$ 20% of patients).

Glycosuria is common with decreased glucose tolerance.

Lactosuria should not be confused with glucose in urine.

Urine porphyrins may be increased.

Urinary gonadotropins (HCG) are increased (see "Pregnancy" Test, pp. 137, 170).

Urine estrogens increase from 6 months to term (≤ 100 μg/24 hours)

Urine 17-ketosteroids rise to upper limit of normal at term.

Serum aldosterone is increased.

ALTERED LABORATORY TESTS DURING MENSTRUATION

Platelet count is decreased by 50–70%; returns to normal by fourth day.

Hemoglobin is unchanged.

Fibrinogen is increased.

Serum cholesterol may increase just before menstruation.

Urine volume, sodium, and chloride decrease premenstrually and increase postmenstrually (diuresis).

Urine protein may increase during premenstrual phase.

Urine porphyrins increase.

Urine estrogens decrease to lowest level 2–3 days after onset.

Infectious Diseases

Table 31-1. Etiology of Bacteremia

Organism	% of Cases	Predisposing Factors
Staphylococcus epidermidis	34	Contaminated IV catheters, heart valve prostheses, shunts
Escherichia coli	22	GU indwelling catheters and instruments, perforated bowel, septic abortion
Staphylococcus aureus	15	Abscess, decubitus ulcer, osteomyelitis, staphylococcal pneumonia
Pseudomonas species	6	Burns, immunosuppressive chemotherapy
Alpha streptococcus	6	Dental procedures, gum disease
Streptococcus pneumoniae	6	Alcoholism, chronic obstructive pulmonary disease (COPD), pneumococcal pneumonia
Bacteroides species	3.5	Trauma, GI or GU tract disease
Hemophilis influenzae	3	*H. influenzae* nasopharyngitis
Candida species	1.5	Burns, immunosuppressive chemotherapy, parenteral alimentation
Streptococcus pyogenes	1.4	Streptococcal pharyngitis/tonsillitis
Clostridium species	1.4	Septic abortion, biliary tract disease/surgery
Salmonella species	0.8	Contaminated food/water

One-third of staphylococcal bacteremias are primary; predisposing factors are decreased immune defenses (e.g., diabetes mellitus, neoplasms, steroid therapy, hemodialysis).

Table 31-2. Etiology of Ear Infections

Organism	% of Cases
External otitis	
Pseudomonas	60
Staphylococcus	15
Proteus	5
Aspergillus	7
Candida	3
Streptococcus, non-Group A	1
Coliform	2
Virus	1
Unidentified	6
Otitis media	
Pneumococcus	30
Hemophilus influenzae	30
Unidentified	25
Staphylococcus	15
Beta streptococcus, Group A	< 1

PNEUMOCOCCAL INFECTIONS

Pneumonia

Increased WBC (usually 12,000–25,000/cu mm) with shift to the left; normal or low WBC in overwhelming infection, in aged patients, or with other causative organisms (e.g., Friedländer's bacillus)

Blood culture positive for pneumococci in 25% of untreated patients during first 3–4 days

Gram stain of sputum—many polynuclear leukocytes, many gram-positive cocci in pairs and singly; direct pneumococcus typing using Neufeld capsular swelling method rarely done now

Pleural effusion in ≅ 5% of patients

Laboratory findings due to complications (endocarditis, meningitis, peritonitis, arthritis, empyema, etc.)

Endocarditis
See pp. 209–210.

Meningitis
See pp. 278, 289.
Laboratory findings due to associated or underlying conditions—pneumococcal pneumonia, endocarditis, otitis, sinusitis, multiple myeloma

Peritonitis
Positive blood culture
Increased WBC
Ascitic fluid—identification of organisms by Gram stain and culture

See section on laboratory findings in body fluids, pp. 176–186.

STREPTOCOCCAL INFECTIONS
(uncommon under age 2)
Group A streptococci showing beta hemolysis
    Upper respiratory infection
    Scarlet fever

WBC is usually increased (14,000/cu mm) early. It becomes normal by end of first week. *(If still increased, look for complication, e.g., otitis.)* Increased eosinophils appear during convalescence, especially with scarlet fever.
Urine may show transient slight albumin, RBCs, casts, without sequelae.
ASO titer (see pp. 140–141)

See sections on rheumatic fever and acute glomerulonephritis, pp. 207–208, 532–533.

Acute glomerulonephritis follows streptococcal infection after latent period of 1–2 weeks; preceding infection may be pharyngeal or of the skin. Latent period prior to onset of acute rheumatic fever is 2–4 weeks; preceding infection is pharyngeal but rarely of the skin.

Group A streptococci are the most frequent type of streptococci causing
    Otitis media, mastoiditis, sinusitis, meningitis, cerebral sinus thrombosis
    Pneumonia, empyema, pericarditis
    Bacteremia, suppurative arthritis
    Puerperal sepsis
    Lymphangitis, lymphadenitis, erysipelas, cellulitis
    Impetigo (in older children, is often mixed infection with staphylococci that overgrow the culture plate)

WBC is markedly increased ($\leq 20,000$–$30,000$/cu mm).
Streptococci appear in smears and cultures from appropriate sites.
Blood culture may be positive.

Streptococcus viridans (alpha-hemolytic streptococci) causes
    Subacute bacterial endocarditis (see pp. 209–210)
Streptococcus faecalis (enterococcus; Group D streptococci) causes
    Bacterial endocarditis
    Urinary tract infection
Anaerobic streptococci
    Associated with coliform bacilli, clostridia, *Bacteroides*
        Compound fractures and soft-tissue wounds
        Puerperal and postabortion sepsis
        Visceral abscesses (e.g., lung, liver, brain)
    Associated with *Staphylococcus aureus*
        Gangrenous postoperative abdominal incision
    Without associated bacteria
        Burrowing skin and subcutaneous infection

STAPHYLOCOCCAL INFECTIONS

Pneumonia—often secondary to measles, influenza, mucoviscidosis, debilitating diseases such as leukemia and collagen diseases or to prolonged treatment with broad-spectrum antibiotics

WBC is increased (usually > 15,000/cu mm).

Sputum contains very many leukocytes with intracellular gram-positive cocci.

Bacteremia occurs in < 20% of patients.

Acute osteomyelitis—due to hematogenous dissemination

Bacteremia occurs in > 50% of early cases.

WBC is increased.

Anemia develops.

Secondary amyloidosis occurs in long-standing chronic osteomyelitis.

Endocarditis—occurs in valves without preceding rheumatic disease and showing little or no previous damage; causes rapid severe damage to valve, producing acute clinical course of mechanical heart failure (rupture of chordae tendineae, perforation of valve, valvular insufficiency) plus results of acute severe infection

Metastatic abscesses occur in various organs.

Anemia develops rapidly.

WBC is increased (12,000–20,000/cu mm); occasionally is normal or decreased.

From 1–13% of cases of bacterial endocarditis are due to coagulase-negative Staphylococcus albus; *bacterial endocarditis due to* Staphylococcus albus *is found following cardiac surgery in one-third and without preceding surgery in two-thirds of patients.*

WBC is increased.

Bacteremia is common.

Teichoic acid antibodies are found in titer ≥ 1:4 in ≅ two-thirds of patients with *Staphylococcus aureus* endocarditis or bacteremia with metastatic infection, ≅ one-half of patients with nonbacteremic staphylococcal infections. May be found in ≅ 10% of other infections or in normal persons. Titer ≥ 1:4 is said to suggest current or recent serious staphylococcal infection; positive result without suppuration at primary site of infection suggests endocarditis or metastatic infection. May also be useful when cultures are negative because of prior antibiotic therapy or when deep-tissue infection is inaccessible to culturing (e.g., osteomyelitis, abscesses of brain, liver, etc.). Major value is to determine length of treatment of bacteremia, since lack of rise of titer during 14 days of therapy makes it unlikely that undetected metastatic seeding has occurred.

Food poisoning—due to enterotoxin

Culture of staphylococci from suspected food (especially custard and milk products and meats)

Necrotizing enterocolitis of infancy as seen in Hirschsprung's disease

Impetigo—especially in infants between ages 3 weeks and 6 months

Meningitis (see pp. 278, 289)

TOXIC SHOCK SYNDROME
(due to toxin-producing strains of *Staphylococcus aureus;* usually associated with use of tampons in healthy menstruating women; may also occur post partum, in postoperative states, or in patients with burns, boils, or abscesses. Fever, shock, and involvement of at least four organ systems are characteristic.)

Anemia is normocytic, normochromic, nonhemolytic, moderate, progressive and may persist for up to 1 month after onset of illness; resolves without treatment; occurs in about 50% of cases.

ESR may be normal or very high.

Moderate leukocytosis with predominance of immature granulocytes in 70% of cases. Usually increases for several days and then rapidly returns to normal.

Thrombocytopenia* (in about 25% of cases) and DIC causing hemorrhage are not significant clinical problems.

Decreased serum protein,* total and ionized calcium,* phosphorus.*

Hypokalemia, hyponatremia, and metabolic acidosis frequently accompany vomiting and diarrhea.*

Sterile pyuria* in 80% of cases, proteinuria, and RBCs resolve within 2 weeks.

Increased prothrombin time and partial thromboplastin time (PTT) in two-thirds of patients.

Increased serum bilirubin, SGOT, LDH, CK, BUN, and creatinine are found in about 60% of cases about the seventh day of illness, at which time clinical improvement begins to occur and these changes rapidly become normal.

No evidence of other infection (bacterial, viral, rickettsial), drug reaction, or autoimmune disorder.

S. aureus need not be isolated to fulfill criteria for diagnosis.

MENINGOCOCCAL INFECTIONS
Meningococcemia

Meningitis (see pp. 278, 289)

Waterhouse-Friderichsen syndrome (see p. 496)

Increased WBC (12,000–40,000/cu mm)

Gram-stained smears of body fluids
> Tissue fluid from skin lesions
> Buffy coat of blood
> Cerebrospinal fluid *(Pyogenic meningitis in which bacteria cannot be found in smear is more likely to be due to meningococcus than to other bacteria.)*
> Nasopharynx

Culture (use chocolate agar incubated in 10% CO_2)—blood, spinal fluid, skin lesions, nasopharynx, other sites of infection

Urine—may show albumin, RBCs; occasional glycosuria

Cerebrospinal fluid (see Table 25-1, pp. 278–284)
> Markedly increased WBC (2500–10,000/cu mm), almost all polynuclear leukocytes
> Increased protein (50–1500 mg/dl)
> Decreased glucose (0–45 mg/dl)
> Positive smear and culture
> Laboratory findings due to complications (e.g., disseminated in-

---

*Abnormalities usually become normal by fifth day of illness.

travascular coagulation, pp. 400, 402–404) and sequelae (e.g., subdural effusion)

GONOCOCCAL INFECTIONS

Genital infection

Gram stain of smear from involved site, especially urethra, prostatic secretions, cervix, pelvic inflammatory disease. *(Smear may become negative within hours of antibiotic therapy.)*

Bacterial culture *(use special media such as Thayer-Martin)* should always be taken at the same time (before beginning antibiotic therapy). In ≅ 2% of male patients, Gram stain of urethral exudate is negative when a simultaneous culture of the same material is positive.

Fluorescent antibody test on smear of suspected material

Beware of concomitant inapparent venereal infection that may be suppressed but not adequately treated by antibiotic therapy of gonorrhea.

Proctitis

Gram-stained smears are not sufficiently reliable.

Bacterial culture on special media (e.g., Thayer-Martin) is required for confirmation.

Rectal biopsy shows mild and nonspecific inflammation. In a few cases, Gram stain of tissue section may reveal small numbers of gram-negative intracellular diplococci after prolonged examination.

Rectal gonorrhea accompanies genital gonorrhea in 20–50% of women and is found without genital gonorrhea in 6–10% of infected women. Therefore rectal cultures for gonococcus should be taken in all suspected cases of gonorrhea.

Arthritis

Synovial fluid (see Table 26-6, pp. 318–319)

Variable; may contain few leukocytes or be purulent

Gonococci identified in about one-third of patients

Gonococcal complement-fixation test for differential diagnosis of other types of arthritis. Not a reliable test in urethritis but may rarely be helpful in arthritis, prostatitis, and epididymitis. Becomes positive at least 2–6 weeks after onset of infection, remains positive for 3 months after cure. If test is negative, it should be repeated; two negative tests help to rule out gonococcus infection. False positive test may occur after gonococcus vaccine has been used. Test is of limited value and is seldom used.

Associated nonbacterial ophthalmitis in ≦ 20% of patients

Rarely, other sites

Ophthalmitis of newborn

Acute bacterial endocarditis (toxic hepatitis common) (see pp. 209–210). *(Gonococcus is the most common bacteria infecting tricuspid or pulmonic valves.)*

Bacteremia—resembles meningococcemia

Peritonitis and perihepatitis following spread from pelvic in-flammatory disease

INFECTIONS WITH COLIFORM BACTERIA
(*Escherichia coli, Enterobacter-Klebsiella* group, paracolon group)
Bacteremia

Secondary to infection elsewhere; occasionally due to transfu-sion of contaminated blood

Secondary to debilitated condition in 20% of patients (e.g., malignant lymphoma, irradiation or anticancer drugs, steroid therapy, cirrhosis, diabetes mellitus)

Gram-negative shock occurs in 25% of patients.
Azotemia
Increased serum potassium
Decreased serum sodium
Metabolic acidosis
Increased SGOT (decreased hepatic perfusion)
Increased serum amylase (decreased renal perfusion)
Other findings due to shock
Shock is most frequently from urinary tract, gastroin-testinal tract, uterus, lung (in that order).
E. coli is the most frequent organism; it causes the lowest mortality (45%) and the lowest incidence of shock. *Pseudomonas aeruginosa* has the highest mortality (85%). *Klebsiella-Enterobacter,* paracolon bacilli, and *Proteus mirabilis* are intermediate, with 70% mortality.
Urinary tract infection (75% of cases due to *E. coli*)
Infections of intestinal tract and biliary tree (e.g., appendicitis, cholecystitis)
Wound infections, abscesses, etc.
Sepsis neonatorum (bacterial infection during the first 30 days of life with primary involvement of blood and, frequently, meninges)
Positive blood culture—*E. coli* and *Klebsiella-Enterobacter* cause ≅ 75% of cases. Group B and Group D streptococci and *Listeria monocytogenes* cause most of the other cases. May also be caused by a large variety of other bacteria. *Incidence of contaminated blood cultures is high in newborns. Negative blood culture does not rule out this condition; should take cultures from umbilical stump, skin lesions, mucous mem-branes, urine.*
Positive culture of cerebrospinal fluid occurs frequently. *There may be no WBC increase early in the course of the disease.*
WBC is variable; leukopenia is often associated with a high mortality.
Anemia and decreased platelets may occur.
Laboratory findings due to involvement of other organs (e.g., kidney, with albumin, cells, or casts increased in urine; liver, with increased direct or indirect bilirubin).
Gastroenteritis in young children and infants—identification of specific enteropathogenic strains by fluorescent antibody tech-nique
Pneumonia—1% of primary bacterial pneumonias due to *Klebsiella* (Friedländer's bacilli), especially in alcoholics
WBC is often normal or decreased.
Sputum is very tenacious; is brown or red. Smear shows encap-

sulated gram-negative bacilli. *(Gram stain of sputum in lobar pneumonia allows prompt diagnosis of this organism and appropriate therapy.)* Bacterial culture confirms diagnosis.

Laboratory findings due to complications (lung abscess, empyema) are present.

Rarely chronic lung infection due to Friedländer's bacilli simulates tuberculosis.

PROTEUS INFECTIONS

Proteus infections usually follow other bacterial infections.

Indolent skin ulcers (decubital, varicose ulcers)

Burns

Otitis media, mastoiditis

Urinary tract infection

Bacteremia

Characteristic spreading growth on culture plate may obscure associated bacteria since Proteus *infection frequently is part of mixed infection; antibiotic sensitivity testing may not be possible.*

PSEUDOMONAS INFECTIONS

Pseudomonas infections occur in various sites.

Due To

Replacement of normal bacterial flora or initial pathogen because of antibiotic therapy (e.g., urinary tract, ear, lung)

Burns

Debilitated condition of patient (e.g., premature infants, the aged, patients with leukemia)

Decreased WBC during bacteremia in patients with leukemia or burns is more frequently due to Pseudomonas *than to other gram-negative rods.*

BACTEROIDES INFECTION

This is usually a component of mixed infection with coliform bacteria, aerobic and anaerobic streptococci or staphylococci.

Local suppuration or systemic infection is secondary to disease of the female genital tract, intestinal tract, or tonsillar region.

Laboratory findings due to complications (e.g., thrombophlebitis, endocarditis, metastatic abscesses of lung, liver, brain, joint) are present.

Laboratory findings due to underlying conditions (e.g., recent surgery, cancer, arteriosclerosis, diabetes mellitus, alcoholism, prior antibiotic treatment, and steroid, immunosuppressive, or cytotoxic therapy) are present.

TYPHOID FEVER

(due to *Salmonella typhosa*)

WBC is decreased—4000–6000/cu mm during first 2 weeks, 3000–5000/cu mm during next 2 weeks; $\geq$ 10,000/cu mm suggests perforation or suppuration.

Decreased ESR is found.

Normocytic anemia is frequent; with bleeding, anemia becomes hypochromic and microcytic.

Blood cultures are positive during first 10 days of fever in 90% of patients and during relapse; < 30% are positive after third week.

Stool cultures are positive after tenth day, with increasing frequency up to fourth or fifth week. Positive stool culture after 4 months indicates a carrier.

Urine culture is positive during second to third week in 25% of patients, even if blood culture is negative.

Widal reaction—H and O agglutinins appear in serum after 7–10 days, increase to peak in third to fifth week, then gradually fall for several weeks; there is no increase during relapse. O appears before H and is usually higher at first; during convalescence H titer becomes higher than O. Positive Widal test may occur on account of typhoid vaccination or previous typhoid infection; nonspecific febrile disease may cause this titer to increase (anamnestic reaction). Rising titer (especially of O) on serial determinations may be necessary for proper evaluation. Usual criteria for serologic diagnosis in unvaccinated patients is fourfold increase in O titer or O titer > 1:50 or 1:100 in a single specimen or during first 2–3 weeks of illness. ≤ 5% of healthy unvaccinated individuals may have O titer of 1:50.

> Early treatment with chloramphenicol or ampicillin may cause titer to remain negative or low.
>
> Increase in O titer may reflect infection with any organism in the Group D salmonellae (e.g., *Salmonella enteritidis, Salmonella panama*) and not just *Salmonella typhosa*.
>
> Because of differences in commercially manufactured antigens, there may be a twofold to fourfold difference in O titers on the same sample of serum tested with antigens of different manufacturers.
>
> H titer is very variable and may show nonspecific response to other infections; it is therefore of little value in diagnosis of typhoid fever.

Laboratory findings due to complications

> Increased serum LDH, alkaline phosphatase, and SGOT are frequent; increased CK occurs in some patients
>
> Intestinal hemorrhage is occult in 20% of patients, gross in 10%; it occurs usually during second or third week. It is less frequent in treated patients.
>
> Intestinal perforation occurs in 3% of untreated patients.
>
> Relapse occurs in ≤ 20% of patients. Blood culture becomes positive again; Widal titers are unchanged.
>
> Secondary suppurative lesions (e.g., pneumonia, parotitis, furunculosis) are found.
>
> Abnormal liver function tests (e.g., serum bilirubin, SGOT) occur in ≅ 25% of patients as an incidental finding. Hepatitis is the chief clinical feature in ≅ 5% of patients.

INFECTIONS DUE TO OTHER *SALMONELLA* ORGANISMS

Enteritis

> Stool culture remains positive for 1–4 weeks, occasionally longer.
>
> WBC is normal.

Paratyphoid fever—usually due to *Salmonella paratyphi A* or *B* or to *Salmonella choleraesuis*

> Cultures of blood and stool and decreased WBC show same values as indicated in preceding section.

Bacteremia—especially due to *Salmonella choleraesuis*
  Blood cultures are intermittently positive.
  Stool cultures are negative.
  WBC is normal. It increases (≦ 25,000/cu mm) with develop-
    ment of focal lesions (e.g., pneumonia, meningitis, pyelone-
    phritis, osteomyelitis).
Local infections
  Meningitis, especially in infants
  Local abscesses with or without preceding bacteremia or en-
    teritis

One-third of patients are predisposed by underlying disease (e.g.,
malignant lymphoma, disseminated lupus erythematosus). Bacteremia and osteomyelitis are more common in patients with
sickle hemoglobinopathy. Bacteremia is more common in patients
with acute hemolytic *Bartonella* infection.

*Agglutination tests on sera from acute and convalescent cases are
often not useful unless present in high titer (≧ 1 : 560) or rising titer
is shown.*

BACILLARY DYSENTERY
(due to *Shigella* species)
Stool culture is positive in > 75% of patients.
  Rectal swab can also be used.
Microscopy of stool shows mucus, RBCs, and leukocytes.
Serologic tests are not useful.
WBC is normal.
Blood cultures are negative.
Laboratory findings due to complications
  Marked loss of fluid and electrolytes
  Intestinal bleeding
  Relapse (in 10% of untreated patients)
  Carrier state
  Acute arthritis—especially untreated disease due to *Shigella
    shigae* (culture of joint fluid negative)

CHOLERA
(due to *Vibrio comma*)
Stool culture is positive. One may also identify organism in stool
  using immunofluorescent techniques.
Laboratory findings due to marked loss of fluid and electrolytes
  Loss of sodium, chloride, and potassium
  Hypovolemic shock
  Metabolic acidosis
  Uremia

CAMPYLOBACTERIOSIS
(due to *Campylobacter fetus*)
Clinical types
  Disseminated form without diarrhea
    Meningitis—occurs in infants less than 2 months old, usu-
      ally premature or with congenital CNS defects; 50% mor-
      tality.
    Pediatric bacteremia—rare disorder, usually secondary to
      malnutrition or diarrhea; usually recover

Disseminated adult infection—commonly have predisposing conditions (e.g., immunosuppression, malignancy, cardiovascular, endocrine disease, etc.). 90% of cases have positive blood culture. Indirect hemagglutination shows antibody titers of 1:1600 to 1:6400 in acute phase and 1:40 to 1:320 six months after cure.

Gastroenteritis

Stool culture using microaerophilic incubation

Microscopic examination of stool shows "seagull" organisms.

Stools become negative in 3–6 weeks even without therapy, but 5–10% of patients have organisms in stool for a year or longer.

Blood culture positive in < 1% of cases

HEMOPHILUS INFLUENZAE INFECTIONS

Clinical types

Upper respiratory tract infections

Lower respiratory tract infections

Otitis media

Empyema

Meningitis

Pyarthrosis, single or multiple

Increased WBC (15,000–30,000/cu mm) and polynuclear leukocytes

Positive blood culture in ≅ 50% of patients with meningitis

Infants less than age 1 commonly have empyema, bacteremia, and meningitis concomitantly; therefore CSF should always be examined in infants with empyema.

PERTUSSIS (WHOOPING COUGH)
(due to *Bordetella pertussis*)

Marked increase in WBC ($\leq$ 100,000/cu mm) and $\leq$ 90% mature lymphocytes

Negative blood cultures

Positive cultures from nasopharynx or cough plate

PARAPERTUSSIS
(due to *Bordetella parapertussis*)

There are increased WBCs (usually 12,000–25,000/cu mm) and lymphocytes.

Isolation of organism by culture from nasopharynx or cough plate differentiates condition from pertussis.

CHANCROID
(due to *Hemophilus ducreyi*)

Biopsy of genital ulcer or regional lymph node is helpful.

Smear of genital ulcer or regional lymph node stained with Unna-Pappenheim method shows bacteria.

Smear of lesion for Donovan bodies is negative.

Dark-field examination of lesion for treponemas is negative.

Serologic tests for syphilis are negative.

Cultures of lymph node aspirate are more frequently positive than cultures from lesion. Culture is of limited practical value.

BRUCELLOSIS

Agglutination reaction becomes positive during second to third week of illness; 90% of patients have titers of $\geqq 1:320$. Rising titer is of diagnostic significance. False negative results are rare. False positive test results may occur with tularemia or cholera or with cholera vaccination or after brucellin skin test. In chronic localized brucellosis, titers may be negative or $\leqq 1:200$. They may remain positive long after infection has been cured.

Multiple blood cultures should be performed. (Brucella abortus *requires 10% CO_2 for culture.*) They are more likely to be positive with high agglutination titer.

Bone marrow culture is occasionally positive when blood culture is negative. It may show microscopic granulomas.

Opsonophagocytic test and complement-fixation test are not generally useful.

WBC is usually < 10,000/cu mm, with a relative lymphocytosis. Decreased WBC occurs in one-third of patients.

ESR is increased in < 25% of patients and usually in nonlocalized type of brucellosis.

Anemia appears in < 10% of patients and usually with localized type of disease.

Biopsy of tissue may show nonspecific granulomas suggesting a diagnosis of brucellosis. Tissue may be used for culture.

Liver function tests may be abnormal.

TULAREMIA
(due to *Pasteurella tularensis*)

Clinical types
> Typhoidal
> Ulceroglandular
> Glandular
> Pneumonic
> Rarely oculoglandular, gastrointestinal, endocardial, meningeal, osteomyelitic, etc.

Agglutination reaction becomes positive in second week of infection. Significant titer is $1:40$; usually it becomes $\geqq 1:320$ by third week. Peaks at 4–7 weeks ($\leqq 1:1000$), then gradually decreases during next year; appreciable titer persists for many years. May cross-react with *Brucella* agglutinins.

Culture and animal inoculation (positive with $\geqq 5$ organisms) of suspected material from appropriate site are performed. (Positive blood culture is rare; regional lymph node and mucocutaneous lesions are usually positive.)

WBC is usually normal.

ESR may be increased in severe typhoidal forms; it is normal in other types.

Biopsy of involved lymph node shows a characteristic histologic picture.

PLAGUE
(due to *Pasteurella pestis*)

Clinical types
> Bubonic
> Primary septicemic
> Pneumonic

Identify bacteria by smear, culture, fluorescent antibody technique, or animal inoculation of suspected material from appropriate site (e.g., lymph node aspirate, blood, sputum).

Serum hemagglutination antibodies are present.

WBC is increased (20,000–40,000/cu mm), with increased polynuclear leukocytes.

INFECTIONS WITH *PASTEURELLA MULTOCIDA*

Clinical types

Localized suppurative infections (e.g., osteomyelitis, cellulitis)

Bacteremia with endocarditis, meningitis, etc.

Respiratory tract infection

Gram stain and culture of bacteria from appropriate sites are performed (e.g., blood, skin, spinal fluid).

WBC is increased.

GLANDERS

(due to *Malleomyces mallei*)

Clinical types

Acute fulminant

Chronic disseminated granulomas and abscesses in skin, respiratory tract, etc.

Culture or animal inoculation of infected material from appropriate sites is performed.

Agglutination and complement-fixation tests are positive in chronic disease.

WBC is variable.

MELIOIDOSIS

(due to *Pseudomonas pseudomallei*)

Clinical types

Acute febrile

Chronic febrile with abscesses in bone, skin, viscera

Infection is occasionally transmitted among narcotic addicts using needles in common.

Culture or animal inoculation of infected material from appropriate sites is performed (e.g., pus, urine, blood, sputum).

Agglutination test is positive in chronic disease; an occasional false positive test occurs.

WBC is normal or increased.

INFECTIONS WITH *MIMAE-HERELLEA*

Clinical types

Bacteremia, bacterial endocarditis, meningitis, pneumonia, etc.

Often associated with intravenous catheters or cutdowns

Bacteria are isolated from appropriate sites (e.g., blood, spinal fluid, sputum).

GRANULOMA INGUINALE

(due to Donovan body)

Wright-stained or Giemsa-stained smears of lesions show intracytoplasmic Donovan bodies in large mononuclear cells in acute stage; they may be present in chronic stages.

Biopsy of lesion shows suggestive histologic pattern and is usually positive for Donovan bodies in acute stage.

Serologic tests for syphilis are negative unless concomitant infection is present.

Dark-field examination for syphilis is negative.

LISTERIOSIS
(due to *Listeria monocytogenes*)

Especially in newborn from antepartum infection of mother
   Findings due to meningitis or disseminated abscesses of viscera are made.
   WBC is increased, and other evidence of infection is found.
   Gram stain of meconium shows gram-positive bacilli. *This should be done whenever mother is febrile before or at onset of labor.*

Infection of adult nonpregnant patients is associated with debilitation (e.g., alcoholism, diabetes mellitus, adrenocorticoid therapy).
   Laboratory findings due to bacteremia, endocarditis, skin infection, etc., are present.

ANTHRAX
(due to anthrax bacillus)

Identification of gram-positive bacillus in material by Gram stain, culture, and animal inoculation from site of involvement (fluid from cutaneous lesions; sputum and pleural fluid from patients with pulmonary disease; stool or vomitus from patients with intestinal disease; blood from patients with bacteremia)

WBC and ESR normal in mild cases; increased in severe cases

With meningeal involvement
   CSF bloody
   CSF smear and culture positive for bacilli

Precipitin antibodies with high or increasing titer sometimes useful in pulmonary or intestinal disease

DIPHTHERIA
(due to *Corynebacterium diphtheriae*)

WBC is increased ($\leq 15,000$/cu mm). If $> 25,000$/cu mm are found, there is probably a concomitant infection (e.g., hemolytic streptococcal).

Smear from involved area stained with methylene blue is positive in $> 75\%$ of patients.

Culture from involved area is positive within 12 hours on Löffler's medium (more slowly on blood agar). *If there has been prior antibiotic therapy, culture may be negative or take several days to grow.* Penicillin G eliminates *C. diphtheriae* within 12 hours; without therapy, organisms usually disappear after 2–4 weeks.

Fluorescent antibody staining of material from involved area provides more rapid diagnosis, with a higher percentage of positive results.

Laboratory findings of peripheral neuritis (see pp. 298–299) are present in 10% of patients, usually during second to sixth week. Increased CSF protein may be of prolonged duration.

Laboratory findings of myocarditis (which occurs in $\leq$ two-thirds of patients) are present.

Albumin and casts are frequently present in urine; blood is rarely found.

Hemagglutination titer assays antitoxin titer of patient's serum. Fourfold increase in titer in acute and convalescent sera confirms diagnosis.

A moderate anemia is common.

Decreased serum glucose occurs frequently.

TETANUS
(due to *Clostridium tetani*)

WBC is normal.

Urine is normal.

CSF is normal.

Identification of organism in local wound is difficult and not usually helpful.

BOTULISM
(due to *Clostridium botulinum*)

CSF is normal.

Usual laboratory tests are not abnormal or useful.

Diagnosis is made by injecting suspected food intraperitoneally into mice, which will die in 24 hours unless protected with specific antiserum.

CLOSTRIDIAL GAS GANGRENE, CELLULITIS, AND PUERPERAL SEPSIS
(due to *Clostridium perfringens, C. septicum, C. novyi,* etc.)

WBC is increased (15,000 to > 40,000/cu mm).

Platelets are decreased in 50% of patients.

In postabortion sepsis, sudden severe hemolytic anemia is common. Hemoglobulinemia, hemoglobinuria, increased serum bilirubin, spherocytosis, increased osmotic and mechanical fragility, etc., may be associated.

Protein and casts are often present in urine.

Renal insufficiency may progress to uremia.

Smears of material from appropriate sites show gram-positive rods, but spores are not usually seen and other bacteria are often also present.

Anaerobic culture of material from appropriate site is positive. *Clostridia are frequent contaminants of wounds caused by other agents. Other bacteria may cause gas formation within tissues.*

LEGIONNAIRES' DISEASE
(due to *Legionella pneumophila,* a gram-negative bacillus that is an aerobic, intracellular, opportunistic pathogen widely disseminated in environment; at least 6 serogroups are known)

Indicators of acute infection

Elevation of liver enzymes

Hematuria, proteinuria

Organism may be cultured on special material from pleural fluid, lung biopsy, transtracheal or bronchial aspirate, blood; isolate can then only be identified by special tests (e.g., direct fluorescent antibody staining).

Direct immunofluorescence may demonstrate the organism in sputum, pleural fluid, or lung tissue within 2–3 days of onset of clinical disease; however, there may be cross reactions with commensal organisms.

Serologic tests
> Titers < 1:128 are found in the general asymptomatic population.
> Standardized antisera are just becoming commercially available for various serologic tests, e.g., indirect fluorescent antibody (allows detection of IgM versus IgG antibody), ELISA, agglutination, etc. A diagnostic rise in titer may be seen 3 weeks after onset *(fourfold titer rise has been reported in other diseases, e.g., tularemia, plague, leptospirosis).*

ANAEROBIC INFECTIONS
Frequently several anaerobic organisms are present simultaneously and are often associated with aerobic bacteria as well. If cultures from suspicious sites are reported as negative, the culturing for anaerobic organisms has not been performed properly.

Mixed aerobic-anaerobic infections are often successfully treated by suppressing only the anaerobes.

The most common anaerobic organisms cultured are *Bacteroides* and *Clostridia* species and streptococci.

The most commonly associated aerobic bacteria are the gram-negative enteric bacteria (*Escherichia coli, Klebsiella, Proteus, Pseudomonas,* enterococci).

Anaerobic organisms should be sought particularly in cultures from intra-abdominal infections (e.g., bowel perforations, acute appendicitis, biliary tract disease), obstetric and gynecologic infections (e.g., pelvic abscess, Bartholin gland abscess, postpartum, post-abortion, posthysterectomy infections), chest infections (e.g., bronchiectasis, lung abscess, necrotizing pneumonia), urinary tract, soft tissue infections, < 5% of endocarditis cases (especially streptococci), 10% of cases of bacteremia.

Bacteremia due to anaerobic organisms is characterized by high incidence of jaundice, septic thrombophlebitis, and metastatic abscesses; the gastrointestinal tract and the female pelvis are the usual portals of entry (in aerobic bacteremia, the urinary tract is the most common portal of entry).

LEPTOSPIROSIS
(most frequently due to *Leptospira icterohaemorrhagiae, L. canicola,* and *L. pomona*)
Normochromic anemia is present.
WBC may be normal or ≦ 40,000/cu mm in Weil's disease.
ESR is increased.
Urine is abnormal in 75% of patients: proteinuria, WBCs, RBCs, casts.
Liver function tests are abnormal in 50% of patients.
> Increased serum bilirubin
> Increased alkaline phophatase
> Increased SGOT and SGPT, but average levels are not as high as in hepatitis

Increased CK in about one-third of patients during first week may help to differentiate condition from hepatitis.

Reversed A/G ratio

CSF is abnormal in cases with meningeal involvement ($\leqq$ two-thirds of patients)

Increased cells ($\leqq$ 500/cu mm), chiefly mononuclear type

Increased protein ($\leqq$ 80 mg/dl)

Glucose and chloride normal

Organisms are not found in CSF.

Blood culture is positive during first 3 days of disease in $\leqq$ 90% of patients.

Urine cultures may be positive only intermittently and are difficult because of contamination and low pH. They are rarely positive after the fourth week.

Of the serologic tests, the hemolysis test is most useful. Agglutination, complement fixation, and hemolysis antibodies reach peaks in 4–7 weeks and may last for many years. An increasing titer is diagnostic. An individual titer of 1:300 is suggestive.

RELAPSING FEVER
(due to *Borrelia recurrentis, B. novyi, B. duttonii*)

Identification of organism by

Wright's or Giemsa stain or dark-field microscopy of peripheral blood smear or buffy coat

Intraperitoneal injection of rats

Agglutination of *Proteus* OX-K

Biologic false positive serologic test for syphilis in $\leqq$ 25% of patients

Increased WBC (10,000–15,000/cu mm)

Protein and mononuclear cells sometimes increased in CSF

Laboratory findings due to complications (e.g., hemorrhage, rupture of spleen, secondary infection)

INFECTIONS WITH *STREPTOBACILLUS MONILIFORMIS* (RAT-BITE FEVER, HAVERHILL FEVER, ETC.)

Clinical types

Rat-bite fever

Febrile rash with multiple joint type of arthritis

Isolation of bacteria from appropriate sites (e.g., blood, pus, joint fluid) during acute febrile stage

Agglutination antibodies in serum during second to third week; rising titer significant

INFECTIONS WITH *BARTONELLA BACILLIFORMIS*

Oroya Fever

Sudden very marked anemia is found.

Blood smears may show gram-negative bacilli in $\leqq$ 90% of RBCs (Giemsa stain); they are also present in monocytes. Bacteria are also present in phagocytes of reticuloendothelial system.

Blood culture is positive. *(Use special enriched media.)*

Beware of secondary Salmonella *infection.*

Verugga Peruana

Moderate anemia is found.

Blood smears and blood cultures are positive for bacilli.

SYPHILIS
(due to *Treponema pallidum*)

Primary Syphilis

Dark-field examination of genital lesion is made; if it is negative, regional lymph node aspirate may be used. *Examination will be negative if there has been recent therapy with penicillin or other treponemicidal drugs.* Can also use immunofluorescent staining of smears from lesion, a procedure that allows properly prepared specimens to be mailed to the laboratory.

Serologic test shows rising titer with or without positive dark-field examination. VDRL does not become positive until 7–10 days after appearance of chancre.

Biopsy of suspected lesion is done for histologic examination.

Secondary Syphilis

Dark-field examination of mucocutaneous lesions is positive.
Serologic tests are almost always positive in high titer.

Latent Syphilis

A positive serologic test is the only diagnostic method.

Congenital Syphilis

Dark-field examination of mucocutaneous lesions or scraping from moist umbilical cord is positive.

Serologic tests are positive and show rising or very high titer. *The serologic test may be positive because of maternal antibodies but without congenital syphilitic infection.* Rising infant's titer or titer higher than mother's establishes diagnosis of congenital syphilis. If mother has been adequately treated, infant's titer falls steadily to nonreactive level in 3 months. If mother acquires syphilis late in pregnancy, infant may be seronegative and clinically normal at birth and then manifest syphilis 1–2 months later.

Only the quantitative VDRL is recommended for the diagnosis of congenital syphilis (performed serially to detect rise or fall in titers).

Late Syphilis

CNS (VDRL on CSF is highly specific but lacks sensitivity)
    Meningitis
        $\leq$ 2000 lymphocytes/cu mm
        Positive serologic test in blood and spinal fluid
    Meningovascular disease
        Increased cell count ($\leq$ 100 mononuclear cells/cu mm) in 60% of cases
        Increased protein (up to 260 mg/dl) in 66% of cases; increased gamma globulin in 75% of cases
        Positive serologic test in blood and spinal fluid
        Laboratory findings due to cerebrovascular thrombosis
    Tabes dorsalis
        Early—increased cell count and protein and positive serologic test in blood and spinal fluid (titer may be low). Increased gamma globulin is less marked than in general paresis.
        Late—$\cong$ 25% of patients may have normal spinal fluid and negative serologic tests in blood and spinal fluid

General paresis (spinal fluid always abnormal in untreated patients)

Increased cell count up to 175 mononuclear cells/cu mm

Increased protein up to 100 mg/dl with marked increase in gamma globulin

Positive serologic test (titer usually high)

CSF cell count should return to normal within 3 months after therapy; otherwise retreatment is indicated.

Asymptomatic CNS lues

May have negative blood and positive spinal fluid serologic test

Increased cell count and protein are index of activity.

Cardiovascular syphilis-VDRL—usually reactive but titer often low

Gummatous lesions-VDRL—almost always reactive, usually in high titer

Cardiovascular, liver, etc., involvement

Biopsy of skin, lymph node, larynx, testes, etc.

Adequately treated primary and secondary syphilis usually show falling titer and become serologically nonreactive in about 9 and 12 months, respectively; 2% of patients remain positive for several years. Therapy causes a negative reagin test in 75% of patients with early latent syphilis in 5 years, but less than 25% of patients with late syphilis become nonreactive although titers may fall steadily over a long period. In contrast to the VDRL, the FTA-ABS remains reactive once it has become reactive, except for early primary syphilis, and cannot be used to confirm a cure.

If late syphilis of any type is suspected, always do FTA-ABS, even if VDRL is nonreactive.

One-third of patients with only weakly reactive VDRL are reactive with more sensitive test (e.g., TPI); weakly reactive VDRL should always be confirmed with FTA-ABS.

VDRL may be nonreactive in undiluted serum in presence of an actual high titer ("prozone" phenomenon) in 1% of patients with secondary syphilis.

See Serologic Tests for Syphilis, pp. 138–140.

YAWS (due to *Treponema pertenue*), PINTA (due to *T. carateum*), BEJEL (due to a treponema indistinguishable from *T. pallidum*)

Positive serologic tests for syphilis

Positive dark-field demonstration of a treponema in smears from appropriate lesions

TUBERCULOSIS

Acid-fast stained smears and cultures (and occasionally guinea pig inoculation) of concentrates of suspected material from involved sites (e.g., sputum, gastric fluid, effusions, urine, CSF, pus) should be performed on multiple specimens. If negative, guinea pig inoculation of this material may be needed.

WBC is usually normal. Granulocytic leukemoid reaction may occur in miliary disease. Active disseminated disease is suggested by more monocytes (10–20%) than lymphocytes (5–10%) in peripheral smear.

ESR is normal in localized disease; increased in disseminated or advanced disease. It is not used as index of activity.

Moderate anemia may be present in advanced disease.

Characteristic histologic pattern appears in random biopsy of lymph node, liver, bone marrow (especially in miliary dissemination), or other involved sites (e.g., bronchus, pleura).

Urine—rule out renal tuberculosis in presence of hematuria (gross or microscopic) or pyuria with negative cultures for pyogenic bacteria.

Laboratory findings due to extrapulmonary tuberculosis

    Tuberculous meningitis

        CSF shows

            100–1000 WBC/cu mm (mostly lymphocytes)

            Increased protein (slight in early stages but continues to increase; > 300 mg/dl associated with advanced disease; much higher levels when block of CSF occurs)

            Decreased glucose (< 50% of blood glucose)

            Decreased chloride—not useful in diagnosis

            Increased tryptophan

            Acid-fast smear and culture from pellicle

        Serum sodium may be decreased (110–125 mEq/L) especially in aged; may also occur in overwhelming tuberculous infection.

    Tuberculous pleural effusion (see pp. 176–185)

        Sputum is positive on culture in 25% of patients; pleural fluid is positive on culture in 25% of patients.

        Fluid is an exudate with increased protein (> 3 gm/dl) and increased lymphocytes.

    Lymph nodes

        Culture is important to rule out infection due to other mycobacteria (atypical or anonymous).

Laboratory findings due to complications (see appropriate separate sections)

    Amyloidosis

    Addison's disease

    Other

Laboratory findings due to underlying diseases (e.g., diabetes mellitus, sickle cell anemia)

LEPROSY (HANSEN'S DISEASE)
(due to *Mycobacterium leprae*)

Mild anemia is found. Sulfone therapy frequently causes anemia, which indicates dosage change is needed.

Serum albumin is decreased, and serum globulin is increased.

ESR is increased.

Serum cholesterol is slightly decreased.

Serum calcium is slightly decreased.

False positive serologic test for syphilis occurs in ≤ 40% of patients.

Acid-fast bacilli are found in smear or tissue biopsy from nasal scrapings or lepromatous lesions. Acid-fast diphtheroids are not infrequently found in nasal septum smears or scrapings in normal persons, and *M. leprae* is not found here in two-thirds of early lepromatous cases. Therefore nasal smear may have very limited diagnostic value. Bacilli may show a typical granulation and fragmentation that precede the clinical improvement due to sulfone therapy. Larger, more nodular lesions are more likely to be posi-

Table 31-3. Stages of Syphilis

Stage	Symptom	Time After Exposure	Laboratory Changes	Response to Treatment	
				VDRL	FTA-ABS/MHA-TP
Primary	Chancre	Average 3 weeks (11–90 days)	Dark-field positive Serologic tests often negative Rising titers VDRL and FTA-ABS	Remains negative	Remains negative
	Lymph nodes	Average 4 weeks	Dark-field positive Rising antibody titers	Usually becomes negative within 6 months	After seroconversion, usually remains positive indefinitely without regard for stage of disease or adequacy of treatment
Secondary		6–20 weeks	Dark-field positive Peak antibody titers CSF abnormal in 25–50% of patients without CNS findings	Usually becomes negative within 12–24 months	

Stage	Duration	Findings	Serology
		Increased alkaline phosphatase (due to pericholangitis) in 20% Proteinuria	
Latent	Early: 3–12 months Late: > 12 months	CSF VDRL negative Serum treponemal test positive Falling VDRL titers	
Neurosyphilis (asymptomatic)	Usually > 4 years	CSF: VDRL positive or increased cells and protein Serum treponemal test positive; nontreponemal test positive or negative Without treatment, CNS disease occurs within 10 years in 20% of patients	
Late (tertiary)			Usually remains positive indefinitely with gradually declining titer
Late (tertiary) Symptomatic	> 4 years	Same as asymptomatic Treatment does not reverse nontreponemal test in 25–75% of patients	

tive. During lepra reactions, enormous numbers of bacilli may be present in skin lesions and may be found in peripheral blood smears. Bacilli are usually very difficult to find in skin lesions of tuberculoid leprosy.

Histologic pattern of the lesions is used for classification of type of leprosy.

Laboratory findings due to complications are noted.

Amyloidosis occurs in 40% of patients in the United States.

Other diseases (e.g., tuberculosis, malaria, parasitic infestation) may be present.

Sterility due to orchitis is very frequent.

SWIMMING-POOL DISEASE
(due to *Mycobacterium balnei*)

Histologic pattern of ulcerated skin lesions on extremities is that of nonspecific granuloma containing acid-fast bacilli.

Cultures from these lesions must be incubated at 31°C rather than 37°C.

ANTIBIOTICS

The summary of the selection of antibiotic drugs presented in Table 31-4 illustrates various approaches to the problems of treating infections rather than being an encyclopedic compendium of antibiotic sensitivity studies. The following points must be remembered when using this table.

Although in many cases an infection may be successfully treated without a culture, a sensitivity test should *always* be performed for the organism cultured in a particular case, since various strains of bacteria may have different antibiotic susceptibility. Tables published in the literature are useful general guides, but they may not be applicable to a specific case. Thus the antibiotic of choice may vary, depending on whether the infection is due to a community-acquired strain or to a hospital-acquired strain of bacteria. Some antibiotics may not be reliable, or they may cause toxic effects or provoke an allergic response.

Cultures should always be taken before antibiotic therapy has been administered. Repeat cultures should be taken if clinical response does not occur.

A smear for Gram's stain should always be taken at the same time as the culture; this is often a useful guide to the choice of antibiotics until the culture results are reported.

Causes of antibiotic treatment failure include

Improper laboratory techniques (e.g., taking the culture after beginning antibiotic treatment, using incorrect culture media, failing to use anaerobic methodology)

Mixed bacterial infections

Inadequate dosage of antibiotic

Interfering pathology (e.g., obstruction with lack of adequate drainage, immunologically compromised patient)

Since there are inherent delays in the publication of a book, the most current information is likely to be found in the periodical literature.

Table 31-4 should be used in conjunction with Table 19-1, pp. 188–193.

Table 31-4. Antibiotic Selection Guide for the More Common Infections

Organism	Major	Minor	Primary Choice[a]	Alternative Choice[a]
Gram-positive				
Staphylococcus aureus	Endocarditis, bacteremia, pneumonia, osteomyelitis		Nafcillin Oxacillin Penicillin G (if sensitive)	Cephalosporin Vancomycin Clindamycin TMP/SMX
		Minor soft tissue	Dicloxacillin Cloxacillin Oxacillin Penicillin G (if sensitive)	Cephalosporin Clindamycin Erythromycin
Staphylococcus epidermidis	Sepsis, GU tract infection, infected CNS shunts		Same as *S. aureus*	
Streptococcus (Diplococcus) pneumoniae	Pneumonia with bacteremia		Penicillin G	Cephalosporin Chloramphenicol Erythromycin
	Meningitis, arthritis		Penicillin G	Chloramphenicol Vancomycin
		Pneumonia Otitis	Penicillin G Penicillin V	Erythromycin
Streptococcus pyogenes (beta-hemolytic Group A)	Osteomyelitis, burns, sepsis		Penicillin G or V	Ampicillin Cephalosporin
		Pharyngitis, otitis, impetigo	Benzathine penicillin or penicillin V	Erythromycin
		Prophylaxis of rheumatic fever	Penicillin G	Sulfadiazine
Streptococcus viridans (alpha-hemolytic, including anaerobic streptococci)	Endocarditis, brain abscess		Penicillin G with/without streptomycin	Cephalosporin Vancomycin
Group D streptococci (enterococci)	Endocarditis, bacteremia		Ampicillin (or penicillin G) + streptomycin or gentamicin	Vancomycin + streptomycin or gentamicin
		GU tract infection	Ampicillin or amoxicillin	Nitrofurantoin
Corynebacterium diphtheriae	Diphtheria		Erythromycin	Penicillin G
		Carrier	Erythromycin	
Bacillus anthracis	Anthrax		Penicillin G	Erythromycin Tetracycline

Table 31-4 (continued)

Organism	Infection Major	Infection Minor	Primary Choice[a]	Alternative Choice[a]
Clostridium perfringens (welchii)	Wound infection		Penicillin G	Clindamycin Tetracycline Metronidazole Chloramphenicol
Clostridium tetani	Tetanus		Penicillin G	Tetracycline
Clostridium difficile	Antibiotic-associated colitis		Vancomycin	Metronidazole Bacitracin
Listeria monocytogenes	Sepsis, meningitis		Ampicillin with/without gentamicin	Tetracycline Erythromycin TMP/SMX Chloramphenicol
Mycoplasma pneumoniae		Pneumonia, bronchitis	Erythromycin or tetracycline	
Ureplasma urealyticum		GU tract infection	Erythromycin	Tetracycline
Actinomyces israelii	Actinomycosis		Penicillin G	Tetracycline
Treponema pallidum	Syphilis		Penicillin G	Tetracycline Erythromycin
Leptospira	Leptospirosis		Penicillin G	Tetracycline
Lyme disease agent	Lyme disease		Tetracycline	Penicillin G
Spirillum minus	Rat bite fever		Penicillin G	Tetracycline Streptomycin
Streptobacillus moniliformis	Rat bite fever (Haverhill fever)		Penicillin G	Tetracycline Streptomycin
Gram-negative				
Neisseria gonorrhoeae	Bacteremia		Penicillin G	Cephalosporin Tetracycline
		Gonorrhea, beta-lactamase negative	Penicillin G or amoxicillin	Ampicillin Tetracycline
		Gonorrhea beta-lactamase positive	Spectinomycin	Cephalosporin
Neisseria meningitidis	Bacteremia		Penicillin G	Cephalosporin
	Meningitis		Penicillin G	Chloramphenicol Sulfa (frequently resistant)
		Carrier state	Rifampin	Minocycline Sulfa (frequently resistant)
Branhamella catarrhalis	Bronchitis, pneumonia		TMP/SMX	Erythromycin Tetracycline Cephalosporin

Table 31-4 (continued)

Organism	Infection Major	Infection Minor	Primary Choice[a]	Alternative Choice[a]
Hemophilus influenzae	Meningitis,[b] pneumonia, epiglottitis		Chloramphenicol	Ampicillin TMP/SMX Cephalosporin[b]
		Otitis	Ampicillin Amoxicillin	TMP/SMX Cephalosporin Tetracycline
Bordetella pertussis	Whooping cough		Erythromycin	Ampicillin TMP/SMX
Escherichia coli	Neonatal sepsis, bacteremia		Ampicillin Aminoglycoside	Kanamycin Cephalosporin TMP/SMX Tetracycline Penicillins (e.g., carbenicillin, ticarcillin, mezlocillin, piperacillin, azlocillin)
		GU tract infection	Ampicillin	Sulfa Amoxicillin
		Enteropathogenic diarrhea	Colistin	Nitrofurantoin Nalidixic acid TMP/SMX Cephalosporin Neomycin
Klebsiella	Bacteremia		Gentamicin	Kanamycin Cephalosporin Tetracycline
		GU tract infection	Cephalosporin	Tetracycline TMP/SMX Nitrofurantoin
Pseudomonas aeruginosa	Sepsis, burns		A penicillin + aminoglycoside	
		GU tract infection	A penicillin	Aminoglycoside Polymyxin
Pseudomonas mallei	Glanders		Streptomycin + tetracycline	Streptomycin + chloramphenicol
Pseudomonas pseudomallei	Melioidosis		TMP/SMX	Chloramphenicol + tetracycline or aminoglycoside Sulfonamide
Enterobacter	Bacteremia		Aminoglycoside	A penicillin Cephalosporin
		GU tract infection	TMP/SMX	Carbenicillin
Proteus mirabilis	Bacteremia		Ampicillin	Aminoglycoside Cephalosporin Chloramphenicol
		GU tract infection	Ampicillin	Cephalosporin TMP/SMX

Table 31-4 (continued)

Organism	Infection Major	Infection Minor	Primary Choice[a]	Alternative Choice[a]
Providencia *(Proteus in-constans)*	Sepsis		Aminogly-coside	A penicillin Cephalosporin TMP/SMX Chloramphenicol
Bacteroides	Bacteremia Abscess		Clindamycin Metronidazole	Penicillin G (except *B. fragilis*) Ampicillin (except *B. fragilis*) A penicillin Chloramphenicol Cefoxitin
Brucella	Brucellosis		Tetracycline with/without strep-tomycin	Chloramphenicol with/without streptomycin TMP/SMX
Campylobacter *(Vibrio)* *fetus*	Diarrhea Sepsis, meningi-tis		Erythromycin Gentamicin	Tetracycline Chloramphenicol Other aminogly-cosides
Francisella *tularensis*	Tularemia		Streptomycin Aminogly-coside	Tetracycline Chloramphenicol
Pasteurella *multocida*	Sepsis Abscesses		Penicillin G	Tetracycline Cephalosporin
Gardnerella *(Hemophi-lus) vagi-nalis*		Vaginitis	Metronidazole	Ampicillin
Hemophilus *ducreyi*	Chancroid		TMP/SMX or erythromy-cin	Tetracycline Streptomycin
Calymmato-bacterium granulo-matis	Granuloma in-guinale		Tetracycline	Streptomycin
Legionella *pneumo-philia*	Legionnaire's disease		Erythromycin with/without rifam-pin	
Serratia	Bacteremia		Aminogly-coside	A penicillin Cephalosporin Chloramphenicol TMP/SMX
Salmonella	Bacteremia		Ampicillin (if susceptible) Chloramphen-icol	Amoxicillin TMP/SMX
		Gastroen-teritis	None unless there is invasion of tissues or blood or high-risk patient (e.g., infant < 2 months, sickle cell disease) Ampicillin for *S. typhi* carriers	

Table 31-4 (continued)

Organism	Infection Major	Infection Minor	Primary Choice[a]	Alternative Choice[a]
Shigella		Gastroen- teritis	TMP/SMX	Chloramphenicol Ampicillin Tetracycline
Vibrio cholerae	Cholera		Tetracycline	TMP/SMX
Yersinia en- terocolitica	Enteritis Arthritis Sepsis		TMP/SMX	Aminoglycoside Cephalosporin Tetracycline
Yersinia pestis	Bubonic plague		Streptomycin	Tetracycline Chloramphenicol
Chlamydia				
C. psittaci	Psittacosis, or- nithosis		Tetracycline	Chloramphenicol
C. tracho- matis	Trachoma		Tetracycline (topical + oral)	Sulfonamide (topical + oral)
	Inclusion conjunctivitis		Erythromycin	Tetracycline Sulfonamide
	Pneumonia		Erythromycin	Sulfonamide Tetracycline
	Urethritis		Tetracycline	Erythromycin
	Lymphogranu- loma ve- nereum		Tetracycline	Erythromycin
Pneumocystis carinii	Pneumonia		TMP/SMX	Pentamidine
Rickettsia	Rocky Mountain spotted fever, Q fever, typhus, scrub typhus, en- demic typhus, rickettsialpox		Tetracycline	Chloramphenicol

TMP/SMX = trimethoprim-sulfamethoxazole.

[a] When more than one antibiotic appears for an infection, only one is to be administered at a time unless combination is denoted by a + sign.

[b] Cephalosporins are not recommended for treatment of meningitis.

These tables are meant only as general guides. For the most accurate and current information, the reader is referred to the recent literature and the manufacturers' inserts. The reader should also be familiar with the antibiogram showing the prevalence of various organisms and their percent of susceptibility *for that particular hospital* or *environment* (see Table 31-6). It must be remembered that antibiotic susceptibility may change. Other factors not included here may cause the selection of a drug other than one included here (e.g., cost, route of administration, time of absorption, frequency of dosage, toxicity, side effects, patient allergies, seasonal preva- lence of disease, patient age, and many more). These tables are never a substitute for taking material for Gram stain, culture, and sensitivity before antibiotic treatment is started but can be useful empiric guides pending the result of such tests.

Source: Data from C. J. Wilkowske and P. E. Hermans, General principles of antimicrobial therapy. *Mayo Clin. Proc.* 58:6, 1983; The choice of antimicrobial drugs. *Med. Lett.* 26:19, 1984; B. R. Meyers, *Antimicrobial Therapy Guide.* Princeton, N.J.: Antimicrobial Prescribing, Inc., 1984; J. D. Nelson, *Pocketbook of Pediatric Antimicrobial Therapy.* Dallas: Jodone, 1983.

Prevalence of Organisms

In addition to becoming familiar with the data in Table 31-4 relating antibiotics to bacteria, the clinician should appreciate that the prevalence of organisms will vary geographically and from one time period to another. It would be useful to be familiar with the prevalence of various bacteria isolated from different sites and the susceptibility or resistance of organisms to antibiotics in *that particular practice environment*. Illustrations of such data are shown in Tables 31-5, 31-6, and 31-7. The clinician should obtain the specific data from the laboratory to which he refers his speci-

Table 31-5. Organisms Isolated from Various Sites (sample)

Urine (600 isolates)	
Escherichia coli	46%
Pseudomonas aeruginosa	15%
Proteus mirabilis	9%
Enterococcus	7%
Klebsiella pneumoniae	7%
All others	16%
Blood (100 isolates)	
E. coli	16%
Staphylococcus epidermidis	15%
Enterococcus	13%
P. aeruginosa	10%
Staphylococcus aureus	10%
All others	36%
Respiratory Tract (450 isolates)	
P. aeruginosa	24%
E. coli	9%
K. pneumoniae	9%
Serratia marcescens	9%
Enterobacter sp.	13%
S. aureus	7%
P. mirabilis	6%
All others	33%
Wound (400 isolates)	
S. aureus	22%
S. epidermidis	15%
Enterococcus	12%
E. coli	10%
P. aeruginosa	9%
All others	32%
Operating Room Specimens (100 isolates)	
P. aeruginosa	16%
E. coli	15%
Enterococcus	13%
S. aureus	12%
S. epidermidis	9%
K. pneumoniae	9%
Enterobacter	7%
All others	19%

Table 31-6. Year 198_ Antibiotic Resistance Data for Gram-Positive Organisms (sample)

Gram-Positive Organism	No. Treated	% Resistant								
		Penicillin	Methicillin, Nafcillin	Vancomycin	Erythromycin	Clindamycin	Gentamicin	Tetracycline	TMP/SMX	Chloramphenicol
Staphylococcus aureus	2400	91	14[a]	0	26	13	11	25	8	3
Staphylococcus epidermidis	380	87	53	0	56	44	40	39	24	15
Pneumococcus	110	0	0	0	0			29	100	0
Beta-streptococcus Group A	15	0	0	0	0	14	0	91		0
Beta-streptococcus Group B	50	0	0			0	74	75	57	
Enterococcus	880	[b]	98	2	60	97	94		55	31
Other gram-positive organisms	140	16	40	0	14	24	27	36	16	4
Total	3975	82	34	1	35	31	34	38	23	10

[a] Methicillin-resistant *S. aureus* is clinically resistant to nafcillin, dicloxacillin, and cephalosporins.
[b] Almost all enterococci are susceptible to penicillin and ampicillin.

Table 31-7. Year 198_ Antibiotic Resistance Data for Gram-Negative Organisms (sample)

Gram-Negative Organisms	No. Treated	% Resistant											
		Ampicillin	Carbenicillin	Piperacillin	Cephalothin	Cefamandole	Cefoxitin	Cefotaxime	Moxalactam	Gentamicin	Tobramycin	Amikacin	TMP/SMX
Escherichia coli	3150	43	40	24	24	6	2	1	1	4	4	1	8
Klebsiella	1500	98	97	30	25	14	4	1	1	21	17	2	22
Enterobacter	580	88	26	11	85	17	74	5	5	7	6	1	8
Serratia marcescens	260	94	48	30	97	71	46	4	8	41	43	10	33
Proteus mirabilis	740	16	12	3	9	2	2	1	1	2	2	0	8
Proteus species	140	87	23	9	88	31	22	1	0	4	2	0	8
Pseudomonas aeruginosa	1280	99	34	19	100	99	99	81	73	52	22	15	95
Pseudomonas species	100	90	71	42	97	91	85	83	42	55	50	37	43
Acinetobacter	400	91	27	8	97	93	89	56	85	7	8	6	16
Providencia	170	82	56	38	86	4	3	2	1	38	35	2	32
Citrobacter	400	92	77	37	53	24	43	11	7	27	25	13	27
Salmonella	220	19	18	19	16	9	1	1	0	0	0	0	2
Shigella	70	52	49	26	11	0	0	2	0	0	0	0	0
Other gram-negative organisms	300	74	56	13	76	33	42	11	15	19	20	13	17
Total	9310	67	47	22	47	29	29	17	17	17	12	5	25

mens; note that these data will refer to the specific previous time period (e.g., 3 or 6 months) and will be periodically updated. Using the data in these various tables, the clinician can initiate antibiotic therapy pending the results of culture and sensitivity studies; these tables are not substitutes for performing such microbiologic studies.

Suggested Antibiotics for Routine Testing Against Certain Bacteria

Bacteria	Antibiotic
Staphylococci	Penicillin, methicillin, cephalothin, clindamycin, vancomycin, erythromycin
Enterococci	Ampicillin, gentamicin, penicillin, streptomycin
Enterobacteria	Ampicillin, chloramphenicol, gentamicin, cephalothin, carbenicillin, tetracycline, TMP/SMX. If gentamicin resistant, test amikacin. If cephalothin resistant, test cefoxitin and cefamandole.
Pseudomonas	Carbenicillin, gentamicin, amikacin, tobramycin, polymyxin
Anaerobes (e.g., clostridia, *Bacteroides,* fusobacteria, anaerobic cocci)	Penicillin, carbenicillin, chloramphenicol, clindamycin, cefoxitin, metronidazole, erythromycin, tetracycline

When these organisms are isolated from the GU tract, add nitrofurantoin, TMP/SMX, nalidixic acid.

All strains of *Streptococcus pyogenes* (Group A streptococci) and *Streptococcus pneumoniae* are very sensitive to penicillin G, so that identification alone is sufficient for choice of therapy. In contrast, therapy for enterococcal Group D streptococcal endocarditis is guided by in vitro susceptibility tests to penicillin, ampicillin, streptomycin, and gentamicin and by serum bactericidal tests.

Enterobacteriaceae should be tested against all aminoglycosides, cephalosporins, and ampicillin, since there are strains resistant to gentamicin that may be sensitive to tobramycin and/or amikacin; when susceptible to ampicillin or a cephalosporin, treatment should be continued with these rather than with the more toxic aminoglycosides.

Pseudomonas aeruginosa strains are not all susceptible to gentamicin; therefore testing against aminoglycosides is necessary.

In vitro testing is not usually useful in *Bacillus fragilis* infections, which should be treated with chloramphenicol, clindamycin, or metronidazole.

Related Drug Susceptibilities

Bacteria Susceptible To	Are Usually Susceptible To
Penicillin	Penicillin G, penicillin V
Methicillin	oxacillin, cloxacillin, dicloxacillin, nafcillin
Ampicillin	Hetacillin, amoxicillin
Carbenicillin	Ticarcillin
Cephalothin	Cephalexin, cefazolin, cefoxitin, cephapirin, cephaloridine, cefamandole, cephradine

Related Drug Susceptibilities

Bacteria Susceptible To	Are Usually Susceptible To
Polymyxin	Polymyxin B, colistin
Tetracycline	Demeclocycline, doxycycline, minocycline
Gentamicin	Tobramycin, amikacin

Not every member of a class of related drugs need be tested.

Sometimes drugs should be tested in combination (e.g., penicillins and aminoglycosides may be synergistic with certain strains of *Pseudomonas aeruginosa* and Group D streptococci).

Certain in vitro susceptibility results are not reliable for clinical use (e.g., *Salmonella typhi* shows in vitro susceptibility to aminoglycosides and polymyxins; enterococci to cephalosporins; *Nocardia* to various antibiotics).

Antibiotic-resistant strains develop in certain species that were previously predictably susceptible and may now require testing (e.g., *Hemophilus influenzae* for ampicillin, *Neisseria gonorrhoeae* for penicillin, *Neisseria meningitidis* for sulfonamide, *S. typhi* for ampicillin and chloramphenicol).

Indications for Use of Antibiotics

*Erythromycin**

Indications

> *Staphylococcus aureus*—minor infections
>
> Infections due to beta-hemolytic streptococci, *Streptococcus pneumoniae, Mycoplasma pneumoniae, Legionella, Campylobacter jejuni*
>
> Diphtheria carriers
>
> Prophylaxis for rheumatic fever
>
> Prophylaxis for subacute bacterial endocarditis in patients allergic to penicillin
>
> Syphilis and gonorrhea in patients allergic to penicillin

Tetracyclines

Indications

> Genitourinary tract infections (not in acute pyelonephritis unless other antimicrobial agents [e.g., aminoglycosides, semisynthetic penicillins] are contraindicated)
>
> Chronic bronchopulmonary infections for long-term, intermittent, suppressive therapy alternated with other broad-spectrum agents (e.g., ampicillin)
>
> Syphilis and gonorrhea in patients allergic to penicillin
>
> Chlamydial and *Ureaplasma urealyticum* urethritis—treatment of choice. Doxycycline for chlamydial cervicitis.
>
> *M. pneumoniae*—treatment of choice
>
> Brucellosis—treatment of choice when combined with tetracycline and streptomycin
>
> Cholera
>
> Prophylaxis for traveler's diarrhea due to toxicogenic *Escherichia coli*
>
> Whipple's disease

*Source: Data from W. R. Wilson and F. R. Cockerill, Tetracyclines, chloramphenicol, erythromycin, and clindamycin. *Mayo Clin. Proc.* 58:92, 1983.

Table 31-8. Organisms for Which Penicillins Are Antimicrobial Drug of Choice

Penicillin Type	Organism	Alternate Drug (penicillin allergy)
Penicillin G	*Streptococcus pneumoniae*	Erythromycin
	Streptococcus pyogenes	Erythromycin
	Streptococcus viridans	Erythromycin
	Streptococcus faecalis (usually with an aminoglycoside)	Vancomycin with an aminoglycoside)
	Anaerobic streptococci	A tetracycline or clindamycin
	Staphylococcus aureus (non-penicillinase-producing)	A cephalosporin
	Neisseria meningitidis	Chloramphenicol
	Neisseria gonorrhoeae	A tetracycline or spectinomycin
	Bacillus anthracis	Erythromycin
	Clostridia	A tetracycline
	Corynebacterium diphtheriae	Erythromycin
	Erysipelothrix insidiosa	Erythromycin
	Pasteurella multocida	A tetracycline
	Streptobacillus moniliformis	A tetracycline
	Bacteroides (not *fragilis*)	Clindamycin or chloramphenicol
	Treponema pallidum	A tetracycline
	Spirillum minor	A tetracycline
	Leptospira	A tetracycline
	Fusospirochetes	A tetracycline
	Actinomyces israelii	A tetracycline
Methicillin, oxacillin, nafcillin, cloxacillin, dicloxacillin	*S. aureus* (penicillinase-producing)	A cephalosporin or vancomycin
Ampicillin	*Proteus mirabilis*	A cephalosporin
	Hemophilus influenzae	Chloramphenicol
	Actinomyces muris ratti	A tetracycline
	Listeria monocytogenes	A tetracycline
	Salmonellae (not *S. typhi*)	Chloramphenicol
	Shigellae	TMP/SMX
Carbenicillin, ticarcillin	*Pseudomonas aeruginosa*	Moxalactam, aminoglycosides
	Escherichia coli	A cephalosporin, aminoglycosides

Source: Data from A. J. Wright and C. J. Wilkowske, The penicillins. *Mayo Clin. Proc.* 58:21, 1983.

Tularemia, plague *(Yersinia pestis), Nocardia asteroides* infections
Rickettsial infections

Chloramphenicol
Indications
Anaerobic infections (especially *Bacteroides fragilis*)
Hemophilus influenzae meningitis
Typhoid fever
Patients allergic to penicillin with meningitis due to pneumococcus or meningococcus
Brain abscess
Rickettsial infection

Clindamycin
Indications (limited because of pseudomembranous enterocolitis that occurs relatively often in association with use of clindamycin)
Anaerobic infection, especially *B. fragilis,* in patients allergic to penicillin
Susceptible aerobic gram-positive cocci—only if other antimicrobial agents are contraindicated

Cephalosporins
First generation
Cephalothin, cephapirin, cephradine, cefazolin: parenteral
Cephaloxin, cephradine, cefadroxil, cefaclor: oral
Second generation
Cefamandole, cefoxitin: parenteral
Third generation
Cefotaxime, moxalactam: parenteral
Indications
Most gram-positive cocci (except enterococci): Second and third generation are less active and should not be used. Penicillin is more active and less expensive and should be used; if patient is allergic to penicillin, first generation cephalosporins may be indicated. Cephalosporins are less toxic and therefore preferable to clindamycin or vancomycin. Methicillin-resistant *S. aureus* should be treated with vancomycin.
Surgical prophylaxis: cephalosporin provides expanded gram-negative activity.
Enterobacteriaceae: Cephalosporins are generally treatment of choice, but bacterial susceptibility is unpredictable; until determined by in vitro tests, only empiric treatment should be moxalactam or an aminoglycoside (e.g., gentamicin, tobramycin, or amikacin).
Anaerobic bacteria: Cephalosporins are active but not treatment of choice, as there are more specific and more active agents (e.g., chloramphenicol, clindamycin, metronidazole).
Moxalactam is an alternative treatment for *H. influenzae* meningitis and rare meningitis due to Enterobacteriaceae with a demonstrated low minimal inhibitory concentration.

Vancomycin
Indications
In patients who cannot tolerate penicillin and cephalosporins or with infections due to antibiotic-resistant organisms (e.g.,

serious staphylococcal infections, *Corynebacterium diphthe-roides* endocarditis, endocarditis due to Group D enterococcal or nonenterococcal or *Streptococcus viridans* infections)
Antibiotic prophylaxis in patients who cannot tolerate penicillin
Antibiotic-induced enterocolitis due to staphylococcus and *Clostridium difficile*
Presence of prosthetic devices and infection due to organisms with multiple antibiotic resistance

*Trimethoprim-Sulfamethoxazole (TMP/SMX)**
Indications
    Genitourinary tract
        Chronic and recurrent infection, acute or chronic prostatitis due to susceptible organisms
        Gonorrhea (especially penicillinase-producing strains)
        Cystitis in females
    Respiratory tract
        Pneumocystis carinii pneumonia—treatment of choice
        Pulmonary prophylaxis—patients with cystic fibrosis
        Acute otitis media and bronchitis due to *S. pneumoniae* and *H. influenzae*
    Gastrointestinal
        Shigella (due to increasing ampicillin resistance)
        Salmonella typhi and *paratyphi* resistant to chloramphenicol
        Infantile diarrhea due to enteropathogenic *E. coli*
    N. asteroides infections

Metronidazole†
Indications
    Trichomonas vaginalis infections
    Amebiasis
    Giardiasis
    Gram-negative obligate anaerobic bacilli (e.g., *Bacteroides, Fusobacterium*) including mixed aerobic and anaerobic infections
    "Nonspecific vaginitis" due to *Gardnerella vaginalis* and various anaerobes

RICKETTSIAL DISEASES
Weil-Felix reaction (see Table 31-9, p. 598)
Complement-fixation or agglutination tests are positive in most cases when group-specific and type-specific rickettsial antigens are used. These tests permit differentiation of various rickettsial diseases. No test is available for trench fever. Rising titer during convalescence is the most important criterion. Early antibiotic therapy may delay appearance of antibodies for an additional 1–4 weeks, and titers may not be as high as when treatment is begun later. Low titers of complement-fixing antibodies may persist for years.

*Source: Data from F. R. Cockerill and S. R. Edson, Trimethoprim-sulfamethox-azole. *Mayo Clin. Proc.* 58:147, 1983.
†Source: Data from J. E. Rosenblatt and R. S. Edson, Metronidazole. *Mayo Clin. Proc.* 58:154, 1983.

Table 31-9. Weil-Felix Reaction*

Disease	Rickettsia	Proteus OX-19	Proteus OX-2	Proteus OX-K	Comments
Spotted fevers					
Rocky Mountain spotted fever	R. rickettsii	1–4+	1–4+	0	
Boutonneuse fever	R. conorii	1–4+	2–3+	0	OX-19 frequently positive only in low titer
Other spotted fevers	E.g., R. australis, R. siberica	1–4+	2–3+	0	
Rickettsialpox	R. akari	0	0	0	
Typhus group					
Endemic (murine) typhus	R. mooseri	3–4+	Usually 0 or 1+	0	
Epidemic typhus	R. prowazekii	3–4+	Usually 0 or 1+	0	
Brill-Zinsser disease (recrudescent latent epidemic typhus)	R. prowazekii	Usually negative, or positive only in very low titer	0	0	
Scrub typhus	R. tsutsugamushi	0	0	3+	OX-K appears late in second week. Positive in ≅ 50% of patients
Q fever	R. burnetii	0	0	0	Usually pneumonitis. Hepatitis in ⅓ of severe cases. Occasional cases of sub-acute endocarditis
Trench fever	R. quintana	0	0	0	Can be grown on blood agar

*Weil-Felix reaction: Rise in titer by comparison of acute and later serum samples is most useful diagnostic procedure. Agglutinins appear in 5–8 days, reach peak in 1 month, then decrease to negative by 5–6 months. Reaction will not detect Q fever and rickettsialpox and is usually negative in Brill-Zinsser disease. May not differentiate epidemic and endemic typhus and spotted fever. Thus, is not useful for *early* diagnosis.

Guinea pig inoculation—scrotal reaction following intraperitoneal injection of blood into male guinea pig

Marked in Rocky Mountain spotted fever and endemic typhus

Moderate in boutonneuse fever

Slight in epidemic typhus and Brill-Zinsser disease

Negative in scrub typhus, Q fever, trench fever, and rickettsialpox

Test is not often used at present.

Microscopic examination of organisms following animal inoculation; test is not often used.

In less severe cases, blood findings are not distinctive.

In *severe cases,* the following changes are found:

Early in disease WBC is decreased and lymphocytes are increased (usually 4000–6000/cu mm; as low as 1200/cu mm in early scrub typhus). Later WBC increases to 10,000–15,000/cu mm with shift to the left and toxic granulation. If count is higher, rule out secondary bacterial infection or hemorrhage.

Mild normochromic normocytic anemia (as low as Hg = 9 gm/dl) appears around tenth day.

ESR is increased.

Total protein and serum albumin are decreased.

BUN may be increased (prerenal).

Serum chloride may be decreased.

Urine shows slight increase in albumin; granular casts.

CSF is normal despite symptoms of meningitis.

Blood cultures for bacteria are negative (to rule out other tick-borne diseases, e.g., tularemia).

Laboratory findings due to specific organ involvement (e.g., pneumonitis, hepatitis) or due to complications (e.g., secondary bacterial infection, hemorrhage) are present.

Acute glomerulonephritis occurs in 78% of patients with epidemic typhus, 50% of patients with Rocky Mountain spotted fever, and 30% of patients with scrub typhus.

VIRAL PNEUMONIA DUE TO EATON AGENT (*MYCOPLASMA PNEUMONIAE*)

WBC is slightly increased (in 25% of patients) or is normal.

ESR is increased in 65% of patients.

Increased cold hemagglutination occurs late in course in 50% of patients ($\leq$ 90% in severe illness); becomes positive at about seventh day, rises to peak at 4 weeks, then declines rapidly and usually is negative by 4 months. May sometimes be present in other conditions (see p. 147).

Increased streptococcal MG agglutination occurs in 25% of patients; higher titer in more severe illness.

Serologic tests

Show fourfold increase in titer in complement-fixation and, less frequently, hemagglutination tests. Complement-fixation titer is the most useful serologic test; increase begins in 7–9 days; peak at 3–4 weeks may last for 4–6 months, then gradual fall for 2–3 years; if only a convalescent serum is available, a titer of > 1:64 is highly suggestive of diagnosis of *Mycoplasma pneumoniae* infection.

Fluorescent antibody test is useful.

Isolation of organism by special techniques on broth media.

Mycoplasma hominis may cause pyelonephritis, pelvic inflammatory disease, and postpartum febrile complications. Mycoplasmas should also be considered in the differential diagnosis of acute arthritis, hemolytic anemia, various dermatologic disorders, myocardial or cerebral disease, as well as severe bilateral pneumonia.

UPPER RESPIRATORY VIRAL INFECTION

Due to respiratory syncytial virus

ESR and WBC may be increased in children.

Pharyngeal smears may reveal many epithelial cells that contain cytoplasmic inclusion bodies.

Rise in titer of complement-fixing and neutralizing antibodies occurs during convalescence. Since complement-fixing antibodies soon disappear but neutralizing antibodies persist longer, the former should be used if reinfection is suspected.

Only virus isolation or rise in antibody titer during convalescence allows specific diagnosis.

Due to adenovirus (may cause at least six clinical syndromes involving pharynx, conjunctiva, and pneumonitis)

WBC is slightly decreased after about 7 days.

ESR is increased.

Complement-fixing and neutralizing antibodies appear after 1 week and peak in 2–3 weeks. Complement-fixing antibody decreases considerably in 2–3 months, but neutralizing antibody may decrease only 2–3 times after 1–2 years. An increase in complement-fixing antibody titer during convalescence is presumptive evidence of infection but does not indicate the type of adenovirus.

Only virus isolation or rise in type-specific neutralizing antibody titer during convalescence allows specific diagnosis.

Due to rhinoviruses

WBC may be slightly increased.

ESR is increased in ≅ 35% of patients.

Serologic confirmation by rise in neutralizing antibody titer during convalescence or virus isolation allows specific diagnosis.

Complement-fixing antibody titer is not specific.

Due to parainfluenza virus

WBC is variable at first; later becomes normal or decreased.

INFLUENZA

WBC is usually normal (5000–10,000/cu mm) with relative lymphocytosis. Leukopenia occurs in 50% of the patients. WBC > 15,000/cu mm suggests secondary bacterial infection.

Influenza virus antibody (hemagglutination inhibition, complement-fixation) titer shows fourfold increase in sera taken during acute phase and 2–3 weeks later.

PARAINFLUENZA

Specific diagnosis requires recovery of virus in tissue-culture preparation.

Serologic tests include hemagglutination inhibition and tissue-culture neutralization; complement-fixation serves only Types II and III. Not useful for routine clinical studies.

CHLAMYDIAE INFECTIONS

Trachoma—see p. 601.

Ophthalmia neonatorum—mothers have genital infection (usually cervicitis), and fathers have urethritis.

Adult form of inclusion conjunctivitis is associated with genital tract infections.

Typical intracytoplasmic inclusions in epithelial cells on Giemsa-stained smears from conjunctival scrapings are found in 50% of cases. Inflammatory response shows both neutrophils and mononuclear cells compared to viral conjunctivitis, which shows predominantly lymphocytes and allergic conjunctivitis that shows predominantly eosinophils. Immunofluorescent stains are commercially available and significantly increase sensitivity.

Tissue culture of *Chlamydia* is the most sensitive and specific, test and positive cultures are usually detectable within 48 hours.

Serologic tests: Microimmunofluorescence titers ($\geqq 1:8$) are positive in nearly all patients, and complement-fixation titers ($\geqq 1:16$) are positive in $\cong$ 50% of patients (antigens not yet commercially available).

Distinctive pneumonia syndrome of infants (afebrile, chronic diffuse lung involvement, increased serum IgG and IgM, slight eosinophilia, distinctive cough) is the major cause of pneumonia before age 6 months with incidence of 8/1000 live births; 70% of infants of infected mothers become infected.

Psittacosis—see below.

Lymphogranuloma venereum—see p. 607.

Genital tract infection—see Nonspecific Urethritis, pp. 555–556.

Reiter's syndrome—*Chlamydia trachomatosis* has been isolated from the urethra in up to 60% of men with Reiter's syndrome, but tetracycline does not change the clinical course, and etiologic role is speculative.

Acute proctitis—see p. 240.

TRACHOMA

Typical cytoplasmic inclusion bodies are in epithelial cells scraped from conjunctiva of upper eyelid.

Secondary bacterial infection is common.

PSITTACOSIS

WBC may be normal or decreased in acute phase and increases during convalescence.

ESR is increased or frequently is normal.

Cold agglutination is negative.

Albuminuria is common.

Sputum smear and culture show normal flora.

Viral serologic tests: Positive complement-fixation test in early stage is presumptive but is not conclusive because of cross reaction with lymphogranuloma venereum and false positive in presence of some other infections (e.g., brucellosis, Q fever). Rising complement-fixation titer is seen between acute-phase and convalescent-phase sera.

COXSACKIEVIRUS AND ECHOVIRUS INFECTIONS
(e.g., epidemic pleurodynia, "grippe," meningitis, myocarditis, herpangina, etc.)

Laboratory findings are not specific.

CSF
> Cell count is $\leq$ 500/cu mm, occasionally $\leq$ 2000/cu mm; predominantly polynuclear leukocytes at first, then predominantly lymphocytes.
> Protein may increase $\leq$ 100 mg/dl.
> Glucose is normal.

WBC varies but is usually normal.

Viral serologic tests show increasing titer of neutralizing or complement-fixing antibodies between acute-phase and convalescent-phase sera.

VIRAL GASTROENTEROCOLITIS
(especially echovirus)

Identified by exclusion by negative tests for other causes of the symptoms (e.g., failure to find *Entamoeba histolytica, Shigella, Salmonella*)

POLIOMYELITIS

CSF
> Cell count is usually 25–500/cu mm; rarely is normal or $\leq$ 2000/cu mm. At first, most are polynuclear leukocytes; after several days, most are lymphocytes.
> Protein may be normal at first; increased by second week (usually 50–200 mg/dl); normal by sixth week.
> Glucose is usually normal.
> GOT is always increased but does not correlate with serum GOT; reaches peak in 1 week and returns to normal by 4 weeks; level of GOT does not correlate with severity of paralysis.

CSF findings are not diagnostic but may occur in many CNS diseases due to viruses (e.g., Coxsackie, mumps, herpes), bacteria (e.g., pertussis, scarlet fever), other infections (e.g., leptospirosis, trichinosis, syphilis), CNS tumors, multiple sclerosis, etc.

Blood shows early moderate increase in WBC ($\leq$ 15,000/cu mm) and polynuclear leukocytes; normal within 1 week.

Laboratory findings of associated lesions (e.g., myocarditis) or complications (e.g., secondary bacterial infection, stone formation in GU tract, alterations in water and electrolyte balance due to continuous artificial respiration) are present. Increased SGOT in 50% of patients is due to the associated hepatitis.

Viral serologic tests show fourfold increase in neutralizing antibody titer between acute-phase and convalescent-phase (after 3 weeks) sera, but titer has already reached peak at time of hospitalization in 50% of patients.

Virus may be cultured from stool up to early convalescence (done by the U.S. Public Health Service's Communicable Disease Center, Atlanta, Ga.).

LYMPHOCYTIC CHORIOMENINGITIS

WBC is slightly decreased at first; normal with onset of meningitis.

ESR is usually normal.

Thrombocytopenia develops during first week.

CSF
> Cell count is increased (100–3000 lymphocytes/cu mm, occasionally $\leq$ 30,000).

Protein is normal or slightly increased.

Glucose is usually normal.

Viral serologic tests show increasing titer between acute-phase and convalescent-phase sera in complement-fixing (after 2 weeks) and neutralizing (after 6–8 weeks) antibodies.

Viral isolation by animal inoculation is not routinely performed.

EASTERN AND WESTERN EQUINE ENCEPHALOMYELITIS

Marked decrease occurs in WBC with relative lymphocytosis.

CSF findings (see Table 25-1, pp. 278–282).

RABIES (HYDROPHOBIA)

WBC is increased (20,000–30,000/cu mm), with increased polynuclear leukocytes and large mononuclear cells.

Urine shows hyaline casts; reaction for albumin, sugar, and acetone may be positive.

CSF is usually normal or has a slight increase in protein and an increased number of mononuclear cells (usually < 100/cu mm).

Brain of suspected animal shows Negri bodies (absent in > 10% of animals with virus isolated from brain).

Fluorescent antibody examination of postmortem brain tissue is fast, accurate, and reliable.

Suspected animal dies within 7–10 days.

ENCEPHALOMYELITIS (VIRAL AND POSTINFECTIOUS)

CSF

Early (first 2–3 days)

Cell count is usually increased (≦ 100/cu mm), mostly polynuclear leukocytes (higher total count and more polynuclear leukocytes in infants).

Protein is usually normal.

Glucose and chloride are normal.

Later (after third day)

Increased cell count is > 90% lymphocytes.

Protein gradually increases after first week (≦ 100 mg/dl).

Glucose and chloride remain normal.

Viral serologic tests are for specific virus identification (fourfold increase from acute-phase sera to convalescent-phase sera in hemagglutination-inhibition, neutralization, or complement-fixation titers).

For additional laboratory tests, see

Cytomegalic inclusion disease (next section)

Mumps (p. 604)

Rabies (preceding section)

Psittacosis (p. 601)

Other

CYTOMEGALIC INCLUSION DISEASE

(limited to salivary gland involvement in 10% of infant autopsies; disseminated in 1–2% of childhood autopsies)

Intranuclear inclusions in epithelial cells in urine sediment and liver biopsy (more useful in infants than adults)

Hemolytic anemia with icterus and thrombocytopenic purpura in infants

Complement-fixation test on acute-phase and convalescent-phase sera

Evidence of damage to liver, kidney, brain

Laboratory findings due to predisposing or underlying conditions (e.g., malignant lymphoma, leukemia, refractory anemia, after renal transplant) or after receiving many transfusions of fresh blood; may be associated with *Pneumocystis carinii* pneumonia in adults

May cause a syndrome of heterophil-negative infectious mononucleosis in immunologically competent adults characterized by

> Hematologic and hepatic test findings identical with those in heterophil-positive infectious mononucleosis due to Ebstein-Barr virus (see p. 364). CMV causes two-thirds of all heterophil-negative mononucleosis-like illness in patients over age 14 years.

> Immunologic findings

>> Increased cold agglutinin titer (same as in heterophil-positive patients)

>> Cryoglobulinemia is common (mixed IgG-IgM).

>> (Increased rheumatoid factors (cold-reactive more common than warm-reactive)

>> Positive direct Coombs' test is common.

>> Polyclonal hypergammaglobulinemia is common.

>> False positive serologic test for syphilis in < 3% of cases

>> Antinuclear antibodies (speckled pattern) commonly present transiently

> Confirmatory tests for CMV

>> Indirect immunofluorescence test for CMV-IgM allows rapid diagnosis using a single test during acute illness ($\geqq 1:32$); titer $1 \geqq 1:16$ may persist for 12 months in 24% of patients; may reappear during reactivation. False positive and false negative rate in newborns each > 20%.

>> Complement-fixing antibody shows fourfold increase in titer in sample taken during convalescence in 50% of cases; titer 1:64 may persist for 12 months in 75% of patients. Rheumatoid factor can cause false positive results.

>> Immunofluorescence test for CMV-IgG parallels complement-fixation test and is of limited usefulness.

>> Virus may be isolated from fresh urine (100% of cases) and throat swabs (50% of cases) during acute phase; virus may be shed in urine for years after onset of illness.

>> Viral inclusions may be seen in cells of urine sediment—results may be negative in a single specimen; such inclusions may be found in other viral infections.

MUMPS

Uncomplicated salivary adenitis

> WBC and ESR are normal; WBC may be decreased, with relative lymphocytosis.

> Serum and urine amylase are increased during first week of parotitis; therefore increase does not always indicate pancreatitis.

> Serum lipase is normal.

> Serologic tests

>> Serum neutralization test becomes positive by fifth day. It is the most reliable and specific index of immunity but also the most cumbersome and time-consuming.

Complement-fixation test becomes positive during second week and remains elevated > 6 weeks; paired sera showing a fourfold increase in titer confirm recent infection. High titer suggests recent infection. Test correlates well with neutralization test.

Hemagglutination-inhibition reaction develops later and persists longer (several months) than complement-fixation test. It is possibly useful for screening only at high titers and is less sensitive and specific than neutralization.

Complications of mumps

Orchitis (in 20% of postpubertal males but rare in children)
WBC is increased, with shift to the left. ESR is increased. Sperm are decreased or absent after bilateral atrophy.

Ovaries are involved in 5% of adult females.

Pancreatitis (pp. 271–272) is much less frequent in children. Serum amylase and lipase are increased. Patient may have hyperglycemia and glycosuria.

Meningitis or meningoencephalitis (p. 289)—mumps causes > 10% of cases of aseptic meningitis. The disease may be clinically identical with mild paralytic poliomyelitis. WBC is usually normal. Serum amylase may be increased even if no abdominal symptoms are present. CSF contains 0–2000 mononuclear cells.

Thyroiditis, myocarditis, arthritis, etc.

MEASLES (RUBEOLA)

WBC shows slight increase at onset, then falls to ≅ 5000/cu mm with increased lymphocyte count. Increased WBC with shift to the left suggests bacterial complication (e.g., otitis media, pneumonia, appendicitis).

Mild thrombocytopenia in early stage.

Wright's stain of sputum or nasal scrapings show measles multinucleated giant cells, especially during prodrome and early rash.

Papanicolaou's stain of urine sediment after appearance of rash shows intracellular inclusion bodies; more specific is fluorescent antibody demonstration of measles antigen in urine sediment cells.

Viral serologic tests: Neutralizing antibody, complement-fixation, and antihemagglutination tests become positive one week after onset, evidencing infection.

Measles encephalitis: There is a marked increase in WBCs. CSF may show slightly increased protein and ≦ 500 mononuclear cells/cu mm. ≦ 10% of all measles patients have a significant increase in cells in CSF.

Measles may cause remission in children with nephrosis.

RUBELLA (GERMAN MEASLES)

It is important to identify exposure to rubella infection and susceptibility status in pregnant women because infection in the first trimester of pregnancy is associated with congenital abnormalities, abortion, or stillbirth in about 30% of patients; during first month up to 80% of patients show this association.

Viral serologic tests: hemagglutination inhibition (HAI), complement-fixation, neutralization

Screening of pregnant women shows lack of susceptibility (i.e., previous rubella infection) if HAI titer is > 1:10–1:20 or if complement-fixation test is positive.

Change in HAI titer from acute-phase to convalescent-phase sera is the most useful technique to demonstrate a rise in antibody titer.

With rubella rash, diagnosis is established if acute sample titer is > 1:10 or if convalescent-phase serum taken 7 days after rash shows a fourfold increase in titer.

If no rash develops in a patient exposed to rubella, a convalescent-phase serum specimen taken 14–28 days after exposure that shows a fourfold increase in titer compared to the earlier sample indicates rubella infection.

Complement-fixing antibodies appear early (within 1 week after rash); therefore acute-phase serum must be collected promptly or the rise in titer may not be detected. They may last for from 8 months to some years. A positive test is useful to indicate recent infection or postinfection immunity. Rate of false positive test is < 2%.

Neutralization antibodies appear within 1–3 days after rash and reach maximum in 2 weeks, and test may remain positive for > 20 years; titer of ≧ 1:8 indicates past infection and therefore present immunity. A titer of 1:32 suggests recent infection. In infants with congenital abnormalities, a high neutralization antibody titer establishes the diagnosis. Test is technically difficult to perform and requires 7–10 days.

EXANTHEMA SUBITUM (ROSEOLA INFANTUM)
WBC is increased during fever, then decreased during rash, with relative lymphocytosis.

ERYTHEMA INFECTIOSUM (FIFTH DISEASE)
WBC is normal. Some patients have slight increase in eosinophils.

CHICKENPOX (VARICELLA)
Microscopic demonstration of very large epithelial giant cells with intranuclear inclusion in fluid or base of vesicle

Similar giant cells may occur in herpes simplex and herpes zoster.

WBC is normal; increased with secondary bacterial infection.
Serum electrophoresis may show decreased albumin with increased beta and gamma globulins.

SMALLPOX (VARIOLA)
Microscopic findings of cytoplasmic elementary bodies (Guarnieri bodies) in scrapings from base of skin lesions
Fluorescent antibody staining of virus from skin lesion
Viral serologic tests

Increased titer of neutralizing antibody in acute-phase and convalescent-phase (2–3 weeks later) sera

Rapid technique using vesicular fluid in hemagglutination, precipitation, or complement-fixation tests

WBC decreased during prodrome, increased during pustular rash

VACCINIA
(vaccine virus skin infection during vaccination against smallpox)
Guarnieri bodies (cytoplasmic inclusions) in skin lesions
Complications
Progressive vaccinia. *Rule out malignant lymphoma, chronic lymphatic leukemia, neoplasms, hypogammaglobulinemia, and dysgammaglobulinemia.*
Superimposed infection (e.g., tetanus)
Postvaccinal encephalitis

HERPES SIMPLEX
WBC is normal.
Scrapings of skin lesions show multinucleated giant cells with intranuclear inclusions (Tzanck smear). Vesicles produce a positive smear in 66% and positive viral culture in 100% of cases; pustules produce a positive smear in 50% and a positive viral culture in 70% of cases; crusted ulcers produce a positive smear in 15% and a positive viral culture in 34% of cases. Permits rapid diagnosis. Also positive in herpes zoster and varicella. (Positive smear refers to multinucleated giant cells not necessarily showing inclusions.)
Culture of skin lesions establishes the diagnosis.
Increased titer of complement-fixation and neutralizing antibodies is shown in convalescent-phase compared with acute-phase sera in primary infections; in recurrent infections, a high titer is present in acute-phase sera and thus has little value.
Findings of encephalitis if this complication occurs. High-titer serologic tests in CSF may be useful to establish the diagnosis.
Causes 5% of cases of aseptic meningitis.

HERPES ZOSTER (SHINGLES)
(reactivation of latent varicella virus)
Skin lesions may show intranuclear inclusions in degenerated epithelial cells or multinucleated giant cells.
40% of patients show increased cells ($\leq$ 300 mononuclear/cu mm) in CSF.

LYMPHOGRANULOMA VENEREUM
WBC is normal or increased $\leq$ 20,000/cu mm. There may be relative lymphocytosis or monocytosis.
ESR is increased.
Slight anemia may be present.
Serum globulin is increased with reversed A/G ratio during period of activity.
Biologically false positive reaction for syphilis that becomes negative in a few weeks appears in 20% of patients. *If titer increases, beware of concomitant syphilitic infection.*
Biopsy of regional lymph node shows stellate abscesses.
High complement-fixation titer (>1:80) and increasing titers or conversion of negative to positive indicate recent infections. Fall in titer evidences therapeutic success in acute stage. Persistent negative in the presence of disease is rare.

See Chlamydiae Infections, p. 600–601.

CAT-SCRATCH DISEASE
Microscopic examination of excised lymph node should be done.

Culture of involved lymph nodes is sterile.
ESR is usually increased.
WBC is usually normal but occasionally is increased $\leq$ 13,000/cu
  mm; eosinophils may be increased.
Frei test is negative.
Skin test with cat-scratch antigen is positive.

YELLOW FEVER
Decreased WBC is most marked by sixth day, associated with de-
  creased leukocytes and lymphocytes.
Proteinuria occurs in severe cases.
Laboratory findings are those due to GI hemorrhage, which is fre-
  quent; there may be associated oliguria and anuria.
Liver function tests are abnormal, but serum bilirubin is only
  slightly increased.
Biopsy of liver is taken for histologic examination.
Serum is positive by mouse intracerebral inoculation $\leq$ the fifth
  day; serum during convalescence protects mice.

DENGUE
WBC decreased (2000–5000/cu mm) with toxic granulation of
  leukocytes in early stage; often increased during convalescence
Children commonly have decreased platelets.

VIRAL EPIDEMIC HEMORRHAGIC FEVER
WBC is increased, with shift to the left.
Platelet count is decreased (< 100,000/cu mm) in 50% of patients.
Laboratory findings due to renal damage
    Proteinuria
    Oliguria with azotemia and hemoconcentration and abnormal
      electrolyte concentrations

Return of normal tubular function may take 4–6 weeks.

*Other viral hemorrhagic fevers (e.g., Philippine, Thailand, Singa-
  pore, Argentinian, Bolivian, Crimean, Omsk, Kyasanur Forest)
  show much less severe renal damage, and WBC is normal (Philippine, Thailand) or decreased.*

COLORADO TICK FEVER
WBC is decreased (2000–4000/cu mm). The number of polynuclear
  leukocytes is decreased, but with shift to the left.
Viral serologic tests show an increase in complement-fixation and
  neutralizing antibodies in sera taken during acute and convalescent phases.
Blood should be inoculated into suckling mice.

PHLEBOTOMUS FEVER (SANDFLY FEVER)
Decreased WBC and lymphocytes with shift to the left of polynu-
  clear leukocytes are most marked when fever ends.
CSF is normal.
Liver function tests are normal.
Urine is normal.

CRYPTOCOCCOSIS
(due to *Cryptococcus neoformans*)
Serologic tests

> Latex slide agglutination on serum and spinal fluid detects specific cryptococcal *antigen*. Use for screening of suspected cryptococcosis, since it is more sensitive than India ink smears of spinal fluid. Serum or cerebrospinal fluid is positive in most cases; when negative, agglutination test may be positive.
>
> Use whole yeast cell agglutination test for presence of *antibodies* in serum and cerebrospinal fluid. It is positive only in early CNS disease or no CNS involvement; may become positive only after institution of therapy. Rising titer may be a favorable prognostic sign.
>
> Culture of CSF for *C. neoformans* on Sabouraud's medium becomes positive in 1–2 weeks (positive in 97% of cases) followed by mouse inoculation; 20% of cases require multiple cultures. One may also get positive cultures from blood (25%), urine (37%), stool (20%), sputum (19%), and bone marrow (13%). Sputum cultures are most often positive when there is no x-ray evidence of pulmonary disease. Urine cultures are commonly positive with little kidney involvement. Positive blood culture indicates extensive disease and an extremely poor prognosis.
>
> India ink slide of CSF is positive in ≅ 50% of patients; thus one-half of cases will be missed if India ink preparations are used as the sole criterion.
>
> CSF cell count is almost always increased to ≦ 800 cells (more lymphocytes than leukocytes). Protein is increased in 90% (<500 mg/dl). Glucose is moderately decreased in ≅ 55% of patients. Relapse is less frequent when increase in protein and cells is marked rather than moderate. Poor prognosis is suggested if initial CSF examination shows positive India ink preparation, low glucose (<20 mg/dl), low WBC count (<20/cu mm).
>
> In biopsy material, mucicarmine stain is positive; also positive on intraperitoneal injection of white mice.
>
> CBC and ESR usually remain normal.
>
> Increased risk of failure of amphotericin B treatment if positive culture from sites other than CSF (e.g., blood, sputum, urine, etc.), anticryptococcal antibodies are absent, CSF or serum cryptococcal antigen titer initially is > 1:32 or posttreatment is ≧ 1:8, concomitant lymphoreticular malignancy or corticosteroid therapy or other immunosuppressed states.
>
> There is evidence of coexisting disease in ≅ 50% of patients (especially those with diabetes mellitus, prior steroid therapy, Hodgkin's disease, lymphosarcoma, leukemia, other immunosuppressed states).

COCCIDIOIDOMYCOSIS
(due to *Coccidioides immitis*)
Serologic tests

> Precipitin antibodies appear early, decrease after the third week, are uncommon after the fifth month. They occur at some stage of the disease in 75% of patients and usually indi-

cate early infection. In primary infection, they are the only demonstrable antibodies in 40% of patients. If tests are negative, repeat 3 times at intervals of 1–2 weeks. *Beware of occasional cross-reaction with primary histoplasmosis and cutaneous blastomycosis.*

Complement-fixing antibodies appear later (positive in 10% of patients in first week), and the number rises with increasing severity. Antibodies decrease after 4–8 months but may remain positive for years. The titer is useful for following the course of the disease; a titer greater than 1:16 suggests dissemination; a fall in titer suggests effective therapy. Less than one-third of cases are positive in the first month; most positive reactions occur between the fourth and fifth weeks. The antibodies are usually present in disseminated disease.

Latex particle agglutination test shows 6% false positive reactions. Chief value is for screening purposes for detection of precipitin antibodies. A positive result should be confirmed with complement-fixation and precipitin antibody tests. A negative test does not rule out coccidioidomycosis.

Agar immunodiffusion and counterimmunoelectrophoresis tests parallel latex particle agglutination test but are somewhat less sensitive. Chief value is for rapid screening purposes.

Smear (wet preparation in 20% KOH) and culture are taken from sputum, gastric contents, cerebrospinal fluid, urine, marrow biopsy, liver biopsy, exudate, skin scrapings, etc., on Sabouraud's medium or intraperitoneal injection of mice.

Biopsy of skin lesions and affected lymph nodes is made.

CSF in meningitis shows 100–200 WBCs/cu mm (mostly mononuclear), increased protein, frequently decreased glucose. Complement-fixing antibodies are present in 75% of meningitis patients.

Eosinophilia is ≦ 35%; > 10% in 25% of patients.

WBC (with shift to the left) and ESR are increased.

HISTOPLASMOSIS
(due to *Histoplasma capsulatum*)

Culture is made (may be difficult) of skin and mucosal lesions, sputum, gastric washings, blood, bone marrow (Sabouraud's medium at room temperature; blood agar at 37°C not specific). Blood and bone marrow cultures are positive in 50% of patients. Culture is positive in < 10% of asymptomatic self-limiting cases, 65% of cavitary pulmonary cases, and 75% of disseminated cases. Mouse inoculation, especially from sputum, may give a positive subculture from spleen on Sabouraud's medium in 1 month. A positive skin test can cause conversion of serologic titers within 1 week.

Complement-fixation titers are positive in 90% of chronic cases and in 50% of acute pulmonary cases. Positive titers persist for months or years if disease remains active. They appear during the third to sixth week. A low titer in known cases may indicate a poor prognosis. Titers may be negative in severe disease.

Latex agglutination titers become positive in 2–3 weeks and revert to negative in 5–8 months, even with persistent disease. There are few false positives. A titer of 1:32 or more indicates active or very recent disease.

False positive serologic tests are reported in ≅ 10% of cases.
Biopsy is made of skin and mucosal lesions, bone marrow, and reticuloendothelial system.
Anemia and leukopenia are nonspecific.

ACTINOMYCOSIS
(due to *Actinomyces israelii*)

Recognition of organism in material (e.g., sinus tracts, abscess cavities, empyema fluid; *may be found normally in sputum*) from sites of involvement (especially jaw, lung, cecum)
Sulfur granules show radial gram-positive bacilli or filaments with central gram-negative zone.
No growth is seen on Sabouraud's medium.
Anaerobic growth on blood agar shows small colonies after 4–6 days.
Animal inoculation is negative.
Anaerobic culture methods (e.g., Brewer's thioglycollate medium) are positive.

Histologic examination is suggestive; the diagnosis may be confirmed if a "ray fungus" is seen.
Serologic tests are not useful.
WBC is normal or slightly increased (≦ 14,000/cu mm); high WBC indicates secondary infection.
ESR is usually increased.
Normocytic normochromic anemia is mild to moderate.

NOCARDIOSIS
(due to *Nocardia asteroides*)

Clinical types
Lung abscess; metastatic brain abscesses in one-third of patients
Maduromycosis
Recognition of organism
Direct smear—gram-positive and acid-fast *(may be over-decolorized by Ziehl-Neelsen stain for tubercle bacilli)*
Positive culture on Sabouraud's medium and blood agar *(Beware of inactivation by concentration technique for tubercle bacillus.)*
Positive guinea pig inoculation

May be saprophytic in sputum or gastric juice.

Rule out underlying pulmonary alveolar proteinosis, Cushing's syndrome.

BLASTOMYCOSIS
(North American blastomycosis due to *Blastomyces dermatitidis*; South American blastomycosis due to *Paracoccidioides brasiliensis*)

Clinical types
South American—involvement of nasopharynx, lymph nodes, cecum
North American—involvement of skin and lungs
Later, visceral involvement may occur in both types.
Recognition of organism in material (e.g., pus, sputum, biopsied tissue)
Wet smear preparation in 20% KOH

Table 31-10. Summary of Laboratory Findings in Fungus Infections

Disease	Causative Organism	Blood	Cerebrospinal fluid	Stool	Urine	Nasopharynx, throat	Sputum, lung	Gastric washings	Vagina, cervix	Exudates, lesions, sinus tracts, etc.	Skin, nails, hair	Bone marrow	Lymph node	Fresh unstained material	Stained material	Culture	Animal inoculation	Serologic tests	Complement-fixation	Agglutination	Precipitin	Histologic examination
											Source of Material				Microscopic Examination				Diagnostic Methods			
Cryptococcosis	*Cryptococcus neoformans*	+	+	+	+		+				+	+			+	+	+			+		+
Coccidioidomycosis	*Coccidioides immitis*		+				+	+			+			+		+	+		+		+	+
Histoplasmosis	*Histoplasma capsulatum*	+					+	+			+	+	+			+	+		+	+	+	+
Actinomycosis	*Actinomyces israelii*						+			+					+	+						+

Disease	Organism											
Nocardiosis	*Nocardia asteroides*	+						+				+
North American blastomycosis	*Blastomyces dermatitidis*	+			+		+	+	+			+
South American blastomycosis	*Paracoccidioides brasiliensis*	+			+		+	+	+		+	
Moniliasis	*Candida albicans*						+				+	+
Aspergillosis	*Aspergillus fumigatus*, others	+					+	+	+	+		
Geotrichosis	*Geotrichum candidum*	+					+			+		
Chromoblastomycosis	*Phialophora pedrosi, compactum*, etc.	+					+	+				
Sporotrichosis	*Sporotrichum schenckii*	+	+	+	+		+	+				
Rhinosporidiosis	*Rhinosporidium seeberi*	+										

Positive culture on Sabouraud's medium at room temperature and blood agar at 37°C; slow growth of *P. brasiliensis* on blood agar ≦ 1 month

Negative animal inoculation

Complement-fixation test is positive in high titer with systemic infection. High titer is correlated with poor prognosis.

WBC and ESR are increased.

Serum globulin is slightly increased.

Mild normochromic anemia is present.

Alkaline phosphatase may be increased with bone lesions.

MONILIASIS
(due to *Candida albicans*)

Positive culture on Sabouraud's medium and on direct microscopic examination of suspected material

In vaginitis, rule out underlying diabetes mellitus.

In skin and nail involvement in children, rule out congenital hypoparathyroidism and Addison's disease.

In septicemia with endocarditis, rule out narcotic addiction.

In GI tract overgrowth, rule out chemotherapy suppression of normal bacterial flora.

In positive blood culture, which is rare, rule out serious underlying disease (e.g., malignant lymphoma), multiple therapeutic antibiotics, and plastic intravenous catheters.

ASPERGILLOSIS
(due to *Aspergillus fumigatus* and other species)

Recognition of organism in material (especially sputum) from sites of involvement (especially lung; also brain, sinuses, orbit, ear)

Positive culture on most media at room temperature or 35°C

Organisms occur as saprophytes in sputum and mouth. Confirm by staining organisms in biopsy specimens.

Laboratory findings due to underlying or primary disease

Superimposed on lung cavities caused by tuberculosis, bronchiectasis, carcinoma

Underlying condition (e.g., malignant lymphoma, irradiation, steroid, or antibiotic therapy)

GEOTRICHOSIS
(due to *Geotrichum candidum*)

Recognition of organisms from material from sites of involvement (respiratory tract; possibly colon)

Positive culture on Sabouraud's medium (room temperature)

Organisms occur as saprophytes in pharynx and colon.

Microscopic visualization of organisms in biopsy material

CHROMOBLASTOMYCOSIS
(due to *Phialophora pedrosi, P. compactum*, etc.)

Recognition of organism from sites of involvement (usually skin; rarely brain abscess)

Wet smear preparation in 10% KOH

Positive culture on Sabouraud's medium (slow growth)

Biopsy of tissue

SPOROTRICHOSIS
(due to *Sporotrichum schenckii*)

Recognition of organism in skin, pus, or biopsy
  Positive culture on Sabouraud's medium from unbroken pustule. Intraperitoneal mouse inoculation of these colonies or of fresh pus produces organism-containing lesions.
  Direct microscopic examination is usually negative.

Serum agglutinins, precipitins, and complement-fixing (titer of $\geq$ 1:16) antibodies can be demonstrated in extracutaneous disease (e.g., pulmonary, disseminated).

RHINOSPORIDIOSIS
(due to *Rhinosporidium seeberi*)

Recognition of organism in biopsy material from polypoid lesions of nasopharynx or eye (*cannot be cultured*)

MUCORMYCOSIS
(due to *Mucorales fungi*)

Clinical types
  Cranial (acute diffuse cerebrovascular disease and ophthalmoplegia in uncontrolled diabetes mellitus with acidosis)
  Pulmonary (findings due to pulmonary infarction)
  In abdominal blood vessels (findings due to hemorrhagic infarction of ileum or colon)

Mycologic cultures from brain and spinal fluid are negative; may be positive from infected nasal sinuses or turbinate.

Laboratory findings of underlying disease (e.g., diabetes mellitus with acidosis, leukemia, irradiation or cytotoxic drugs, uremic acidosis) are present.

Laboratory findings due to complications (e.g., visceral infarcts) are present.

MALARIA
(due to *Plasmodium vivax, P. malariae, P. falciparum, P. ovale*)

Identification of organism is made in thin or thick smears of peripheral blood or bone marrow.

Anemia (average 2.5 million RBCs/cu mm in chronic cases) is usually hypochromic; may be macrocytic in severe chronic disease. Reticulocyte count is increased.

Monocytes are increased in peripheral blood; there may be pigment in large mononuclear cells occasionally.

WBC is decreased.

There is increased serum indirect bilirubin and other evidence of hemolysis.

Bone marrow shows erythroid hyperplasia, RBCs containing organisms, and pigment in RE cells. Marrow hyperplasia may fail in chronic phase. Agranulocytosis and purpura may occur late.

Serum globulin is increased (especially euglobulin fraction); albumin is decreased.

ESR is increased.

Biologic false positive test of syphilis is frequent.

Osmotic fragility of RBCs is normal.

Acute hemorrhagic nephritis due to *P. malariae*
  Albuminuria
  Hematuria

Table 31-11. Serologic Tests in Diagnosis of Parasitic Diseases

Disease	Indirect Hemagglutination	Complement Fixation	Direct Agglutination	Indirect Immunofluorescence	Bentonite Flocculation	Counterimmunoelectrophoresis	ELISA (enzyme-linked immunosorbent assay)	Tests are performed by CDC, Atlanta, Ga. (titers are expressed as ≧)
Malaria				1:64				
Chagas' disease	+	1:8	+					
Leishmaniasis	+	1:8	1:64					
Toxoplasmosis	+			1:256				IgM-IFA ≧ 1:16
Pneumocystis carinii				+				

Amebiasis	1:256			+	
Ascariasis	+		+		
Toxocariasis					+
Strongyloidiasis	+				
Trichinosis			1:5	+	
Filariasis	1:128		+		
Schistosomiasis	+	1:16			+
Paragonimiasis	+				
Cysticercosis	1:64		+		
Echinococcosis	1:256		+		

Source: Data from D. D. Despommier, The immune system and parasitism. *Infect. Dis.* 9:4, June 1979; W. L. Drew, Serologic tests—Diagnosing viral, fungal, and parasitic infections. *Consultant*, March 1983, pp. 123–141.

Table 31-12. Summary of Laboratory Findings in Protozoan Diseases

Disease	Causative Organism	Blood	Cerebrospinal fluid	Stool	Urine	Vagina	Urethra	Exudates, ulcers, skin lesions	Bone marrow	Spleen	Lymph node aspirate	Fresh unstained material	Stained material	Culture	Animal inoculation	Xenodiagnosis	Serologic tests	Complement-fixation	Others	Histologic examination	Anemia	WBC decreased	Monocytosis	Serum globulin increased	Cerebrospinal fluid abnormalities	Renal function abnormalities	Liver function abnormalities	Skeletal muscle abnormalities	Cardiac abnormalities	Other
Malaria	*Plasmodium* species	+							+				+						+		+	+	+	+	+	+	+			
Trypanosomiasis Acute sleeping sickness	*T. rhodesiense*	+	+						+		+		+	rare	+						+		+	+	+					
Chronic sleeping sickness	*T. gambiense*	+	+						+		+		+		+			+			+		+	+	+					
Chagas' disease	*T. cruzi*	+											+	+		+		+		a					+			+	+	

Disease	Organism															
Leishmaniasis																
Kala-azar	L. donovani	+					+			+						+[d]
American muco-cutaneous	L. brasiliensis		+ + +		+ +					+ +	+		+		+	
Oriental sore	L. tropica			+		+ +										
Toxoplasmosis	T. gondii	+		+	+	+		+ [b] [c] +					+			
Interstitial plasma cell pneumonia	Pneumocystis carinii						+ +									
Amebiasis	Entamoeba histolytica				+		÷ + + [e]									
Giardiasis	G. lamblia	+ [f]			+											
Balantidiasis	B. coli	+			+											
Coccidiosis	Isospora hominis or belli	+			+											
Trichomoniasis	T. vaginalis	+ + +			+											

[a] Liver, lymph node.
[b] Hemagglutination, Sabin-Feldman dye test.
[c] Lymph node, muscle.
[d] Special stains.
[e] Rectum.
[f] Also duodenal washings.

Serologic tests can be performed at the Centers for Disease Control (Atlanta, Ga.) on specimens submitted through state health department laboratories that do not perform such tests.

Blackwater fever (massive intravascular hemolysis) due to *P. falciparum*

>   Severe acute hemolytic anemia (1–2 million RBCs/cu mm) with increased bilirubin, hemoglobinuria, etc.

>   May be associated with acute tubular necrosis with hemoglobin casts, azotemia, oliguria to anuria, etc.

>   Parasites absent from blood

Laboratory findings due to involvement of organs

>   Liver—vary from congestion to fatty changes to malarial hepatitis or central necrosis; moderate increase in SGOT, SGPT, and alkaline phosphatase

>   Pigment stones in gallbladder

>   Cerebral malaria

Serologic tests (performed in special reference laboratories, e.g., at the Centers for Disease Control, Atlanta, Ga.)

>   Indirect fluorescent antibody test shows high sensitivity and specificity and is useful for diagnostic purposes.

>   Indirect hemagglutination can detect antibody many years after infection and is useful for prevalence studies.

TRYPANOSOMIASIS

Sleeping sickness

>   Acute (Rhodesian) due to *Trypanosoma rhodesiense*

>   Chronic (Gambian) due to *Trypanosoma gambiense*

>>   Identification of organism in appropriate material (blood, bone marrow, lymph node aspirate, CSF) by thick or thin smears or concentrations, animal inoculation, rarely culture

>>   Anemia

>>   Increased serum globulin producing increased ESR, positive flocculation tests, etc.

>>   Increased monocytes in peripheral blood

>>   Cerebrospinal fluid

>>>   Increased number of cells (mononuclear type)—$\leqq$ 30/cu mm during second month; later 100–400/cu mm.

>>>   Increased protein (use as index to severity of disease and to therapeutic response)—60–100 mg/dl with considerable increase in gamma globulin.

>>   Organisms may be identified by microscopic examination of CSF sediment.

>>   Complement-fixation test specific for *T. gambiense*

Chagas' disease (American trypanosomiasis) due to *Trypanosoma cruzi*

>   Identification of organism

>>   Blood concentration technique during acute stage

>>   Biopsy of lymph node or liver (shows leishmanial forms)

>>   Culture on blood broth at 28°C from lymph node aspirate

>>   Xenodiagnosis (laboratory-bred bug fed on patient develops trypanosomes in gut in 2 weeks)

>   Complement-fixation test positive in 50% of acute cases; specific and positive in > 90% of chronic cases. In the acute infection the indirect hemagglutination test is more reliable.

>   Laboratory findings due to organ involvement (e.g., heart, central nervous system, skeletal muscle)

LEISHMANIASIS
Kala-azar (due to *Leishmania donovani*)
> Organism identified in stained smears from spleen, bone marrow, peripheral blood, liver biopsy, lymph node aspirate
>
> Culture (incubate at 26°C) from same sources
>
> Complement-fixation test usually positive but also positive in tuberculosis
>
> Anemia due to hypersplenism and decreased marrow production
>
> Leukopenia
>
> Thrombocytopenia
>
> Markedly increased serum globulin (IgG) with decreased albumin and reversed A/G ratio
>
> Increased ESR, etc., due to increased serum globulin
>
> Frequent urine changes
>> Proteinuria
>>
>> Hematuria
>
> Laboratory findings due to amyloidosis in chronic cases

American mucocutaneous leishmaniasis (due to *Leishmania brasiliensis*)
> Organism identification by direct microscopy, culture, or histologic examination in scrapings from lesions often fails.
>
> Anemia sometimes present

Oriental sore (cutaneous leishmaniasis) (due to *Leishmania tropica*)
> Organisms identified by direct microscopy and culture in scrapings from lesion

TOXOPLASMOSIS
(due to *Toxoplasma gondii*)
Recognition of trophozoite in appropriate material (CSF, lymph node, muscle). Cysts may be incidental finding of chronic asymptomatic infection.
> Smears stained with Wright's or Giemsa stain
>
> Mouse inoculation or tissue culture from blood or CSF
>
> Histologic examination of tissue (e.g., lymph node, muscle)

Serology
> Sabin-Feldman dye test is benchmark for evaluating new tests but is superseded by other tests due to complexity. Dye test detects antibodies 1–2 weeks after onset of infection, and titer rapidly rises to $\geq 1:1000$ in the next few weeks, then declines during months or years to low level $(1:4–1:64)$ for life of patient; false positive or false negative tests are rare. Indirect hemagglutination titer follows the same course but lags by a few days.
>
> IgM-indirect fluorescent antibody appears in first week of infection, peaks within 1 month, disappears within several months (as early as 1 month). A negative test rules out infection of $<$ 3 weeks' duration but does not exclude infection of longer duration. A single high titer or serial rise in titer (more than 2 dilutions, run in parallel) indicates recent new or reactivated infection. (High titer $\geq 1:80$, low titer $\leq 1:20$, negative titer $< 1:10$.)
>
> IgG-indirect fluorescent antibody test (major test currently in use), Sabin-Feldman dye test, indirect hemagglutination test, or complement-fixation test that shows a 2-dilution rise in

titer at 3-week interval when tested in parallel indicates acute infection. IgG peak occurs within 1–2 months, so initial specimen must be drawn early to demonstrate the rise in titer. Titers will eventually reach 1:1000; IgG or dye test is rarely < 1:1000 in acute toxoplasmosis.

IgM test should be done if the IgG or dye test is positive at any titer in a pregnant woman; if not available, do serial IgG or dye tests. If IgM is negative and IgG < 1:1000, further evaluation is unnecessary.

Antinuclear antibodies and rheumatoid factor may cause false positive IgM-indirect fluorescent antibody test; complement-fixation and dye tests do not show false positive reactions.

Adult Patients

WBC varies from leukopenia to leukemoid reaction; atypical lymphocytes may be found.

Anemia is present.

Serum gamma globulins are increased.

Heterophil agglutination is negative, but hematologic picture may exactly mimic infectious mononucleosis; eosinophilia in 10–20% of patients.

Laboratory findings are those due to involvement of various organ systems.

> Lymph node shows distinctive marked hyperplasia; organism may be identified in histologic section.
>
> Central nervous system shows CSF changes, and organism can be identified in smear of sediment.
>
> Disseminated form is an important complication of the immunologically compromised patient (e.g., lymphoma, leukemia, immunosuppressive drugs), but positive or changing titers may not be present.
>
> If ocular findings are the only clinical disease, many patients show only very low titers that are not useful.

Pregnancy

25–45% of women 20–39 years old in the U.S. have chronic toxoplasmosis, which therefore will not cause spontaneous abortion or infection of fetus. Fetal infection only occurs if mother acquires toxoplasmosis after conception (2–6 cases/1000 pregnancies/year in U.S.; >3000 congenital infections/year in U.S.).

Repeat testing of pregnant patients with negative titers or high titers are best done just before 20th week and just before delivery to identify recent antibody converter to determine therapy (e.g., therapeutic abortion at 20th week, treatment during rest of pregnancy, or treatment of infant after delivery).

With IgG = 1:2000 and negative IgM titers and no rise in titers, it is not possible to tell if infection occurred at or after conception.

Unchanging immunofluorescent or dye tests and IgM or complement-fixation that is negative or low titer or falling titer indicates infection occurred more than a few months ago (i.e., prior to conception), and fetal infection will not occur.

Presence of antibodies before pregnancy probably assures protection against congenital toxoplasmosis in the child.

Sabin-Feldman dye and indirect fluorescent antibody test titers are usually the same in the newborn and in the mother for the first 30 days of the infant's life. In diagnosis of congenital toxoplasmosis, these tests are useful when a persistently elevated or rising titer is found in the infant 2–3 months after birth.

Maternal transfer of IgM occurs in < 1% of newborns; therefore presence of IgM antibody allows presumptive diagnosis; rapid decay of IgM causes marked decrease if due to maternal transfer, but persistent level 2 weeks later confirms diagnosis.

Indirect hemagglutination and complement-fixation tests may be negative in congenital toxoplasmosis and therefore are not recommended in this condition; the dye test titer is high.

PNEUMOCYSTIS PNEUMONIA
(due to *Pneumocystis carinii*)

There are no specific laboratory tests.

No culture techniques are available.

No serologic techniques are available.

Lung biopsy is necessary to make a definite diagnosis. The organism is rarely found in sputum or bronchial washings.

Organisms are found in postmortem histologic preparations.

The morphology of the lung lesions suggests the diagnosis.

Organism does not stain with routine H & E stains; requires special stains (e.g., Giemsa, Schiff).

Laboratory findings are those of associated diseases (especially cytomegalic inclusion disease, systemic bacterial infections, especially *Pseudomonas* or *Staphylococcus*) or of underlying diseases (malignant lymphoma, leukemia, tuberculosis, cryptococcosis, premature or debilitated infants, immunoglobulin defects), administration of cytotoxic drugs and corticosteroids. These findings are present in 25% of patients who die after renal transplant.

Leukopenia indicates a poor prognosis.

Serologic tests are not useful. Complement-fixation is positive in < 20% of patients, and indirect fluorescent antibody is positive in 30%.

AMEBIASIS
(due to *Entamoeba histolytica*)

Microscopic examination of stool for *E. histolytica*. Six daily consecutive stools concentrated and stained will identify 90% of positive cases. *(Beware of interfering substances in feces, e.g., bismuth, kaolin, barium sulfate, soap or hypertonic-salt enema solutions, antacids and laxatives, sulfonamides; antibiotic, antiprotozoal, and antihelmintic agents.) Abundant RBCs but minimal WBCs on microscopic examination of stool helps to differentiate condition from bacillary dysentery (see pp. 172–3, 571).*

Biopsy of rectum for *E. histolytica*

Serologic tests

Indirect hemagglutination test is sensitive and specific; associated with current or previous infection. A negative test is unlikely if amebic infection (especially hepatic) is present. Significant positive titer is ≧ 1:128.

Complement-fixation test is usually positive only during active (especially hepatic) disease. Usually reverts to normal 6 months after cure. Significant positive titer is ≧ 1:16.

Agar-gel diffusion test parallels complement-fixation test.
Height of titer above significant levels or changing titers are not clinically significant.
Also enzyme-linked immunosorbent assay (ELISA), counterimmunoelectrophoresis (CIE), double diffusion precipitin test.
When severe diarrhea is due to *E. histolytica,* serologic tests will be positive in > 90%; when diarrhea has never been present, <50% of carriers will have positive serologic tests.
Serologic tests are positive in > 95% of all patients with extraintestinal infection, but cysts or trophozoites cannot usually be found in stools.

Liver abscess
Normochromic, normocytic anemia
Leukocytosis (5000–33,000/cu mm)
Eosinophilia is not usually present.
ESR is markedly increased.
Increased SGOT and SGPT (2–6 times normal)
Increased alkaline phosphatase (usually 2–3 times normal)
Serum albumin may be decreased and globulin increased.
Total bilirubin may be increased if complications occur.
Liver scanning

GIARDIASIS
(due to *Giardia lamblia*)
Recognition of organism is achieved in stools or duodenal washings stained with iodine. Chronic infection may cause malabsorption syndrome.

BALANTIDIASIS
(due to *Balantidium coli*)
Recognition of organisms in stool *(Intermittent appearance requires repeated examinations.)*

COCCIDIOSIS
(due to *Isospora hominis* or *I. belli*)
Recognition of organism in $ZnSO_4$-concentrated stool specimens

TRICHOMONIASIS
(due to *Trichomonas vaginalis*)
Recognition of organism in material from vagina
Wet-mount preparation of freshly examined vaginal fluid (sensitivity 50–70% compared to culture)
Frequently an incidental finding in routine urinalysis
Frequently found in routine Papanicolaou smears (sensitivity about same as wet mount but less specific). The organism is often not identified but may be associated with characteristic concomitant cytologic changes.
Culture is the most definitive and sensitive test; special media must be freshly prepared.

Douching within 24 hours decreases sensitivity of tests.

Occasionally detected in material from male urethra in cases of nonspecific urethritis.

ASCARIASIS
(due to *Ascaris lumbricoides*)
Stools contain ova.
Eosinophils are increased during symptomatic phase, especially
  pulmonary phase.

TRICHURIASIS
(due to whipworm—*Trichuris trichiura*)
Stools contain ova.
Increased eosinophils ($\leqq 25\%$), leukocytosis, and microcytic hypochromic anemia may be present.

PINWORM INFECTION
(due to *Enterobius vermicularis*)
Ova and occasionally adults are found on Scotch tape swab of
  perianal region. *Swab should be taken on first arising early in
  morning.*
Stool is usually negative for ova and adults.
Eosinophil count is usually normal; may be slightly increased.

VISCERAL LARVA MIGRANS
(due to *Toxocara canis* or *T. cati*)
WBC is increased; increased eosinophils are vacuolated and contain
  fewer than normal granules.
Serum gamma globulin is often increased.
Indirect hemagglutination and bentonite flocculation tests may be
  insensitive and nonspecific.
Disease may cause Löffler's syndrome.
Biopsy of liver showing granulomas containing larvae is best proce-
  dure for definite diagnosis.

TRICHOSTRONGYLOSIS
(due to *Trichostrongylus* species)
Stools contain ova. *Usually a concentration technique is required;
  worm may be mistaken for hookworm.*
There is an increase in WBC and eosinophils ($\leqq 75\%$) when patient
  is symptomatic.

STRONGYLOIDIASIS
(due to *Strongyloides stercoralis*)
Stools contain larvae. Larvae may also be found in duodenal washings. Larvae appear in sputum with pulmonary involvement.
Leukocytosis is common.
Increase in eosinophils is almost always present, but the number
  usually decreases with chronicity. Leukopenia and absence of
  eosinophilia are poor prognostic signs.

*Condition is especially common in orphanages and mental institu-
  tions.*

HOOKWORM DISEASE
(due to *Necator americanus* or *Ancylostoma duodenale*)
WBC is normal or slightly increased, with 15–30% eosinophils; in
  early cases, $\leqq 75\%$ eosinophils are present.

Table 31-13. Identification of Parasites

Organism	Stool	Other Body Sites
Nematodes		
Ascaris lumbricoides	O, A	Rarely L in sputum early
Trichuris trichiura	O	
Enterobius vermicularis	Usually neg.; A after enema	Scotch tape, perianal region—O and A
Strongyloides stercoralis	L	Occasionally L in sputum and duodenal contents
Ancylostoma duodenale	O, rarely L	
Necator americanus	O, rarely L	
Trichinella spiralis	Occasionally A and/or L	
Wuchereria bancrofti, W. malayi	None	Microfilariae in blood
Loa loa	None	Microfilariae in blood; adult under conjunctiva
Onchocerca volvulus	None	Adult in subcutaneous nodules
Dracunculus medinensis	None	L in fluid from ulcer
Cestodes		
Taenia solium	G, O, S; A after treatment	
Taenia saginata	G, O, S	Scotch tape, perianal region—O
Hymenolepis nana, H. diminata	O	
Diphyllobothrium latum	O	
Echinococcus multilocularis	Not found	Histologic examination of biopsy specimen
Trematodes		
Schistosoma mansoni, S. japonicum,	O	See p. 629
S. haematobium	None	O in urine
Clonorchis sinensis	O	O in duodenal contents
Opisthorchis felineus	O	O in duodenal contents
Paragonimus westermani	O	O in sputum
Fasciola hepatica	O	
Fasciolopsis buski	O, occasionally A	

O = ova; A = adult; L = larvae; G = gravid segments; S = scolex.

Anemia due to blood loss is hypochromic microcytic. When anemia is more severe, eosinophilia is less prominent.

Hypoproteinemia may occur with heavy infestation.

Stools contain hookworm ova. Stools are usually positive for occult blood. Charcot-Leyden crystals are present in > 50% of patients.

Laboratory findings are those due to frequently associated diseases (e.g., malaria, beriberi).

TRICHINOSIS
(due to *Trichinella spiralis*)

Eosinophilia appears with values of $\leq$ 85% on differential count and 15,000/cu mm on absolute count. It occurs about 1 week after the eating of infected food and reaches maximum after third week. It usually subsides in 4–6 weeks but may last up to 6 months and occasionally for years. Occasionally it is absent; it is usually absent in fatal infections.

Stool may contain adults and larvae *only* during the first 1–2 weeks after infection (during the stage of enteritis and invasion).

Identification of larvae is made in suspected meat by acid-pepsin digestion followed by microscopic examination.

Muscle biopsy may show the encysted larvae beginning 10 days after ingestion. Direct microscopic examination of compressed specimen is superior to routine histologic preparation.

Serologic tests become positive 1 week after onset of symptoms in only 20–30% of patients and reach a peak in 80–90% of patients by fourth to fifth week. Rise in titer in acute- and convalescent-phase sera is diagnostic. Titers may remain negative in overwhelming infection. False positive results may occur in polyarteritis nodosa, serum sickness, penicillin sensitivity, infectious mononucleosis, malignant lymphomas, and leukemia.

> *Trichinella* complement-fixation test becomes positive $\cong$ 2 weeks after occurrence of eosinophilia. It may remain positive for 6 months.

> Bentonite flocculation test may remain strongly positive for 6 months; less strongly positive for another 6 months; becomes negative in 2–3 years. It is the best single test for diagnosis.

> Precipitin tests are also used.

Decrease in serum total protein and albumin occurs in severe cases between 2 and 4 weeks and may last for years.

Increased (relative and absolute) gamma globulins parallel titer of serologic tests and of thymol turbidity. The increase occurs between 5 and 8 weeks and may last 6 months or more.

ESR is normal or only slightly increased.

Decreased serum cholinesterase often lasts 6 months.

Some serum enzymes may be increased (e.g., aldolase).

Urine may show albuminuria with hyaline and granular casts in severe cases.

With meningoencephalitis, CSF may be normal or up to 300 lymphocytes/cu mm with increased protein.

FILARIASIS
(due to *Wuchereria bancrofti* or *W. malayi*)

Microfilariae appear in peripheral blood smear (Wright's or Giemsa stain) or wet preparation.

Eosinophils are increased.

Biopsy of lymph node may contain adult worms.

Complement-fixation test may not be reliable.

Chyluria may occur.

Tropical eosinophilia due to filaria

Eosinophilia is extreme (usually >3000/cu mm) and persists for weeks.

Serum IgE levels are markedly elevated (usually >1000 units/ml).

High titers of antifilarial antibodies are detected by complement-fixation, hemagglutination, and other techniques.

No microfilaria can be found in blood but may be found in enlarged lymph nodes when adenopathy is present.

Other laboratory abnormalities (e.g., elevated ESR) are not diagnostically significant.

LOAIASIS
(due to *Loa loa*)

Marked increase of eosinophils (50–80%) may occur.

TAPEWORM INFESTATION

Due to *Taenia saginata* (beef tapeworm)

In stool, ova cannot be distinguished from those of *Taenia solium.*

Proglottids establish diagnosis. Stool examination is positive in 50–75% of patients.

Scotch tape swab of perianal region is positive in ≦ 95% of patients.

Eosinophils may be slightly increased.

Due to *T. solium* (pork tapeworm)

Stool and Scotch tape swab of perianal region are examined.

Eosinophils may be slightly increased.

CSF may show increased eosinophils with cysticercal meningoencephalitis.

Due to *Hymenolepis nana* (dwarf tapeworm)

Stool shows ova, occasionally proglottids, etc.

Due to *Diphyllobothrium latum* (fish tapeworm)

Stool shows ova.

Macrocytic anemia (see p. 329) occurs when worm is in proximal small intestine.

Increased eosinophils and leukocytes are found.

Due to *Echinococcus granulosus (multilocularis)*

Cystic lesion appears, especially in liver (see Metastatic or Infiltrative Disease of Liver, p. 262). 65% of cysts occur in lung, and the remaining 10% of cysts are widely scattered.

Identification of scolices and hooklets is made in cyst fluid and histologic examination.

Eosinophils are occasionally increased; the number rises dramatically in cyst leaks.

Stool examination is not helpful.

Serologic tests: High titers (≧1024), indirect hemagglutination, and bentonite flocculation (>5) usually indicate disease; low titers are equivocal and may be found with collagen disease or cirrhosis. The tests often cross-react with cysticercosis antibody. They are more sensitive in presence of liver cysts (85%) than lung cysts (<50%).

SCHISTOSOMIASIS
(due to *Schistosoma mansoni, S. japonicum, S. haematobium*)
Acute
> Eosinophilia occurs; may be 20–60%.
> ESR is increased.
> Serum globulin is increased.

Chronic
> Ova appear in stools; only viable eggs indicate active infection.
>> Quantification by egg count per gram of feces or per 10 ml of urine gives some indication of severity of infection.
>
> Unstained rectal mucosa examined microscopically may show living or dead ova when stools are negative.
>
> Serologic tests are particularly useful for chronic infections when stools contain no ova; they are not useful to assess chemotherapeutic cure.
>> Fluorescent antibody test requires additional standardization.
>>
>> Cercarial slide flocculation test has some technical shortcomings and difficulties; some cross reaction to other infestations.
>>
>> Bentonite flocculation test is somewhat less sensitive than cercarial slide test; some cross reaction to other infestations.
>>
>> Complement-fixation test is the best serologic procedure (100% specific and 95% sensitive).
>>
>> Circumoval precipitin test is particularly useful for testing spinal fluid since it is specific for involvement of central nervous system; intestinal involvement alone causes positive reaction with serum but negative reaction with spinal fluid.
>>
>> Cercarienhullen reaction test is performed with living infectious cercariae and therefore is not useful as a routine procedure.
>>
>> Indirect hemagglutination test is more often used for epidemiologic studies.
>
> Rectal biopsy of mucosal fold may show parasites and granulomatous lesions.
>
> Multiple granulomatous lesions appear in uterine cervix.
>
> Changes appear that are secondary to clay pipestem fibrosis of liver with portal hypertension, esophageal varices, splenomegaly, etc. Liver function changes are quite minimal; increased serum bilirubin is rare, even with advanced cirrhosis. Increased serum globulin is frequent. Serum alkaline phosphatase is elevated in 50% of adult patients but is not useful in children.
>
> Changes secondary to pulmonary hypertension are seen.
>
> Ova appear in urine sediment and in biopsy of vesical mucosa in infection with *S. haematobium*.

PARAGONIMIASIS
(due to *Paragonimus westermani*)
Eosinophilia is usual.
Ova appear in sputum, which may contain blood.

CLONORCHIASIS
(due to *Clonorchis sinensis*)
Ova appear in stool or duodenal contents.

Complement-fixation test may be positive.

Clonorchiasis may cause laboratory findings due to biliary obstruction or recurrent cholecystitis.

OPISTHORCHIASIS
(due to *Opisthorchis felineus*)
Ova appear in stool or duodenal contents.

FASCIOLIASIS
(due to *Fasciola hepatica*)
Ova appear in stool or duodenal contents.
Eosinophils are increased.
Liver function tests are abnormal.

FASCIOLOPSIASIS
(due to *Fasciolopsis buski*)
Ova appear in stool.

OPPORTUNISTIC INFECTIONS
Laboratory findings due to underlying diseases (e.g., malignant lymphoma and leukemia, diabetes mellitus, immunoglobulin defects, following renal transplant, uremia, hypoparathyroidism, hypoadrenalism, AIDS)

Laboratory findings due to administration of drugs (antibiotics, corticosteroids, cystotoxic and immunosuppressive drugs)

Associated with other factors (e.g., plastic intravenous catheters, narcotic addiction)

Laboratory findings due to particular organism (see appropriate separate sections)

> *Cryptococcus neoformans*
> *Candida albicans*
> *Aspergillus*
> *Mucorales fungi*
> *Staphylococcus aureus*
> *Staphylococcus albus, Bacillus subtilis, Bacillus cereus,* and other saprophytes
> Enteric bacteria (*Pseudomonas aeruginosa, Escherichia coli, Klebsiella-Enterobacter, Proteus*)

Table 31-14. Commonly Associated Pathogens in Patients with Immunosuppression (for Organ Transplantation or Treatment of Malignancies)

Immune Response Depressed	Underlying Condition	Commonly Associated Pathogens
Humoral	Lymphatic leukemia Lymphosarcoma Multiple myeloma Congenital hypogammaglobulinemias Nephrotic syndrome Treatment with cytotoxic or antimetabolite drugs	Pneumococci *Hemophilus influenzae* Streptococci *Pseudomonas aeruginosa* *Pneumocystis carinii*
Cellular	Terminal cancers Hodgkin's disease Sarcoidosis Uremia Treatment with cytotoxic or antimetabolite drugs or corticosteroids	Tubercle bacillus *Listeria* *Candida* species *Toxoplasma* *Pneumocystis carinii*
Leukocyte bactericidal	Myelogenous leukemia Chronic granulomatous disease Acidosis Burns Treatment with corticosteroids Granulocytopenia due to drugs	Staphylococci *Serratia* *Pseudomonas* species *Candida* species *Aspergillus* *Nocardia*

Table 31-15. Some Human Diseases That May Be Transmitted by Animal Pets

	Dogs	Cats	Birds	Farm animals	Poultry	Rodents	Reptiles	Monkeys
Bacterial								
Salmonella infections	+	+	+	+	+	+	+	+
Bacillary dysentery								+
Pasteurella infections	+	+		+	+	+		
Anthrax	+			+				
Brucellosis	+	+		+	+	+		
Tularemia	+	+				+		
Leptospirosis	+		+	+		+		
Tuberculosis	+	+		+				
Viral								
Rabies	+	+		+				
Cat-scratch disease		+						
Psittacosis			+		+			
Encephalomyelitis			+	+				
Lymphocytic choriomeningitis	+					+		
Fungal								
Ringworm	+	+		+		+		
Parasitic								
Roundworm infestation	+	+						
Tapeworm infestation	+	+		+				
Visceral larva migrans	+	+						
Cutaneous larva migrans	+	+						
Scabies	+	+						
Toxoplasmosis	+	+						

Miscellaneous Diseases

SYSTEMIC LUPUS ERYTHEMATOSUS (SLE)
(see discussion of serologic tests for SLE and LE cell test, p. 141,
Nephritis of Systemic Lupus Erythematosus, p. 550)
Criteria for classification of SLE (American Rheumatism Association, 1982)

1. Malar rash
2. Discoid lupus
3. Oral/nasopharyngeal ulcers
4. Photosensitivity
5. Arthritis
6. Proteinuria (>0.5 gm/day) or cellular casts
7. Seizures or psychosis
8. Pleuritis or pericarditis
9. Cytopenia
   Autoimmune hemolytic anemia
   Neutropenia
   Lymphopenia
   Thrombocytopenia
10. Anti-nDNA antibodies
    Anti-Sm antibodies
    LE cells
    Chronic false positive VDRL
11. Positive FANA

LE cell preparation detects only 60% of patients with SLE. May be converted by steroids but is not useful to monitor response to therapy. LE cells occur in 70–90% of SLE patients at some time during the course of disease and in 100% of drug-induced lupus. Found in up to 10% of rheumatoid arthritis cases and occasional patients with scleroderma. Specificity in SLE is as low as 80%.

FANA is the most sensitive laboratory test for SLE (detects up to 95% of cases); specificity is as low as 50% in rheumatic disease in general. Negative ANA in patient with active multisystem disease is strong (but not absolute) evidence against SLE; positive ANA without other manifestations is not diagnostic. Pattern of ANA immunofluorescence is of limited value in discriminating SLE from other collagen vascular diseases. Persistently negative ANA tests occur in about 5% of SLE patients due to congenital deficiency of early complement component (usually C4 or C2); detected by absent total hemolytic complement (CH50). These patients tend to have prominent skin disease and low incidence of serious renal and CNS disease. ANA may also become negative during remission.

Anti-ENA (extractable nuclear antigen) (passive hemagglutination assay) detects only 2 ENAs: RNP (ribonucleoprotein) and Sm.

Data from N. Kramer and P. R. Krey, SLE: Use of laboratory tests in diagnosis and management. *J. Med. Soc. N.J.* 80:344, 1983.

Anti-RNP is found in 25–30% of SLE, 10% of rheumatoid arthritis, 22% of scleroderma, 100% of MCTD (mixed connective tissue disease) patients.

Anti-Sm is found in 25–30% of SLE patients and is the most specific diagnostic test for SLE (speckled immunofluorescence pattern).

Anti-DNA (native double-stranded DNA) is found in 40–80% of SLE patients and rarely in other diseases; high specificity is almost same as anti-Sm (rim or peripheral nodular immunofluorescence pattern).

Lupus band test (LBT) (direct immunofluorescence on biopsy of normal skin in SLE patients) is positive in 50% of all SLE patients and up to 80% with active multisystem (especially renal) disease. Appears specific for SLE, especially when IgG is major immunoglobulin deposited. Is diagnostically useful (1) in patients without sufficient clinical manifestations (e.g., only renal or CNS findings), (2) in patients whose symptoms and other laboratory tests show remission due to steroid therapy, or (3) in differentiation of early SLE from rheumatoid arthritis.

DNA-histone (deoxyribonucleoprotein) antibodies are found in drug-induced SLE due to procainamide, hydralazine, phenytoin, and other drugs and many connective tissue diseases.

Anemia of chronic disease (normochromic, normocytic) correlates with disease activity; autoimmune hemolytic type with positive Coombs' test in 2% of cases. Coombs' test may be positive in absence of frank anemia.

ESR typically reflects disease activity.

Leukopenia (<4000/cu mm) and especially lymphocytopenia (<1500/cu mm) may reflect disease activity. Marked leukocytosis (>25,000/cu mm) occurs occasionally.

Traditional parameters of disease activity—hemoglobin, WBC, ESR, urinalysis, serum creatinine—do not distinguish activity from superimposed infection or drug toxicity and may not be sensitive enough to detect early exacerbation.

Current parameters of disease activity

Decrease in early complement components (C3; C4 is most sensitive)

Increasing titers of anti-DNA

Presence of circulating immune complexes

Presence of cryoglobulins (see pp. 404–405) correlates well with disease activity.

Monoclonal rheumatoid factor assay

Raji cell assay (recognizes immune complexes that contain C3b)

C1q binding

These parameters do not predict which manifestations are likely to become active or the time interval (may be weeks to months), and some patients with these laboratory abnormalities never manifest active disease. The strongest correlation is with active nephritis, but these tests may be normal in 10–25% of cases and in any case do not substitute for renal biopsy.

Combination of positive ANA test, positive dsDNA antibodies, and hypocomplementemia has diagnostic specificity for SLE of virtually 100%.

SLE may present as "idiopathic" thrombocytopenic purpura.

CRP may be increased.

Serum gamma globulin is increased in 50% of patients; a continuing rise may indicate poor prognosis. Alpha$_2$ globulin is increased; albumin is decreased. Immunoglobulins may be abnormal on immunoelectrophoresis.

Abnormal serum proteins frequently occur.

Biologically false positive (BFP) test for syphilis is very common—occurs in < 20% of patients. *(This may be the first manifestation of SLE and may precede other features by many months; 7% of asymptomatic individuals with BFP test for syphilis ultimately develop SLE.)*

An inhibitor to extrinsic coagulation pathway is found in 20% of SLE patients, and 80% of these are associated with a BFP. Should be suspected if patient has prolonged PTT; diagnosis is made by 50:50 mixture of patient and normal serum not correcting PTT.

Laboratory findings reflecting specific organ involvement

Urine findings indicate acute nephritis, nephrotic syndrome, chronic renal impairment, secondary pyelonephritis. Patients with azotemia and marked proteinuria usually die in 1–3 years. Sediment is the same as in chronic active glomerulonephritis. With uremia, nephrotic syndrome, or active nephritis, the LE test may become negative. High antibody titer to native DNA associated with decreased serum complement indicates lupus nephritis.

CSF findings are of aseptic meningitis (increased protein and pleocytosis are found in 50% of these patients.) *(Rule out complicating tuberculosis and cryptococcosis.)*

Cardiovascular, pulmonary, etc., findings may be present.

Joint involvement occurs in 90% of patients.

Laboratory findings reflecting frequently associated diseases

Hashimoto's thyroiditis (see p. 458)

Sjögren's syndrome (see p. 321)

Myasthenia gravis (see p. 302)

Tissue biopsy of skin, muscles, kidney, and lymph node may be useful.

Drug-induced lupus syndromes (see pp. 666–667) are due to prolonged administration of

Procainamide

Hydralazine

Isoniazid

Various anticonvulsants (e.g., Dilantin)

Differ from spontaneous SLE in their lower incidence of renal findings and of anemia and leukopenia. About two-thirds of patients receiving these drugs develop serologic abnormalities (see p. 141) even though clinical findings and other laboratory changes are absent. May also occur as allergic reaction to certain drugs (e.g., sulfonamides, methyldopa, birth control pills).

POLYARTERITIS NODOSA

WBC is increased ($\leq$ 40,000/cu mm), and polynuclear leukocytes are increased. A rise in eosinophils takes place in 25% of patients, sometimes very marked; it usually occurs in patients with pulmonary manifestations.

ESR is increased.

Mild anemia is frequent; may be hemolytic anemia with positive
  Coombs' test.
Urine is frequently abnormal.
    Albuminuria (60% of patients)
    Hematuria (40% of patients)
    "Telescoping" of sediment (variety of cellular and noncellular
      casts)
Uremia occurs in 15% of patients.
Tissue biopsy
    Random skin and muscle biopsy is confirmatory in 25% of pa-
      tients; most useful when taken from area of tenderness; if no
      symptoms are present, pectoralis major is the most useful
      site.
    Testicular biopsy is useful when local symptoms are present.
    Lymph node and liver biopsies are usually not helpful.
    Renal biopsy is not specific; often shows glomerular disease.
Serum globulins are increased.
Abnormal serum proteins occasionally occur. BFP test occurs for
  syphilis, circulating anticoagulants, cryoglobulins, macroglobulins, etc.
Laboratory findings due to organ involvement by arteritis may be
  present—genitourinary system, nervous system, pulmonary etc.

WEGENER'S GRANULOMATOSIS
**(necrotizing granulomatous vasculitis affecting respiratory tract;
disseminated form shows renal involvement)**
Diagnosis is established by tissue biopsy.
Normochromic anemia is common.
Mild leukocytosis is common; 50% of patients show eosinophilia.
ESR is increased, often to very high levels.
Serum globulins (IgG and IgA) are often increased.
C3 and C4 complement levels may be increased.
Rheumatoid factor may be present.
ANA and lupus preparations are normal.
Laboratory findings reflecting specific organ involvement
    Renal—hematuria, proteinuria, azotemia. Nephrosis or chronic
      nephritis may occur. Most patients develop renal insuffi-
      ciency. Biopsy most frequently shows focal necrotizing glo-
      merulonephritis with crescent formation; coarse granular
      pattern with immunofluorescent staining. Biopsy is impor-
      tant to define extent of disease.
    Central nervous system
    Respiratory tract
    Heart

TEMPORAL ARTERITIS
WBC is usually slightly increased with shift to the left.
Usually moderate normocytic normochromic anemia is present.
Serum protein electrophoresis may show increased gamma globu-
  lins. Rouleaux may occur.
ESR is increased.
Laboratory findings reflecting specific organ involvement
    Kidney
    Central nervous system
    Heart and great vessels

Biopsy of involved segment of temporal artery is diagnostic.
Intracerebral artery involvement may cause increased CSF protein.

SCLERODERMA
Laboratory findings reflect specific organ involvement.
> Malabsorption syndrome due to small intestine involvement
> Abnormal urinary findings, renal function tests, and uremia
>   due to renal involvement
> Myocarditis, pericarditis, secondary bacterial endocarditis
> Pulmonary fibrosis, secondary pneumonitis
> Other

Biopsy of skin, esophagus, intestine, synovia may establish diagnosis.

ESR is normal in one-third of patients, mildly increased in one-third of patients, markedly increased in one-third of patients.

Mild hypochromic microcytic anemia may be present in 10% of patients.

Serum gamma globulins are increased in 25% of patients (usually slight increase).

Abnormal serum proteins occasionally occur, as revealed by BFP test for syphilis (5% of patients), positive LE test, positive RA test (35% of patients), cold agglutinins, cryoglobulins, etc.

Antinuclear antibodies in titer of $\geq 1:16$ are found in 60% of patients.

SCLEREDEMA
WBC, ESR, and other laboratory tests are usually normal.

WEBER-CHRISTIAN DISEASE (RELAPSING FEBRILE NODULAR NONSUPPURATIVE PANNICULITIS)
Biopsy is taken of involved area of subcutaneous fat.
WBC may be increased or decreased.
Mild anemia may occur.

DISCOID LUPUS
Some patients may show
> Decreased WBC
> Decreased platelet count
> Increased ESR

Increased serum gamma globulins
Positive LE cell test ($< 10\%$ of patients)

SARCOIDOSIS
Kveim reaction (skin biopsy 4–6 weeks after injection of human sarcoid tissue shows histologic picture of sarcoid at that site) is positive in 80% of patients with sarcoidosis; many false negatives are seen in patients who are later proved to have sarcoidosis; a positive reaction is less frequent if there is no lymph node involvement, if the disease is of long standing and inactive, and during steroid therapy; false positive reactions occur in 2–5% of patients. Positive Kveim tests may occur in other diseases with enlarged lymph nodes (e.g., tuberculosis, leukemia). Kveim test material is not available commercially; a few medical centers have limited quantities with variable specificities.

Tissue biopsy may be taken at several sites; shows noncaseous granulomas for which a specific cause (e.g., fungal, acid-fast bacillus infection, or berylliosis) has been excluded.

Needle biopsy of liver shows granulomas in 75% of patients even if there is no impairment of liver function.

Lymph node biopsy is likely to be positive if lymph node is enlarged.

Muscle biopsy is likely to be positive if arthralgia or muscle pain is present.

Skin lesions occur in 35% of cases.

Other sites of biopsy are synovium, eye, lung, minor salivary glands of lower lip.

Serum angiotensin-converting enzyme (ACE) is increased in 85% of patients with active pulmonary sarcoidosis but only 11% with inactive disease (normal <57 units/ml by radioassay). May also be increased in youth, diabetes mellitus, hyperthyroidism, Gaucher's disease, leprosy, up to 50% of patients with primary biliary cirrhosis, amyloidosis, myeloma. Is primarily useful to monitor activity of disease and response to therapy.

Bronchioalveolar lavage and radioactive gallium (^{67}Ga) scans of lung have also been used to assess disease activity.

Serum globulins are increased in 75% of patients, producing reduced A/G ratio and increased total protein (in 30% of patients).

Serum protein electrophoresis shows decreased albumin and increased globulin (especially gamma) with characteristic "sarcoid-step" pattern.

WBC is decreased in 30% of patients. Eosinophilia occurs in 15% of patients.

Mild normocytic, normochromic anemia occurs.

ESR is increased.

Increased urine calcium occurs twice as often as hypercalcemia and may be found even with normal serum calcium. Increased frequency of renal calculi is found and of nephrocalcinosis in some series of patients.

Serum calcium is increased in > 16% of patients.

Serum and urine calcium abnormalities are frequently corrected by cortisone.

Increased sensitivity to vitamin D is often present.

Serum phosphorus is normal.

Increased serum uric acid may occur even with normal renal function in ≦ 50% of patients.

Mumps complement-fixation test, which is positive in presence of negative mumps skin test (due to dissociation between normal circulating antibodies and defective cellular antibody response), supports the diagnosis but is not specific.

Laboratory findings reflect specific organ involvement.

Liver—serum alkaline phosphatase is increased (see p. 262).

Spleen—hypersplenism may occur (anemia, leukopenia, thrombocytopenia).

Central nervous system—CSF may be normal or may show moderate to marked increase in protein and pleocytosis (chiefly lymphocytes). Sugar is sometimes decreased.

Pituitary—diabetes insipidus is evident.

Kidney—renal function is decreased (because of hypercalcemia or increased uric acid with resultant nephrocalcinosis or renal calculi).

Lung—PO_2 and PCO_2 are decreased.

Other

AMYLOIDOSIS

Biopsy of tissue may be done at several sites.

Gingival biopsy is positive in one-half to two-thirds of patients.

Rectal biopsy is positive in one-half to two-thirds of patients.

Needle biopsy of kidney is useful when gingival and rectal biopsies are not helpful and there is a differential diagnosis of nephrosis.

Needle biopsy of liver is often positive, but beware of intractable bleeding or rupture.

Skin biopsy is taken from sites of plaque formation.

Other areas of involvement include GI tract, spleen, respiratory tract.

One should use Congo red stain of tissue under polarized light (apple-green birefringence) as well as transmitted light.

Electron microscopy is the most specific diagnostic method.

Congo red test is positive in one-third of patients with primary amyloidosis and approximately two-thirds of patients with secondary amyloidosis.

Evans blue dye is retained in serum.

Classification

Light-chain amyloid (AL)

One-third of cases show overt myeloma; occurs in 4% of cases of multiple myeloma. Primary when there is no evidence of myeloma. May also be associated with Waldenstrom's macroglobulinemia, heavy-chain disease, etc.

One organ usually shows predominant involvement.

Cardiovascular system—involved in almost all cases; presenting symptom in 26% of cases

Proteinuria and azotemia occur in most cases; nephrotic syndrome occurs in 25% of cases.

Tongue is enlarged in 20% of cases.

Peripheral neuropathy in 16% of cases; CNS is not involved by amyloidosis.

Respiratory system is usually involved, but decreased pulmonary function is rare.

Others

Serum protein electrophoresis shows hypogammaglobulinemia in 40% and an abnormal immunoglobulin in another 56% of cases.

Urine contains free light chains in 95% of cases, two-thirds of these are lambda-type Bence Jones proteins. In primary type, free light chains may be detected only if urine is concentrated 100–500 times prior to immunoelectrophoresis, and marrow may show 10–15% plasma cells. See Multiple Myeloma (pp. 370–374) for findings in that disease.

Mild anemia in 50% of cases.

Platelet count may be elevated.

WBC is frequently increased.

ESR is increased.

Reactive systemic protein A amyloid (AA)

Rheumatoid arthritis (10–15% of cases)

Juvenile rheumatoid arthritis (9–15% of cases)

Ankylosing spondylitis (9–15% of cases)

Chronic infections
> Osteomyelitis, burns, decubital ulcers (25% of cases)
> Leprosy (6–31% of cases)
> **Tuberculosis (was most common cause prior to antibiotic era)**
Hodgkin's disease
Nonlymphoid solid tumors (e.g., renal and bladder adenocarcinoma)
Heredofamilial systemic amyloidosis
> Familial Mediterranean fever (25% of cases) (AA type)
> Neuropathic types (I, II, III, IV)—serum protein electrophoresis and immunoelectrophoresis are normal.
Local amyloidosis
> Senile cardiac amyloid (formed from prealbumin)
> Tumor amyloid (due to neoplastic production of a protein product; usually asymptomatic)
Laboratory findings due to associated diseases (see above)
Laboratory findings due to involvement of specific organs (e.g., liver, kidney, GI system, endocrine, skin; see appropriate separate sections)

SYSTEMIC MAST CELL DISEASE (MASTOCYTOSIS)
This is a rare condition of disseminated mast cell tumor with functional secretion or abnormal proliferation of tissue mast cells.

Progressive anemia and thrombocytopenia are present.
WBC may be increased or (rarely) decreased.
Peripheral blood contains ≤ 10% mast cells.
Eosinophilia and occasionally basophilia may occur.
Histamine is increased in blood, urine, and tissues. Increased levels of metabolites of histamine in random and 24-hour urine specimens. Is more specific and sensitive than determination of histamine itself.
Gastric acid is increased; there is a higher incidence of peptic ulcer. Hypochlorhydria and achlorhydria have been reported.
Urinary 5-HIAA (hydroxyindole acetic acid) is normal.
Many mast cells appear in bone marrow smears and in metastatic sites.

BASAL CELL NEVUS SYNDROME
Rare disease that shows
> Multiple basal cell tumors of skin
> Odontogenic cysts of jaw
> Bone anomalies (especially of ribs, vertebrae, and metacarpals) and defective dentition
> Neurologic abnormalities (calcification of dura, etc.)
> Ophthalmologic abnormalities (abnormal width between the eyes, lateral displacement of inner canthi, etc.)
> Sexual abnormalities (frequent ovarian fibromas; male hypogonadism, etc.)
> Normal karyotyping by chromosomal analysis
> Hyporesponsiveness to parathormone (Ellsworth-Howard test)

Rule out presence or development of occult neoplasms (e.g., ovarian fibroma, medulloblastoma).

MALIGNANT NEOPLASMS
(see appropriate separate sections for analytes below)

Decreased
Serum glucose

Increased
Serum uric acid

Serum LDH

Serum calcium—occurs in $\cong$ 20% of cancer patients, usually due to bone metastases, which sometimes cannot be detected. > 14 mg/dl indicates cancer rather than hyperparathyroidism.

Serum globulin (e.g., multiple myeloma)

Serum alkaline phosphatase and GGPT in liver metastases; increase is predictive of positive liver scan but not of positive bone scan for metastases from breast cancer.

Serum acid phosphatase in carcinoma of prostate

Serum alpha-fetoprotein (see p. 91)

Serum carcinoembryonic antigen (CEA) (see p. 92)

Serum gastrin (gastrinoma, gastric carcinoma)

Serum calcitonin (medullary carcinoma of thyroid)

Specific products of hormone-producing tumor (e.g., renin-producing tumor of kidney, insulinoma, parathormone, urine VMA and catecholamines, urinary 17-ketosteroids)

Serum thyroglobulin in patients with total thyroidectomy; detectable level indicates recurrent thyroid cancer.

Beta-HCG subunit (in blood or urine) for early detection of hydatidiform mole or choriocarcinoma as well as early detection of tumor recurrence

Hemorrhage

Anemia

Malnutrition

Hypoproteinemia

Development of autoantibodies, hemolytic anemia, increased ESR, etc.

Tumor cells in bone marrow, liver biopsy, etc.

Metastatic tumor masses (e.g., liver, brain)

Obstruction (e.g., ureters, bile ducts, intestine)

Functional changes due to metastases that interfere with endocrine secretion (e.g., adrenal, pituitary)

Secretion of active hormonal substances by nonendocrine tumors (e.g., bronchogenic carcinoma)

Diseases that occur with particular frequency in association with neoplasms (e.g., polymyositis)

BIOCHEMICAL DETECTION OF CANCER
(changes in blood not including those due to complications such as hemorrhage, obstruction, infection, changes in fluid and electrolyte balance, metastases, etc.)

These changes in blood are more likely to be useful to monitor effect of therapy or recurrence of lesion, to follow the clinical course or to pinpoint the tissue of origin than to establish a definite diagnosis or be useful screening tests. May sometimes be useful to assess the extent of tumor and to estimate prognosis. (See appropriate separate sections for each.)

Carcinoembryonic antigen (CEA)
Alpha-fetoprotein (AFP)
Human chorionic gonadotropin (HCG)
Calcitonin
Thyroglobulin
Gastrin
Ferritin
Casein
Prostatic acid phosphatase
Alkaline phosphatase
General metabolic changes
    Increased LDH
    Hyperuricemia
    Hypoglycemia
    Hypercalcemia
    Hyperlactacidemia
Primary neoplastic endocrinopathies due to synthesis of hormones appropriate to cell of origin (including carcinoid, trophoblastic cancers, paraneoplastic erythrocytosis, medullary thyroid carcinoma)
Paraneoplastic syndromes
    One-third of these patients show ectopic hormone production.
    One-third show evidence of connective tissue (e.g., polymyositis, dermatomyositis) and dermatologic (e.g., acanthosis nigricans) disorders.
    One-sixth show psychiatric and neurologic syndromes.
    Remainder show immunologic, gastrointestinal (e.g., malabsorption), renal (e.g., nephrotic syndrome), hematologic (e.g., anemia of chronic disease, DIC), paraproteinemias (e.g., multiple myeloma), amyloidosis.
Complications of anticancer therapy
    Blood dyscrasias including secondary leukemia
    Bladder cancer after prolonged Cytoxan therapy
    Cardiotoxicity (e.g., doxorubicin hydrochloride [Adriamycin])
    Pulmonary fibrosis (e.g., methotrexate, bleomycin)
    Sterility
    Teratogenic effects

ACUTE TUMOR LYSIS SYNDROME
Caused by effective induction chemotherapy of rapidly growing neoplasms (e.g., acute leukemia, malignant, lymphoma, Burkitt's lymphoma). Associated with very large tumors, inadequate urine output, high pretreatment serum LDH levels that rise further. Occurs in one-third of nonazotemic and virtually all azotemic patients.
    Hyperuricemia
    Hyperkalemia
    Hypocalcemia
    Severe hyperphosphatemia—occurs only after chemotherapy; is criterion for dialysis to avoid renal failure. Pretreatment with allopurinol and diuresis may prevent syndrome unless there is concomitant renal failure.

OCCULT NEOPLASIA
(e.g., pheochromocytoma, hypernephroma, breast carcinoma, and various benign tumors)
Rule out presence or development of occult neoplasia in

Neurofibromatosis
Sturge-Weber syndrome
Lindau-von Hippel disease
Tuberous sclerosis
Basal cell nevus syndrome
Polymyositis
Acanthosis nigricans

BREAST CANCER
Indications for administration of adrenal hormones
> Hypercalcemia
> Metastases
>> To brain or liver
>> Diffuse pulmonary

STEROID RECEPTOR ASSAYS
Useful in prognosis and treatment of breast carcinoma
When estrogen receptor assay (ERA) is negative, there is $< 10\%$ chance of obtaining a favorable response to any endocrine therapy; thus chemotherapy would be the primary approach. There is a greater likelihood of visceral metastases ($>50\%$) with ER-negative than with ER-positive patients ($<6\%$).
When ERA is positive, there is 55–60% chance of favorable response (i.e., tumor shrinkage and/or clinical improvement).
Predictive value of positive ERA is increased if
> ERA titer > 100 fmol/mg protein (femtomoles/mg)
> PRA (progesterone receptor assay) is also positive.
> Estrogen receptors are demonstrated in nuclear portion of cancer cells as well as the cytosol.
Prognostic value
> Recurrence rate is significantly greater for ERA-negative tumors, both Stage I (negative axillary lymph nodes) and Stage II (positive axillary lymph nodes).
Overall response rate to endocrine therapy is about 50%.

	Response Rate to Endocrine Therapy
ERA > 100 fmol/mg protein	$\cong 75\%$
ERA < 100 fmol/mg protein	$\cong 40\%$
ERA < 3 fmol/mg protein	$\cong 12\%$
ERA positive/PRA positive (60% total group)	$\cong 80\%$
ERA negative/PRA negative (31% of total group)	$\cong 5\%$
ERA positive/PRA negative	$\cong 26\%$
ERA negative/PRA positive (4% of total group; this small group may be due to inaccuracy in assay procedures)	$= 50\%$

Receptor assay should also be performed on recurrent carcinoma even when the original tumor has been previously assayed to substantiate the generally valid assumption that the receptor is still present.
Receptor assay may sometimes be useful in differential diagnosis of metastatic undifferentiated carcinoma in women.

Conditions Due to Physical and Chemical Agents

NARCOTICS ADDICTION
(usually heroin)

Persistent absolute and relative lymphocytosis occurs, with lymphocytes, often bizarre and atypical, that may resemble Downey cells.

Eosinophilia is seen in 25% of patients.

Liver function tests commonly show increased serum SGOT and SGPT (increased in 75% of patients) and/or increased cephalin flocculation and thymol turbidity tests. Higher frequency of positive tests is evident on routine periodic repeat of these tests. (This probably represents a mild, chronic, intermittently active, usually anicteric serum hepatitis.) Serum protein electrophoresis is usually normal.

Liver biopsy shows abnormal morphology in 25% of patients, and foreign particles are particularly suggestive.

HB$_s$Ag is found in 10% of patients.

Laboratory findings due to preexisting glucose-6-PD deficiency may be precipitated (by quinine, which is often used to adulterate the heroin).

Laboratory findings due to malaria transmitted by common syringes may occur. *(Malaria is not frequent; may be suppressed by quinine used for adulteration of heroin.)*

Laboratory findings due to active duodenal ulcer may occur.

Laboratory findings due to tuberculosis, which develops with increased frequency in narcotics addicts, may be present.

Laboratory findings due to staphylococcal pneumonia or septic pulmonary emboli secondary to skin infections or bacterial endocarditis (conditions that are more frequent in narcotics addicts) may be present.

Laboratory findings due to endocarditis
> Right-sided—usually *Staphylococcus aureus* affecting previously normal tricuspid valve
> Left-sided—may be due to *Candida* superimposed on previously normal valve

Oral and IV glucose tolerance curves are often flat (explanation for this finding is not known).

Urinalysis is usually normal unless renal failure due to endocarditis occurs.

Laboratory findings due to syphilis, which occurs with increased frequency in narcotics addicts, may occur. BFP tests for syphilis also occur with increased frequency.

Laboratory findings due to tetanus (which occurs with increased frequency in narcotics addicts because of "skin-popping") may occur. *(Tetanus causes 5–10% of addicts' deaths in New York City.)*

Laboratory findings due to concomitant use of sedative, especially alcohol, barbiturates, and glutethimide (Doriden), may occur.

BARBITURATE OVERDOSAGE

Correlation between serum concentrations of barbiturates and state of intoxication in patients who have taken only a short-acting barbiturate, who are not habitual drug users, and who have no medical complications:

<6	Alert
6–10 µg/ml	Drowsy
11–17 µg/ml	Stuporous
16–20 µg/ml	Coma 1
20–24 µg/ml	Coma 2
24–28 µg/ml	Coma 3
28–40 µg/ml	Coma 4

If the serum drug level is less than expected for the state of intoxication, look for medical complications (e.g., aspiration pneumonia, head trauma) or presence of other drugs.

ALCOHOLISM

Laboratory findings due to alcohol ingestion

Blood alcohol level > 300 mg/dl at any time or > 100 mg/dl in routine examination. *(Blood alcohol level > 150 mg/dl without gross evidence of intoxication suggests alcoholic patient's increased tolerance.)* In high-dose coma, blood alcohol should be > 300 mg/dl; otherwise rule out other etiologies, especially diabetic acidosis and hypoglycemia.

Rules of thumb to estimate blood alcohol level

Peak is reached ½ to 3 hours after last drink.

Each ounce of whisky, glass of wine, or 12 ounces of beer raises blood alcohol 15–25 mg/dl.

Women absorb alcohol much more rapidly than do men and show a 35–45% higher blood alcohol level. During premenstrual period, peak occurs more rapidly and reaches a higher peak. Birth control pills cause a higher, more sustained level.

Elderly become intoxicated more quickly than young persons.

Serum osmolality (reflects blood alcohol levels)—every 22.4 increment > 200 mOsm/L reflects 50 mg/dl alcohol.

Results of alcohol ingestion

Hypoglycemia

Hypochloremic alkalosis

Low magnesium level

Increased lactic acid

Thrombocytopenia

Anemia most often due to folic acid deficiency; less frequently due to iron deficiency, hemorrhage, etc. (see appropriate separate sections)

Alcohol is the most common cause of ring sideroblasts

Three types of hemolytic syndromes may occur (spur cell anemia, acquired stomatocytosis, Zieve syndrome).

Increased blood values with no other known cause that should arouse suspicion of alcoholism

MCV (e.g., >97) (26% of cases) with round macrocytosis

Uric acid (10% of cases)

SGPT, SGOT (48% of cases)

Table 33-1. Stages of Acute Alcoholic Intoxication

Blood Alcohol Concentration (% w/v)	Stage of Alcohol Influence
0.01–0.05	Sobriety
0.03–0.12	Euphoria
0.09–0.25	Excitement
0.18–0.30	Confusion
0.27–0.40	Stupor
0.35–0.50	Coma
0.45 +	Death

Alkaline phosphatase (16% of cases)
Bilirubin (13% of cases)
Triglycerides
In alcoholic hepatitis, SGOT is rarely > 300 IU/l but is higher than
SGPT, in contrast to drug or viral hepatitis. Severity of alcoholic
hepatitis does not correlate with elevation of SGOT, which is normal in 15% of cases. Serum bilirubin level > 5 mg/dl and prothrombin time 3 seconds longer than control time that do not
respond to IV vitamin K indicate poor prognosis. Serum alkaline
phosphatase is often increased, but if > 2 times normal, suggests
complicating biliary obstruction. Serum GGTP is increased in
many types of liver disease; in alcoholism, is most useful to monitor abstinence; returns to normal 6–8 weeks after drinking stops.
Declining serum potassium level to hypokalemia during alcohol
withdrawal is said to be a reliable predictor of delirium tremens.
Laboratory findings due to major alcohol-associated illnesses (see
appropriate separate sections)
Fatty liver, alcoholic hepatitis (see above), cirrhosis, esophageal
varices, peptic ulcer, chronic gastritis, pancreatitis, malab-
sorption, vitamin deficiencies
Head trauma, Korsakoff's syndrome, delirium tremens, periph-
eral neuropathy, myopathy
Cardiac myopathy
Various pneumonias, lung abscess, tuberculosis
Associated addictions
Others

SALICYLATE INTOXICATION
(due to aspirin, sodium salicylate, oil of wintergreen, methyl salicylate)
Increased serum salicylate
> 10 mg/dl when symptoms are present
> 40 mg/dl when hyperventilation is present
At $\cong$ 50 mg/dl, severe toxicity with acid-base imbalance and
ketosis
At 45–70 mg/dl, death
When awaiting laboratory measurement, can estimate peak salicy-
late levels:

$$\text{mg/dl of salicylate} = \frac{\text{mg of salicylate ingested}}{70\% \text{ of body weight in gm*}} \times 100$$

*Total body water.

Table 33-2. Differentiation of Acidosis in Salicylate Intoxication and Diabetes Mellitus

Measurement	Salicylate Intoxication	Diabetes Mellitus
Ferric chloride test on urine	Remains positive after boiling	Becomes negative after boiling (volatile acetoacetic acid is removed)
Nitroprusside test for acetoacetic acid in urine	Negative	Positive
Urinary reducing substances	May be due to glucose or other reducing substances (e.g., salicylglucuronide)	Due to glucose
Serum ketone level	Usually < 20 mg/dl	Often > 50 mg/dl
Prothrombin time	Increased	Normal
Serum salicylate level	> 40 mg/dl	Negative or increased to nontoxic level

In older children and adults, serum salicylate level corresponds well with severity; in younger children, correlation is more variable.

Gastric lavage may increase salicylate level $\leqq 10$ mg/dl.

Early, serum electrolytes and CO_2 are normal.

Later, progressive decrease in serum sodium and PCO_2 occurs. There is combined respiratory alkalosis and metabolic acidosis; change in blood pH reflects the net result. *(Infants may show immediate metabolic acidosis with the usual initial respiratory alkalosis. In older children and adults, the typical picture is respiratory alkalosis.)*

Hypokalemia accompanies the respiratory alkalosis. Dehydration occurs.

Urine shows paradoxic acid pH despite the increased serum bicarbonate.

    Ferric chloride test is positive on boiled as well as unboiled urine (thus differentiating salicylate from ketone bodies); it may have a false positive result because of phenacetin.

    Tests for glucose (e.g., Clinistix), reducing substances (e.g., (Clinitest), or ketone bodies (e.g., Ketostix) are positive.

    RBCs may be present.

    Number of renal tubular cells is increased because of renal irritation

Hypoglycemia occurs, especially in infants on restricted diet and in diabetics.

Serum SGOT and SGPT may be increased.

Hypoprothrombinemia after some days of intensive salicylate therapy is temporary and occasional; rarely causes hemorrhage.
Hydroxyproline is decreased in serum and urine.

PHENACETIN—CHRONIC EXCESSIVE INGESTION

Laboratory findings due to increased incidence of peptic ulceration, especially of stomach, often with bleeding, may be present.
Laboratory findings associated with increased incidence of papillary necrosis and interstitial nephritis may be present.

> Proteinuria is slight or absent.
> Hematuria is often present in active papillary necrosis.
> WBC is increased in urine in absence of infection.
> Papillae are passed in urine.
> Creatinine clearance is decreased.
> Renal failure may occur.

Anemia is common and frequently precedes azotemia.

ACETAMINOPHEN POISONING

Blood levels

> 200 μg/ml within 4 hours after ingestion or > 50 μg/ml at 12 hours forecasts severe liver damage, and treatment with acetylcysteine should begin.
> < 150 μg/ml at 4 hours or < 30–35 μg/ml at 12 hours indicates no liver damage will occur.
> *Liver toxicity cannot be predicted from blood levels earlier than 4 hours.*
> *Exact time of ingestion is often difficult to ascertain.*
> *Patients taking other drugs or with concomitant cirrhosis may develop liver toxicity at different blood levels.*
> *Toxicity is less common in children < 5 years old, and changes in liver function tests may be mild when serum drug levels are in toxic range.*

With hepatotoxicity

> During first 12–24 hours, no other laboratory test abnormalities are found, and serum drug levels are the chief guide to therapy; this is the only stage when treatment can prevent liver damage.
> During next 24–48 hours, SGOT, SGPT, serum bilirubin, prothrombin time are increased.
> Third to fourth day, liver function abnormalities peak; hypoglycemia, secondary renal failure may occur.

BROMISM

Bromism should always be ruled out in the presence of mental symptoms or psychosis.

Serum and urine bromide levels are increased.
CSF protein is increased in acute bromide psychosis.
Serum "chloride" is increased, as indicated by AutoAnalyzer.

If result of chloride determination with AutoAnalyzer is increased out of proportion to result with Cotlove coulimetric titrator, bromism should be ruled out.

SOME POSSIBLE SIDE EFFECTS OF STEROID THERAPY THAT CAUSE LABORATORY CHANGES

Endocrine effects (e.g., adrenal insufficiency after prolonged use, suppression of pituitary or thyroid function, development of diabetes mellitus)

Increased susceptibility to infections

Gastrointestinal effects (e.g., peptic ulcer, perforation of bowel, infarction of bowel, pancreatitis)

Musculoskeletal effects (e.g., osteoporosis, pathologic fractures, arthropathy, myopathy)

Decreased serum potassium, increased WBC, glycosuria, ecchymoses, etc.

PROCAINAMIDE THERAPY

Procainamide therapy may induce the findings of systemic lupus erythematosus (SLE).

Positive serologic tests for SLE are very frequent, especially in dosage of $\geq$ 1.25 gm/day, and may precede clinical manifestations.

LE cell tests become positive in 50% of patients.

Anti-DNP (anti-deoxyribonucleoprotein) tests become positive in 65% of patients.

Anti-DNA tests become positive in 35% of patients.

One of these tests becomes positive in 75% of patients.

Perform serologic tests for SLE on all patients receiving procainamide.

APRESOLINE REACTION
(in hypertension therapy)

Anemia and pancytopenia occur infrequently.

Prolonged use causes a syndrome resembling lupus erythematosus (microscopic hematuria, leukopenia, increased ESR, presence of LE cells, altered serum proteins with increased gamma globulin). After cessation of drug, remission is aided by administration of ACTH.

ENTERIC-COATED THIAZIDE POTASSIUM CHLORIDE

Laboratory findings due to small-intestine ulceration, obstruction, or perforation.

COMPLICATIONS OF PHENYTOIN SODIUM (DILANTIN) THERAPY

Megaloblastic anemia may occur. It is completely responsive to folic acid (even when Dilantin therapy is continued) but not always to vitamin B_{12}. This is the most common hematologic complication.

Rarely there may occur pancytopenia, thrombocytopenia alone, or leukopenia, including agranulocytosis.

Laboratory findings of hepatitis may be present.

Laboratory findings resembling those of malignant lymphomas may be present.

Laboratory findings resembling those of infectious mononucleosis may occur, but heterophil agglutination is not increased.

Increased T-3 uptake, but RAIU, serum cholesterol, etc., are normal (because of competition for binding sites of thyroxin-binding globulin).

Dilantin therapy may induce a lupus-like syndrome.

LABORATORY CHANGES AND SIDE EFFECTS FROM LIPID-LOWERING DRUGS

Nicotinic acid may cause

Dramatic lowering (often) of blood triglyceride in hyperlipid-
emia, Types II and IV and probably also Types III and V
Increased blood sugar
Increased blood uric acid
Abnormal liver function tests
Jaundice (rarely)
Cholestyramine in the form of a chloride salt may cause
Lowering of cholesterol in familial Type II hyperlipidemia
Mild hyperchloremic acidosis

HYPERVITAMINOSIS A
Increased serum vitamin A level ($\leqq$ 2000 µg/dl)
May also show
Increased ESR
Increased serum alkaline phosphatase
Decreased serum albumin
Increased serum bilirubin
Decreased hemoglobin
Slight proteinuria
Slightly increased serum carotene
Increased prothrombin time

CHRONIC ARSENIC POISONING
**(from insecticides, rat poisons, or therapeutic arsenic, e.g., Fowler's
solution)**
Increased arsenic appears in urine (usually > 0.1 mg/L; in acute
cases may be > 1.0 mg/L).
Increased arsenic appears in hair (normal = 0.05 mg/100 gm of
hair; chronic toxicity = 0.1–0.5 mg/100 gm of hair; acute toxicity
= 1–3 mg/100 gm of hair).
Increased arsenic appears in nails 6–9 months after exposure.
Moderate anemia is present.
Moderate leukopenia occurs (2000–5000/cu mm), with mild
eosinophilia.
Liver function tests show mild abnormalities.
Urine shows slight proteinuria.
CSF is normal.

*Arsine gas (hydrogen arsenide) causes hemolysis with hemoglo-
binuria; may cause oliguric renal failure.*

LEAD POISONING
Delta-aminolevulinic acid is increased in urine. Since it is increased
in 75% of asymptomatic lead workers who have normal coropor-
phyrin in urine, it can be used to detect early excess lead absorption.
Recently, rapid micromethods have been developed for measurement of zinc protoporphyrin (hematofluorometer) and free erythrocyte protoporphyrin, and these have been recommended as
more sensitive indicators of lead poisoning than delta-
aminolevulinic acid in urine.
Increased coproporphyrin in urine is a reliable sign of intoxication
and is often demonstrable before basophilic stippling (but one
should rule out a false positive reaction due to drugs such as
barbiturates and salicylates). This is the most useful rapid screening test.

Confirm diagnosis with determination of
> Blood lead
>> < 20 μg/dl is considered normal.
>> 25–40 μg/dl is evidence of increased lead exposure.
>> > 50 μg/dl is a treatable level.
>> 80 μg/dl in children is an indication for emergency treatment.
>
> Urine lead
>> < 80 μg/10 dl is normal for children.
>> < 150 μg/10 dl is normal for adults.

Anemia is common, is usually mild (rarely < 9 gm/dl). Is usually normochromic and normocytic but may be hypochromic and microcytic, especially in children. MCHC is reduced only moderately.

Anisocytosis and poikilocytosis may be found, and a few nucleated RBCs may be seen. Some polychromasia is usual.

Stippled RBCs occur later. Basophilic stippling is not pathognomonic of lead poisoning.

Bone marrow shows erythroid hyperplasia, and 65% of erythroid cells show stippling, some of which are ringed sideroblasts (thus this may be considered a secondary sideroblastic anemia).

Osmotic fragility is decreased, but mechanical fragility is increased.

Hematologic changes of lead poisoning are more marked in patients with iron deficiency.

Urine urobilinogen and uroporphyrin are increased. Porphobilinogen is normal or slightly increased in urine.

Renal tubular damage occurs, with Fanconi's syndrome (hypophosphatemia, aminoaciduria, and glycosuria), usually in very severe or very chronic cases. Albuminuria may occur.

CSF protein is increased, and frequently up to 100 mononuclear cells/cu mm are present in encephalopathy.

MERCURY POISONING

Levels of mercury in serum, urine, and CSF are increased.

95% of asymptomatic normal people (not exposed to mercury) have a urine value < 20 μg/L and blood level < 3 μg/L. Urine and blood levels are nondiagnostic, in that they vary among patients with symptoms, and daily urine levels vary in the same patient. Thus in one epidemic, urine levels ≦ 1000 μg/L occurred in asymptomatic patients whereas other patients had symptoms at levels of 200 μg/L. The above values apply to mercury vapor and inorganic mercury salts.

Organic mercury (e.g., ethyl and methyl mercury) is more toxic; accumulates in RBCs and CNS. Most is slowly excreted in feces with half-life of 70 days. Only 10% is excreted in urine; urine levels may be normal even with significant exposure. Phenyl and methoxyethyl mercuries are less toxic and show higher urine levels.

Clinical correlation with organic mercury

	Whole Blood Total Mercury, in μg/L (or ng/ml or ppm)
Safe level	< 100
Probably no symptoms	100–200
Symptoms occasionally present	> 650
Symptoms usually present	> 1000

ACUTE IRON POISONING
(occurs in children who have ingested medicinal iron preparations)

Increased serum iron and TIBC. Serum iron < 350 µg/dl is rarely significant clinically. With severe intoxication, serum iron is > 500 µg/dl within 6 hours of ingestion. TIBC measurement itself is not useful. Poor prognostic sign when serum iron greatly exceeds TIBC. Serum should be obtained after absorption is complete and before peak serum level falls due to protein-binding and tissue distribution. If the first sample was taken 1–2 hours after ingestion, a second sample should be obtained several hours later.

Renal changes may occur (e.g., acute renal failure, nephrotic syndrome, specific tubular defects).

ORGANIC PHOSPHATE (INSECTICIDES—PARATHION, MALATHION, ETC.) POISONING

Decreased RBC and plasma cholinesterase by ≧ 50% due to inhibition of cholinesterase by organic phosphate pesticides)

In industrial exposure, worker should not return to work until these values rise to 75% of normal. RBC cholinesterase regenerates at rate of 1%/day. Plasma cholinesterase regenerates at rate of 25% in 7–10 days.

MOTHBALLS (CAMPHOR, PARADICHLOROBENZENE, NAPHTHALENE) POISONING

Paradichlorobenzene inhalation may cause liver damage.

Naphthalene ingestion may cause hemolytic anemia in patients with RBCs deficient in glucose-6-PD (see p. 353).

YELLOW PHOSPHORUS POISONING
(rat poison ingestion)

Acute yellow atrophy of liver occurs.

Vomitus may glow in the dark.

PHENOL AND LYSOL POISONING

Severe acidosis often occurs.

Acute tubular necrosis may develop.

OXALATE POISONING
(due to ingestion of stain remover or ink eradicator containing oxalic acid)

Hypocalcemic tetany (due to formation of insoluble calcium oxalate)

METHYL ALCOHOL POISONING

Onset is 12–24 hours after ingestion.

Severe acidosis

Frequent concomitant acute pancreatitis

MILK SICKNESS ("TREMBLES")
(poisoning from goldenrod, snakeroot, richweed, etc., or from eating poisoned animals)

Acidosis

Hypoglycemia

Increased nonprotein nitrogen (particularly guanidine)

Acetonuria

HEAT STROKE

Uniformly increased SGOT (mean is 20 times normal), SGPT (mean is 10 times normal), and LDH (mean is 5 times normal) reach peak on third day and return to normal by 2 weeks. Very high levels are often associated with lethal outcome. Consecutive normal values rule out diagnosis of heat stroke.

Cerebrospinal fluid GOT, GPT, and LDH are normal.

Serum potassium varies from decreased levels associated with hyperventilation and respiratory alkalosis to increased levels associated with lactic acidosis or skeletal muscle damage.

Evidence of kidney damage may vary from mild proteinuria and slight abnormalities of urine sediment to acute oliguric renal insufficiency.

Disseminated intravascular coagulation is common in severe cases.

ACCIDENTAL HYPOTHERMIA

Acid-base disturbances are very common.

Initial hyperventilation causes respiratory alkalosis followed by respiratory acidosis due to CO_2 retention.

Metabolic acidosis due to lactate accumulation. During rewarming, metabolic acidosis may become worse as lactic acid is mobilized from poorly perfused tissues.

Hemoconcentration is common.

WBC frequently falls, but differential is usually normal.

DIC may occur during rewarming.

"Cold diuresis," glycosuria, and natriuresis may occur; oliguria suggests complicating hypovolemia, acute tubular necrosis, rhabdomyolysis, or drug overdose.

Pancreatitis is a frequent complication.

Marked abnormalities in liver function tests are unusual.

DROWNING AND NEAR-DROWNING

Hypoxemia (decreased PO_2)

Metabolic acidosis (decreased blood pH)

In severe freshwater aspiration
Decreased serum sodium and chloride
Increased serum potassium
Increased plasma hemoglobin

In severe seawater aspiration
Hypovolemia
Increased serum sodium and chloride
Normal plasma hemoglobin

Above-mentioned changes follow aspiration of very large amounts of water. Electrolytes return toward normal within 1 hour following survival, even without therapy.

In near-drowning in fresh water, often
Normal serum sodium and chloride
Variable serum potassium
Increased free plasma hemoglobin; hemoglobinuria may occur
Oliguria with transient azotemia and proteinuria may develop.
Fall in RBC, hemoglobin, and hematocrit in 24 hours

In near-drowning in seawater, often
Moderate increase in serum sodium and chloride

Normal or decreased serum potassium
Normal hemoglobin, hematocrit, and plasma hemoglobin

Blood count may appear normal even when considerable hemolysis is present because usual methodology does not distinguish between hemoglobin within RBC and free hemoglobin in serum. Fall in hemoglobin and hematocrit may be delayed 1–2 days.

ACUTE CARBON MONOXIDE POISONING
Arterial PO_2 is normal, although O_2 is significantly decreased.
Arterial PCO_2 may be normal or slightly decreased.
Blood pH is markedly decreased (metabolic acidosis due to tissue hypoxia).
Symptoms are correlated with the percentage of carbon monoxide in hemoglobin:

% COHb	Symptoms
0–2%	Asymptomatic
2–5%	Found in moderate cigarette smokers; usually asymptomatic but may be slight impairment of intellect
5–10%	Found in heavy cigarette smokers; slight dyspnea with severe exertion
10–20%	Dyspnea with moderate exertion; mild headache
20–30%	Marked headache, irritability, disturbed judgment and memory, easy fatiguability
30–40%	Severe headache, dimness of vision, confusion, weakness, nausea
40–50%	Headache, confusion, fainting, ataxia, collapse, hyperventilation
50–60%	Coma, intermittent convulsions
>60%	Respiratory failure and death if exposure is long continued
80%	Rapidly fatal

INJURY DUE TO ELECTRIC CURRENT (INCLUDING LIGHTNING)
Increased WBC with large immature granulocytes
Albuminuria; hemoglobinuria in presence of severe burns
CSF sometimes bloody
Myoglobinuria and increased SGOT, serum CK, etc., indicate severe tissue damage.

BURNS
Decreased plasma volume and blood volume. This decrease follows (and therefore is not due to) marked drop in cardiac output. Greatest fall in plasma volume occurs in the first 12 hours and continues at a much slower rate for only 6–12 hours more. In a 40% burn, plasma volume falls to 25% below preburn levels.
Infection
Burn sepsis: Gram-positive organisms predominate until the third day, when gram-negative organisms become dominant. By fifth day, untreated infection is active. *Fatal burn-wound sepsis shows no noteworthy spread of bacteria beyond wound in half the cases. Before antibiotic therapy, this caused 75% of deaths due to burns; it now causes 10–15% of deaths.*

Laboratory findings due to pneumonia, which now causes most deaths that result from infection. Two-thirds of pneumonia cases are airborne infections. One-third are hematogenous infections and are often due to septic phlebitis at sites of old cutdowns.

Local and systemic infection due to *Candida* and *Phycomycetes.*

Laboratory findings due to renal failure. Reported frequency varies—1.3% of total admissions to 15% of patients with burns involving > 15% of body surface.

Laboratory findings due to Curling's ulcer. Occurs in 11% of burn patients. *Gastric ulcer is more frequent in general, but duodenal ulcer occurs twice as often in children as in adults. Gastric lesions are seen throughout the first month with equal frequency in all age groups, but duodenal ulcers are most frequent in adults during the first week and in children during the third and fourth weeks after the burns.*

Blood viscosity rises acutely; remains elevated for 4–5 days although hematocrit has returned to normal.

Fibrin split products are increased for 3–5 days.

Other findings that may occur in all types of trauma

Platelet count rises slowly, lasting for 3 weeks. Platelet adhesiveness is increased.

Fibrinogen falls during first 36 hours, then rises steeply for up to 3 months.

Factors V and VIII may be 4–8 times normal level for up to 3 months.

CONVULSIVE THERAPY
(e.g., electroshock therapy)

Increased cerebrospinal fluid GOT and LDH peak (3 times normal) in 12 hours; return to normal by 48 hours.

SNAKEBITE

Pit vipers (rattlesnake, copperhead, water moccasin)

Increased WBC (20,000–30,000/cu mm)

Platelets decreased to approximately 10,000/cu mm within an hour; return to normal in about 4 hours

Burrs on almost all RBCs

Clotting caused by some venoms; normal coagulation prevented by others, which destroy fibrinogen so that fibrin split products are detected, fibrinogen levels are very low or absent, and PT and PTT are very high. As a screening test, blood drawn into a modified Lee-White clotting tube that fails to clot within a few minutes of constant agitation is a reliable indication of envenomization.

Albuminuria

Elapidae (coral snakes, kraits, cobras)

Hemolytic manifestations

SPIDER BITE

Black widow spider *(Latrodectus mactans)*

Moderately increased WBC

Findings of acute nephritis

Brown spider *(Loxosceles reclusa)*

Hemolytic anemia with hemoglobinuria and hemoglobinemia
Increased WBC
Thrombocytopenia
Proteinuria

INSECT BITE
(due to ticks, lice, fleas, bugs, beetles, ants, flies, bees, wasps, etc.)
No specific laboratory findings unless secondary infection occurs.

SERUM SICKNESS
Decreased WBC due to decreased polynuclear neutrophils; occasion-
ally WBC is increased.
Eosinophils are usually normal.
ESR is normal.
Heterophil agglutination test is often positive and is decreased by
guinea pig kidney absorption (see p. 137).

Effects of Drugs on Laboratory Test Values

Alteration of Laboratory Test Values by Drugs

With the coincident ingestion of a large number of drugs and the performance of many laboratory tests (many of which are unsolicited), test abnormalities may be due to drugs as often as to disease. Correct interpretation of laboratory tests requires that the physician be aware of all drugs that the patient is taking. It is important to remember that patients often do not tell their physician about medications they are taking (prescribed by other doctors or by the patients themselves). In addition, there is environmental exposure to many drugs and chemicals.

The classes of drugs most often involved include the anticoagulants, anticonvulsants, antihypertensives, anti-infectives, oral hypoglycemics, hormones, and psychoactive agents.

The following lists of the more frequently performed laboratory test values that may be altered by commonly used drugs are only a general guide to the direction of increase or decrease, not an all-inclusive collection of such information. The selection and arrangement of data by clinical groups provide the most useful, most rapid, and simplest summary of a very complex subject. Only generic names for drugs are used.

The frequency of such modified laboratory test values is variable. A number of causative mechanisms may operate, sometimes simultaneously. Thus some changes are due to interference with the chemical reaction used in the testing procedure. Other changes reflect damage to a specific organ, such as the liver or kidney. In some cases, specific metabolic alterations are induced, such as accelerated or retarded formation or excretion of a specific chemical, competition for binding sites, stimulation or suppression of degradative enzymes, etc. Often the mechanism of these altered laboratory test values is not known.

This chapter is meant only as an illustration of various possible mechanisms of such alterations and as a list of some of the more common responsible drugs. It is not to be considered a complete or exhaustive list, nor should it be used to rule out drug-caused effect on a laboratory test by virtue of a drug's not appearing on the lists. For the most specific information, the reader should consult more detailed sources about an individual drug, such as the manufacturer's insert sheets and data, computer-file based data, and the most current literature available published since this and other compilations.

DRUGS THAT MAY CAUSE MARKED ELEVATION OF URINE SPECIFIC GRAVITY
Dextran
Radiopaque contrast media
Sucrose

DRUGS THAT MAY ALTER URINE COLOR

Urine coloration due to drugs may mask other abnormal colors (e.g., due to blood, bile, porphyrins) as well as interfere with various chemical determinations (fluorometric, colorimetric, photometric)

Drug	Resulting Color
Acetophenetidin	Hematuria or pink-red due to metabolite
Aminosalicylic acid (PAS)	Discoloration abnormal but not distinctive
Amitriptyline	Blue-green
Anisindione (indandione)	Orange (alkaline urine), pink-red-brown (acid urine)
Anthraquinones	Pink to brown
Anticoagulants	Pink to red to brown (due to bleeding)
Cascara	Brown (acid urine), yellow-pink (alkaline urine), black on standing
Chloroquine	Brown
Chlorzoxazone (metabolite)	Purple, red, pink, rust
Cinchophen	Red-brown
Dihydroxyanthraquinone	Pink to orange (alkaline urine)
Emodin	Pink to red to red-brown (alkaline urine)
Ethoxazene	Orange, red, pink, rust
Furazolidone	Brown
Indomethacin	Green (due to biliverdin)
Iron sorbitol	Brown
Methocarbamol	Dark brown, black, blue or green on standing
Methyldopa	Red darkens on standing, pink or brown
Methylene blue	Greenish-yellow to blue
Metronidazole (metabolite)	Dark brown
Nitrofurantoin and derivatives	Brown, yellow
Pamaquine	Brown
Phenacetin	Dark brown
Phenazopyridine	Orange to red
Phenindione	Red-orange in alkaline urine
Phenolphthalein	Pink to red to magenta (alkaline urine), orange, rust (acid)
Phenothiazines	Pink, red, purple, orange, rust
Phensuximide	Pink, red, purple, orange, rust
Primaquine	Rust yellow to brown
Quinacrine (mepacrine)	Deep yellow on acidification
Quinine and derivatives	Brown to black
Rhubarb	Yellow-brown (acid), yellow-pink (alkaline), darkens
Riboflavin	Yellow
Rifampin	Red-orange
Salicylates	Pink to red to brown (due to bleeding)
Salicylazosulfapyridine	Pink, red, purple, orange, rust
Senna	Red (alkaline urine), yellow-brown (acid urine)
Sulfonamides	Rust, yellow, or brown
Thiazolsulfone	Pink, red, purple, orange, rust

Drug	**Resulting Color**
Tolonium	Blue, green
Triamterene	Green, blue with blue fluorescence

DRUGS THAT MAY CAUSE FALSE POSITIVE TEST FOR URINE PROTEIN

Drugs with nephrotoxic effect (e.g., gold, arsenicals, antimony compounds)

Drugs that may interfere with sulfosalicylic acid methods
    Cephaloridine
    Cephalothin
    Sulfamethoxazole
    Tolbutamide
    Tolmetin sodium
    Other

Drugs that may cause false positive turbidity tests
    Chlorpromazine, promazine
    Penicillin (massive doses)
    Radiopaque contrast media (for up to 3 days)
    Sulfisoxazole
    Thymol
    Other

Drugs that react with Folin-Ciocalteu reagent of Lowry procedure
    Aminosalicylic acid (PAS)
    Dithiazine
    Other

Drugs that cause false positive reaction with Labstix because of high pH
    Sodium bicarbonate
    Acetazolamide
    Other

DRUGS THAT MAY CAUSE POSITIVE TEST FOR URINE GLUCOSE

Drugs that may cause hyperglycemia with secondary glycosuria (e.g., corticosteroids, indomethacin, isoniazid)

Drugs that cause renal damage (e.g., degraded tetracycline)

Vaginal powders that contain glucose, causing artifactual false positive (e.g., furazolidone)

Drugs that cause false positive test by reducing action with Benedict's solution and Clinitest but not with Clinistix or Testape
    Acetylsalicylic acid
    Aminosalicylic acid (PAS)
    Cephaloridine (abnormal dark color)
    Cephalothin (brown-black color)
    Chloral hydrate
    Cinchophen
    Nitrofurantoin
    Streptomycin
    Sulfonamides
    Other

DRUGS THAT MAY CAUSE FALSE NEGATIVE TEST FOR URINE GLUCOSE
(glucose oxidase method, e.g., Clinistix, Testape)

Ascorbic acid

Levodopa (with Clinistix but not Testape)
Phenazopyridine

DRUGS THAT MAY CAUSE FALSE POSITIVE URINE ACETONE TEST

Ketostix or Acetest Methods **Labstix, Bili-Labstix, etc.**
PSP   Levodopa
Inositol or methionine
Metformin, phenformin

DRUGS THAT MAY CAUSE FALSE POSITIVE URINE DIACETIC ACID TEST
(Gerhardt ferric chloride test; Phenistix)
Aminosalicylic acid (PAS)
Chlorpromazine
Phenothiazines
Levodopa
Salicylates

DRUGS THAT MAY CAUSE POSITIVE TEST FOR URINE AMINO ACIDS
ACTH and cortisone
Tetracyclines (degraded) and other nephrotoxic agents
Gentamicin, neomycin, and kanamycin cause spurious spots on thin-layer chromatograms (ninhydrin reaction)

DRUGS THAT MAY ALTER URINE TESTS FOR OCCULT BLOOD
Guaiac   **Benzidine**
False positive   False positive
    Bromides   Bromides
    Copper   Copper
    Iodides   Iodides
    Oxidizing agents   Permanganate

False negative
    Ascorbic acid (high doses)

DRUGS THAT MAY CAUSE POSITIVE TESTS FOR HEMATURIA OR HEMOGLOBINURIA
Drugs that cause nephrotoxicity (e.g., amphotericin B, bacitracin)
Drugs that cause actual bleeding (e.g., phenylbutazone, indomethacin, coumarin)
Drugs that cause hemolysis (e.g., acetylsalicylic acid, acetophenetidin, acetanilid)

DRUGS THAT MAY CAUSE POSITIVE TESTS FOR BILE IN URINE
Drugs that cause cholestasis
Drugs that are hepatotoxic
Drugs that interfere with testing methods
    Acriflavine (yellow color when urine is shaken)
    Chlorpromazine (interferes with Bili-Labstix)
    Ethoxazene (atypical red color with Bili-Labstix and Ictotest)

Mefenamic acid
Phenazopyridine (false positive with Bili-Labstix and Ictotest)
Phenothiazines (may interfere with Bili-Labstix)
Thymol (affects Hay's test for bile acids)

DRUGS THAT MAY CAUSE INCREASED OR DECREASED URINE UROBILINOGEN

Increased
Drugs that interfere with
   testing methods
      Aminosalicylic acid (PAS)
      Antipyrine
      Bromsulfalein (BSP)
      Cascara
      Chlorpromazine
      Phenazopyridine
      Phenothiazines
      Sulfonamides
      5-Hydroxyindoleacetic acid
         Bananas
Drugs that cause hemolysis

Decreased
Drugs that cause cholestasis
Drugs that reduce the bacterial flora
   in the gastrointestinal tract (e.g.,
   chloramphenicol)

DRUGS THAT MAY CAUSE POSITIVE TESTS FOR URINE PORPHYRINS (FLUOROMETRIC METHODS)

Drugs that produce fluorescence
      Acriflavine
      Ethoxazene
      Phenazopyridine
      Sulfamethoxazole
      Tetracycline
      Other
Drugs that may precipitate porphyria
      Antipyretics
      Barbiturates
      Phenylhydrazine
      Sulfonamides
      Other

DRUGS THAT MAY CAUSE INCREASED OR DECREASED URINE CREATINE

Increased	Decreased
Caffeine	Androgens and anabolic steroids
Methyltestosterone	Thiazides
PSP	

DRUGS THAT MAY CAUSE INCREASED OR DECREASED URINE CREATININE

Increased	Decreased
Ascorbic acid	Androgens and anabolic steroids
Corticosteroids	Thiazides
Levodopa	
Methyldopa	
Nitrofurans	
PSP	

DRUGS THAT MAY CAUSE INCREASED OR DECREASED URINE CALCIUM

Increased
Androgens and anabolic
  steroids
Cholestyramine
Corticosteroids
Dihydrotachysterol, vitamin D
  parathyroid injections
Viomycin

Decreased
Sodium phytate
Thiazides

DRUGS THAT MAY CAUSE FALSE POSITIVE PSP TEST IN URINE

Kaolin
Magnesium
Methylene blue
Nicotinic acid
Quinacrine (mepacrine)
Quinidine
Quinine

DRUGS THAT MAY CAUSE INCREASED OR DECREASED URINE 17-KETOSTEROIDS

Increased
Ampicillin
Cephaloridine
Cephalothin
Chloramphenicol
Chlorpromazine
Cloxacillin
Dexamethasone
Erythromycin
Ethinamate
Meprobamate
Nalidixic acid
Oleandomycin
Penicillin
Phenaglycodol
Phenazopyridine
Phenothiazines
Quinidine
Secobarbital
Spironolactone

Decreased
Chlordiazepoxide
Estrogens
Meprobamate
Metyrapone
Probenecid
Promazine
Reserpine

DRUGS THAT MAY CAUSE INCREASED OR DECREASED URINE 17-HYDROXYCORTICOSTEROIDS

Increased
Acetazolamide
Chloral hydrate
Chlordiazepoxide
Chlorpromazine
Colchicine
Erythromycin
Etryptamine
Meprobamate
Oleandomycin

Decreased
Estrogens and oral
  contraceptives
Phenothiazines
Reserpine

Increased	Decreased
Paraldehyde	
Quinine and quinidine	
Spironolactone	

DRUGS THAT MAY INTERFERE WITH DETERMINATION OF URINE CATECHOLAMINES
(by producing urinary fluorescence)
Ampicillin
Ascorbic acid
Chloral hydrate
Epinephrine
Erythromycin
Hydralazine
Methenamine
Methyldopa
Nicotinic acid (large doses)
Quinine and quinidine
Tetracycline and derivatives
Vitamin B complex

DRUGS THAT MAY CAUSE DECREASED URINE CATECHOLAMINES
Guanethidine
Phenothiazines
Reserpine

DRUGS THAT MAY CAUSE INCREASED OR DECREASED URINE VMA (VANILLYLMANDELIC ACID)

Increased	Decreased
Aspirin	(Values are usually not de-
Aminosalicylic acid	pressed to normal in patients
(PAS)	with pheochromocytoma)
Bromsulfalein (BSP)	Chlorpromazine
Glyceryl guaiacolate	Clofibrate
Mephenesin	Guanethidine analogs
Methocarbamol	Imipramine
Nalidixic acid	Methyldopa
Oxytetracycline	Monoamine oxidase (MAO)
Penicillin	inhibitors
Phenoazopyridine	Reserpine
PSP	
Sulfa drugs	

DRUGS THAT MAY CAUSE INCREASED OR DECREASED URINE 5-HIAA (5-HYDROXYINDOLEACETIC ACID)

Increased	Decreased
Acetanilid	Chlorpromazine, promazine
Acetophenetidin	Imipramine
Glyceryl guaiacolate	Isoniazid
Mephenesin	MAO inhibitors
Methocarbamol	Methenamine
Reserpine	Methyldopa
	Phenothiazines
	Promethazine

DRUGS THAT MAY CAUSE A FALSE POSITIVE URINE PREGNANCY TEST
Chlorpromazine (frog, rabbit, immunologic)
Phenothiazines (frog, rabbit, immunologic)
Promethazine (Gravindex)

DRUG THAT MAY CAUSE A FALSE NEGATIVE URINE PREGNANCY TEST
Promethazine (DAP test)

DRUGS THAT MAY CAUSE INCREASED OR DECREASED ERYTHROCYTE SEDIMENTATION RATE (ESR)

Increased	Decreased
Dextran	Quinine (therapeutic effect)
Methyldopa	Salicylates (therapeutic effect)
Methysergide	Drugs that cause a high blood
Penicillamine	glucose level
Theophylline	
Trifluperidol	
Vitamin A	

DRUGS THAT MAY CAUSE A POSITIVE DIRECT COOMBS' TEST
Acetophenetidin
Cephalosporins (most common with cephalothin; less frequent with cefazolin and cephapirin; reported in 3–50% of patients)
Chlorpromazine
Chlorpropamide
Dipyrone
Mefenamic acid
Melphalan
Oxyphenisatin
Penicillin (with daily IV dose of 20 million units/day for several weeks)
Phenacetin (low incidence)
Phenylbutazone
Phenytoin sodium
Ethosuximide
Hydralazine
Isoniazid
Levodopa
Procainamide
Quinidine, quinine
Rifampin (rare)
Streptomycin
Sulfonamides
Tetracyclines
Tolbutamide (rare)

Illustrative information: For methyldopa, a positive direct Coombs' test occurs in 10–20% of patients on continued therapy. Occurs rarely in first 6 months of treatment. If not found within 12 months, is unlikely to occur. Is dose-related, with lowest incidence in patients receiving $\leq$ 1 gm daily. Reversal may take weeks to months after the drug is discontinued.

DRUGS THAT MAY CAUSE POSITIVE TESTS FOR LUPUS ERYTHEMATOSUS CELLS AND/OR ANTINUCLEAR ANTIBODIES
Acetazolamide
Aminosalicylic acid (PAS)
Birth control pills
Chlorprothixene
Chlorothiazide
Griseofulvin
Hydralazine
Penicillin
Phenylbutazone
Phenytoin sodium
Procainamide
Streptomycin
Sulfonamides
Tetracyclines

Isoniazid	Thiouracil
Methyldopa	Trimethadione

DRUGS THAT MAY CAUSE INCREASED BLEEDING TIME
Acetylsalicylic acid
Dextran
Pantothenyl alcohol and derivatives
Streptokinase-streptodornase

DRUGS THAT MAY CAUSE INCREASED OR DECREASED COAGULATION TIME

Increased	**Decreased**
Anticoagulants	Corticosteroids
Tetracyclines	Epinephrine

DRUGS THAT POTENTIATE COUMARIN ACTION
(increase prothrombin time)

Anabolic steroids	Oxyphenbutazone
Chloral hydrate	Phenylbutazone
Chloramphenicol	Phenyramidol
Clofibrate	Phenytoin sodium
Glucagon	Quinidine
Indomethacin	Salicylates
Mefenamic acid	D-Thyroxine
Neomycin	

DRUGS THAT MAY POTENTIATE COUMARIN ACTION
(increase prothrombin time)

Acetaminophen	Monoamine oxidase (MAO)
Allopurinol	inhibitors
Diazoxide	Nalidixic acid
Disulfiram	Northriptyline
Ethacrynic acid	Sulfinpyrazone
Heparin	Sulfonamides (long-acting)
Mercaptopurine	Thyroid drugs
Methyldopa	Tolbutamide
Methylphenidate	

DRUGS THAT INHIBIT COUMARIN ACTION
(decrease prothrombin time)
Barbiturates
Ethchlorvynol
Glutethimide
Griseofulvin
Heptabarbital
Vitamin K

DRUGS THAT MAY INHIBIT COUMARIN ACTION
(decrease prothrombin time)
Adrenocortical steroids
Birth control pills
Cholestyramine
Colchicine
Meprobamate
Rifampin

Patients on long-term coumarin treatment should not take barbiturates, chloral hydrate, chloramphenicol, ethchlorvynol, glutethimide, phenylbutazone (or its congeners), phenyramidol, quinidine, or salicylates. Patients on long-term coumarin treatment should not take any other drugs without consideration of possible drug interaction.

DRUGS THAT MAY INHIBIT HEPARIN
Antihistamines
Digitalis
Nicotine
Penicillin (intravenous)
Protamine
Tetracycline
Tranquilizers (phenothiazine)

DRUGS THAT MAY CAUSE THROMBOCYTOPENIA BY DEPRESSION OF BONE MARROW
Doxorubicin hydrochloride (Adriamycin)
Alkylating agents
Antipurines
Antipyrimidines
Bleomycin
D-Asparaginase

DRUGS THAT MAY CAUSE IDIOSYNCRATIC THROMBOCYTOPENIA
Antibacterial agents
  Isoniazid (INH)
  Sulfonamides
Antibiotics
  Chloramphenicol
  Streptomycin
Anticonvulsant drugs
  Ethosuximide (Zarontin)
  Methylhydantoin
  Paramethadione
  Phenacemide
  Trimethadione
Antirheumatic drugs
  Colchicine
  Gold salts
  Indomethacin
  Phenylbutazone

Hypoglycemic agents
  Carbutamide
  Chlorpropamide
  Tolbutamide
Tranquilizers
  Chlordiazepoxide
  Chlorpromazine
  Meprobamate
  Promazine
Miscellaneous
  Acetazolamide
  Chlorothiazide
  Hydralazine
  Quinacrine
  Tripelennamine
  Quinidine
  Acetaminophen

DRUGS THAT MAY CAUSE ALLERGIC VASCULAR PURPURA WITH NORMAL PLATELET FUNCTION AND NUMBERS
Acetophenetidin
Aspirin
Carbromal
Camphenazine
Chloral hydrate
Chlorothiazide
Chlorpromazine

Griseofulvin
Iodides
Isoniazid
Meprobamate
Oxytetracycline
Phenothiazines
Procaine penicillin

Colchicine
Coumarin congeners
Diphenhydramine (Benadryl)
Erythromycin

Quinidine
Sulfonamides
Tetracycline
Trifluoperazine

DRUGS THAT MAY CAUSE COLOR CHANGES IN STOOL

Drug	Resulting Color
Alkaline antacids and aluminum salts	White discoloration or speckling
Anticoagulants (excess)	Due to bleeding
Anthraquinones	Brown staining
Bismuth salts	Black
Charcoal	Black
Dithiazine	Green to blue
Indomethacin	Green (due to biliverdin)
Iron salts	Black
Mercurous chloride	Green
Phenazopyridine	Orange-red
Phenolphthalein	Red
Phenylbutazone and oxyphenbutazone	Black (due to bleeding)
Pyrvinium pamoate	Red
Rhubarb	Yellow
Salicylates	Due to bleeding
Santonin	Yellow
Senna	Yellow to brown
Tetracyclines in syrup (due to glucosamine)	Red

DRUGS THAT MAY CAUSE FALSE NEGATIVE TEST FOR OCCULT BLOOD IN STOOL
Vitamin C (usually > 500 mg/day)

DRUGS THAT MAY CAUSE INCREASED SERUM GLUCOSE AND/OR IMPAIRED GLUCOSE TOLERANCE
Hormones (e.g., oral contraceptives, thyroid hormone, glucocorticoids, progestins)
Anti-inflammatory agents (e.g., indomethacin)
Diuretic and antihypertensive drugs (e.g., thiazides, furosemide, clonidine)
Neuroactive drugs (e.g., phenothiazines, tricyclics, lithium carbonate, haloperidol, adrenergic agonists)
Others (e.g., isoniazid, heparin, cimetidine, nicotinic acid)

DRUGS THAT MAY CAUSE INCREASED SERUM UREA NITROGEN

Due To
Nephrotoxic effect (see Table 34-1, pp. 672–677)
Methodologic interference
    Nesslerization (chloral hydrate, chloramphenicol, ammonium salts)
    Berthelot (aminophenol, asparagine, ammonium salts)
    Fearon (acetohexamide, sulfonylureas)

DRUGS THAT MAY CAUSE DECREASED SERUM UREA NITROGEN

Due To
Methodologic interference—Berthelot (chloramphenicol, streptomycin)

DRUGS THAT MAY CAUSE INCREASED SERUM CREATININE

Due To
Interference with tubular secretion of creatinine
    Acetohexamide
    Cephalosporins
    Cimetidine
    Trimethoprim
Methodologic interference (e.g., ascorbic acid, PSP, para-aminohippurate, levodopa)

DRUGS THAT MAY CAUSE INCREASED SERUM URIC ACID

Due To
Cytotoxic effect causing increased turnover rate of nucleic acids (e.g., antimetabolite and chemotherapeutic agents in neoplastic diseases [e.g., methotrexate, busulfan, vincristine, azathioprine, prednisone])
Decreased renal clearance or tubular secretion (e.g., various diuretics [thiazides, furosemide, mercurials])
Nephrotoxic effect (e.g., mitomycin C)
Other effects (e.g., levodopa, phenytoin sodium)
Methodologic interference (e.g., ascorbic acid, levodopa, methyldopa)

DRUGS THAT MAY CAUSE DECREASED SERUM URIC ACID

Due To
Decreased production (allopurinol [xanthine oxidase inhibition])
Uricosuric effect (e.g., probenecid, high doses of salicylates, cinchophen, corticotropin, coumarins, thiazide diuretics, acetohexamide)
Other effects (e.g., corticosteroids, indomethacin)

DRUGS THAT MAY CAUSE INCREASED SERUM BILIRUBIN

Due To
Hepatotoxic effect
Cholestatic effect
Hemolysis and hemolytic anemia (e.g., antimalarials, streptomycin)
Hemolysis in glucose-6-PD deficiency (e.g., primaquine, sulfa drugs)
Methodologic interference
    Evelyn-Malloy (dextran, novobiocin)
    Diazo reaction (ethoxazene, histidine, indican, phenazopyridine, rifampin, theophylline, tyrosine)
    SMA 12/60 (aminophenol, ascorbic acid, epinephrine, isoproterenol, levodopa, methyldopa, phenelzine)
    Spectrophotometric methods (drugs that cause lipemia)

FACTORS THAT MAY CAUSE DECREASED SERUM BILIRUBIN

Presence of hemoglobin
Exposure to sunlight or fluorescent light
Barbiturates (in newborns)

DRUGS THAT MAY CAUSE INCREASED SERUM CHOLESTEROL

Due To

Hepatotoxic effect (e.g., phenytoin sodium)
Cholestatic effect (e.g., androgens and anabolic steroids, thiazides, sulfonamides, promazines, chlorpropamide, cinchophen)
Hormonal effect (e.g., corticosteroids, birth control pills)
Methodologic interference (Zlatkis-Zak reaction) (e.g., bromides, iodides, chlorpromazine, corticosteroids, viomycin, vitamin C, vitamin A)
10% of patients on long-term levodopa therapy

DRUGS THAT MAY CAUSE DECREASED SERUM CHOLESTEROL

Due To

Hepatotoxic effect (e.g., allopurinol, tetracyclines, erythromycin, isoniazid, MAO inhibitors)
Synthesis inhibition (e.g., androgens, chlorpropamide, clomiphene, phenformin)
Diminished synthesis (probable mechanism) (e.g., clofibrate)
Other mechanisms (e.g., azathioprine, kanamycin, neomycin, estrogens, chlorestyramine)
Methodologic interference (Zlatkis-Zak reaction) (e.g., thiouracil, nitrates, nitrites)

DRUGS THAT MAY CAUSE INCREASED SERUM TRIGLYCERIDES

Estrogens and birth control pills, cholestyramine

Due To

Methodologic interference (enzyme reaction) (glyceraldehyde)

DRUGS THAT MAY CAUSE DECREASED SERUM TRIGLYCERIDES

Ascorbic acid	Clofibrate	Phenformin
Asparaginase	Metformin	Other

DRUGS THAT MAY CAUSE INCREASED SERUM SODIUM

Due To

Retention of salt and water (e.g., corticosteroids, guanethidine, phenylbutazone)
Alkalosis (e.g., bicarbonates)
Mineralocorticoid effect (e.g., anabolic steroids, cortisone)
Effect on renal tubules (e.g., clonidine, methoxyflurane, tetracycline)

DRUGS THAT MAY CAUSE DECREASED SERUM SODIUM

Due To

Diuretic effect (e.g., ethacrynic acid, furosemide, thiazides, triamterene, mannitol, ammonium chloride, spironolactone)

Table 34-1. Effects of Various Drugs on Laboratory Test Values

Drugs	Hepatotoxic and/or cholestatic	Nephrotoxic	Intestinal malabsorption	Serum iron	Serum TIBC	Serum folate (inhibit *L. casei*)	Creatinine	BUN	Uric acid	Calcium	Bilirubin	SGOT/SGPT	Glucose
Antihistamines													
Antimony compounds	+	+											
Arsenicals	+	+											
Caffeine											D		I
Cholinergics											I	I	
Cinchophen	+								D				
Clofibrate	+								D				
Coumarins	+								D				
Cyclophosphamide	+												
Dextran				I				I	I		I		I
Phenytoin sodium	+		+			D							I
Heparin										a			
Levodopa									I				
Methotrexate	+					+			I[a]				
Procainamide	+												
Propylthiouracil	+								I[a]				
Quinacrine	+												
Quinine, Quinidine													
Radiopaque contrast media		+							D		+		
Theophylline									I		I		
Vitamins Ascorbic acid							I		I		I	I	I
Nicotinic acid (large doses)	+										I		
Vitamin A											I		
Vitamin D		a											
Vitamin K													
Hormones ACTH				D	D				D				I
Anabolic steroids and androgens	+												
Corticosteroids									D	D			I
Estrogens	+					D							I
Birth control pills (estrogens + progestin)	+			I	I	D							
D-Thyroxine													I

See footnotes on p. 677.

Glucose tolerance	Cholesterol	T-3 uptake	T-4	^{131}I uptake	Amylase/lipase	Sodium	Potassium	Chloride	Prothrombin time	Comments
									D	
I										
				I						Changes due to spasm of sphincter of Oddi
	D								I	D–triglycerides, total lipids, LDH
									I	
										I–protein
D		I	D							D–IgA
		I	D						I	[a]Alters turbidity tests and lipoprotein electrophoresis pattern. May interfere with calcium
			I							[a]In gout
		D	D	D					I	[a]SMA methodology
									I	
										I–protein. Serum protein electrophoresis pattern cannot be interpreted.
				D						I–ESR
										D–LDH
	I									
	I									[a]With hypervitaminosis D
									D	
D			D	D	I	I	D	D		
D		D	I							
	I					I	D	I		
D	D	D	I	I						
									D	
	D	I	I						I	

Table 34-1. (continued)

Drugs	Hepatotoxic and/or cholestatic	Nephrotoxic	Intestinal malabsorption	Serum iron	Serum TIBC	Serum folate (inhibit *L. casei*)	Creatinine	BUN	Uric acid	Calcium	Bilirubin	SGOT/SGPT	Glucose
Anti-inflammatory anti-gout, anti-arthritis													
Allopurinol	+								D				
Colchicine	+		+										
Gold	+	+											
Indomethacin	+												
Phenylbutazone	+												
Probenecid	+	+							D				
Salicylates	+	+							I^a				
Psychoactive Agents													
Chloral hydrate							I^a						
Chlordiazepoxide	+												
Imipramine	+												
Lithium		+											
Phenobarbital	+					D							
Phenothiazines													
Chlorpromazine	+								D				I
Chlorprothixene	+								D				
Fluphenazine													
Thiothixene	+												
Narcotics													
Codeine											I	I	
Meperidine (Demerol)											I	I	
Morphine (heroin)											I	I	
Marihuana								I	D				D
Antidiabetic (oral)													
Acetohexamide (sulfonylurea)	+							I					
Chlorpropamide	+												
Tolbutamide	+												I^a
Antihypertensives													
Guanethidine analogs								I				I	D
Hydralazine									I	I		I	I
MAO inhibitors	+		+										
Methyldopa	+						I		I				
Reserpine													I

See footnotes on p. 677.

Glucose tolerance	Cholesterol	T-3 uptake	T-4	^{131}I uptake	Amylase/lipase	Sodium	Potassium	Chloride	Prothrombin time	Comments
									D[a]	[a]On coumarins
										[a]With some methods
									I	
		I		D					I	
		I	D							[a]High doses decrease uric acid
									D	[a]React with Neisler's reagent
		D		D						
										D–VMA and 5-HIAA
		D		D						I–TSH. Mild to moderate I in WBC
									D	
D										D–5-HIAA. May cause false positive pregnancy test
					I					⎫ I–LDH. Laboratory changes
					I					⎬ due to spasm of sphincter
					I					⎭ of Oddi
						I	I	I		
										[a]SMA methodology
I						I		I	I	D–VMA
										D–VMA and 5-HIAA
									I	D–5-HIAA
			D							I–5-HIAA

Table 34-1. (continued)

Drugs	Hepatotoxic and/or cholestatic	Nephrotoxic	Intestinal malabsorption	Serum iron	Serum TIBC	Serum folate (inhibit *L. casei*)	Creatinine	BUN	Uric acid	Calcium	Bilirubin	SGOT/SGPT	Glucose
Diuretics													
Acetazolamide									I				
Chlorthalidone		+											I
Ethacrynic acid	+								I				I
Furosemide								I	I				I
Thiazides	+								I	I			I
Antibiotics, etc.													
Aminosalicylic acid (PAS)	+					D							
Amphotericin B	+	+											
Ampicillin		+				D							
Cephaloridine		+											
Cephalothin													
Chloramphenicol	+			I	D	D		I or D^a					
Colistin		+											
Erythromycin	+					D						I^a	
Gentamicin	+	+											
Griseofulvin	+	+											
Isoniazid	+	+										I^a	
Kanamycin	+	+	+										
Lincomycin	+					D							
Methicillin		+											
Nalidixic acid	+	a											I^b
Neomycin		+	+										
Nitrofurantoin	+	+											
Novobiocin	+												
Oleandomycin	+												
Oxacillin	+	+											
Penicillin						D							
Polymyxin B		+											
Rifampin	+	+											
Streptomycin		+						D					
Sulfonamides	+	+						I		D			
Tetracyclines	+	+				D							

Table 34-1. (continued)

Glucose tolerance	Cholesterol	T-3 uptake	T-4	131I uptake	Amylase/lipase	Sodium	Potassium	Chloride	Prothrombin time	Comments
D									I	
D						D	D	D	I	
D						D	D	D		
D					I	D	D	D		D–PSP and creatinine tolerance
										aDepends on method
										aColorimetric method
			D							aSMA method. D–5-HIAA
										aNitrogen retention bCopper reduction method
										With massive dosage D–PSP
			D							I–PAH clearance

+ = presence of laboratory test changes due to drug effect on organ; I = values may be increased, elevated, or falsely positive; D = values may be decreased, lowered, or falsely negative.

a and b See last column on right.

Hepatotoxic refers to liver damage that may alter one or more laboratory tests of liver function, including alkaline phosphatase, bilirubin, transaminase. When this column is marked with a + sign, the individual columns (e.g., bilirubin, SGOT) are not also marked with a + sign.

Nephrotoxic refers to renal damage that may cause changes in BUN, creatinine, urine protein, casts, or cells. When this column is marked with a + sign, the individual columns (e.g., BUN, creatinine) are not also marked with a + sign.

DRUGS THAT MAY CAUSE INCREASED SERUM POTASSIUM

Due To

Effect on renal tubules (e.g., spironolactone)
Renal toxicity (e.g., amphotericin B, methicillin, tetracycline)
Antineoplastic agents due to rapid lysis of cells, especially in leukemia and lymphoma
Potassium contents (e.g., 1 million units of penicillin G potassium contains 1.7 mEq of potassium)
Others (e.g., triamterene)

DRUGS THAT MAY CAUSE DECREASED SERUM POTASSIUM

Due To

Diuretic effect (e.g., ethacrynic acid, furosemide, thiazides)
Increased renal excretion (e.g., corticosteroids, IV EDTA)
Other loss (e.g., chronic laxative abuse, aldosterone, licorice)
Alkalosis (e.g., bicarbonates)
Potassium shift into cells (e.g., glucose, insulin)

DRUGS THAT MAY CAUSE INCREASED SERUM CHLORIDE

Due To

Hyperchloremic alkalosis during prolonged treatment
    Chlorothiazide
    Hydrochlorothiazide
Retention of salt and water (e.g., corticosteroids, guanethidine, phenylbutazone)

DRUGS THAT MAY CAUSE DECREASED SERUM CHLORIDE

Due To

Alkalosis (e.g., bicarbonates, aldosterone, corticosteroids)
Diuretic effect (e.g., ethacrynic acid, furosemide, thiazides)
Other loss (e.g., chronic laxative abuse)

DRUGS THAT MAY CAUSE INCREASED SERUM CARBON DIOXIDE

Due To

Alkalosis (e.g., bicarbonates, aldosterone, hydrocortisone, thiazides, ethacrynic acid)
Diuretic effect (e.g., metolazone)

DRUGS THAT MAY CAUSE DECREASED SERUM CARBON DIOXIDE

Due To

Nephrotoxic effect (e.g., methicillin, nitrofurantoin, tetracycline, triamterene
Acidosis (e.g., dimercaprol, paraldehyde, phenformin)

DRUGS THAT MAY CAUSE INCREASED SERUM AMYLASE

Due To

Spasm of sphincter of Oddi (e.g., codeine, morphine, meperidine, methacholine, cholinergics)
Liver damage (e.g., birth control pills)

Induced acute pancreatitis (e.g., aminosalicylic acid, azathioprine, corticosteroids, dexamethasone, ethacrynic acid, furosemide, thiazides, mercaptopurine, phenformin, triamcinolone)

Methodologic interference (e.g., pancreozymin [contains amylase], chloride and fluoride salts [enhance amylase activity], lipemic serum [turbidimetric methods])

DRUGS THAT MAY CAUSE DECREASED SERUM AMYLASE

Due To

Methodologic interference (e.g., citrate and oxalate—decrease activity by binding calcium ions)

DRUGS THAT MAY CAUSE INCREASED SERUM LIPASE

Due To

Spasm of sphincter of Oddi (e.g., codeine, morphine, meperidine, methacholine, cholinergics)

Induced acute pancreatitis (see preceding section on serum amylase)

Cholestatic effect (e.g., indomethacin)

Methodologic interference (e.g., pancreozymin [contains lipase], deoxycholate, glycocholate, taurocholate [prevent inactivation of enzyme], bilirubin [turbidimetric methods])

FACTORS THAT MAY CAUSE DECREASED SERUM LIPASE

Due To

Methodologic interference (e.g., presence of hemoglobin, calcium ions)

DRUGS THAT MAY CAUSE INCREASED
OR DECREASED T-4

Increased	**Decreased**
By increasing TBG	By decreasing TBG
Estrogens	Anabolic steroids, androgens
Methadone	Aspirin (high doses)
Phenothiazines	Chlorpropamide
Progestins	Corticotropin, cortisone, predni-
By altering T-4 peripheral	sone
conversion	Sulfonamides
L-Thyroxine	By decreasing T-4 synthesis
	Aminosalicylic acid
	Iodides
	Liothyronine sodium
	Lithium
	Methimazole
	Thiouracil
	Sulfonamides
	Sulfonylureas
	By displacing T-4 from binding sites
	Aspirin
	Heparin
	Phenytoin
	Tolbutamide
	By increasing T-4 hepatic metabolism
	Chlorpromazine
	Phenytoin
	Reserpine

DRUGS THAT MAY CAUSE INCREASED PLASMA RENIN ACTIVITY

Diazoxide
Estrogens
Furosemide
Guanethidine
Hydralazine
Minoxidil
Nitroprusside
Saralasin
Spironolactone
Thiazides

DRUGS THAT MAY CAUSE DECREASED PLASMA RENIN ACTIVITY

Clonidine
Methyldopa (slight)
Propranolol
Reserpine

Bibliography

Baum, G. L., and Wolinsky, E. (Eds.). *Textbook of Pulmonary Diseases* (3rd ed.). Boston: Little, Brown, 1983.

Bloodworth, J. M., Jr. *Endocrine Pathology* (2nd ed.). Baltimore: Williams & Wilkins, 1982.

Conn, R. B., Jr. (Ed.). *Current Diagnosis*. Philadelphia: Saunders, 1985.

Early, L. E., and Gottschalk, C. W. (Eds.). *Strauss and Welt's Diseases of the Kidney* (3rd ed.) Boston: Little, Brown, 1979.

Henry, J. B. (Ed.). *Todd-Sanford-Davidson Clinical Diagnosis by Laboratory Methods* (17th ed.). Philadelphia: Saunders, 1984.

International Committee for Nomenclature and Nosology of Renal Disease. *A Handbook of Kidney Nomenclature and Nosology*. Boston: Little, Brown, 1975.

Isselbacher, K. J., et al. (Eds.). *Harrison's Principles of Internal Medicine* (9th ed.). New York: McGraw-Hill, 1980.

Mandell, H. N., and Johnson, M. *Laboratory Medicine in Clinical Practice*. Boston: Wright-PSG, 1983.

Miale, J. B. *Laboratory Medicine: Hematology* (6th ed.). St. Louis: Mosby, 1982.

Sonnenwirth, A. C., and Jarrett, L. (Eds.). *Gradwohl's Clinical Laboratory Methods and Diagnosis* (8th ed.). St. Louis: Mosby, 1980.

Stanbury, J. B., Wyngaarden, J. B., and Fredrickson, D. S. (Eds.). *The Metabolic Basis of Inherited Disease* (5th ed.). New York: McGraw-Hill, 1982.

Stein, J. H., et al. (Eds.). *Internal Medicine*. Boston: Little, Brown, 1983.

Tietz, N. W., and Finley, P. R. *Clinical Guide to Laboratory Tests*. Philadelphia: Saunders, 1983.

Wallach, J. *Interpretation of Pediatric Tests*. Boston: Little, Brown, 1983.

Wilkins, R. W., and Levinsky, N. G. (Eds.). *Medicine: Essentials of Clinical Practice* (3rd ed.). Boston: Little, Brown, 1983.

Wintrobe, M. M., Lee, G. R., Boggs, D. R., et al. (Eds.). *Clinical Hematology* (8th ed.). Philadelphia: Lea & Febiger, 1981.

Ziai, M. (Ed.) *Pediatrics* (3rd ed.). Boston: Little, Brown, 1984.

Appendix

Tables for Conversion of Conventional Units to SI (Système International) Units for Some Common Clinical Tests

These tables are provided to assist the gradual transition to the use of SI units.* As of July 1, 1986, all laboratory data published in the journals of the American Medical Association will have the traditional values given first with SI values in parentheses. As of July 1, 1987, SI units will be given first with traditional values in parentheses. After July 1, 1988, SI units alone will be used.

*Data from Campbell, J. M., and Campbell, J. B. *Laboratory Mathematics. Medical and Biological Applications.* St. Louis: Mosby, 1984.

Table A-1. Current Units and SI Units for Hematologic Tests

Test	Kind of Quantity	Current Units	SI Units	Conversion Factors Current to SI Units	Conversion Factors SI Units to Current Units
Leukocytes (total WBC count)	Particle concentration	per μl (cu mm) (mm^3)	$\times 10^9$/L	0.001	1000
Thrombocytes (platelet count)	Particle concentration	per μl (cu mm) (mm^3)	$\times 10^9$/L	0.001	1000
Reticulocytes	Particle fraction	% (per 100 RBC)	$\times 10^{-3}$	0.01	100
Erythrocytes (RBC count)	Particle concentration	millions per μl (millions per cu mm or per mm^3)	$\times 10^{12}$/L	1	1
Hematocrit (packed cell volume, PCV)	Volume fraction	percent (%)	L/L Symbol may be omitted	0.01	100

	Volume (mean)	μ^3 (cu microns)	fl	1	1
Mean cell volume (MCV, volume index)	Volume (mean)	μ^3 (cu microns)	fl	1	1
Mean cell hemoglobin (MCH, color index)	Mole rate (mean)	$\mu\mu$g	fmol	0.06205	16.12
Mean cell hemoglobin concentration (MCHC, saturation index)	Molar concentration (mean)	gm/dl (%)	mmol/L	0.6205	1.612
Hemoglobin (Fe)	Molar concentration	gm/dl	mmol/L	0.6205	1.612
Fetal hemoglobin	Mole fraction of Hb (F total)	percent	mol/mol Symbol may be omitted	0.01	100
Haptoglobin	Molar concentration	mg/dl	μmol/L (Hb[Fe])	0.6205	1.612
Fibrinogen	Mass concentration	mg/dl	gm/L	0.01	100
CSF cells	Particle concentration	per μl (cu mm) (mm^3)	$\times 10^6$/L	1	1

Table A-2. Conversion of One Conventional Enzyme Unit to International Units per Liter (IU/L)

Enzyme Unit	IU/L Equivalent
Acid phosphatase	
Bodansky	5.37
Shinowara-Jones-Reinhart	5.37
King-Armstrong	1.77
Bessey-Lowry-Brock	16.67
Aldolase	
Sibley-Lehninger	0.74
Alkaline phosphatase	
Bodansky	5.37
Shinowara-Jones-Reinhart	5.37
King-Armstrong	7.1
Bessey-Lowry-Brock	16.67
Babson	1.0
Amylase	
Somogyi (saccharogenic)	1.85
Somogyi	20.6
Cholinesterase	
de la Huerga	16.7
Hydroxybutyric dehydrogenase	
Rosalki-Wilkinson	0.482
Isocitrate dehydrogenase	
Wolfson-Williams-Ashman	0.0167
Taylor-Friedman	0.0167
Lactate dehydrogenase	
Wroblewski	0.482
Lipase	
Cherry-Crandal	277.0
Malic dehydrogenase	
Wacker-Ulmer-Valee	0.482
Transaminases	
Reitman-Frankel	0.482
Karmen	0.482

Table A-3. Current Units and SI Units for Chemistry Tests*

Test	Kind of Quantity	Units	SI Units	Conversion Factors Current to SI Units	Conversion Factors SI Units to Current Units
Albumin (S)	Mass concentration	gm/dl	gm/L	10	0.1
(CSF)	Mass concentration	mg/dl	gm/L	0.01	100
Ammonia	Molar concentration	μg/dl	μmol/L	0.5872	1.703
Bilirubin, total	Molar concentration	mg/dl	μmol/L	17.1	0.05847
Calcium (S)	Molar concentration	mg/dl, mEq/L	mmol/L	0.5	2
(U)	Mole rate	mg/day, mEq/day	mmol/day	0.5	2
Carbon dioxide pressure, tension (PCO₂)	Partial pressure	mm Hg	mbar	0.1333	7.502
Carbonate (total + CO₂, bicarbonate, alkali reserve, combined CO₂ capacity)	Molar concentration	volume percent	mmol/L	0.4492	2.226
Standard bicarbonate (PCO₂) (hydrogen carbonate)	Molar concentration	mEq/L	mmol/L	1	1
Chloride (S)	Molar concentration	mg/dl, mEq/L	mmol/L	1	1
(U)	Mole rate	mg/day, mEq/day	mmol/day	1	1

Table A-3. (continued)

Test	Kind of Quantity	Units	SI Units	Conversion Factors	
				Current to SI Units	SI Units to Current Units
Cholesterol, total	Molar concentration	mg/dl	mmol/L	0.02586	38.66
Copper	Molar concentration	μg/dl	μmol/L	0.1574	6.354
Coproporphyrins (I and III) (U)	Mole rate	μg/day	nmol/day	1.527	0.6548
Creatinine (S)	Molar concentration	mg/dl	mmol/L	0.0884	11.31
(U)	Mole rate	gm/day	mmol/day	8.840	0.1131
(clearance)	Clearance	ml/min	ml/sec	0.01667	60
Cyanocobalamin (vitamin B_{12})	Molar concentration	μμg/ml	pmol/L	0.7367	1.357
Glucose	Molar concentration	mg/dl	mmol/L	0.0551	18.02
17-Hydroxycorticosteroids (17-ketogenic steroids) (U)	Mole rate	mg/day	μmol/day	2.766	0.3615
17-Ketosteroids (as androsterone) (U)	Mole rate	mg/day	μmol/day	3.443	0.2904
Iron (iron ion, Fe, transferrin bound)	Molar concentration	μg/dl	μmol/L	0.1791	5.585
Lead (Pb)	Molar concentration	μg/dl	μmol/L	0.04826	20.72
Lipids, total (fat)	Mass concentration	mg/dl	gm/L	0.01	100

	Present Units	Conversion Type	SI Units	Factor	Factor
Magnesium ion (Mg)	mg/dl, mEq/L	Molar concentration	mmol/L	0.5	2.0
Phosphate (inorganic phosphorus)	mg/dl	Molar concentration	mmol/L	0.3229	3.097
pH	pH	pH	cHnmol/L	9 − pH	
Porphobilinogen (U)	µg/day	Mole rate	µmol/day	0.00442	226.2
Potassium (S)	mg/dl, mEq/L	Molar concentration	mmol/L	0.2558, 1	3.910, 1
(U)	mg/day, mEq/day	Mole rate	mmol/day	0.02558, 1	39.1, 1
Protein (S)	gm/dl	Mass concentration	gm/L	10	0.1
(U)	mg/day	Mass rate	mg/day	10	0.1
Sodium (S)	mg/dl, mEq/L	Molar concentration	mmol/L	0.435, 1	2.299, 1
(U)	mg/day, mEq/day	Mole rate	mmol/day	0.0435, 1	22.99, 1
Transferrin (Fe) (total iron binding capacity, TIBC)	µg/dl	Molar concentration	µmol/L	0.1791	5.583
Uric acid	mg/dl	Molar concentration	mmol/L	0.05948	16.81
Urea nitrogen (S)	mg/dl	Molar concentration	mmol/L	0.1665	6.006
(U)	gm/day	Mole rate	mmol/day	16.65	0.06006
(clearance)	ml/min	Clearance	ml/sec	0.01667	60
Vitamin C (ascorbic acid)	mg/dl	Molar concentration	mmol/L	56.78	0.01761

*All are serum (S) specimens unless otherwise specified; U = urine; CSF = cerebrospinal fluid.

Index

Flail chest, hypoxemia in, 51
Fluid. *See also specific fluids*
  ascitic, 26, 176
  cerebrospinal, 25, 277–285
  duodenal, 174–175
  gastric, 174–175
  pericardial, 26, 176
  pleural, 26
  serous, 26, 176–186
  synovial, 27
    in joint diseases, 318–319
Flukes, liver, biliary infestation of, 270
Fluorescence of tissue, in porphyrias, 437,
    438
Fluorescent antibodies. *See* Antibodies,
    fluorescent
Fluorescent light exposure, and bilirubin in
    serum, 671
Fluorescent treponemal antibody absorbed
    test in syphilis, 138, 139–140, 580
Fluorometric tests, for porphyrins in urine,
    drugs affecting, 663
Fluphenazine, and laboratory test values,
    674–675
Folic acid
  antagonists of
    and FIGLU excretion in urine, 167
    and folic acid levels in serum, 128
  deficiency of
    in alcoholic hepatitis, 251
    in cirrhosis, 256
    in Crohn's disease, 234
    and FIGLU excretion in urine, 167
    laboratory tests in, 337
    in malabsorption, 237
    small intestine biopsy in, 239
    and vitamin B_{12} levels, 127, 128, 129
  in red blood cells, 37
  serum levels, 8, 37, 128–129
    drugs affecting, 128, 672, 674, 676
    and FIGLU excretion in urine, 128, 167
    in pernicious anemia, 335
    in pregnancy, 560
  therapy with
    in anemia from phenytoin, 649
    and folic acid levels in serum, 129
Follicle-stimulating hormone
  serum levels, 33
    in anorexia nervosa, 506
    in Stein-Leventhal syndrome, 498
  in urine, 171
Food poisoning, staphylococci in, 565
Foodborne gastroenteritis, 234–235
Forbes' disease, 442, 443–444
Foreign bodies
  in airways
    hypoxemia in, 52
    respiratory acidosis in, 415
  and osteomyelitis, 309
  in stomach, 231
Formiminoglutamic acid excretion, 128, 167
Fowler's solution, arsenic poisoning from,
    650
Fractures
  and alkaline phosphatase serum levels, 58
  and creatine urine levels, 166
  fat embolism in, 287, 314
  of femur, and avascular necrosis of, 315
  of long bones, cerebral embolism in, 287
  in osteoectasia, familial, 312
  pathologic, from corticosteroids, 649

and phosphorus levels, 57
  of skull, 286
    meningitis in, 289
Fragility, osmotic, of red blood cells, 7. *See
    also* Erythrocytes, osmotic fragility of
Francisella tularensis, antibiotics affecting, 588
Frei test, in cat-scratch disease, 608
Friedländer's bacillus. *See Klebsiella, pneu-
    moniae*
Friedreich's ataxia
  hyperglycemia in, 472
  hypertension in, 201
Fröhlich's syndrome, 507
  hypothalamic disease in, 507
Fructose
  intolerance to
    congenital, 435–436
      glucose serum levels in, 42
      renal tubular acidosis in, 521
    lactic acidosis from, 413
  in test for glycogenoses, 443, 444
  tolerance test in malabsorption, 237, 238
  in urine, 160
Fructose-1,6-diphosphatase deficiency, lactic
    acidosis in, 413
Fructose 1-phosphate aldolase serum levels,
    in Tay-Sachs disease, 74
Fructosuria, 160
  benign, 436
Fruits, and vanillylmandelic acid in urine,
    168
FSH. *See* Follicle-stimulating hormone
FTA-ABS test in syphilis, 138, 139–140, 580
α-Fucosidase deficiency, 447
Fucosidosis, 447
Function tests, 96–109
  adrenal, 273, 478–479
  of kidney, 30–31. *See also* Kidney, function
    tests
  of liver, 29. *See also* Liver, function tests
  of thyroid, 455–457. *See also* Thyroid,
    function tests
Fungi
  in blood, 191
  in cerebrospinal fluid, 283
  in pleura, 193
Fungicides, renal failure from, acute, 524
Fungus infections, 609–615
  arthritis in, 316
  brain abscess in, 297
  calcium levels in, 56
  and eosinophilia
    in pleural fluid, 178
    pulmonary infiltrations with, 222
  endocarditis in, 209
  laryngeal, 217
  meningeal, 289
  meningitis in, recurrent, 291
  NBT test in, 115
  oral manifestations of, 230
  pericardial effusion in, 213
  pleural effusion in, 179, 181
  pneumoconiosis in, 222
  pneumonia in, 220, 221
  sputum in, 179
  transmission by animals, 632
"Funny-looking kid" syndrome, chromosome
    analysis in, 194
Furazolidone
  and false positive test for urine glucose, 661
  urine coloration from, 660